Particle and Fibre Toxicology

Particle and Fibre Toxicology

Editor: Hailey Kennedy

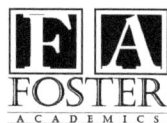

FA FOSTER ACADEMICS

www.fosteracademics.com

www.fosteracademics.com

FA
FOSTER
ACADEMICS

Cataloging-in-Publication Data

Particle and fibre toxicology / edited by Hailey Kennedy.
        p. cm.
Includes bibliographical references and index.
ISBN 978-1-63242-908-7
1. Particles--Toxicology. 2. Pulmonary toxicology. 3. Fibers--Toxicology. I. Kennedy, Hailey.
RC720 .P37 2020
616.200 471--dc23

© Foster Academics, 2020

Foster Academics,
118-35 Queens Blvd., Suite 400,
Forest Hills, NY 11375, USA

ISBN 978-1-63242-908-7 (Hardback)

Contents

Chapter 9   **Group II innate lymphoid cells and microvascular dysfunction from pulmonary titanium dioxide nanoparticle exposure** 120
Alaeddin Bashir Abukabda, Carroll Rolland McBride, Thomas Paul Batchelor,
William Travis Goldsmith, Elizabeth Compton Bowdridge, Krista Lee Garner,
Sherri Friend and Timothy Robert Nurkiewicz

Chapter 10   **Vasomotor function in rat arteries after ex vivo and intragastric exposure to food-grade titanium dioxide and vegetable carbon particles** 133
Ditte Marie Jensen, Daniel Vest Christophersen, Majid Sheykhzade,
Gry Freja Skovsted, Jens Lykkesfeldt, Rasmus Münter, Martin Roursgaard,
Steffen Loft and Peter Møller

Chapter 11   **The unrecognized occupational relevance of the interaction between engineered nanomaterials and the gastro-intestinal tract** 151
Antonio Pietroiusti, Enrico Bergamaschi, Marcello Campagna, Luisa Campagnolo,
Giuseppe De Palma, Sergio Iavicoli, Veruscka Leso, Andrea Magrini,
Michele Miragoli, Paola Pedata, Leonardo Palombi and Ivo Iavicoli

Chapter 12   **Effects of urban coarse particles inhalation on oxidative and inflammatory parameters in the mouse lung and colon** 174
Cécile Vignal, Muriel Pichavant, Laurent Y. Alleman, Madjid Djouina,
Florian Dingreville, Esperanza Perdrix, Christophe Waxin, Adil Ouali Alami,
Corinne Gower Rousseau, Pierre Desreumaux and Mathilde Body-Malapel

Chapter 13   **Detection of titanium particles in human liver and spleen and possible health implications** 187
M. B. Heringa, R. J. B. Peters, R. L. A. W. Bleys, M. K. van der Lee, P. C. Tromp,
P. C. E. van Kesteren, J. C. H. van Eijkeren, A. K. Undas, A. G. Oomen and
H. Bouwmeester

Chapter 14   **Suppression of PTPN6 exacerbates aluminum oxide nanoparticle-induced COPD-like lesions in mice through activation of STAT pathway** 196
Xiaobo Li, Hongbao Yang, Shenshen Wu, Qingtao Meng, Hao Sun, Runze Lu,
Jian Cui, Yuxin Zheng, Wen Chen, Rong Zhang, Michael Aschner and Rui Chen

Chapter 15   **Cardiovascular and inflammatory mechanisms in healthy humans exposed to air pollution in the vicinity of a steel mill** 209
Premkumari Kumarathasan, Renaud Vincent, Erica Blais, Agnieszka Bielecki,
Josée Guénette, Alain Filiatreault, Orly Brion, Sabit Cakmak, Errol M. Thomson,
Robin Shutt, Lisa Marie Kauri, Mamun Mahmud, Ling Liu and Robert Dales

    Permissions

    List of Contributors

    Index

Preface

The main aim of this book is to educate learners and enhance their research focus by presenting diverse topics covering this vast field. This is an advanced book which compiles significant studies by distinguished experts in the area of analysis. This book addresses successive solutions to the challenges arising in the area of application, along with it; the book provides scope for future developments.

Airborne particles when inhaled, can lead to pathological changes in the respiratory tract. Therefore, toxicological studies on the effects of inhalable fibers and particles involve an assessment of the histopathological alterations in the trachea, lungs and the upper respiratory tract. The pathology of particle and fibre toxicology depends on the exposure source, duration, concentration and individual predisposition. Particles such as combustion-derived particles, engineered nanoparticles, ultrafine particles, silica, asbestos, etc. can induce an inflammatory response. There may be long term effects of chronic particle exposure, such as allergic airway inflammation, chronic obstructive pulmonary disease, fibrosis or neoplasms. The extent of tissue damage and pulmonary inflammation can be addressed and studied via pulmonary histopathology as well as diverse histopathological inflammatory parameters. This book unfolds the innovative aspects of particle and fibre toxicology which will be crucial for the progress of this field in the future. It will also provide interesting topics for research which interested readers can take up. It attempts to assist those with a goal of delving into toxicology.

It was a great honour to edit this book, though there were challenges, as it involved a lot of communication and networking between me and the editorial team. However, the end result was this all-inclusive book covering diverse themes in the field.

Finally, it is important to acknowledge the efforts of the contributors for their excellent chapters, through which a wide variety of issues have been addressed. I would also like to thank my colleagues for their valuable feedback during the making of this book.

Editor

Silica nanoparticles inhibit the cation channel TRPV4 in airway epithelial cells

Alicia Sanchez[1], Julio L. Alvarez[1], Kateryna Demydenko[1,5], Carole Jung[2], Yeranddy A. Alpizar[1], Julio Alvarez-Collazo[1], Stevan M. Cokic[3], Miguel A. Valverde[2], Peter H. Hoet[4] and Karel Talavera[1]* (iD)

Abstract

Background: Silica nanoparticles (SiNPs) have numerous beneficial properties and are extensively used in cosmetics and food industries as anti-caking, densifying and hydrophobic agents. However, the increasing exposure levels experienced by the general population and the ability of SiNPs to penetrate cells and tissues have raised concerns about possible toxic effects of this material. Although SiNPs are known to affect the function of the airway epithelium, the molecular targets of these particles remain largely unknown. Given that SiNPs interact with the plasma membrane of epithelial cells we hypothesized that they may affect the function of Transient Receptor Potential Vanilloid 4 (TRPV4), a cation-permeable channel that regulates epithelial barrier function. The main aims of this study were to evaluate the effects of SiNPs on the activation of TRPV4 and to determine whether these alter the positive modulatory action of this channel on the ciliary beat frequency in airway epithelial cells.

Results: Using fluorometric measurements of intracellular Ca^{2+} concentration ($[Ca^{2+}]_i$) we found that SiNPs inhibit activation of TRPV4 by the synthetic agonist GSK1016790A in cultured human airway epithelial cells 16HBE and in primary cultured mouse tracheobronchial epithelial cells. Inhibition of TRPV4 by SiNPs was confirmed in intracellular Ca^{2+} imaging and whole-cell patch-clamp experiments performed in HEK293T cells over-expressing this channel. In addition to these effects, SiNPs were found to induce a significant increase in basal $[Ca^{2+}]_i$, but in a TRPV4-independent manner. SiNPs enhanced the activation of the capsaicin receptor TRPV1, demonstrating that these particles have a specific inhibitory action on TRPV4 activation. Finally, we found that SiNPs abrogate the increase in ciliary beat frequency induced by TRPV4 activation in mouse airway epithelial cells.

Conclusions: Our results show that SiNPs inhibit TRPV4 activation, and that this effect may impair the positive modulatory action of the stimulation of this channel on the ciliary function in airway epithelial cells. These findings unveil the cation channel TRPV4 as a primary molecular target of SiNPs.

Keywords: silica nanoparticles, TRPV4, GSK1016790A, epithelial cells, ciliary beat frequency

Background

Synthetic amorphous SiNPs are extensively used due to its interesting physico-chemical properties, low cost and relatively easy production. This material has many applications in industrial manufacturing, cosmetics, biotechnology, medicine, and food, pharmaceutical and chemical industries [1–4]. SiNPs are widely used in consumer products and as a consequence, human exposure to this nanomaterial has highly increased. However, there is very little information available about the risks associated to the exposure to this nanomaterial [5].

It is known that SiNPs can penetrate cells, interacting with the plasma membrane, intracellular structures and organelles, thereby posing potential health threats [6–8]. The toxicity generated by nanoparticles has been related to an increased generation of reactive oxygen species (ROS) [9, 10]. This results in oxidative stress, mitochondrial perturbation and the generation of inflammatory mediators leading to cell dysfunction and apoptosis [2, 3, 11–19].

* Correspondence: karel.talavera@kuleuven.be
[1]Department of Cellular and Molecular Medicine, Laboratory of Ion Channel Research, KU Leuven; VIB Center for Brain & Disease Research, Leuven, Belgium
Full list of author information is available at the end of the article

One of the main entry pathways of nanoparticles into the body is the epithelium of the airways. In addition to its function in gas exchange, the respiratory epithelium protects the body against hazardous environmental substances and pathogens, constituting an active diffusion barrier, and supporting the mechanisms of mucociliary clearance and recruitment of inflammatory cells [20–22]. Several cellular responses to SiNPs in the airways have been reported. Rabiolli et al. demonstrated that SiNPs induce lung inflammation through the stimulation of IL-1β production by alveolar macrophages [23]. Skuland et al. showed evidence of pro-inflammatory responses induced by amorphous SiNPs in lung epithelial cells [24]. Delaval et al. reported that SiNPs pre-exposure in pneumonia induced by *Pseudomonas aeruginosa* increases lung permeability and enhance mortality [25], and Kasper et al. showed inflammatory and cytotoxic responses such as DNA damage, hypoxia and ER-stress induced by SiNPs in an alveolar-capillary co-culture model [18].

However, little is known about the influence of SiNPs on specific molecular targets and cell signaling events, especially at the level of the plasma membrane. In this study we hypothesized that SiNPs may affect the function of TRPV4, a Ca^{2+}-permeable cation channel expressed in airway epithelial cells. This channel plays a role in the transduction of physical and chemical stimuli into Ca^{2+} signals that regulate ciliary beat frequency and mucociliary transport [26, 27]. Moreover, TRPV4 contributes to the barrier integrity in the lung and to the regulation of endothelial and epithelial permeability [28, 29], and has been implicated in the modulation of the respiratory function and proposed as target for the treatment of respiratory diseases such chronic obstructive pulmonary disease and asthma [30–33].

We used intracellular Ca^{2+} imaging and patch-clamp to evaluate the effects of SiNPs on TRPV4 activation. We found that SiNPs inhibit the activation of native TRPV4 channels in human and mouse airway epithelial cells, as well as recombinant TRPV4 in the heterologous expression system HEK293T. Furthermore, SiNPs inhibited the TRPV4-mediated increase in ciliary beat frequency in mouse airway epithelial cells. TRPV4 emerges therefore as a defined molecular target of SiNPs, with possible deleterious consequences for epithelial barrier function.

Methods

Ludox® SiNPs
SM30 Ludox® SiNPs were purchased from Sigma-Aldrich (Bornem, Belgium) as the commercial source of 30% wt suspension in H_2O. For the biological experiments the nanoparticle suspension was diluted to the desired concentrations in Krebs solution containing (in mM): 150 NaCl, 6 KCl, 1 $MgCl_2$, 1.5 $CaCl_2$, 10 glucose, 10 4-

(2-hydroxyethyl)-1-piperazineethanesulfonic acid (HEPES) and titrated to pH 7.4 with NaOH.

Dynamic Light Scattering (DLS) and Zeta potential
The stock suspension of SiNPs particles was diluted in water to 30 μg/ml. DLS and Zeta potential measurements were performed with a Brookhaven 90 Plus/ZetaPlus instrument (Brookhaven Instruments Ltd, Redditch, UK). DLS measurements were performed using a NanoParticle Size Distribution Analyser (scattering angle 90 u, wavelength 659 nm, power 15 mW). Correlation functions were analyzed using the Clementine package (maximum entropy method) for Igor Pro 6.02A (WaveMetrics, Portland, OR, USA).

Zeta potential measurements were done by applying electrophoretic light scattering. A primary and reference beam (659 nm, 35 mW), modulated optics and a dip-in electrode system were used. The frequency shift of scattered light (relative to the reference beam) from a charged particle moving in an electric field is related to the electrophoretic mobility of the particle. The Smoluchowski limit was used to calculate the Zeta potential from the electrophoretic mobility.

Transmission Electron Microscopy (TEM)
Suspensions (5 μl of stock suspension and 30 μg/ml) of the SiNPs particles were applied on formvar-coated cupper mesh grids (drop on grid). After drying overnight (25 °C in the dark), the particles were characterized by TEM (JEOL JEM-1200 EX-II, Tokyo, Japan).

Endosafe-PTS
We used the Endosafe-PTS LAL assay for FDA-licensed endotoxin detection. The cartridges contained four channels to which LAL reagent and a chromogenic substrate were applied. Two of these channels contained also an endotoxin spike that served as positive control. The sensitivity of the assay was 0.05 EU/ml.

Cell culture
Human bronchial epithelial cell line, 16HBE, were grown in Dulbecco's modified Eagle's medium: nutrient mixture F-12 (DMEM/F-12) containing 5% (v/v) fetal calf serum (FCS), 2 mM L-glutamine, 2 U/ml penicillin and 2 mg/ml streptomycin at 37 °C in a humidity-controlled incubator with 5% CO_2 and were seeded on 18-mm glass cover slips coated with poly-L-lysine (0.1 mg/ml).

Human embryonic kidney cells, HEK293T, were grown in Dulbecco's modified Eagle's medium (DMEM) containing 10% (v/v) fetal calf serum (FCS), 2 mM L-glutamine, 2 U/ml penicillin, 1% non-essential amino acids (Invitrogen, Erembodegem - Aalst, Belgium) and 2 mg/ml streptomycin at 37 °C in a humidity-controlled incubator with 10% CO_2 and were seeded on 18-mm glass cover slips coated with poly-L-lysine (0.1 mg/ml). For intracellular Ca^{2+} imaging and patch-clamp experiments, HEK293T cells were transiently transfected with mouse TRPV4 in the CAGGSM2/Ires/GFP/R1R2 vector, using Mirus TransIT-293 (Mirus Corporation; Madison, WI, USA). In all experiments, transfected cells were identified by green fluorescent protein (GFP) expression.

Animals

C57Bl/6J male mice from 8-12 weeks old were used for the experiments. The animals were maintained under standard conditions with a maximum of four animals per cage on a 12-h light/12-h dark cycle and with food and water ad libitum.

Culture of mouse tracheal epithelial cells

Mouse tracheal epithelial cells (mTEC) were isolated following the protocol described by Lam et al. [32], and seeded on 18-mm glass cover slips coated with collagen solution containing 50 µg/ml collagen (type I solution from rat tail, Sigma-Aldrich). Cells were grown for 2-3 days in the appropriate proliferation medium and maintained at 37 °C in a humidity-controlled incubator with 5% CO_2.

Intracellular Ca^{2+} imaging experiments

Ca^{2+}-imaging experiments were conducted with the ratiometric fluorescent indicator Fura-2 acetoxymethyl (AM) ester. Cells were incubated with 2 µM Fura-2 AM for 30 min at 37 °C. Bath solutions were perfused by gravity via a multi-barreled pipette tip with a single outlet of 0.8 mm inner diameter. This system allows full exchange of the medium bathing the recorded cell in less than 2-4 s. For recording in control condition cells were rinsed with Krebs solution. The $[Ca^{2+}]_i$ was monitored through the ratio of fluorescence measured upon alternating illumination at 340 and 380 nm using an MT-10 illumination system and the xcellence pro software (Olympus, Planegg, Germany). All experiments conducted in the native 16HBE and mTEC cells were performed at 35 °C. Experiments in HEK293T cells were performed at 25 °C because at 35 °C the TRPV4-transfected cells were heavily overloaded with Ca^{2+} in basal condition.

The concentration-dependent effects of SiNPs on basal $[Ca^{2+}]_i$ of 16HBE cells was fit with a Hill function of the form:

$$\Delta\left[Ca^{2+}\right] = \Delta\left[Ca^{2+}\right]_{Max} \frac{[SiNPs]^H}{[SiNPs]^H + EC_{50}^H}$$

where $\Delta[Ca^{2+}]_{Max}$ is the maximal amplitude of the response to SiNPs, [SiNPs] is the concentration of SiNPs, EC_{50} is the effective concentration and H is the Hill coefficient.

The concentration-dependent effects of SiNPs on the Ca^{2+} responses to the TRPV4 agonist GSK1016790A were fit with a Hill function of the form:

$$\Delta\left[Ca^{2+}\right] = \left(\Delta\left[Ca^{2+}\right]_{Max} - \Delta\left[Ca^{2+}\right]_{Inf}\right) \frac{[SiNPs]^H}{[SiNPs]^H + IC_{50}^H} + \Delta\left[Ca^{2+}\right]_{Inf}$$

where $\Delta[Ca^{2+}]_{Max}$ is the amplitude of the response in the absence of SiNPs, $\Delta[Ca^{2+}]_{Inf}$ is the amplitude of the response the presence of saturating concentrations of SiNPs, [SiNPs] is the concentration of SiNPs, IC_{50} is the effective inhibitory concentration and H is the Hill coefficient.

Patch-clamp experiments

Whole-cell voltage-clamp recordings were performed at 35 °C with standard patch pipettes (2-3 MΩ resistance) pulled using a DMZ-Universal puller (Zeitz Instruments, Augsburg, Germany). The pipette solution contained (in mM): 2 ATPNa$_2$, 5 EGTA, 10 HEPES, 1 MgCl$_2$, 135 CsCl$_2$ (292 mOsm/kg; pH 7.2, adjusted with CsOH). For perforated patch experiments, 250 µg/ml of Amphotericin B was added to the pipette solution and data were collected after the access resistance reached stable values of ~15 MΩ.

An Ag-AgCl wire was used as reference electrode. The cover slips with cells were placed in the stage of an inverted microscope (Olympus IX70, Tokyo, Japan) and stabilized for a few minutes in Krebs solution, containing (in mM): 150 NaCl, 6 KCl, 1 MgCl$_2$, 1.5 CaCl$_2$, 10 glucose, and 10 HEPES and titrated to pH 7.4 with NaOH. The control bath solution was kept at room temperature and contained (in mM): 140 NaCl, 1.3 MgCl$_2$, 2.4 CaCl$_2$, 10 HEPES, 10 glucose and (311 mOsm/kg; pH 7.4, adjusted with NaOH). Bath solutions were perfused by gravity via a multi-barreled pipette. A bath solution in which all cations were isotonically substituted by NMDG$^+$ (N-methyl-D-glucamine) was used to monitor the size of the leak currents during the patch-clamp recordings [34]. Current signals were recorded using the patch-clamp technique by using an EPC-7 (LIST Electronics, Darmstadt, Germany) amplifier and the Clampex 9.0 software program (Axon instruments, Sunnyvale, CA, USA). Currents were acquired at 10 kHz, filtered at 2 kHz, and stored for off-line analysis on a personal computer. In order to minimize voltage errors, the series resistance was compensated by 30-50% and the capacitance artifact was reduced using the amplifier circuitry. Membrane TRPV4 currents were elicited by a 600 ms long voltage ramp from -100 mV to +100 mV every 5 s with a holding potential of 0 mV.

Patch-clamp data was analyzed with the WinASCD software written by Dr. Guy Droogmans and Origin 7.0 (OriginLab Corporation, Northampton, MA, USA). The concentration dependence of TRPV4 current amplitude was fit with a Hill function of the form:

$$\Delta I = \left(\Delta I_{Max} - \Delta I_{Inf}\right)\frac{[SiNPs]^H}{[SiNPs]^H + IC_{50}^H} + \Delta I_{Inf}$$

where ΔI_{Max} is the current density increase in the absence of SiNPs, ΔI_{Inf} is the current density increase in the presence of saturating concentrations of SiNPs, [SiNPs] is the concentration of SiNPs, IC_{50} is the effective inhibitory concentration and H is the Hill coefficient.

Ciliary beat frequency (CBF) measurements

CBF was measured in primary cultures ciliated cells using with a high-speed digital imaging system as previously described [26]. Briefly, phase-contrast images (512 × 512 pixels) were collected at 120–135 frames per second with a high speed CCD camera using a frame grabber (Infaimon, Barcelona, Spain) and recording software from Video Savant (IO Industries, London, ON, Canada). The ciliary beat frequency was determined from the frequency of variation in light intensity of the image as a result of repetitive motion of cilia.

Reagents

All chemicals were purchased from Sigma-Aldrich (Bornem, Belgium).

Statistics

Data are given as mean ± standard error of the mean. Comparisons tests are indicated in the text were appropriate. Statistical significance were taken at $P < 0.05$ or $P < 0.01$.

Results

Characterization of the SM30 Ludox® SiNPs

Analysis of the SiNPs by DLS showed a single population of average size 10.2 nm (P10: 8.1 nm - P90: 11.8). The particles had a Zeta-potential of 20 ± 3 mV. TEM analysis of undiluted samples showed large aggregates, but in the diluted samples only a few aggregates could be found, and the particles appeared as spherical entities. No endotoxin contamination was detected in 30 µg/ml SiNPs dilutions.

Silica NPs inhibit TRPV4 activation in cultured human airway epithelial cells

To determine whether SiNPs modulate native human TRPV4 channels we used fluorometric measurements of $[Ca^{2+}]_i$ in cultured human bronchial epithelial 16HBE cells, which were reported to express this channel [34–37]. We found that 10 nM GSK1016790A induced intracellular Ca^+ responses in 100% (n = 333) of these cells, indicating for a prevalent functional expression of TRPV4 (Fig. 1a).

Extracellular application of SiNPs increased the basal $[Ca^{2+}]_i$ in a concentration-dependent manner (Fig. 1b-d), which was characterized by an EC_{50} of 99 ± 13 µg/ml, a Hill coefficient of 0.71 ± 0.07 and a maximal response of 0.6 ± 0.1 µM (Fig. 1e). To evaluate the effect of SiNPs on TRPV4 activation we compared the amplitude of the $[Ca^{2+}]_i$ responses measured 2 min after application of 10 nM GSK1016790A, in the absence and in the presence of nanoparticles. SiNPs induced a concentration-dependent inhibition of the responses to GSK1016790A, with an IC_{50} of 130 ± 40 µg/ml and a Hill coefficient of -1.2 ± 0.4 (Fig. 1f). Of note, SiNPs failed to completely abolish the response to GSK1016790A up to a concentration of 3000 µg/ml, leaving ~30% of the response to the channel agonist.

SiNPs increase basal $[Ca^{2+}]_i$ in a TRPV4-independent manner

It has been previously suggested that TRPV4 is implicated in intracellular Ca^{2+} responses to SiNPs in a cell subpopulation of the GT1-7 neuron-derived cell line [38]. Thus, we tested whether TRPV4 is involved in the $[Ca^{2+}]_i$ increases triggered by SiNPs in 16HBE cells. First, we determined whether the amplitude of the responses to SiNPs correlated with the amplitude of the responses to GSK1016790A, i.e., with the level of functional expression of TRPV4 in each cell. We found that this was not the case, with correlation values (R) of 0.074 (Fig. 2a). This value is lower than those we have previously found for the correlation between the amplitudes of responses to very low and high concentrations of GSK1016790A [39]. The average increase in basal $[Ca^{2+}]_i$ elicited by 300 µg/ml SiNPs in 16HBE was not significantly different in the absence (0.40 ± 0.04 µM) and in the presence of the specific TRPV4 blocker HC067047 [40] (0.43 ± 0.05 µM; P = 0.64; Fig. 2b). These data demonstrate that TRPV4 does not mediate the basal Ca^{2+} responses triggered by SiNPs.

An increase in basal $[Ca^{2+}]_i$ does not inhibit a subsequent TRPV4 activation

Next, we determined if an increase in basal $[Ca^{2+}]_i$ such as that induced by SiNPs could cause a decrease in TRPV4 activation. For this we tested the effect of extracellular application of ATP on a subsequent response of 16HBE cells to 10 nM GSK1016790A. We found that ATP triggered a robust intracellular Ca^{2+} signal, and that this did not reduced, but rather increased the amplitude of the TRPV4 response measured at 2 min of GSK1016790A application (0.54 ± 0.05 vs. 0.82 ± 0.08 in control and after ATP application, respectively, P = 0.005; Fig. 3a, b).

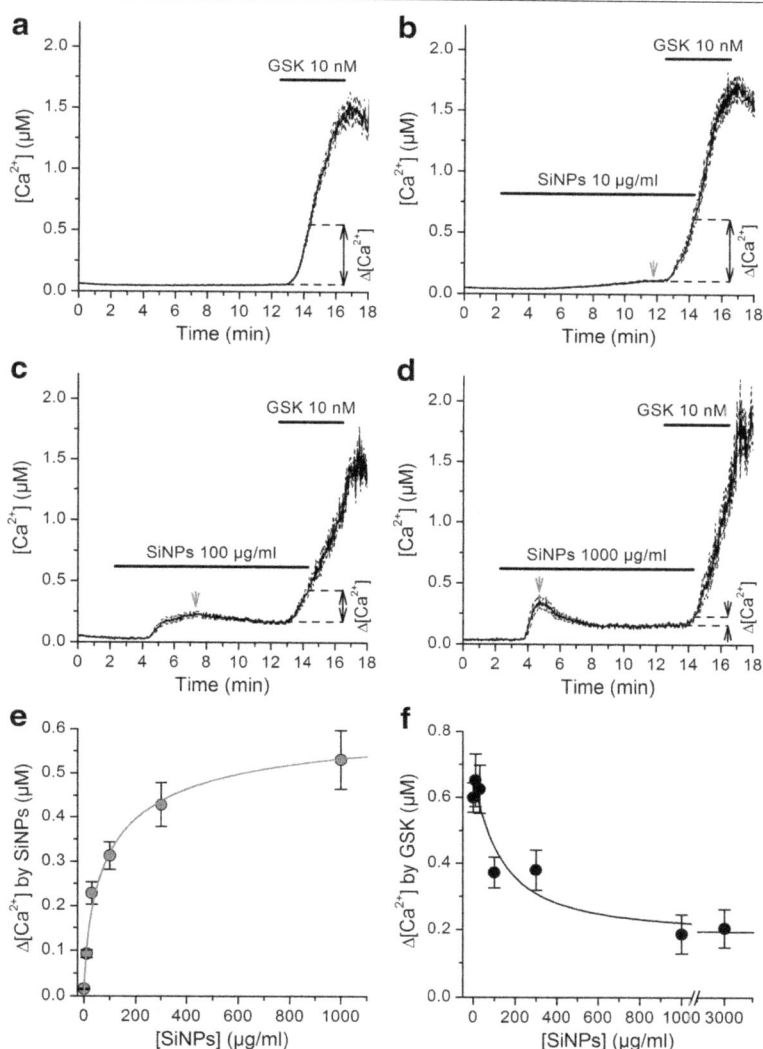

Fig. 1 SiNPs inhibit TRPV4 activation in 16HBE cells. **a, b, c, d** Effects of the TRPV4 agonist GSK1016790A on the $[Ca^{2+}]_i$ in the absence (**a**, $n = 333$) or in the presence of SiNPs 10 µg/ml (**b**, $n = 234$), 100 µg/ml (**c**, $n = 163$) and 1000 µg/ml (**d**, $n = 114$). The thick continuous traces correspond to the average responses and the thin dashed traces correspond to the mean plus/minus the standard errors. The dashed lines and black arrows indicate the amplitude of the average Ca^{2+} responses recorded after 2 min application of GSK1016790A, with respect to the immediate previous basal $[Ca^{2+}]_i$. The gray arrows point to the peak of basal Ca^{2+} responses to SiNPs. **e** Concentration dependence of the maximal amplitude of basal Ca^{2+} responses induced by the application of SiNPs. **f** Average amplitude of responses to 10 nM GSK1016790A when applied in the presence of SiNPs at different concentrations. In (**e**) and (**f**) the solid lines represent fits with Hill functions (see Methods)

SiNPs inhibit TRPV4 activation in mouse tracheal epithelial (mTEC) cells

In order to determine whether the effect of SiNPs is conserved for native mouse TRPV4 we used primary cultured mouse tracheal epithelial cells. Application of 10 nM GSK1016790A triggered intracellular Ca^{2+} signals in 94.4% (187 out of 198) of these cells (Fig. 4a), consistent with a previous report on the functional expression of TRPV4 channels in these cells [26]. SiNPs induced a concentration-dependent inhibition of the responses to GSK1016790A, with an IC_{50} of 1.2 ± 0.2 µg/ml and a Hill coefficient of -1.1 ± 0.3 (Fig. 4b-d).

As observed in 16HBE cells, application of SiNPs at high concentrations did not abolish the response to the TRPV4 agonist, but left ~20% of the maximal response.

SiNPs inhibit activation of recombinant TRPV4

To test whether SiNPs inhibit activation of TRPV4 in a heterologous expression system we performed intracellular Ca^{2+} imaging experiments in HEK293T cells transiently transfected with the mouse channel isoform. These cells showed a wide spectrum of basal $[Ca^{2+}]_i$, a fact that we ascribe to the variable efficacy of TRPV4

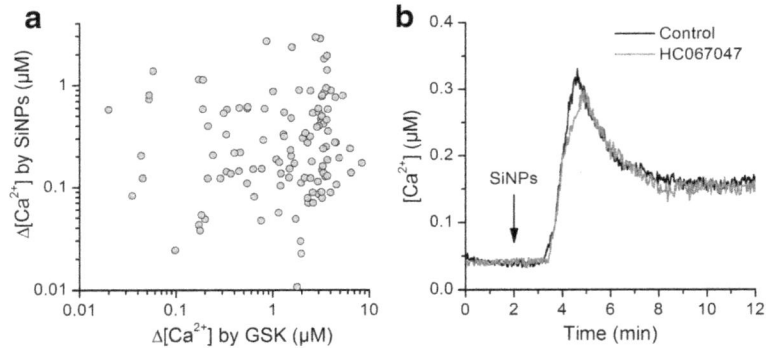

Fig. 2 TRPV4 does not mediate the increase in basal $[Ca^{2+}]_i$ induced by SiNPs in 16HBE cells. **a** Lack of correlation of the amplitudes of the intracellular Ca^{2+} responses to 300 µg/ml SiNPs and to the TRPV4 agonist GSK047067 (10 nM). **b** Effect of 300 µg/ml SiNPs in the absence (Control) and in the presence of the TRPV4 inhibitor HC067047 (10 µM). The lines represent average responses of 120 and 164 cells in control and HC067047, respectively

transfection in each cell and the constitutive activity of this Ca^{2+}-permeable channel. Analysis of the distribution of these values suggested the presence of two cell populations, which could be divided using a cutoff value of 250 nM. Both groups of cells responded robustly to 10 nM GSK1016790A (Fig. 5a).

Application of SiNPs induced a concentration-dependent increase of $[Ca^{2+}]_i$ in cells with low basal $[Ca^{2+}]_i$ (Fig. 5b, c), an effect reminiscent of that we observed in 16HBE cells (Fig. 1b-e). In contrast, SiNPs reduced $[Ca^{2+}]_i$ in cells with high basal Ca^{2+} levels (Fig. 5b, c), which may be an indicative of an inhibitory effect of the SiNPs on the basal activity of TRPV4. In both groups SiNPs reduced the response to GSK1016790A with an IC_{50} of 1.44 ± 0.06 µg/ml and a Hill coefficient of -2.0 ± 0.16 (Fig. 5d). Again, we found that application of SiNPs at high concentrations left ~30% of the response to the TRPV4 agonist.

Next, we determined whether SiNPs inhibit the activation of TRPV4 by another synthetic chemical agonist, 4α-phorbol 12,13-didecanoate (4αPDD). We found that

SiNPs (300 µg/ml) strongly inhibited the response to 4αPDD (Fig. 5e, f), showing that their effect is not exclusive for channel activation with GSK1016790A.

In all experiments described above we allowed sufficient time for the SiNPs effects on basal $[Ca^{2+}]_i$ to roughly reach a steady-state (~10 min). However, we were also interested in estimating the time required for these particles to reduce TRPV4 activation. Thus, we performed a series of experiments in which we varied the time of application of SiNPs before stimulating TRPV4 with 10 nM GSK1016790A. This time varied from zero (simultaneous application of SiNPs and GSK1016790A) to 10 min. We found that TRPV4 responses were significantly smaller in the presence of SiNPs ($P < 0.05$) and that the strength of inhibition was not significantly different when comparing across the various pre-application times tested (Tukey's Multiple Comparison Test; Fig. 6). This indicates that the inhibitory action of these particles on TRPV4 activation was prior to the full activation of TRPV4 by GSK1016790A (~2 - 3 min).

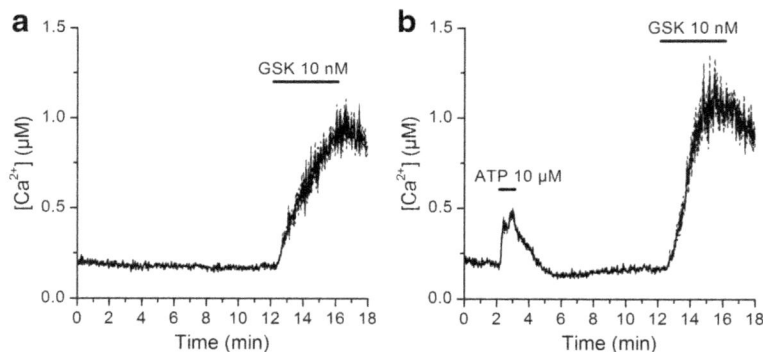

Fig. 3 Stimulation of 16HBE cells with ATP potentiates a subsequent activation of TRPV4. **a, b** Effects of the TRPV4 agonist GSK1016790A on the $[Ca^{2+}]_i$ of HEK293T cells transfected with mouse TRPV4, in control (**a**, $n = 253$) or after extracellular perfusion of ATP (**b**, $n = 266$). The thick continuous traces correspond to the average responses and the thin dashed traces correspond to the mean plus/minus the standard errors

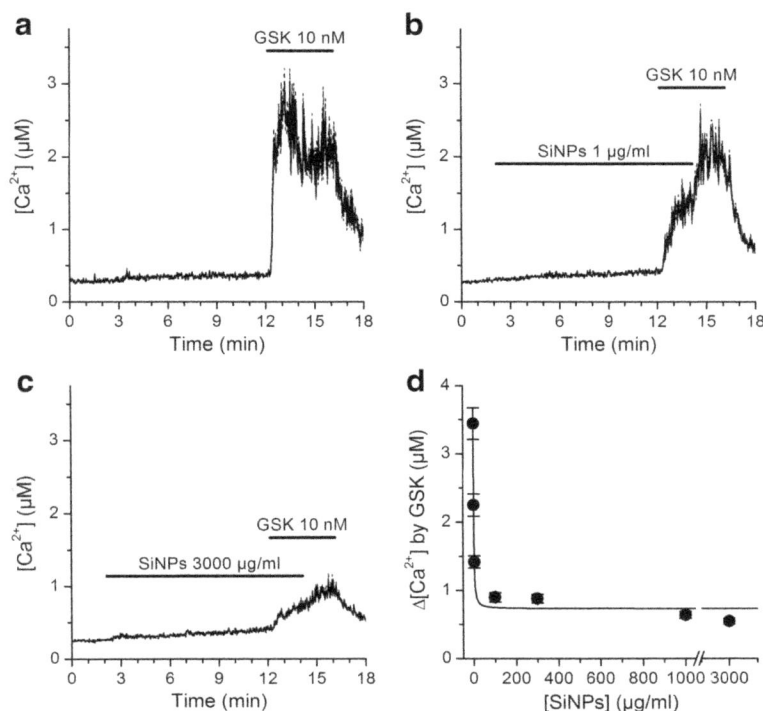

Fig. 4 SiNPs inhibit TRPV4 activation in mTEC. **a, b, c, d** Effects of the TRPV4 agonist GSK1016790A on the $[Ca^{2+}]_i$ in the absence (**a**, $n = 127$) or in the presence of SiNPs 1 µg/ml (**b**, $n = 243$) and 3000 µg/ml (**c**, $n = 349$). The thick continuous traces correspond to the average responses and the thin dashed traces correspond to the mean plus/minus the standard errors. **d** Average amplitude of responses to 10 nM GSK1016790A when applied in the presence of SiNPs at different concentrations. The solid line represents a fit with a Hill function (see Methods)

To directly test the effects of SiNPs on TRPV4 we performed whole-cell patch-clamp experiments (Fig. 7a, b). We recorded currents during the application of repetitive voltage ramps applied from -100 to +100 mV. Application of SiNPs at increasing concentrations had a tendency to augment the amplitude of basal currents, but this was statistically significant only at 300 µg/ml (Fig. 7c). To evaluate the effect of SiNPs on TRPV4 we compared the amplitude of the current responses measured 1 min after application of 10 nM GSK1016790A, in the absence and in the presence of nanoparticles (Fig. 7a and b). The response to GSK1016790A was significantly reduced when this compound was applied in the presence of SiNPs. This effect was dependent on the concentration of SiNPs, and was characterized by an IC_{50} of 2.4 ± 0.5 µg/ml, a Hill coefficient of -0.54 ± 0.07 and minimum value of 0.7 ± 0.2 pA/pF, for the currents measured at -75 mV (Fig. 7d).

To test whether the inhibition of TRPV4 activation is observed also in experimental conditions in which the intracellular milieu is better preserved we performed perforated patch-clamp experiments using Amphotericin B in the patch pipette (Fig. 8a, b). We found that extracellular application of SiNPs (30 µg/ml) significantly reduced the response of TRPV4 current to 10 nM GSK1016790A (Fig. 8c).

Effects of SiNPs on the capsaicin receptor TRPV1

Next, we performed intracellular Ca^{2+} imaging experiments to determine the effects of 300 µg/ml SiNPs on the response of TRPV1 to its specific agonist capsaicin (1 µM). TRPV1 is the founding member of the vanilloid subfamily of TRP channels, and its amino acid sequence has 42.3% identity and 58.9% similarity with that of TRPV4 (EMBOSS Needle application for Protein Alignment; http://www.ebi.ac.uk/Tools/psa/emboss_needle/help/index-protein.html). We found that the responses of HEK293T cells transfected with mouse TRPV1 to capsaicin were increased by 44% in the presence of SiNPs (P = 0.0011; Fig. 9).

SiNPs inhibit TRPV4-mediated increase of ciliary beat frequency in airway epithelial cells

The cilia of airway epithelial cells are considered to be sensory organelles with the ultimate function of sweeping mucous loaded with pollutants and pathogens out of the airways. TRPV4 is expressed in the cilia, and has been proposed to regulate mucociliary transport by transducing physical and chemical stimuli such as viscosity or fluid tonicity into a Ca^{2+} signal that enhances ciliary beat frequency [26, 27, 41, 42]. Thus, to determine whether the inhibition of TRPV4 by SiNPs has a

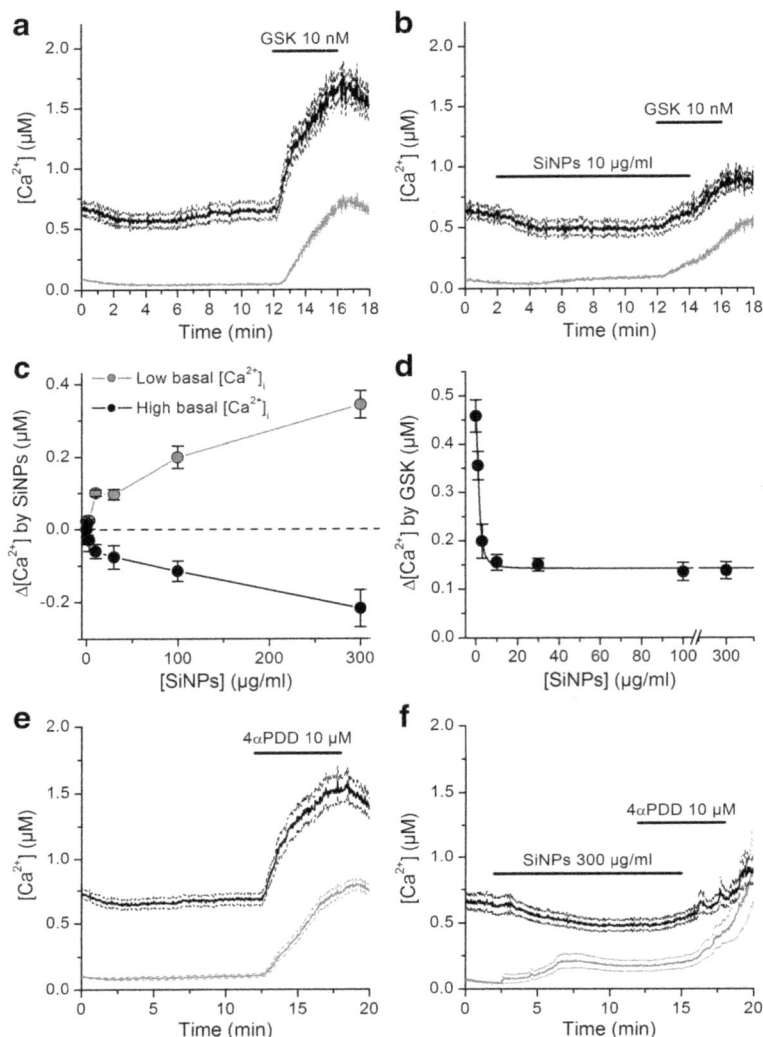

Fig. 5 SiNPs inhibit activation of mouse TRPV4 heterologously expressed in HEK293T cells. **a, b** Effects of the TRPV4 agonist GSK1016790A on the $[Ca^{2+}]_i$ in the absence (**a**, $n = 127$) or in the presence of 10 μg/ml SiNPs (**b**, $n = 243$). The thick continuous traces correspond to the average responses and the thin dashed traces correspond to the mean plus/minus the standard errors. The black and grey traces correspond to cells with high or low basal $[Ca^{2+}]_i$, respectively (see text). **c** Concentration-dependent effects on SiNPs on the intracellular Ca^{2+} levels in cells with low and high basal Ca^{2+}. **d** Average amplitude of responses to 10 nM GSK1016790A when applied in the presence of SiNPs at different concentrations. The solid line represents a fit with a Hill function (see Methods). **e, f** Effects of the TRPV4 agonist 4αPDD on the $[Ca^{2+}]_i$ in the absence (**a**, $n = 347$) or in the presence of SiNPs (**b**, $n = 164$). The traces are color-coded as in panels (**a**) and (**b**)

correlate at the level of a cellular function, we determined the effects of these nanoparticles on the response of cilia to GSK1016790A. Application of 10 nM GSK1016790A in control condition induced a significant 26 ± 3% increase in CBF ($n = 22$; $P < 10^{-4}$; paired t test; Fig. 10a). This effect was very similar to that reported by Alenmyr et al. in human nasal epithelial cells [43]. Application of 300 μg/ml SiNPs modestly reduced the basal CBF (~10%; n = 34; $P < 10^{-4}$; paired t test; Fig. 10b) and fully abrogated the response to GSK1016790A ($n = 34$; $P = 0.41$; paired t test between CBF immediately before and after 3 min application of the TRPV4 agonist).

Washout of SiNPs in the presence of the TRPV4 agonist led to an increase in CBF ($n = 34$; $P = 0.014$; paired t test). Because SiNPs reduced the basal CBF only slightly and fully inhibited the response to GSK1016790A we argue that the latter effect was mainly mediated by inhibition of TRPV4, and not by an unspecific effect of the nanoparticles on other mechanisms regulating the CBF.

Discussion

Despite the current advances in the characterization of the toxicological properties of SiNPs, little is known about how this material interacts with specific cellular

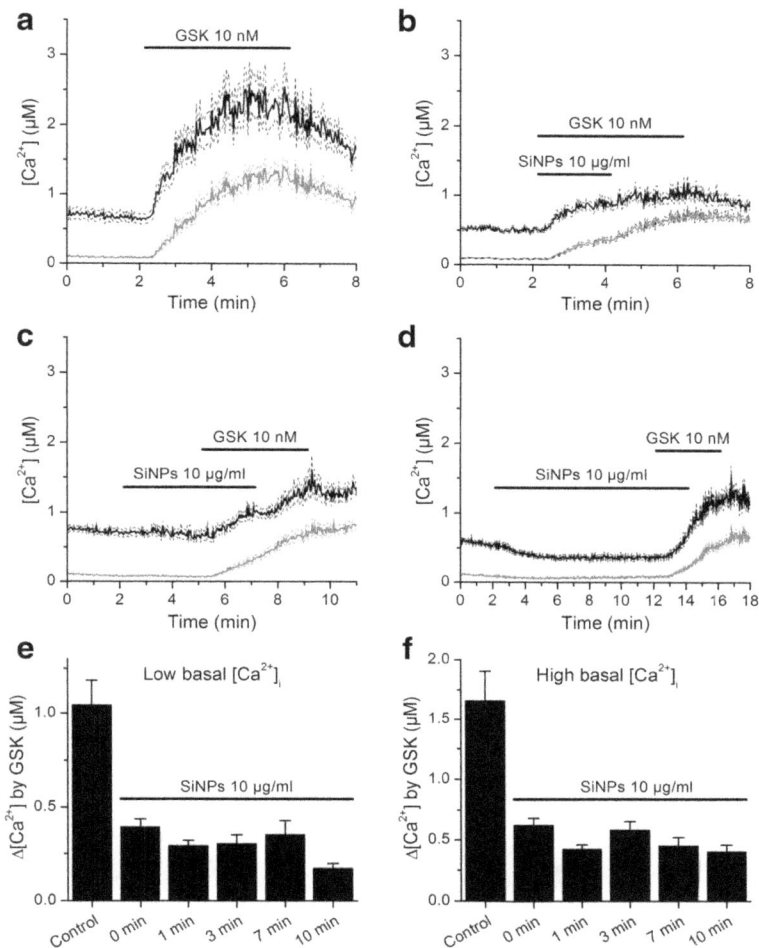

Fig. 6 The pre-application time of SiNP has no significant effect on the magnitude of inhibition of TRPV4 response to GSK1016790A. **a** Effects of the TRPV4 agonist GSK1016790A on the [Ca²⁺]ᵢ of HEK293T cells transfected with mouse TRPV4. **b, c, d** TRPV4 responses to GSK1016790A after pre-application of SiNPs during different periods (0, 3 and 10 min for panels **b, c** and **d**, respectively). The thick continuous traces correspond to the average responses and the thin dashed traces correspond to the mean plus/minus the standard errors. The black and grey traces correspond to cells with high or low basal [Ca²⁺]ᵢ, respectively (see text). **e, f** Average amplitude of responses to 2 min applications of GSK1016790A in control and after pre-application of SiNPs for different periods (n = 105 - 385)

components. Under the plausible assumption that SiNPs interact primarily with the plasma membrane of epithelial cells, in this study we evaluated the effects on TRPV4, a cation-permeable channel that is highly enriched in these cells.

In essence, we found that SiNPs inhibit intracellular Ca²⁺ signals triggered by activation of native TRPV4 channels in human and mouse airway epithelial cells. TRPV4 inhibition by SiNPs was confirmed with Ca²⁺ imaging and direct measurements of TRPV4 currents in the heterologous expression system HEK293T. In sharp contrast to these results, we show that SiNPs enhanced the activation of TRPV1, demonstrating that these particles have a specific inhibitory action on TRPV4 channels. Finally, we found that SiNPs abrogate the increase

in ciliary beat frequency induced by TRPV4 activation in mouse airway epithelial cells.

The comparison of the data obtained in mTEC and HEK293T cells transfected with mouse TRPV4 indicate that SiNPs have very similar effects on the responses to GSK1016790A, with IC_{50} values around 1 µg/ml. In contrast, SiNPs appeared to be much less effective in 16HBE cells, with a 100-fold higher IC_{50} value. This may indicate that human TRPV4 is less sensitive than the mouse isoform. Nevertheless, the SiNPs concentrations required to inhibit TRPV4 mediated responses in the human-derived cells (100 - 3000 µg/ml) are in the same range or lower than those used in cytotoxicity and cytokine release *in vitro* experiments performed in previous studies (25 - 6000 µg/ml [18, 23, 24]. Moreover, we

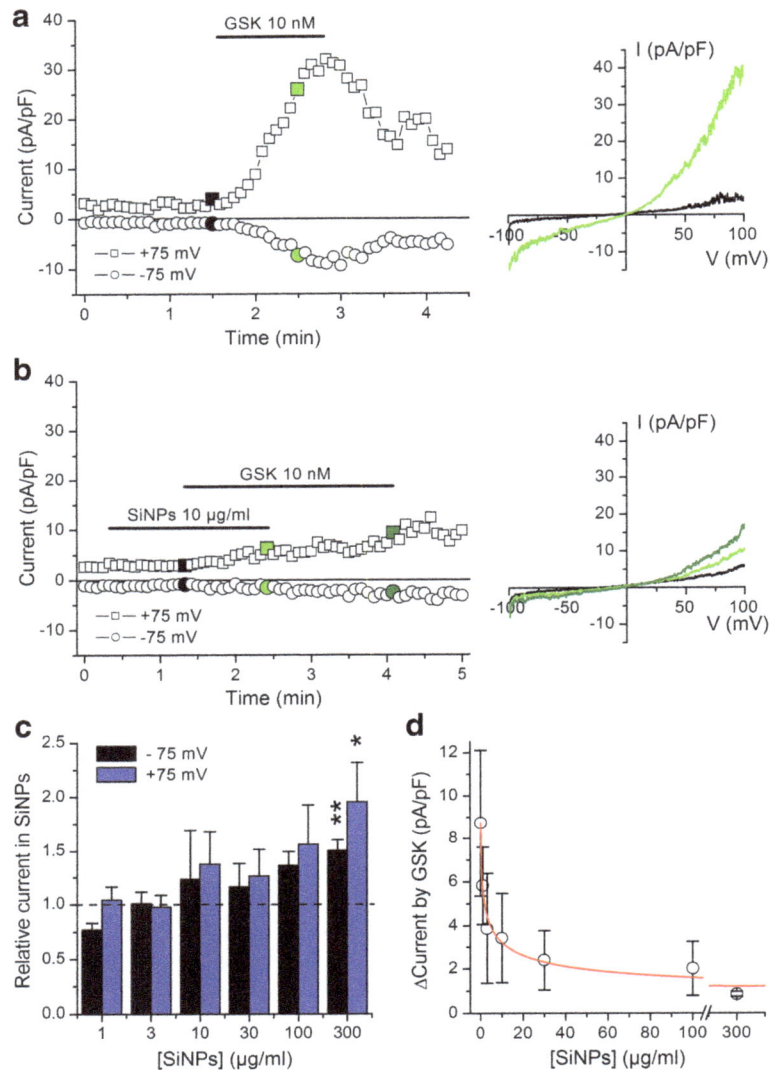

Fig. 7 SiNPs inhibit activation of TRPV4 currents in whole-cell patch-clamp recordings. **a, b)** Experiments in TRPV4-transfected HEK293T cells showing the effects of the TRPV4 agonist GSK1016790A in the absence (**a**) and in the presence (**b**) of SiNPs. The data points represent the amplitude of the currents measured at -75 and +75 mV. The colored data points correspond to the current traces displayed on the panels shown on the right. **c** Average amplitude of currents recorded at -75 and +75 mV during application of SiNPs. For every cell these values were normalized to the amplitude measured in control condition ($n = 3 - 10$; * and ** indicate $P < 0.05$ and $P < 0.01$, respectively; t test for comparison to 1). **d** Concentration-dependent inhibitory effect of SiNPs on the amplitude of TRPV4 currents measured at -75 mV during 1 min application of GSK1016790A. The solid line represents the fit with a Hill function (see Methods)

observed the inhibitory effect on TRPV4 in a matter of minutes, which represents a time scale 3- to 150-fold shorter than that of those previous reports. This strongly suggests TRPV4 as a primary and sensitive target of SiNPs.

As for the mechanism underlying the effects of SiNPs, it may be speculated that these particles somehow disrupt the binding site of GSK1016790A. SiNPs are roughly the same size of the whole channel protein, and more than twice the size of the length of the channel's transmembrane segments. So, it is unlikely that these

nanoparticles interact directly with a relatively small binding pocket for GSK1016790A, unless this would be located on the channel's outer interface. However, to the best of our knowledge, the binding site for GSK1016790A is not yet known. On the other hand, we gained some insight into this issue from the result that SiNPs also strongly inhibit TRPV4 activation by 4αPDD, a compound that was reported to interact with an internal pocket of the channel formed between transmembrane segments 3 and 4 [44]. Notably, SiNPs also altered the response of TRPV1 to capsaicin, which was reported to bind to an

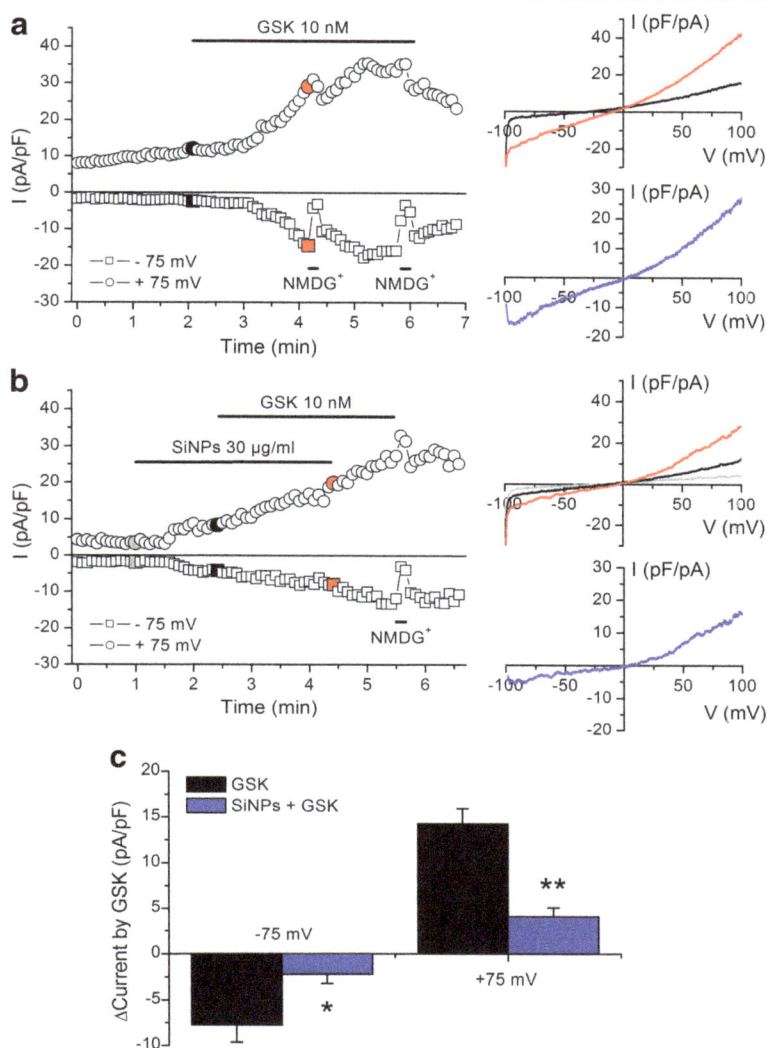

Fig. 8 SiNPs inhibit activation of TRPV4 currents in perforated patch-clamp recordings. **a, b** Experiments in TRPV4-transfected HEK293T cells showing the effects of the TRPV4 agonist GSK1016790A in the absence (**a**) and in the presence (**b**) of SiNPs. The data points represent the amplitude of the currents measured at -75 and +75 mV. The colored data points correspond to the current traces displayed on the panels shown on the right. **c** Average increase in the amplitude of currents (recorded at -75 and +75 mV) induced by the application of 10 nM GSK1016790A during 2 min, in the absence (n = 5) and in the presence (n = 6) of 30 µg/ml SiNPs. The * and ** symbols indicate P < 0.05 and P < 0.01; unpaired t test

occluded region of this channel [45]. Thus, according to our reasoning above, SiNPs seem not to act on TRPV4 and TRPV1 activation mechanisms by competitive inhibition. At this point we may just speculate that SiNPs induce mechanical perturbations in the plasma membrane that may disrupt activation of TRPV4 and enhance activation of TRPV1.

An interesting observation was that the SiNPs failed to completely inhibit TRPV4 activation. This could result from the presence of two channel populations with distinct sensitivities to SiNPs. This might be the case for the HEK293T cells, in which an endogenous human TRPV4 channel population may co-exist with the transfected mouse TRPV4 channels. However, we observed

the lack of complete inhibition also in native 16HBE and mTEC, for which there is no evidence for separate populations of TRPV4. Although further studies are required to address this point, we may also consider that if SiNPs inhibit channel activation by inducing mechanical perturbations in the plasma membrane, these might not be sufficient to completely silence channel activity.

A concomitant finding in our experiments was that SiNPs induce an increase in basal $[Ca^{2+}]_i$ in the human-derived cells. However, our data demonstrates that TRPV4 channels are not involved in this effect (e.g., lack of inhibitory effect of the TRPV4 blocker HC067047). This is different from what was previously suggested by Gilardino et al., who found that the unspecific TRPV

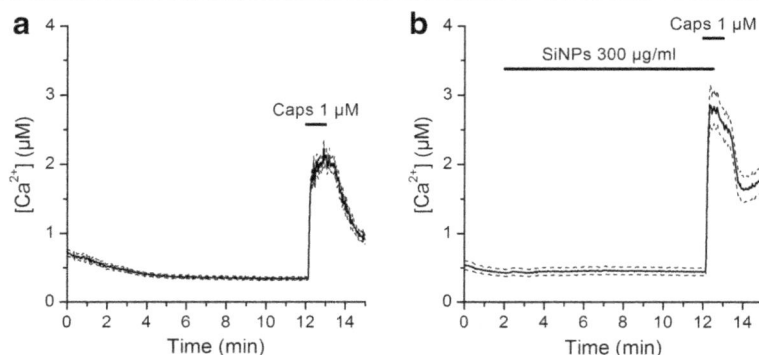

Fig. 9 Effects of SiNPs on the capsaicin receptor TRPV1. **a, b** Effects of the TRPV1 agonist capsaicin on the $[Ca^{2+}]_i$ of HEK293T cells transfected with mouse TRPV1, in the absence (**a**, $n = 200$) or in the presence of SiNPs (**b**, $n = 68$). The thick continuous traces correspond to the average responses and the thin dashed traces correspond to the mean plus/minus the standard errors

channel blocker ruthenium red inhibited intracellular Ca^{2+} responses to SiNPs [38]. A possible cause for this is that these authors used particles of 50 nm in diameter, which represents about a 170-fold larger volume than that of the ones we used here. Considering that TRPV4 can be activated by mechanical stress at the plasma membrane [39, 46], it is conceivable that only the larger particles may induce TRPV4 activation. On the other hand, Gilardino et al. [38] did find TRPV4-independent responses to SiNPs, which could be triggered via mechanisms similar to those underlying the responses we found in 16HBE cells and in HEK293T cells displaying low basal Ca^{2+} concentration. Of note, for some yet unclear reasons mTEC did not display Ca^{2+} responses upon SiNPs application.

Other features of our results are also qualitatively comparable to those obtained by Gilardino et al. [38]. For instance, the intracellular Ca^{2+} responses to SiNPs occurred after a significant delay and showed a transient initial phase (Fig. 2b). The mechanisms underlying these responses remain fully unknown, but could be related to Ca^{2+} release from intracellular stores. However, the fact that we found SiNPs to increase inward and outward

basal currents in HEK293T cells is more consistent with enhanced activities of Ca^{2+}-permeable channels in the plasma membrane (e.g., the ubiquitously expressed TRPM7 channels) [47]. These mechanisms should be addressed in future studies because they may bare relevance for the toxic effects of SiNPs (Ca^{2+} overload) in airway epithelial cells.

Conclusions

Our results show that SiNPs inhibit TRPV4 activation, and that this effect may impair the positive modulatory action of the stimulation of this channel on the ciliary function in airway epithelial cells. It has been proposed that inhibition of TRPV4 could have therapeutic benefits in several respiratory conditions, such as chronic heart failure, hypoxia-induced pulmonary hypertension, acute lung injury, chronic obstructive pulmonary disease and cough [48–51]. However, TRPV4 activity has been shown to underlie protective responses in airway epithelial cells, including the increase in CBF [26, 43]. In addition, TRPV4 function was reported to be important for essential functions in other cells that are direct targets of polluting SiNPs. These include the enhancement

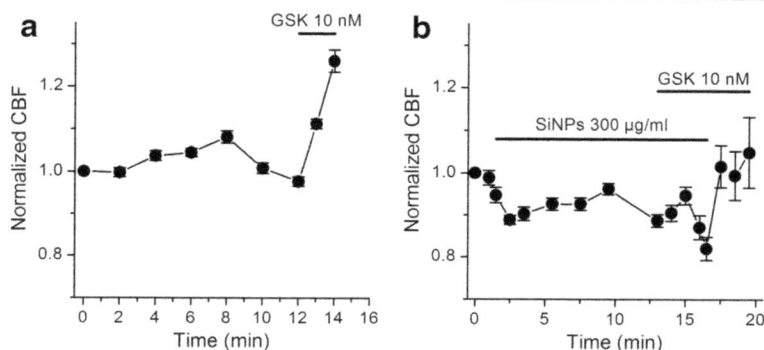

Fig. 10 SiNPs inhibit the increase in ciliary beat frequency induced by activation of TRPV4 in mTEC. **a** Increase of CBF induced by application of the TRPV4 agonist GSK1016790A. **b** Lack of effect of GSK1016790A on the CBF in the presence of SiNPs

of barrier function is skin keratynocytes [52, 53], endothelium-dependent vasorelaxation in pulmonary arteries [54], and ATP release from oesophageal keratynocytes [55]. Thus, inhibition of TRPV4 by SiNPs is expected to have complex effects on airway pathophysiology and rather certain detrimental effects on several epithelial cell functions. Our findings unveil TRPV4 and TRPV1 as defined molecular targets of SiNPs, and prompt for further exploration of the role of these channels in the cellular effects of other types of particulate matter.

Acknowledgements
The authors would like to thank Prof. Bernd Nilius and the members of the LICR laboratory for helpful discussions and to Melissa Benoit for the maintenance of the cell cultures.

Funding
Y.A.A. held a Postdoctoral Mandate of the KU Leuven and is currently a Postdoctoral Fellow of the Fund for Scientific Research Flanders (FWO). Research was supported by grants from the Research Foundation Flanders FWO (G076714), the Research Council of the KU Leuven (Grants GOA/14/011 and PF-TRPLe), The Spanish Ministry of Economy and Competitiveness (SAF2015-69762R and María de Maeztu Programme for Units of Excellence in R&D MDM-2014-0370), and the FEDER Funds.

Authors' contributions
AS, KD and YAA performed Ca^{2+} imaging experiments; AS, JLA and JAC performed the patch-clamp experiments; CJ performed the CBF measurements; SMC performed the characterization of the particles; MAV, PHH and KT supervised the project; AS and KT wrote the manuscript. All authors edited the manuscript, and have given approval to its final version.

Competing interests
The authors declare that they have no competing interests.

Author details
[1]Department of Cellular and Molecular Medicine, Laboratory of Ion Channel Research, KU Leuven; VIB Center for Brain & Disease Research, Leuven, Belgium. [2]Department of Experimental and Health Sciences, Laboratory of Molecular Physiology and Channelopathies, Universitat Pompeu Fabra, Barcelona, Spain. [3]KU Leuven BIOMAT, Department of Oral Health Sciences, KU Leuven & Dentistry University Hospitals Leuven, Leuven, Belgium. [4]Department of Public Health and Primary Care, KU Leuven, Leuven, Belgium. [5]Present address: Department of Cardiovascular Sciences, Laboratory of Experimental Cardiology, Leuven, KU, Belgium.

References
1. Fede C, Selvestrel F, Compagnin C, Mognato M, Mancin F, Reddi E, et al. The toxicity outcome of silica nanoparticles (Ludox®) is influenced by testing techniques and treatment modalities. Anal. Bioanal. Chem. 2012; 404:1789–802.
2. Fede C, Millino C, Pacchioni B, Celegato B, Compagnin C, Martini P, et al. Altered gene transcription in human cells treated with ludox® silica nanoparticles. Int. J. Environ. Res. Public Health. 2014;11:8867–90.
3. Napierska D, Thomassen LCJ, Rabolli V, Lison D, Gonzalez L, Kirsch-Volders M, et al. Size-dependent cytotoxicity of monodisperse silica nanoparticles in human endothelial cells. Small. 2009;5:846–53.
4. Napierska D, Quarck R, Thomassen LCJ, Lison D, Martens J. a, Delcroix M, et al. Amorphous silica nanoparticles promote monocyte adhesion to human endothelial cells: size-dependent effect. Small. 2012;9:1–9.
5. Vance ME, Kuiken T, Vejerano EP, McGinnis SP, Hochella MF, Rejeski D, et al. Nanotechnology in the real world: Redeveloping the nanomaterial consumer products inventory. Beilstein J. Nanotechnol. 2015;6:1769–80.
6. Kettiger H, Schipanski A, Wick P, Huwyler J. Engineered nanomaterial uptake and tissue distribution: from cell to organism. Int. J. Nanomedicine. 2013;8:3255–69.
7. Al-Rawi M, Diabaté S, Weiss C. Uptake and intracellular localization of submicron and nano-sized SiO_2 particles in HeLa cells. Arch. Toxicol. 2011;85:813–26.
8. Thomassen LCJ, Rabolli V, Masschaele K Alberto G, Tomatis M, Ghiazza M, et al. Model system to study the influence of aggregation on the hemolytic potential of silica nanoparticles. Chem. Res. Toxicol. 2011;24:1869–75.
9. Yu P, Li J, Jiang J, Zhao Z, Hui Z, Zhang J, et al. A dual role of transient receptor potential melastatin 2 channel in cytotoxicity induced by silica nanoparticles. Sci. Rep. 2015;5:18171.
10. Ahmad J, Ahamed M, Akhtar MJ, Alrokayan SA, Siddiqui MA, Musarrat J, et al. Apoptosis induction by silica nanoparticles mediated through reactive oxygen species in human liver cell line HepG2. Toxicol. Appl. Pharmacol. Elsevier Inc. 2012;259:160–8.
11. Kim I-Y, Joachim E, Choi H, Kim K. Toxicity of silica nanoparticles depends on size, dose, and cell type. Nanomedicine Nanotechnology, Biol. Med. Elsevier Inc. 2015;11:1407–16.
12. Sun L, Li Y, Liu X, Jin M, Zhang L, Du Z, et al. Cytotoxicity and mitochondrial damage caused by silica nanoparticles. Toxicol. Vitr. Elsevier Ltd. 2011;25:1619–29.
13. Nagakura C, Negishi Y, Tsukimoto M, Itou S, Kondo T, Takeda K, et al. Involvement of P2Y11 receptor in silica nanoparticles 30-induced IL-6 production by human keratinocytes. Toxicology. Elsevier Ireland Ltd. 2014;322:61–8.
14. Corbalan JJ, Medina C, Jacoby A, Malinski T, Radomski MW. Amorphous silica nanoparticles trigger nitric oxide/peroxynitrite imbalance in human endothelial cells: inflammatory and cytotoxic effects. Int. J. Nanomedicine. 2011;6:2821–35.
15. Stępnik M, Arkusz J, Smok-Pieniążek A, Bratek-Skicki A, Salvati A, Lynch I, et al. Cytotoxic effects in 3T3-L1 mouse and WI-38 human fibroblasts following 72 hour and 7 day exposures to commercial silica nanoparticles. Toxicol. Appl. Pharmacol. 2012;263:89–101.
16. Guo C, Xia Y, Niu P, Jiang L, Duan J, Yu Y, et al. Silica nanoparticles induce oxidative stress, inflammation, and endothelial dysfunction in vitro via activation of the MAPK/Nrf2 pathway and nuclear factor-κB signaling. Int. J. Nanomedicine. 2015;10:1463–77.
17. Ariano P, Zamburlin P, Gilardino A, Mortera R, Onida B, Tomatis M, et al. Interaction of spherical silica nanoparticles with neuronal cells: Size-dependent toxicity and perturbation of calcium homeostasis. Small. 2011;7:766–74.
18. Kasper J, Hermanns MI, Bantz C, Maskos M, Stauber R, Pohl C, et al. Inflammatory and cytotoxic responses of an alveolar-capillary coculture model to silica nanoparticles: comparison with conventional monocultures. Part. Fibre Toxicol. BioMed Central Ltd. 2011;8:6.
19. Hofmann F, Bläsche R, Kasper M, Barth KA. Co-culture system with an organotypic lung slice and an immortal alveolar macrophage cell line to quantify silica-induced inflammation. PLoS One. 2015;10:e0117056.
20. Marchiando AM, Graham WV, Turner JR. Epithelial barriers in homeostasis and disease. Annu. Rev. Pathol. 2010;5:119–44.
21. Ganesan S, Comstock AT, Sajjan US. Barrier function of airway tract epithelium. Tissue barriers. 2013;1:e24997.
22. Satir P, Sleigh MA. The physiology of cilia and mucociliary interactions. Annu. Rev. Physiol. 1990;52:137–55.
23. Rabolli V, Badissi A, Devosse R, Uwambayinema F, Yakoub Y, Palmai-Pallag M, et al. The alarmin IL-1α is a master cytokine in acute lung inflammation induced by silica micro- and nanoparticles. Part. Fibre Toxicol. 2014;11:69.
24. Skuland T, Ovrevik J, Låg M, Schwarze P. Refsnes M. Silica nanoparticles induce cytokine responses in lung epithelial cells through activation of a p38/TACE/TGF-α/EGFR-pathway and NF-κB signalling. Toxicol. Appl. Pharmacol. Elsevier Inc. 2014;279:76–86.
25. Delaval M, Boland S, Solhonne B, Nicola M-A, Mornet S, Baeza-Squiban A, et al. Acute exposure to silica nanoparticles enhances mortality and increases lung permeability in a mouse model of Pseudomonas aeruginosa pneumonia. Part. Fibre Toxicol. 2015;12:1.

26. Lorenzo IM, Liedtke W, Sanderson MJ, Valverde MA. TRPV4 channel participates in receptor-operated calcium entry and ciliary beat frequency regulation in mouse airway epithelial cells. Proc. Natl. Acad. Sci. U. S. A. 2008;05:12611–6.

27. Andrade YN, Fernandes J, Lorenzo IM, Arniges M, Valverde MA. The TRPV4 channel in ciliated epithelia. In: TRP Ion Channel Function in Sensory Transduction and Cellular Signaling Cascades. Liedtke WB, Heller S, editors. Boca Raton: CRC Press/Taylor & Francis; 2007. Chapter 30.

28. Alvarez DF, King JA, Weber D, Addison E, Liedtke W, Townsley MI. Transient receptor potential vanilloid 4-mediated disruption of the alveolar septal barrier: A novel mechanism of acute lung injury. Circ. Res. 2006;99:988–95.

29. Cioffi DL, Lowe K, Alvarez DF, Barry C, Stevens T. TRPing on the lung endothelium: calcium channels that regulate barrier function. Antioxid. Redox Signal. 2009;11:765–76.

30. Li J, Kanju P, Patterson M, Chew W-L, Cho S-H, Gilmour I, et al. TRPV4-mediated calcium influx into human bronchial epithelia upon exposure to diesel exhaust particles. Environ. Health Perspect. 2011;119:784–93.

31. Nilius B, Owsianik G, Voets T, Peters J A. Transient receptor potential cation channels in disease. Physiol. 2007; Vol.87.

32. Bhargave G, Woodworth BA, Xiong G, Wolfe SG, Antunes MB, Cohen NA. Transient receptor potential vanilloid type 4 channel expression in chronic rhinosinusitis. Am. J. Rhinol. 22:7–12.

33. Goldenberg NM, Ravindran K, Kuebler WM. TRPV4: physiological role and therapeutic potential in respiratory diseases. Naunyn. Schmiedebergs. Arch. Pharmacol. 2014;388:421–36.

34. Meseguer VM, Denlinger BL, Talavera K. Methodological considerations to understand the sensory function of TRP channels. Curr. Pharm. Biotechnol. 2011;12:3–11.

35. Andrade YN, Fernandes J, Vázquez E, Fernández-Fernández JM, Arniges M, Sánchez TM, et al. TRPV4 channel is involved in the coupling of fluid viscosity changes to epithelial ciliary activity. J. Cell Biol. 2005;168:869–74.

36. Fernández-Fernández JM, Nobles M, Currid A, Vázquez E, Valverde MA, Maxi K⁺ channel mediates regulatory volume decrease response in a human bronchial epithelial cell line. Am. J. Physiol. Cell Physiol. 2002;283:C1705–14.

37. Fernández-Fernández JM, Andrade YN, Arniges M, Fernandes J, Plata C, Rubio-Moscardo F, et al. Functional coupling of TRPV4 cationic channel and large conductance, calcium-dependent potassium channel in human bronchial epithelial cell lines. Pflügers Arch. 2008;457:149–59.

38. Gilardino A, Catalano F, Ruffinatti FA, Alberto G, Nilius B, Antoniotti S, et al. Interaction of SiO₂ nanoparticles with neuronal cells: Ionic mechanisms involved in the perturbation of calcium homeostasis. Int. J. Biochem. Cell Biol. Elsevier Ltd. 2015;66:101–11.

39. Alpizar YA, Sanchez A, Radwan A, Radwan I, Voets T, Talavera K. Lack of correlation between the amplitudes of TRP channel-mediated responses to weak and strong stimuli in intracellular Ca²⁺ imaging experiments. Cell Calcium. Elsevier Ltd. 2013;54:362–74.

40. Everaerts W, Zhen X, Ghosh D, Vriens J, Gevaert T, Gilbert JP, et al. Inhibition of the cation channel TRPV4 improves bladder function in mice and rats with cyclophosphamide-induced cystitis. J. Urol. 2011;186:753.

41. Fernandes J, Lorenzo IM, Andrade YN, Garcia-Elias A, Serra SA, Fernández-Fernández JM, et al. IP3 sensitizes TRPV4 channel to the mechano-and osmotransducing messenger 5'-6'-epoxyeicosatrienoic acid. J. Cell Biol. 2008;181:143–55.

42. Balakrishna S, Song W, Achanta S, Doran SF, Liu B, Kaelberer MM, et al. TRPV4 inhibition counteracts edema and inflammation and improves pulmonary function and oxygen saturation in chemically induced acute lung injury. Am. J. Physiol. Lung Cell. Mol. Physiol. 2014;307:L158–72.

43. Alenmyr L, Uller L, Greiff L, Högestätt ED, Zygmunt PM. TRPV4-mediated calcium influx and ciliary activity in human native airway epithelial cells. Basic Clin. Pharmacol. Toxicol. 2014;114:210–6.

44. Vriens J, Owsianik G, Janssens A, Voets T, Nilius B. Determinants of 4 alpha-phorbol sensitivity in transmembrane domains 3 and 4 of the cation channel TRPV4. J Biol Chem. 2007;282:12796–803.

45. Cao E, Liao M, Cheng Y, Julius D. TRPV1 structures in distinct conformations reveal activation mechanisms. Nature. 2013;504:113–8.

46. Watanabe H, Vriens J, Janssens A, Wondergem R, Droogmans G, Nilius B. Modulation of TRPV4 gating by intra- and extracellular Ca²⁺. Cell Calcium. 2003;33:489–95.

47. Fleig A, Chubanov V. TRPM7. In: Mamm. Transient Recept. Potential Cation Channels Vol. I. Nilius B, Flockerzi V, editors. Berlin, Heidelberg: Springer Berlin Heidelberg; 2014. pp. 521–46.

48. Bonvini SJ, Birrell MA, Smith JA, Belvisi MG, Targeting TRP. channels for chronic cough: From bench to bedside. Naunyn. Schmiedebergs. Arch. Pharmacol. 2015;388:401–20.

49. Goldenberg N, Wang L, Ranke H, Tabuchi A, Kuebler WM. TRPV4 Channel Activity Is Required For Hypoxic Pulmonary Vasoconstriction. Anesthesiology. 2005;122(6):1338–48.

50. Grace MS, Baxter M, Dubuis E, Birrell MA, Belvisi MG. Transient receptor potential (TRP) channels in the airway: Role in airway disease. Br. J. Pharmacol. 2014;171:2593–607.

51. Loot AE, Popp R, Fisslthaler B, Vriens J, Nilius B, Fleming I. Role of cytochrome P450-dependent transient receptor potential V4 activation in flow-induced vasodilatation. Cardiovasc. Res. 2008;80:445–52.

52. Sokabe T, Fukumi-Tominaga T, Yonemura S, Mizuno A, Tominaga M. The TRPV4 channel contributes to intercellular junction formation in keratinocytes. J. Biol. Chem. 2010;285:18749–58.

53. Kida N, Sokabe T, Kashio M, Haruna K, Mizuno Y, Suga Y, et al. Importance of transient receptor potential vanilloid 4 (TRPV4) in epidermal barrier function in human skin keratinocytes. Pflugers. Arch. Eur. J. Physiol. 2012; 463:715–25.

54. Sukumaran SV, Singh TU, Parida S, Narasimha Reddy CE, Thangamalai R, Kandasamy K, et al. TRPV4 channel activation leads to endothelium-dependent relaxation mediated by nitric oxide and endothelium-derived hyperpolarizing factor in rat pulmonary artery. Pharmacol. Res. Elsevier Ltd. 2013;78:18–27.

55. Mihara H, Boudaka A, Sugiyama T, Moriyama Y, Tominaga M. Transient receptor potential vanilloid 4 (TRPV4)-dependent calcium influx and ATP release in mouse oesophageal keratinocytes. J. Physiol. 2011;589:3471–82.

Grouping of nanomaterials to read-across hazard endpoints: from data collection to assessment of the grouping hypothesis by application of chemoinformatic techniques

L. Lamon[†], D. Asturiol[*†] [iD], A. Richarz, E. Joossens, R. Graepel, K. Aschberger and A. Worth

Abstract

Background: An increasing number of manufactured nanomaterials (NMs) are being used in industrial products and need to be registered under the REACH legislation. The hazard characterisation of all these forms is not only technically challenging but resource and time demanding. The use of non-testing strategies like read-across is deemed essential to assure the assessment of all NMs in due time and at lower cost. The fact that read-across is based on the structural similarity of substances represents an additional difficulty for NMs as in general their structure is not unequivocally defined. In such a scenario, the identification of physicochemical properties affecting the hazard potential of NMs is crucial to define a grouping hypothesis and predict the toxicological hazards of similar NMs. In order to promote the read-across of NMs, ECHA has recently published "Recommendations for nanomaterials applicable to the guidance on QSARs and Grouping", but no practical examples were provided in the document. Due to the lack of publicly available data and the inherent difficulties of reading-across NMs, only a few examples of read-across of NMs can be found in the literature. This manuscript presents the first case study of the practical process of grouping and read-across of NMs following the workflow proposed by ECHA.

Methods: The workflow proposed by ECHA was used and slightly modified to present the read-across case study. The Read-Across Assessment Framework (RAAF) was used to evaluate the uncertainties of a read-across within NMs. Chemoinformatic techniques were used to support the grouping hypothesis and identify key physicochemical properties.

Results: A dataset of 6 nanoforms of TiO_2 with more than 100 physicochemical properties each was collected. In vitro comet assay result was selected as the endpoint to read-across due to data availability. A correlation between the presence of coating or large amounts of impurities and negative comet assay results was observed.

Conclusion: The workflow proposed by ECHA to read-across NMs was applied successfully. Chemoinformatic techniques were shown to provide key evidence for the assessment of the grouping hypothesis and the definition of similar NMs. The RAAF was found to be applicable to NMs.

Keywords: Grouping, Nanomaterials, Read-across, Nano-TiO_2, Comet assay, RAAF, REACH, Hazard, Chemoinformatics

* Correspondence: david.asturiol-bofill@ec.europa.eu
[†]L. Lamon and D. Asturiol contributed equally to this work.
European Commission, Joint Research Centre, Ispra, Varese, Italy

Background

Chemicals safety assessment is addressed in Europe by the Regulation (EC) No 1907/2006 concerning the Registration, Evaluation, Authorisation and Restriction of Chemicals (REACH) [1] which requires companies to assess the risks posed by marketed chemicals. This implies the generation of toxicological data as it is required in risk assessment to address any identified hazard. It is stated in the REACH legislation that all available in vitro, in vivo and historical human data, data from valid (Q)SARs and data from structurally related similar substances (read-across approach), must be assessed before carrying out any test.

The use of non-testing strategies like read-across is key for nanomaterials (NMs) as estimations suggest that between 500 and 2000 NMs with < 10 nanoforms[1] per NM type are/will be manufactured or imported in Europe in quantities greater than 1 t/annum [2, 3].

Read-across is regarded as a technique for predicting endpoint information for one or more substances (target substance(s)) by using data from the same endpoint from (an)other substance(s) provided that these substances are similar, i.e. have similar physicochemical, toxicological and ecotoxicological properties, or follow a regular pattern as a result of structural similarity that allows them to be considered a group (REACH Annex XI). The identification of structurally similar substances is more challenging for NMs than regular chemicals because NMs do not have a uniquely defined structure. The European Chemicals Agency (ECHA) has recently released guidance on how to justify grouping for read-across between nanoforms of the same substance [4]. This guidance proposes a revised version of a strategy presented earlier [5] and considers properties beyond chemical composition (e.g. aspect ratio, particle size, shape, or solubility), and reaffirms the similarity rules from REACH Annex XI for NMs.

In spite of the efforts put to favour the use of read-across between nanoforms [5–10] only a few examples of read-across for NMs are found in the literature. One of this examples corresponds to the cytotoxicity of metal oxides for E. coli and HaCaT cell line (human keratinocytes), which uses physicochemical properties like the enthalpy of formation of the metal oxide nanocluster and Mulliken's electronegativity to determine similarity [11]. Another study proposes a NM ranking based on solubility and band gap [12]. These case studies are illustrative for the fact that available studies mostly use physicochemical properties that are not specific to NMs to support grouping based on similarity. Other examples available in the literature are exemplified by the application of the DF4nanoGrouping framework to 24 NM of different types (carbon based, metal and metal oxide, silica, organic) [13], which groups NM into 4 subgroups (soluble, biopersistent, passive, and active) for further read-across. This framework takes into consideration NM-specific physicochemical properties like particle morphology and composition, dissolution rate, surface reactivity, dispersibility.

In this manuscript, we present a case study of grouping and read-across of TiO_2 nanoforms where we apply a simplified version of the grouping framework proposed by ECHA to predict the in vitro comet assay results of the target substances. One key step in read-across is the determination of the physicochemical properties that define the groups and similarities between analogues of the same category, which was achieved with the help of chemoinformatic techniques such as hierarchical clustering (HC), principal component analysis (PCA), and random forest variable selection. Evaluation of uncertainties in the similarity and read-across justifications is an important part of a read-across exercise. ECHA developed the Read-Across Assessment framework (RAAF) as guidance for systematic analysis of uncertainties in read-across justifications submitted for REACH. In this case study, the confidence in the read-across argumentation was evaluated following the RAAF also in view of assessing whether the RAAF is, with the given scenarios, applicable to NMs. Considering that the RAAF is based on chemical structural similarity and consistent with the REACH definition of similarity for read-across, it is expected that the main difficulties for its application to NMs will be related to their characterisation and to the properties associated to the toxicological effect.

Methods
Workflow for grouping and read-across
The present case study follows a simplified version of the workflow proposed by ECHA [4], as illustrated in Fig. 1.

Step 1 of the framework corresponds to the *identification of the nanoforms of the substance* including source (analogues) and target substances, i.e. "what they are" [14], where NMs are identified through properties like composition, impurities, surface chemistry, size, shape. Step 2 on *gathering of data for each group member and evaluate the data for adequacy and reliability* consists in collecting data for each analogue on "where they go", including properties like solubility, hydrophobicity, zeta potential, size distribution, dispersibility, dustiness, and "what they do", including properties related to redox activity. A matrix reports the collected information for analysis. Step 3 *grouping of nanoforms* consists in the analysis to identify similarities between analogues and to build the grouping hypothesis. Step 4 *assess the applicability of the approach, and fill data gaps* consists in the justification of the grouping hypothesis by means of chemoinformatic techniques and the read-across prediction; this step involves also an assessment of the robustness of the grouping hypothesis by supporting it with mechanistic evidence and uncertainty analysis.

1 **Identification of the (nano)forms of the substance**
- Identification of the target analogues
- Identification of the source analogues
  The different nanoforms are identified by their basic physicochemical parameters ("what they are")

2 **Gather the available data for each group member and evaluate the data for adequacy and reliability; build a data matrix**
- *Physicochemical properties*
  Data collection on "where they go" and "what they do"; any other physicochemical property of relevance for the endpoint of interest can be included
- *(Eco) toxicology*
  More data on toxicological endpoints are collected to support the grouping hypothesis
- All the collected information on physicochemical properties and on the toxicological endpoint to read-across is presented in a matrix, including the target analogues

3 **Grouping of nanoforms**
- Develop a grouping hypothesis for the endpoint considering all the collected information on the physicochemical properties and on the available endpoint values· to identify similarity between the source analogues
- Assign the source analogues to the groups

4 **Assess the applicability of the approach and fill data gaps**
- Assessment of the grouping hypothesis
  This may be verified by application of unsupervised computational methods like e.g. clustering techniques, principal component analysis, or supervised computational methods like, e.g. random forest
- Fill data gaps
  If enough data are available, then the prediction can be made by including target analogues in suitable computational techniques (e.g. clustering, PCA, random forest); otherwise the target NMs can be assigned to each group by weight of evidence
- Is the group robust enough?
  Robust mechanistic evidence supports the grouping hypothesis; uncertainty analysis may be included

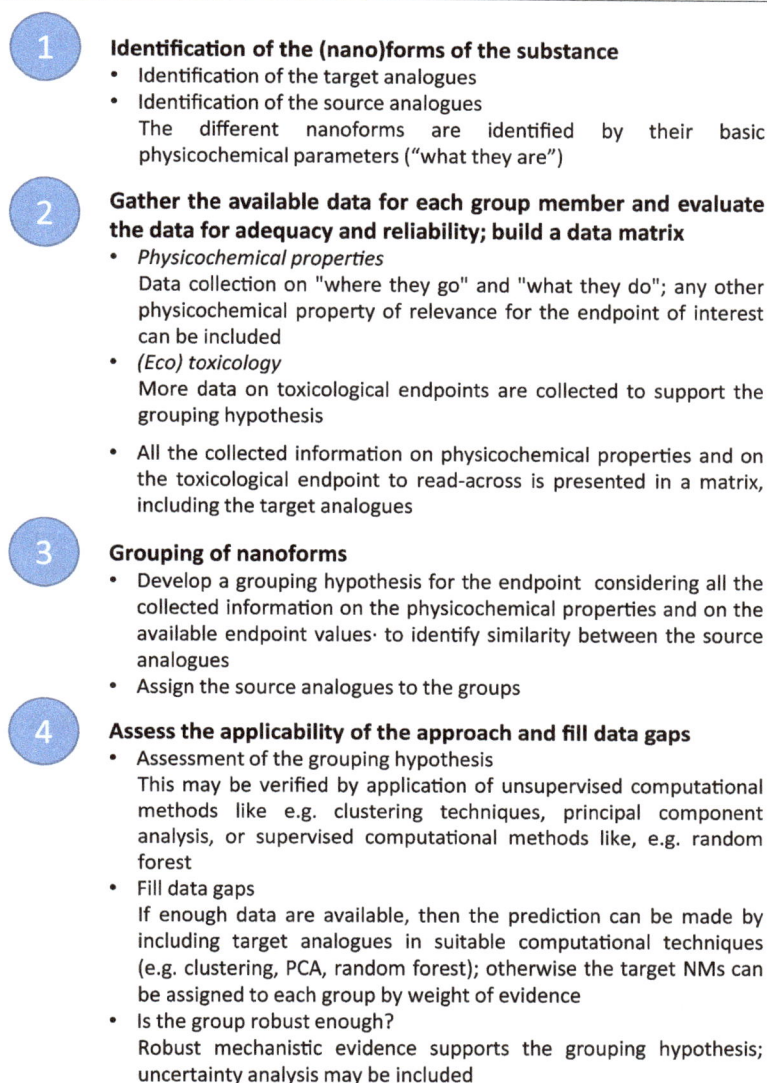

Fig. 1 Framework for grouping and read-across for reporting the nano-TiO$_2$ case study. A simplified version from the framework proposed by ECHA [4]

In the case of NMs, the definition of analogues is not as straightforward as for e.g. organic chemicals, because the influence that the different properties (e.g. size, coating, composition, or solubility) can have on their behaviour (activity) is not yet well understood. If enough data is available, chemoinformatics may also be used to identify the relevant properties for a specific endpoint.

Computational methods

A set of statistical methods often used in chemoinformatics were applied using R 3.2.5 [15] to identify the most relevant (physicochemical) properties to determine similarity between analogues and support the grouping hypothesis. These techniques were:

(1) Hierarchical clustering (HC) [16]: was applied to identify possible clusters or groups of analogues in the dataset, i.e. similar NMs

(2) Principal component analysis (PCA) [17]: was applied to determine the physicochemical properties that differentiate the NMs and to observe possible clusters of NM and properties

(3) Random forest variable selection [18]: was applied to determine the most relevant properties in predicting in vitro comet assay results. Unlike hierarchical clustering and PCA this is a supervised technique and, therefore, makes use of physicochemical properties to *predict* a given outcome, which in this case was genotoxicity as determined by the comet assay.

Data treatment

Our initial dataset on toxicological endpoints was collected from the OECD dossier on TiO_2 [19] that, although not aimed specifically at hazard assessment, is considered an updated NMs data repository. This toxicological dataset was expanded for the selected endpoint to be read-across by searching available studies in the literature. The final dataset consisted mainly of tests carried out within the Nanogenotox Joint Action [20]. A reliability assessment of the collected studies was performed according to the criteria defined by the French agency for food, environmental and occupational health and safety (ANSES) [21], which states that reliable studies must contain:

(1) NMs characterisation (at least size, crystallinity and coating) and a description of the dispersed materials (particle size distribution, zeta potential, polydispersity index)
(2) Observed NM uptake and/or non-cytotoxicity
(3) Positive and negative controls as well as replicates

Due to the lack of standard operating procedures (SOPs) for NMs, the collected data for nano-TiO_2 was found to contain the same measures with different techniques (e.g. Dynamic Light Scattering for particle size distribution and Transmission Electron microscope for particle size), data measured in different solvents (e.g. MilliQ water, Fetal Bovine Serum, Phosphate-Buffered Saline), or with different pre-treatments (e.g. not sonicated, 1 min sonication with tip sonication, 20 min bath sonication). In such a situation, two options can be considered: a) each technique, instrument, media, and pre-treatment is considered as a different property or b) data from different origins is merged into a common value. Both options present advantages and disadvantages. Keeping each value as a different measure leads to a dataset with a number of data gaps, which is unusable for modelling or read-across as the properties are not considered comparable. Therefore, it becomes almost impossible to compare two substances. In order to avoid this scenario, the data obtained from different sources was merged. A detailed explanation of how the data was merged for each property can be found in Section 1.2 of the Additional file 1.

Read-across assessment framework

The ECHA RAAF [22] was used as guidance for a structured evaluation of uncertainties in the read-across argumentation. It distinguishes six scenarios defined by the read-across approach taken (analogue or category approach), whether the effect is caused by identical or different compounds for the source(s) and target(s) – which can be either the parent or metabolites formed by biotransformation, respectively – and whether the predicted property is following a trend in the category or not changing across source structures. For each scenario a set of Assessment Elements (AEs), comprising multiple considerations and questions, has to be addressed. They evaluate amongst others the similarity hypothesis, availability and quality of data, and the postulated mechanism of toxicity. The outcome of the analysis and conclusions on the scientific robustness and validity of the read-across justification are scored with Assessment Options, i.e. scores from one to five indicating whether the information provided is not acceptable at all (1), or in its current form (2), or acceptable with just sufficient (3), medium (4) or high (5) confidence.

From the six RAAF scenarios, scenario 6 was chosen as best describing the present case of nano-TiO_2 read-across. It corresponds to a category approach, with different compounds (i.e. nanoforms) considered to have the same type of effect, and no variations in the effect, i.e. the comet assay result is either positive or negative, but has no varying potency following a trend. The read-across hypothesis is judged via assessment elements C.1-C.6, common to all RAAF scenarios, and 6.1–6.5 as specific AEs for scenario 6.

Results

This section is structured following the workflow of Fig. 1.

Step 1: Identification of the (nano)forms of the substance

According to ECHA's guidance [4], and following the workflow presented in Fig. 1, analogues were identified through the following physicochemical parameters ("what they are"): chemical composition, crystalline structure, impurities, surface chemistry, particle size, shape, surface area, and porosity.

Identification of the target analogues

According to the physicochemical properties [23] (see Table 1) the target materials consist of TiO_2 nanopowders of rutile (TiO_2 R) and anatase (TiO_2 A), respectively. TiO_2 A has a specific surface area of 149 m²/g, is uncoated, and 99.5% w/w pure; while TiO_2 R has a specific surface area of 177 m²/g, is coated, and 87% w/w pure. According to the producer, TiO_2 R nano may contain up to 5% w/w of SiO_2 as surface coating (see Sigma-Aldrich ref. 637,262).

Identification of source analogues

The data gathered for the source analogues was mainly obtained from the SCCS report and the OECD WPMN dossier on nano-TiO_2 [19, 24] (version published online in March 2016). The final dataset consisted of 6 TiO_2 nanoforms with adequate data (see Table 1). The 6 nanoforms mainly vary in size (from 5 to 93 nm), coating (two of them are declared coated by the manufacturer and the others are declared without a coating), crystal type (anatase and rutile) and composition of the coating

Table 1 Physicochemical properties ("what they are") of the source and target analogues [19, 23]

Property	NM-100	NM-101	NM-102	NM-103	NM-104	NM-105	TiO$_2$ R nano	TiO$_2$ A nano
Crystal type	Anatase	Anatase	Anatase	Rutile	Rutile	83% anatase 17% rutile	Rutile	Anatase
Total non-TiO$_2$ content including coating and impurities (% w/w)	1.5	9	5	11	11	0.11	13	0.50
Surface chemistry (as declared by manufacturer)[f]	uncoated	uncoated	uncoated	Al$_2$O$_3$, (C$_2$H$_6$OSi)$_n$ and C$_6$H$_{16}$O$_2$Si	Al$_2$O$_3$, (C$_2$H$_6$OSi)$_n$ and C$_3$H$_8$O$_3$	uncoated	SiO$_2$ (< 5%) Na$_2$SO$_4$ SO$_4^{-2}$	uncoated
Surface coating (% w/w)	0	0	0	8	8	0	11	0
Primary particle diameter (TEM) (nm)	93 ± 23	5 ± 1	22 ± 10	24 ± 2	24 ± 2	20 ± 3	10 nm diameter 62 nm length	14
Crystallite size (XRD) (nm)[a]	117 ± 40	7 ± 2	24 ± 5	24 ± 4	25 ± 4	22 ± 5	–	–
Particle Size Distribution (nm)	210 ± 10[b]	278[b]	440 ± 37[b]	135 ± 25[b]	145 ± 35[b]	177 ± 39[b]	125[c]	145[c]
Shape	Spheroidal	Spheroidal	Spheroidal	Spheroidal	Spheroidal	Spheroidal	Rod	Sphere
Aspect ratio	1.53	1.53	1.53	1.7	1.53	1.36	–	–
Specific surface area (m^2/g)	9[d]	242 ± 73[d]	77 ± 10[d]	54 ± 4[d]	54 ± 2[d]	47 ± 0.5[d]	177[e]	149[e]
Total pore volume (ml/g)	0.0324	0.319	0.2996	0.2616	0.1935	0.1937	–	–

[a]values averaged from different instruments and principles (Peak fit, TOPAS, Fullprof, Scherrer eq., TOPAS, IB, TOPAS FWHM)
[b]value from DLS
[c]values averaged from ICP-MS and DLS experiments
[d]values averaged from SAXS/USAXS and BET
[e]value from BET
[f](C$_2$H$_6$OSi)$_n$ indicates presence of dimethicone, C$_6$H$_{16}$O$_2$Si of dimethoxydimethylsilane, and C$_3$H$_8$O$_3$ of glycerol

(hydrophobic or hydrophilic). NM- 100 is the largest of the NM with a primary particle diameter of size of 93 nm, anatase type, and uncoated. NM-101, instead is the smallest of the source analogues with a primary particle size diameter of 5 nm, of type anatase, declared uncoated and with a large amount of organic matter as impurities (8% w/w). NM-103 and NM-104 were very similar in size (24 nm), coating (both coated with Al$_2$O$_3$, dimethicone (C$_2$H$_6$OSi)$_n$ and silane), and type (rutile). The main difference between them is the surface coating as NM-103 is hydrophobic (dimethoxydimethylsilane), while NM-104 is hydrophilic (glycerol). NM-102 has a particle size diameter of 22 nm, is uncoated, and of type anatase. NM-105 is also uncoated, has primary particle size of 20 nm, and is 83% anatase and 17% rutile.

Step 2: Gather the available data for each group member and evaluate the data for adequacy and reliability; build a data matrix

The data collected for each source analogue can be found in Table SM4 and contains two clearly differentiated blocks of information: a) physicochemical characterisation, fundamental behaviour and reactivity; and b) toxicological data of the endpoint to read-across (comet assay in vitro genotoxicity).

The choice of properties to capture in the database was informed by the templates proposed by Schultz et al. [25], with adaptation to include specific NM properties [4, 14]. The properties collected corresponded to:

(1) **What they are**: Name, JRC nanomaterials repository number, chemical composition, impurities, crystal type, crystal size, surface coating, porosity, basic morphology, primary particle diameter, average particle diameter, average length (TEM), aspect ratio, particle size distribution, pour density (weighing), specific surface area

(2) **Where they go:** Agglomeration, dustiness, solubility(ies), dispersibility, (bio)persistence, redox potential, zeta potential, soelectric point, abiotic transformation, toxicokinetics,

(3) **What they do**: Redox potential

Toxicological studies

A literature review on available genotoxicity studies was carried out. The references and corresponding reliability call assigned according to the ANSES criteria [21] can be found in Table SM5.

Table 2 shows the collected genotoxicity tests, specifically the comet in vitro tests of interest to this case study, in which the results are expressed as the number of positives out of the total number of (reliable) studies. The genotoxicity call for each source analogue was defined by the majority call with respect to the in vitro comet assays, i.e. a value of 1 was assigned when the majority of tests were positive, and 0 when the majority were negative. Results from bacterial mutagenicity test (Bacterial reverse mutation assay; Ames test) were not included in the count, as this test is not considered

Table 2 Summary of genotoxicity results for the source NMs. The number of positives results over the total number of tests performed is indicated

	in vivo		in vitro		
	Micronucleus assay	Comet assay	Micronucleus assay	**Comet assay**	Genotoxicity (1/0)[a]
NM-100	–	–	–	**2/2**	1
NM-101	0/3	1/5	–	**2/6**	0
NM-102	0/6	2/13	3/10	**5/8**	1
NM-103	0/5	1/12	3/8	**0/6**	0
NM-104	0/5	2/12	3/8	**0/6**	0
NM-105	2/9	4/15	4/18	**10/14**	1

[a] 1: NM is considered genotoxic in the in vitro comet assay; 0: NM is considered not genotoxic in the in vitro comet assay. The column highlighted in bold presents data used to determine the genotoxicity (1, 0) of each NM

applicable to NMs in its current form [26, 27]. The in vitro micronucleus test is considered applicable to NMs after modification, and the in vitro comet assay is considered applicable to NMs [28, 29] but it is not a validated test in regulatory toxicology [30].

Physicochemical parameters

The total non-TiO_2 content of the source analogues varies from 0.11 to 11%, where the highest values are justified by the presence of coating. NM-103 and NM-104 contain 6% of Al_2O_3 and 2% of organic functionalisation (dimethicone, silanes, and dimethoxydimethylsilane for NM-103 making it hydrophobic; and tetramethyl silicate glycerol, silanes, hexadecanoic acid, methyl ester, octadecanoic acid for NM-104 making it hydrophilic) [20, 31]. NM-101 is a particular case in the sense that it was not declared as coated by the manufacturer [32], but which was found to have 9% of "organic impurities" consisting of silane, hexadecanoic acid, methyl ester, and octadecanoic acid [20]. This difference is reflected in Table 3 and Table SM4, where the presence of (declared) surface coating is represented by its % w/w and where the "Total non-TiO_2" content accounts for the amount of matter that is not TiO_2, thus including coating and impurities.

The influence of the biological matrix on the particle size distribution of the NM is taken into consideration in our dataset by including NM particle size distribution, zeta potential and polydispersity index measured in different biological media (e.g. MilliQ water, Dulbecco's modified eagle medium - DMEM - with and without L-glutamine, fetal bovine serum - FBS, and phosphate-buffered saline medium - PBS) and with different treatments (e.g. untreated, 1 min probe sonication, and 20 min ultrasound bath sonication). Solubility and redox potential are measured in Gamble's solution (representing a lung fluid) and Caco2 medium (representing the intestinal environment). Inputs on solubility and biodurability were deducted by elemental analysis of the particle-free tested media [33]. For more information on the data analysis behind the values reported in Table SM4, please refer to section 1.2 in the Additional file 1.

Construct a matrix to identify available data

Table 1 summarises the information available on the source and target analogues in our case study, including also the genotoxicity based on the in vitro comet assay.

Step 3: Grouping of nanoforms
Development of grouping hypothesis

The analysis of the literature and the data gathered in Table 3 yields the following grouping hypothesis:

Nano-TiO_2 in its uncoated form has the potential to damage DNA, but this can be masked by the presence of coating or large amounts of impurities on the surface of the NM.

It can be readily seen in the dataset of analogues that the coated NMs turn out negative in the comet assay while the ones without coating and organic impurities turn out positive. This can be explained by both, direct genotoxicity or indirect primary genotoxicity [34]: The conduction band of TiO_2 falls in the range of biological redox potentials [35], meaning that TiO_2 with or without the presence of UV light can generate reactive species that react with cell constituents such as proteins or DNA. In both genotoxic mechanisms physical interaction between NM and DNA (i.e. direct) or another cellular component (e.g. enzyme mediated a redox reaction) that generates reactive oxygen species (ROS) (i.e. indirect) is necessary for the DNA damage to occur. The NM coating may act as a physical barrier that can prevent this contact between the surface of TiO_2 and DNA or other cellular components [36]. Therefore following this rationale, coated nano-TiO_2 will not turn out positive in the comet assay as there will be no physical interaction between the surface of the NM and DNA or cellular components. If NM aggregate/agglomerate, the deposition of NM in in vitro tests is higher. If the deposition is higher, the amount of NM and concentration seen by the cells is "de facto" higher than for an

Table 3 Grouping hypothesis and read-across of comet assay results. TiO$_2$ R and TiO$_2$ A are the two target NMs. According to the grouping hypothesis based on the presence or absence of the coating, the two target NMs are assigned to the negative and positive group, respectively. Missing values are indicated with a dash (−)

Name		NM-100	NM-101	NM-102	NM-103	NM-104	NM-105	TiO$_2$ R	TiO$_2$ A
In vitro comet assay[b]		1	0	1	0	0	1	*0*	*1*
What they are	Total non-TiO$_2$ content including coating and impurities (% w/w)	1.5	9	5	11	11	0.11	13	0.5
	Surface coating (%)	0	0	0	8	8	0	11	0
	Organic matter (% w/w)	0	8	0	2	2	0	9	0
	Crystal type (Anatase)	1	1	1	0	0	0.84	0	1
	Crystal type (Rutile)	0	0	0	1	1	0.16	1	0
	Crystal type (Cubic)	0	0	0	0	0	0	0	0
	Crystallite size (mean) (nm)	117.81	7.69	23.93	24.32	24.71	22.44	−	−
	Shape (elongated = 1, spherical = 0)	0	0	0	1	0	1	1	0
	Aspect ratio	1.53	1.53	1.53	1.7	1.53	1.36	6.2	1
	Primary particle diameter (mean) (nm)	93.45	5.25	22.00	24.00	24.50	20.13	62 × 10	14
	Specific surface area (m^2/g)	9.23	316.07	77.87	53.98	54.33	47	177	149
Where they go	Isoelectric Point (Mean) (pH)	−	5.5	6	8.3	8.5	6.8	−	−
	Density (g/ml)	3.84	3.99	3.84	4.02	4.09	4.05	−	−
	Mean of total pore volume (ml/g)	0.032	0.319	0.300	0.262	0.194	0.194	−	−
	Micro surface area (m^2/g)	0	13.625	1.108	0	0	0	−	−
	Micropore volume (ml/g)	0	0.00179	0.00034	0	0	0	−	−
	Dustiness-Respirable(mg/kg)	1500	5600	9200	19,000	6400	11,000	−	−
	Biodurability 24 h 0.05% BSA (Ti content) (μg/l)	5.2	0	0	0	0	0	−	−
	Biodurability 24 h Gambles solution (Ti content) (μg/l)	0	0	3388	0	0	0	−	−
	Biodurability 24 h Caco2 (Ti content) (μg/l)	796	3414	1741	222	3386	2724	−	−
What they do	Redox Caco2 medium[a]	1	-1	-1	1	-1	-1	−	−
	Redox Gamble's solution[a]	1	0	-1	1	-1	-1	−	−
	Redox BSA[a]	0	0	0	0	0	0	−	−

[a]values obtained from deliverable 4.7 of Nanogenotox [33] determined by measuring the content of O$_2$. Oxidising properties (1), neutral (0), reducing (−1)
[b]1: NM is considered genotoxic in the in vitro comet assay; 0: NM is considered not genotoxic in the in vitro comet assay. In vitro comet results are predicted for TiO$_2$ R and TiO$_2$ A (characters in italics in the last two columns)

analogous situation with less deposition. Therefore, it seems evident that the effect of coating may in one way or another affect the outcome of an in vitro assay.

Step 4: Assess the applicability of the approach and fill data gaps

Assess the grouping hypothesis

The applicability of the approach can be assessed by determining the robustness of the grouping hypothesis, i.e. assess the similarity within each group of NMs. Due to the lack of a uniquely defined structure, the similarity was defined by the physicochemical properties obtained for each nanoform in Table SM4. Different chemoinformatic techniques, two unsupervised and one supervised, were used to assess the grouping hypothesis.

Data reduction - The initial dataset included 6 source analogues with approximately 147 properties for each of

them (Table SM4). Two properties, crystal type cubic and redox activity in BSA, were discarded because their values were constant for all nanoforms. No correlation filter was applied to the dataset because the limited number of data points for each property (6 points) would overestimate the correlations and the filtering. However, some filtering was necessary because the dataset was biased towards Dynamic Light Scattering (DLS) measured properties, as it contained a total of 62 related properties that were measured in slightly different conditions, i.e. different media and treatments (see Step 2, physicochemical parameters). Consequently, the dataset had a high amount of particle size distribution, zeta potential, and polydispersibility index (PdI) measures. In order to reduce the weight of such measures and obtain a more balanced dataset, these properties were reduced to 4 measures each by using a hierarchical clustering of the transposed dataset (see section 1.2 of the Additional file 1).

This allowed the determination of groups of similar properties from which one property for each set was randomly selected as representative of the rest.

Hierarchical clustering (HC) - The HC of the obtained dataset, which contained 50 variables, is presented in Fig. 2 and shows that NM-103 and NM-104 form a very solid group ($p < 0.01$). The other 4 NMs form another group as they are clustered together [16] with high significance according to the approximately unbiased (AU) p-value that is computed by multiscale bootstrap resampling. It is worth mentioning that the clusters obtained here must be only considered from an exploratory point of view and in a weight of evidence context. This information alone cannot be used to define clusters of NMs but must be complemented with other techniques and rationales (e.g. PCA, variable selection, mechanistic information) to be used in read-across.

Principal component analysis (PCA) - While the hierarchical clustering indicates possible groups of NMs by taking into account all physicochemical properties and forming subsequent groups of 2 substances, PCA is a dimensionality reduction technique that shows the properties that account

for the maximum variance between individuals, i.e. the source NM in this case. PCA also uses all properties to determine each of the principal components (PC) but are weighted in such a way that a minimum number of properties can be used to explain the differences between the NMs.

PCA of the dataset of source analogues shows a similar picture to the one obtained in the HC (see Fig. 2). The NMs are placed in the plot by using the PC1 and PC2 scores. The loadings of each property with respect to PC1 and PC2 are indicated as arrows. NMs that appear close to each other indicate similarity in the space defined by PC1 and PC2. Long and light blue arrows indicate high contribution of that specific property to one of the PCs. The closer the arrow is to an axis, i.e. to a PC, the higher correlation with that PC. It is necessary to remember that PCA plots are simplifications of the whole picture and that the fact that NMs appear close to each other only indicates that these NMs are similar to each other in that reduced representation of reality given by 2 variables, i.e. PC1 vs PC2. PC1 and PC2 typically account for a rather large variance and their components indicate what the variables that differentiate NMs the most are. The fact that these variables be related with the endpoint of interest cannot be assured and is not the purpose of PCA or other unsupervised techniques. In Fig. 3, NM-103 and NM-104 appear close to

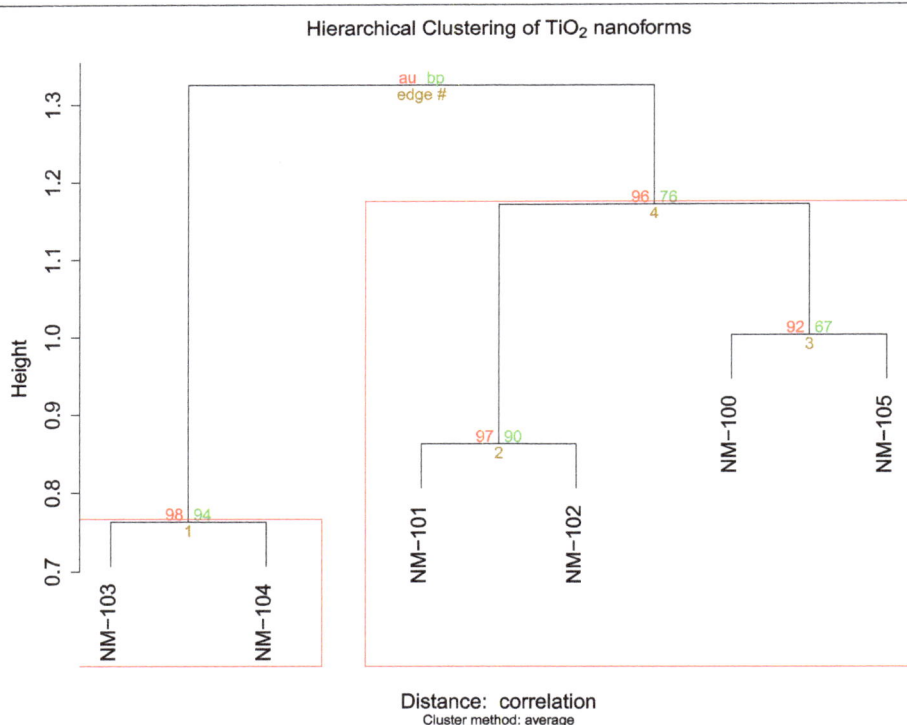

Fig. 2 Hierarchical clustering of the TiO$_2$ analogues. The numbers in red correspond to the "Approximately Unbiased" (AU) p-value that is computed by multiscale bootstrap resampling, and the ones in green to "Bootstrap Probability" p-value (BP), which is computed by normal bootstrap resampling. The height in the Y-axis indicates the distance between clusters computed as average linkage. AU p-value will be used for the interpretation as it is usually a better approximation to the real p-value

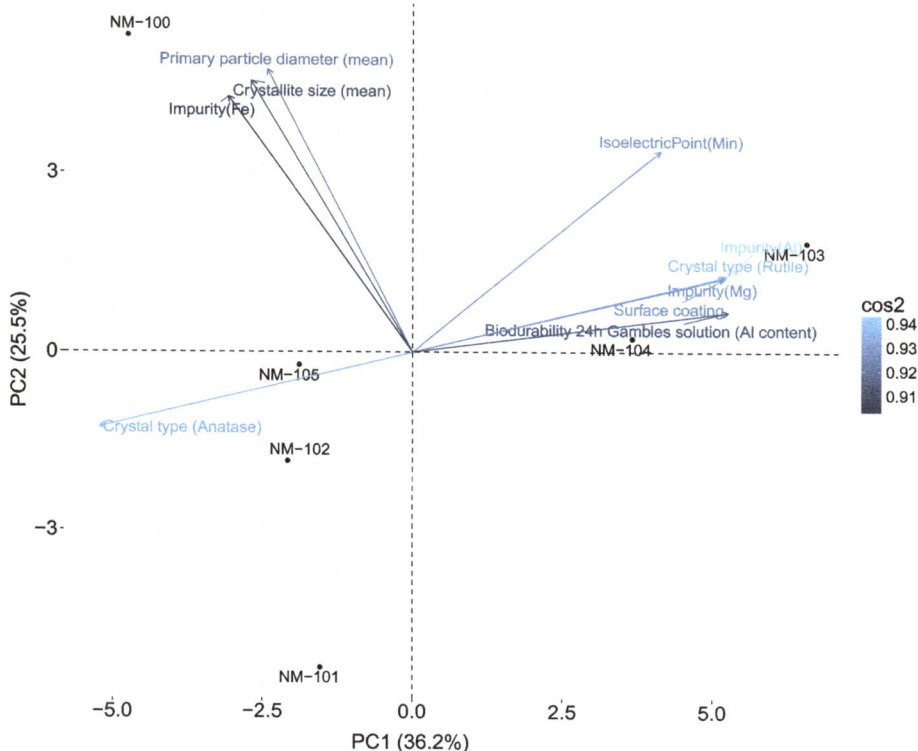

Fig. 3 Principal component analysis (PCA) of the dataset of 6 TiO$_2$ analogues. The position of the analogues (individuals) on the space of PC1 vs PC2 are indicated as black dots. Arrows correspond to the 10 variables with higher contribution to the PCs. The colours are defined by the squared loadings (cos^2) and indicate their contributions to the PCs

each other at the positive side of PC2. The arrows show that these positions are mainly driven by the properties related to impurities of Al (Biodurability 24 h in Gambles solution - Al content), Mg, by the crystal type rutile, and % of surface coating. NM-100 appears at the top part of the plot mainly driven by particle primary diameter and crystallite size, which matches the fact that NM-100 is the biggest NM of the series (~ 93 nm, which can be considered as bulk material). For the same reason, NM-101 appears at the bottom of the plot as it is the smallest NM, and NM-102 and NM-105 appear next to each other on the negative side of PC1, mainly driven by crystal type anatase and by not having surface coating.

The squared loadings of the two first principal components are given in Table 4 and show that the properties with the higher contributions to PC1 are the biodurability 24 h Gambles solution (Al content) and impurity (Al), which are similar properties; crystal type (anatase and rutile), and % of surface coating and Mg impurity. For PC2 the main contributors are the specific surface area, total pore volume, primary particle diameter, crystallite size, and Fe impurities.

The loadings also show that other properties like zeta potential, PdI, or particle size distribution have less influence.

Random forest variable selection - The random forest variable selection algorithm is a supervised technique and uses the physicochemical properties to predict a given outcome, in this case positive or negative results in comet assays. It can provide a measure of relative importance of the variables for the prediction based on the times the variables were selected in the different trees. In this case, the Gini index was used as the target variable to optimise the trees [37].

The variable importance plot of the source analogues (Fig. 4) clearly shows that the most important variables to predict the comet assay results for the 6 analogues are the content of organic matter and total non-TiO$_2$. The properties that follow in the list correspond to the biodurability measures (Al content) after 24 h of incubation in different media (Caco2, Gamble's solution, and BSA). All these measures are directly or indirectly related to the presence of coating as the Al content and organic are mainly found on the coating.

Fill data gaps

HC, PCA and random forest variable selection algorithms supported the grouping hypothesis for the nano-TiO$_2$genotoxicity tested with the in vitro comet assay.

Table 4 Squared loadings of PC1 and PC2 of the PCA of the source analogues

Property	(PC1 loadings)^2	Property	(PC2 loadings)^2
Biodurability 24 h Gambles solution (Al content)	0.90	Specific surface area (mean)	0.77
Impurity(Al)	0.89	Mean of total pore volume (ml/g)	0.74
Crystal type (Rutile)	0.89	Primary particle diameter (mean)	0.73
Crystal type (Anatase)	0.89	Crystallite size (mean)	0.67
Surface coating	0.87	Micropore volume (ml/g)	0.63
Impurity(Mg)	0.87	Impurity(Fe)	0.63

The identification of the two target NMs in Table 3 includes the coating of the two nanoforms. According to the physicochemical properties of the identified target NMs, we can assume that they are included in the same variable space as the source NMs: primary particle size, shape, total non-TiO$_2$ content, organic matter, crystal type, and specific surface area are included in the range of the source analogues. Because of the lack of some physicochemical data for the target NMs, it was not possible to include them in the PCA analysis or in the clustering exercise. However, it is possible to assign the two target NMs to a class according to some of their characteristics. Since the presence of coating or high amount of non-TiO$_2$ content on the surface of nano-TiO$_2$ appears to prevent NM to cause DNA damage, it is possible to group TiO$_2$ R nano with the analogues NM-103, NM-104 and NM-101,

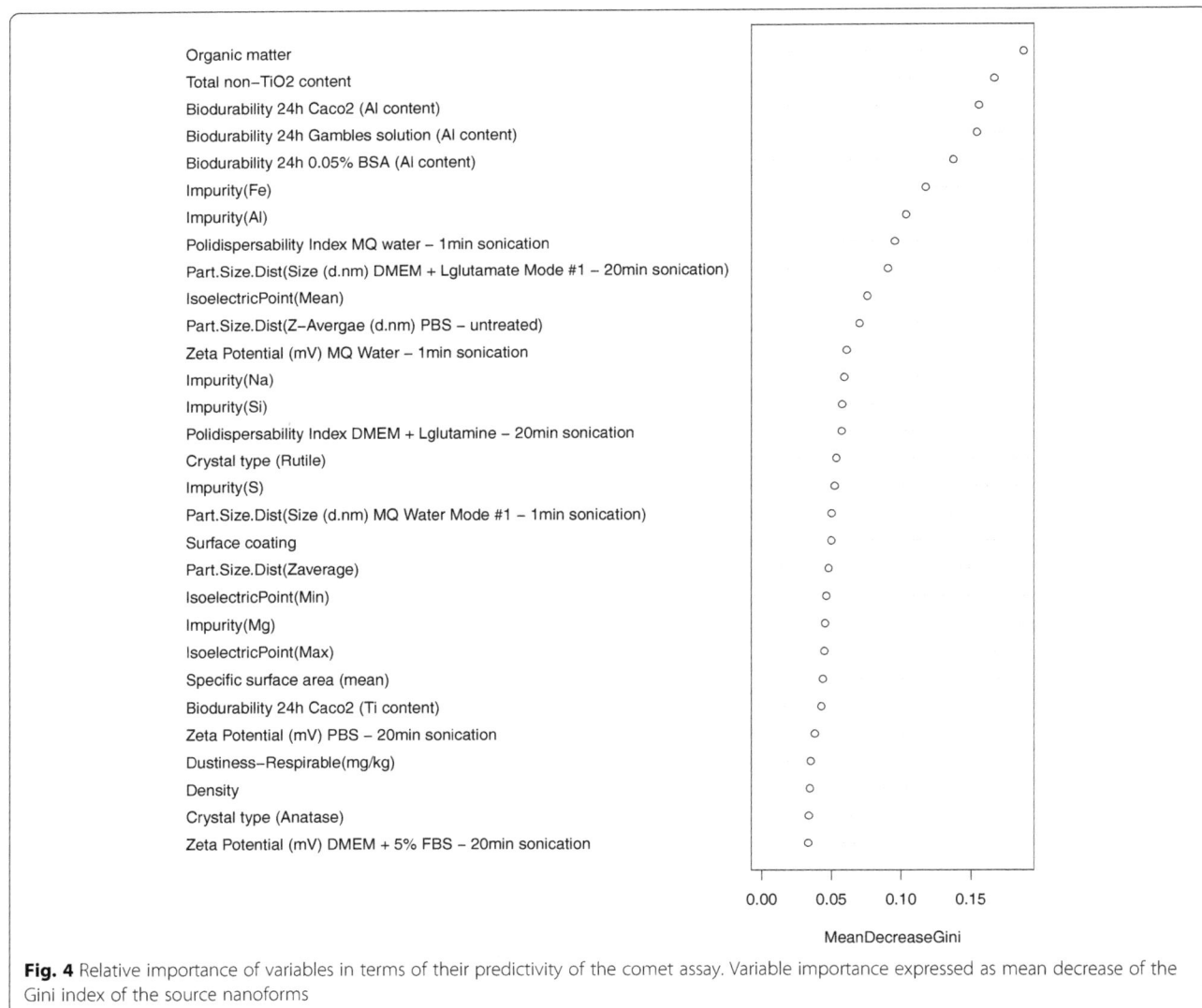

Fig. 4 Relative importance of variables in terms of their predictivity of the comet assay. Variable importance expressed as mean decrease of the Gini index of the source nanoforms

which give negative results in the in vitro comet assay, and TiO$_2$ A nano with NM-100, NM-102 and NM-105, which cause DNA damage. In fact, as shown in Table 1, TiO$_2$ R has a coating, and thus it is predicted to have a negative outcome in the in vitro comet assay. TiO$_2$ A, instead, has a relatively low level of impurities and no coating, for which we thus predict a positive result in the in vitro comet assay. The fact that TiO$_2$ R has a rod-shape (62 × 10 nm) while the source analogues are rather spherical is not expected to influence the result. The aspect ratio is too small to consider that TiO$_2$ R could cause an asbestos-like effect, and although the shape may influence the reactivity, it would still be masked by the coating which is the main driver of the toxic effect. The outcome of the read-across is confirmed by the in vitro comet assay carried out by Guichard et al. [23] which shows that TiO$_2$ A is positive in the in vitro comet assay while TiO$_2$ R is not.

Is the group robust enough?
DNA damage caused by nano-TiO$_2$ may be classified as direct primary genotoxicity, indirect primary damage, or secondary genotoxicity [34, 38]. Direct genotoxicity assumes that DNA and NM are in contact [39]. Indirect primary genotoxicity may be elicited by interaction of NMs with nuclear proteins (involved in replication, transcription, and repair), disturbance of cell cycle checkpoint functions, ROS arising from the NM surface, release of toxic metal ions from the NM surface, ROS produced by cell components, and inhibition of antioxidant defence [40]. Finally, secondary genotoxicity may be elicited by ROS production in inflammatory cells via an inflammation signalling pathway [41, 42]. Most experimental studies point towards a mechanism of action for indirect primary genotoxicity via ROS [38], but other studies could not find a clear correlation between the level of ROS production and DNA damage (similar level of ROS at different concentrations of nanomaterials but increased DNA damage [43], or no correlation between amount of ·OH and ^{1}O$_2$ and DNA damage [44]).

Another relevant aspect in determining the validity of the grouping hypothesis is supporting evidence for the way in which the coating can prevent DNA damage, as the mode-of-action is not entirely clear. For instance, it was shown [45, 46] that the addition of PEG coating to nano-TiO$_2$ increased the dispersion of NMs which resulted in lower cytotoxicity and genotoxicity. Magdolenova et al. [47] showed that the degree of dispersion of TiO$_2$ NMs had an influence on the DNA damage in three cell lines. Agglomerates of less than 200 nm had no effect on genotoxicity while larger ones showed positive results. These results could be due to larger agglomerates precipitate and deposit on the cells increasing the actual exposure to the NM or even covering them completely and suffocating them. Another consideration is the effect that the use of media with

proteins (e.g. BSA, FBS) can have on the results. If the NMs are surrounded by proteins, they are more dispersed, less prone to aggregation and deposition, and also less toxic as the "reactive" part is encapsulated ("hidden") behind the protein corona. Another aspect that cannot be ignored when analysing the in vitro results of TiO$_2$ is its photocatalytic activity, which can be even triggered by a simple fluorescent tube [48]. Thus, it is obvious that the mechanism of genotoxicity of TiO$_2$ is not well defined and that there might be more than one that could even take place simultaneously. Probably the truth is the combination of all factors that have as common source the presence of coating either by preventing aggregation of NMs, deposition, and therefore reducing exposure, or by preventing physical contact with DNA and/or other cell components after uptake. However, what is relevant in this case is that the majority of studies agree with the hypothesis presented here which is the fact that coated nano-TiO$_2$ show fewer positive results in the in vitro comet assay than the uncoated ones, therefore it can be fairly concluded that the presence of coating reduces the genotoxic effects of nano-TiO$_2$. It is important to keep in mind that the present coatings are mainly not "charged" as could be coatings with reactive or non-neutral groups such as terminal –COOH or –NH$_2$, in which cases the grouping hypothesis might change.

Uncertainty evaluation
The AEs of the RAAF scenario 6 were used to systematically identify uncertainties in the grouping and read-across process. Uncertainties related to some aspects of the case study are discussed in more detail below.

Table 5 provides a summary structured according to the RAAF AEs, and also highlights the nanospecific considerations to be taken into account when applying the RAAF to NMs. Overall, the uncertainties were related to the i) complexity of nanostructures, affecting the definition of similarity and category boundaries; ii) nanomaterial identification and physicochemical characterisation, due to high measurement variability; iii) a limited dataset, iv) quality and inconsistency as well as reproducibility of study data due to missing SOPs protocols or uncertainty in their applicability to nanomaterials; v) finding correlations and identifying the physicochemical properties driving the toxicity; vi) limited knowledge about the mechanism of action (MoA).

Discussion
Nano-TiO$_2$ was selected as case study because of its importance in the market [49], data availability [9, 19, 24, 50, 51], and in-house experience from related projects (ENPRA, NanoMILE, NanoTEST, ENRHES).

A simplified version of the workflow proposed by ECHA [4] for the read-across of NMs was applied in this manuscript (see Fig. 1). This simplified workflow collects all the

Table 5 Evaluation of the uncertainties of the TiO$_2$ read-across case study according to the ECHA RAAF scenario 6

RAAF Assessment Element (Scenario 6)	Uncertainties in the TiO$_2$ case study	Nanospecific issues
C.1 Substance characterisation	• Measured physicochemical characteristics of the NMs vary: measurement uncertainty. Is there an influence on other properties of the nanomaterials? • Impurity information not always available or inconsistent	• Physicochemical characterisation of NMs: high variability of measurements (influence of different experimental conditions)
C.2 Structural similarity and category hypothesis	• NM-101 is not declared as coated, but has 9% organic impurities that could be considered as a coating. • Different composition of the coatings/impurities (e.g. some containing Al$_2$O$_3$, dimethoxydimethylsilane, or glycerol) • Uncertainty of reading across a spherical particle to a rod-shaped particle	• For NMs, the similarity cannot be based on chemical (e.g. molecular) structure as for conventional chemicals, but should consider physical form and key physicochemical properties
C.3 Link of structural similarities and structural differences with the proposed property	• Little is known about the mechanisms of toxic action, making it challenging to link similarity to the endpoint (genotoxicity) considered	
C.4 Consistency of effects in the data matrix	• Uncertainty in applying existing testing protocols to nanomaterials and thus uncertainty in assessment of quality, reliability and relevance to human health endpoints of measured toxicity data	• Artefacts affecting the results of toxicity assessment of NMs are discussed in the literature
C.5 Reliability and adequacy of the source study(ies)		
C.6 Bias that influences the prediction	• Selection of analogues based only on data availability	
6.1 Compounds the test organism is exposed to	• The mechanism of genotoxicity of TiO$_2$ is not well defined. It is also possible that several effects take place at the same time.	• For conventional chemicals, either the parent molecule or (bio)transformation products are the indirect/direct toxicants; for NMs the considerations extend to coating, released metals etc.
6.2 Common underlying mechanism, qualitative aspects		
6.3 Common underlying mechanism, quantitative aspects		
6.5 Occurrence of other effects than covered by the hypothesis and justification		
6.4 Exposure to other compounds than to those linked to the prediction	• For example the presence of reactive transition metals may also contribute to oxidative DNA damage induction.	

available data in the first steps and avoids the generation of grouping hypothesis with insufficient data.

The read-across was documented by providing mechanistic interpretation of the available data, where possible, and according to the state of the art in the field. Chemoinformatic techniques such as HC, PCA, and random forest variable selection were used to support the grouping hypothesis of NMs.

Genotoxicity of TiO$_2$ nanoforms as determined by in vitro comet assay was selected as endpoint to read-across. Although nano-TiO$_2$ are well studied and data rich NMs, only 6 NMs with full data could be gathered. In vitro comet assay was deemed as the more suitable/relevant endpoint for the read-across case study, unlike the other endpoints, it provided two groups of NMs (genotoxic vs non-genotoxic) and a relatively high amount and diverse set of NMs.

Different issues arise when trying to read-across NMs with data collected from different sources. Data quality and variability are significant challenges in the field of nanotechnology [52]. As it is reported in the next paragraph, identification of nanoforms can be controversial [53, 54] as in the nano-TiO$_2$ case different amounts of impurities and different sizes are reported for the same target substance and this contributes to increase uncertainty on the first step of the grouping for read-across procedure, consisting of the NM identification. Furthermore, the fact that the mode-of-action of nano-TiO$_2$ genotoxicity is not (yet) well understood [55] complicates the formulation and assessment of grouping hypothesis, the basis of read-across. The necessary modifications to adapt the RAAF [22] to the read-across of nanomaterials were identified, and this is a key step to increase the use and certainty when reading-across nanomaterials.

The issues mentioned above together with the lessons learnt are discussed next.

Data variability

Data variability in the reported parameters was mainly due to the lack of SOPs that leads to the application of different tools or approaches in the measurement of the same property (e.g. crystallite size). In the particular case of NM-100, four different values were collected: 141, 61, 168, and 100 nm. In order to transform ranges of values into single values suitable for read-across analysis, some data treatment was necessary. In general, if the distribution of values is normal, the mean values are a good representation of the reality, but if the distribution is not normal and there are extremes, then the median is a better option. For some parameters (e.g. primary particle size) the variability was rather low and, therefore where possible, it was decided to use the average values. In cases in which different techniques with varying precision provided significantly different results (e.g. specific surface area determined by BET or SAXS), the values provided by the most precise techniques were preferred (see section 1.2 of the Additional file 1 for further details on the data treatment).

The variability in the measurements can be misleading for the characterisation of nanoforms and thus in identifying similar analogues. For example, the physicochemical properties of the target substances showed that the measured ones were slightly different from those reported by the manufacturer. Guichard et al. [23] found for TiO_2 R nano 11% w/w of impurities corresponding mainly to SiO_2 (manufacturer declared up to 0.5%), the measured particle size corresponded to a rod of 62×10 nm (manufacturer declared 40×10 nm), and the surface area to 177 m^2/g (manufacturer declared 50 m^2/g). For the purpose of this study it was assumed that the substance tested in Guichard et al. corresponded to a coated TiO_2 manufactured by Sigma. It is not clear though where is the limit to consider that two substances are the same.

Determining similar NMs

One of the challenges of the case study was the identification of similar analogues as it had to be based on the physicochemical properties. The task was rather easy for some of the properties. For instance, NM-102, NM-103, NM-104, and NM-105 had particle diameter (TEM) of 22 ± 10 nm, specific surface areas between 77 and 47 m^2/g, crystal types of rutile, anatase or combination of both (83% anatase 17% rutile for the case of NM-105). However, it resulted highly complex for properties such as particle size distribution (see Annex IX in Worth et al. [56]) or impurities.

The case of impurities was unexpectedly challenging. Impurities are defined as "an unintended constituent present in a substance as manufactured" [57], while surface coating consists in the surface chemistry purposely added to the NM. The measurement of the elements present on the surface of the NM does not distinguish between the two. In the present case, NM-103 and NM-104 were declared coated and were found to contain 6% of Al_2O_3 and 2% of organic functionalisation (dimethicone, silanes and dimethoxydimethylsilane for NM-103 making it hydrophobic; tetramethyl silicate, glycerol, silanes, hexadecanoic acid, methyl ester, octadecanoic acid for NM-104 making it hydrophilic). NM-101 was not declared coated but it was found to contain a high amount of impurities accounting for around 9% of the total weight. The composition of these impurities (silane, hexadecanoic acid, methyl ester, and octadecanoic acid) was very similar to the coating of the other NMs. In fact, the Nanogenotox project considered them as coating [32], but it was not deemed appropriate in this work as it would contradict the definition of impurities [57]. Since it was impossible to determine whether these impurities were added on purpose and in order to reflect its presence, we defined a new property named "Total non-TiO_2 content including coating and impurities (% w/w)" which corresponded to the sum of all materials that were detected in the NM other than the core material, thus going beyond the surface coating declared by the manufacturer. This measure included also the coating, which was separately declared by the supplier and was also reported separately in our dataset as "Surface chemistry (as declared by manufacturer)" and "Surface coating (%)" indicating the quantity of coating with respect to the total weight of the NM. This way, 2 groups of NMs could be clearly identified, those with a high amount of non-TiO_2 content (> 9% w/w), and those with lower or no amount of non-TiO_2 content (≤ 5% w/w).

Validity of the grouping hypothesis

Chemoinformatic tools such as HC and PCA can be used to process and extract knowledge from large amounts of data. We applied HC, PCA, and a variable selection algorithm based on random forest to support the grouping hypothesis of the read-across exercise.

HC and PCA of the source analogues showed that two groups of NMs can be clearly defined based on their physicochemical properties (see Fig. 2 and Fig. 3). HC can be used to determine similar NM with respect to their properties without biasing the similarity or weighting any of the properties. Following this principle, HC showed that NM-103 and NM-104 (negative in the in vitro comet assay) formed a very strong group ($p < 0.01$). In fact, both NMs were almost identical, of rutile type with a size of ~ 24 nm, and coated. The "only" difference was on the surface chemistry, which in one case was hydrophobic, and in the other hydrophilic. Thus, the analysis of the HC results shows that NMs are clustered according to crystal type, size and presence of coating.

Unlike HC, the PCA can show clusters of similar NMs as well as the properties that define their (dis)similarity. The properties that contribute the most to the PC are those that determine the main differences between the groups of NMs. The main contributors to the PCs were mainly related to the presence of impurities, biodurability, coating, crystal type (anatase vs rutile), particle size, and pore volume (see Table 4). The fact that crystal type variables appeared so high in the list is partially due to the values used to code each crystal type. Since most of the particles were either 100% anatase or 100% rutile, the differences between the anatase and rutile NMs (100% vs 0%) were highly significant. Primary particle diameter was also found to be one of the main differences between NMs as the biggest one was 93 nm and the smallest 5 nm. Biodurability 24 h Gambles solution (Al content) and impurity(Al), both highly related to coating, are very similar properties as the former one corresponds to the quantity of Al dissolved in media after 24 h, and the second one corresponds to the quantity of Al found after calcination of the NMs.

The PCA showed a cluster formed by NM-102 and NM-105. Both are positive in the comet assay and both correspond to uncoated anatase TiO_2 (100% and 84%, respectively) with ~ 23 nm and low amount of impurities. NM-100 does not cluster together with any of the other NMs in the PCA because it corresponds to a relatively large "NM" (~ 98 nm), which makes it significantly different from the rest. In fact, PC2 has a strong component of particle size what pushes NM-100 at the higher part of the plot. However, if only the crystal type and coating were considered, NM-100 would group with NM-102 and NM-105 as it is uncoated, and 100% anatase. Such a classification would match the toxicological profile of these NMs as they all turn out positive in the comet assay. However, this classification would not hold for the other NMs, as NM-101 is also anatase but negative in the comet assay. As mentioned above, NM-101 is a complex case and it is difficult to classify. It is the smallest of all NMs with a diameter of 5 nm (lower part of the PCA), it is of anatase type, and although it is declared uncoated by the producer, it contains a high amount of impurities (9%), which are of similar composition to the coating of NM-103 and NM-104. The results from PCA show that the NMs differences are mainly driven by presence of impurities, biodurability, coating, crystal type, particle size, and pore volume.

Finally, the random forest analysis supports our grouping hypothesis. The variable importance plot in Fig. 5 shows that the properties organic matter and Total non-TiO_2 content are the most discriminating properties to predict in vitro comet assay results. Both properties are related to the presence of coating or impurities, thus, it is clear that there is a correlation between the NMs that have coating and/or organic impurities and the result of the in vitro comet assay. The fact that the presence of coating and/or organic impurities can explain the result of the in vitro assay does not imply that they are the only ones that are relevant. In fact, the chemoinformatic techniques have shown several properties that account for the similarity and clustering of these NMs and that may also be important to understand the outcome of the in vitro comet assay.

One valuable question is what would be the outcome for a NM of type rutile and uncoated. We do not dispose of such a NM in the group of source analogues, therefore, such a read-across would be more uncertain than the current one. Following the present grouping hypothesis, uncoated rutile would also be predicted as positive in the in vitro comet assay because the grouping hypothesis is based on the presence of coating. It would be desirable to dispose of data for this type of nanoform before performing such a read-across so as to have a prediction with less uncertainty.

Uncertainty evaluation according to the ECHA RAAF
The case study shows that the RAAF is applicable to NMs. A few nanospecific issues were identified which should be accommodated when applying the RAAF to NMs. First of all, the consideration of similarity should be extended from being based on the chemical structural to other appropriate parameters such as the physical form and key physicochemical properties. Additional sources of uncertainty to be considered for NMs are the high variability of measurements for NM characterisation as well as the uncertainty of adequate application of testing protocols to NMs, including possible NM-specific artefacts, and thus uncertainty of reliability and relevance of toxicity assay data. In the RAAF scenarios, the toxicant is either the parent chemical or a biotransformation product, for NM additional possibilities might be considered, including for example the coating or release of metals. For defining identical or different compounds – as basis for differentiating RAAF scenarios – factors such as surface coating and size should also be considered. With the knowledge on NMs further increasing in the future, possible identified NM-specific mechanisms of toxicity should also be taken into account.

Conclusions
In this work, we successfully applied a simplified version of the workflow for grouping and read-across proposed by ECHA [4] to read-across nanoforms of TiO_2. We collected and curated all public information available for

nano-TiO$_2$. In vitro comet assay was selected as the endpoint to read-across as it turned out to be the endpoint with the largest number of NMs that could be assigned to either a positive or negative outcome. The final dataset that was used for the read-across was composed of 6 nano-TiO$_2$ with more than 100 physicochemical properties. Two groups of nano-TiO$_2$ were identified based on their physicochemical properties. A grouping hypothesis that reads: "*Nano-TiO$_2$ in its uncoated form has the potential to damage DNA, but this can be masked by the presence of coating or by the large amounts of impurities on the surface of the NM*" was used to successfully read-across the in vitro comet assay results of two nano-TiO$_2$. In order to extend this hypothesis to be able to determine whether nano-TiO$_2$ is genotoxic, it would be necessary to repeat the exercise considering other genotoxicity tests, as the in vitro comet assay has been shown to be prone to give false positives [58].

It was shown how chemoinformatic techniques such as HC, PCA, and random forest may be used to support or evaluate a grouping hypothesis by determining (dis)-similar NMs as well as the properties that differentiate them the most. Furthermore, it was shown that the ECHA RAAF to evaluate the confidence in a read-across argument is also applicable to NMs provided some modifications are made in order to take into consideration NM specificities such as the extension of the basis for similarity beyond chemical structure.

The main challenges that were faced during the read-across exercise were: i) identification of the (non-)nanoforms, ii) experimental variability associated with the physicochemical and toxicological information, iii) lacking measurement protocols, iv) the lack of knowledge on the mechanisms of genotoxic action of NMs. Current efforts in the scientific community are ongoing to address knowledge gaps and availability of SOPs [59–61]. These developments will support nanosafety assessments, including the development of read-across case studies.

Endnotes

[1]In the context of this paper, a nanoform is a form of a substance which fulfils the EC recommended definition of nanomaterial and is characterised also by shape and surface chemistry [62].

Acknowledgements
The authors would like to thank Peter Baricic and in general the Nanocomput steering group with representatives from DG GROW, DG Environment and the European Chemicals Agency (ECHA) for the constructive feedback provided during the project and specifically on the current case study.

Funding
This work was part of the Nanocomput project, carried out by the European Commission Joint Research Centre (JRC) for the Directorate-General (DG) for Internal Market, Industry, Entrepreneurship and SMEs (DG GROW) under the terms of an Administrative Arrangement between JRC and DG GROW.

Authors' contributions
LL adapted the workflow for grouping and read-across, built the dataset, and carried out data analysis. DA selected and applied chemoinformatic techniques and carried out data analysis. RG helped in the compilation of the dataset and participated in the discussions. EJ gave support and supervision on the data analysis and the data treatment. AR applied and adapted the RAAF to the case study. KA and AW participated in all the discussions and helped in the preparation of the manuscript. LL, DA, and AR wrote the manuscript. All authors participated in the discussions on the data treatment, on the definition of the grouping hypothesis, provided feedback on the uncertainty analysis, read, gave feedback, and approved the final manuscript.

Competing interests
The authors declare that they have no competing interests.

References
1. European Parliament and Council. Regulation (EC) No 1907/2006 of the European Parliament and of the Council of 18 December 2006 concerning the Registration, Evaluation, Authorisation and Restriction of Chemicals (REACH), establishing a European Chemicals Agency, amending Directive 1999/4. EC, EC: Official Journal of the European Union; 2006. http://eur-lex.europa.eu/LexUriServ/LexUriServ.do?uri=OJ:L:2006:396:0001:0849:EN:PDF.
2. BiPRO. Examination and assessment of consequences for industry, consumers, human health and the environment of possible options for changing the REACH requirements for nanomaterials. Final Report. 2013. http://ec.europa.eu/environment/chemicals/nanotech/pdf/Final_Report.pdf.
3. KEMI. Impact Assessment of Further Regulation of Nanomaterials at a European Level. 2014.
4. ECHA. Appendix R. Helsinki: 6–1 : Recommendations for nanomaterials applicable to the Guidance on QSARs and Grouping; 2017. https://echa.europa.eu/documents/10162/23036412/appendix_r6_nanomaterials_en.pdf/71ad76f0-ab4c-fb04-acba-074cf045eaaa
5. RIVM, JRC, ECHA. Usage of (eco) toxicological data for bridging data gaps between and grouping of nanoforms of the same substance. Elements to consider 2016. https://doi.org/10.2823/982046.
6. Arts J, Hadi M, Irfan M-A, Keene AM, Kreiling R, Lyon D, et al. A decision-making framework for the grouping and testing of nanomaterials (DF4nanoGrouping). Regul Toxicol Pharmacol. 2015;71:S1–27. https://doi.org/10.1016/j.yrtph.2015.03.007.
7. Kuempel ED, Castranova V, Geraci CL, Schulte PA. Development of risk-based nanomaterial groups for occupational exposure control. J Nanoparticle Res. 2012;14:1029. https://doi.org/10.1007/s11051-012-1029-8.
8. Oomen AG, Bos PMJ, Fernandes TF, Hund-Rinke K, Boraschi D, Byrne HJ, et al. Concern-driven integrated approaches to nanomaterial testing and assessment–report of the NanoSafety cluster working group 10. Nanotoxicology. 2014;8:334–48. https://doi.org/10.3109/17435390.2013.802387.
9. Sellers K, Deleebeeck N, Messiaen M, Jackson, M, Bleeker E, Sijm D, et al. Grouping nanomaterials a strategy towards grouping and read-across. 2015. http://www.rivm.nl/bibliotheek/rapporten/2015-0061.html. Accessed 5 June 2015.
10. Lamon L, Aschberger K, Asturiol D, Richarz AN, Worth A. (n.d.). Grouping of nanomaterials to read-across hazard endpoints: a review. Nanotoxicology. https://www.tandfonline.com/doi/full/10.1080/17435390.2018.1506060.
11. Gajewicz A, Cronin MTD, Rasulev B, Leszczynski J, Puzyn T. Novel approach for efficient predictions properties of large pool of nanomaterials based on limited set of species: nano-read-across. Nanotechnology. 2015;26:15701. https://doi.org/10.1088/0957-4484/26/1/015701.
12. Zhang H, Ji Z, Xia T, Meng H, Low-Kam C, Liu R, et al. Use of metal oxide nanoparticle band gap to develop a predictive paradigm for oxidative stress and acute pulmonary inflammation. ACS Nano. 2012;6:4349–68. https://doi.org/10.1021/nn3010087

13. Arts JHE, Hadi M, Irfan M-A, Keene AM, Kreiling R, Lyon D, et al. Case studies putting the decision-making framework for the grouping and testing of nanomaterials (DF4nanoGrouping) into practice. Regul Toxicol Pharmacol. 2016;76:234–61. https://doi.org/10.1016/j.yrtph.2015.03.007.

14. Stone V, Pozzi-Mucelli S, Tran L, Aschberger K, Sabella S, Vogel U, Poland C, Balharry D, Fernandes T, Gottardo S, Hankin S, Hartl MGJ, Hartmann N, Hristozov D, Hund-Rinke K, Johnston H, Marcomini A, Panzer O, Roncato D, Saber AT, Wallin H, Scott-Fordsmand JJ. ITS-NANO–prioritising nanosafety research to develop a stakeholder driven intelligent testing strategy. Part. Fibre Toxicol. 2014;11:9. https://doi.org/10.1186/1743-8977-11-9.

15. R CoreTeam. R: a language and environment for statistical computing. 2016. https://www.r-project.org/.

16. Suzuki R, Shimodaira H. Pvclust: an R package for assessing the uncertainty in hierarchical clustering. Bioinformatics. 2006;22:1540–2.

17. Husson F, Lê S, Pagès J. Exploratory multivariate analysis by example using R. CRC Press; 2011. https://www.crcpress.com/Exploratory-Multivariate-Analysis-by-Example-Using-R/Husson-Le-Pages/p/book/9781439835814. Accessed 4 July 2017.

18. Liaw A, Wiener M. Classification and regression by randomForest. R News. 2002;2(3):18–22.

19. OECD. Titanium dioxide dossier (NM100-NM105). Paris; 2015. http://www.oecd.org/chemicalsafety/nanosafety/titanium-dioxide-nm100-nm105-manufactured-nanomaterial.htm.

20. NanoGenoTox Joint Action. NANOGENOTOX Final report. Facilitating the safety evaluation of manufactured nanomaterials by characterising their potential genotoxic hazard. 2013. https://www.anses.fr/en/content/nanogenotox-documents.

21. ANSES. CLH report Proposal for Harmonised Classification and Labelling Substance Name : Titanium dioxide. 2016. http://echa.europa.eu/harmonised-classification-and-labelling-previous-consultations/-/substance-rev/13832/term.

22. ECHA. Read-Across Assessment Framework (RAAF). 2017. https://doi.org/10.2823/546436.

23. Guichard Y, Schmit J, Darne C, Gaté L, Goutet M, Rousset D, et al. Cytotoxicity and genotoxicity of nanosized and microsized titanium dioxide and iron oxide particles in Syrian hamster embryo cells. Ann Occup Hyg. 2012;56:631–44. https://doi.org/10.1093/annhyg/mes006.

24. SCCS. Opinion SCCS/1489/12 on titanium dioxide (nano form); COLIPA S75. Brussels: Scientific Committee on Consumer Safety; 2013.

25. Schultz TW, Amcoff P, Berggren E, Gautier F, Klaric M, Knight DJ, et al. A strategy for structuring and reporting a read-across prediction of toxicity. Regul Toxicol Pharmacol. 2015; https://doi.org/10.1016/j.yrtph.2015.05.016.

26. Clift MJD, Raemy DO, Endes C, Ali Z, Lehmann AD, Brandenberger C, et al. Can the Ames test provide an insight into nano-object mutagenicity? Investigating the interaction between nano-objects and bacteria. Nanotoxicology. 2012;7 February:1–13. https://doi.org/10.3109/17435390.2012.741725.

27. OECD. Genotoxicity of manufactured nanomaterials: Report of the OECD expert meeting. Series on the safety of manufactured nanomaterials No. 43. 2014.

28. Rasmussen K, González M, Kearns P, Sintes JR, Rossi F, Sayre P. Review of achievements of the OECD working party on manufactured nanomaterials' testing and assessment Programme. From exploratory testing to test guidelines. Regul Toxicol Pharmacol. 2016;74:147–60. https://doi.org/10.1016/j.yrtph.2015.11.004.

29. Huk A, Collins AR, El Yamani N, Porredon C, Azqueta A, de Lapuente J, et al. Critical factors to be considered when testing nanomaterials for genotoxicity with the comet assay. Mutagenesis. 2015;30:85–8. https://doi.org/10.1093/mutage/geu077.

30. Azqueta A, Dusinska M. The use of the comet assay for the evaluation of the genotoxicity of nanomaterials. Front Genet. 2015;6:239. https://doi.org/10.3389/fgene.2015.00239.

31. Kirsten R, Jan M, Pieter-Jan DT, Eveline V, Nadia W, Frederic VS, et al. Titanium dioxide, NM-100, NM-101, NM-102, NM-103, NM-104, NM-105: characterisation and Physico-chemical properties. 2014. https://doi.org/10.2788/79554 (online).

32. Birkedal R, Shivachev B, Dimova L, Petrov O, Nikolova R, Mast J, et al. Nanogenotox deliverable 4.3: Crystallite size, mineralogical and chemical purity of NANOGENOTOX nanomaterials. Copenhagen; 2012. https://www.anses.fr/en/system/files/nanogenotox_deliverable.3.pdf.

33. Jensen KA, Kembouche Y, Nielsen SH. Nanogenotox deliverable 4.7: Hydrochemical reactivity, solubility, and biodurability of NANOGENOTOX nanomaterials. Copenhagen; 2013. https://www.anses.fr/en/system/files/nanogenotox_deliverable.7.pdf

34. Magdolenova Z, Collins A, Kumar A, Dhawan A, Stone V, Dusinska M. Mechanisms of genotoxicity. A review of in vitro and in vivo studies with engineered nanoparticles. Nanotoxicology. 2014;8:233–78. https://doi.org/10.3109/17435390.2013.773464.

35. Burello E, Worth AP. A theoretical framework for predicting the oxidative stress potential of oxide nanoparticles. Nanotoxicology. 2011;5:228–35. https://doi.org/10.3109/17435390.2010.502980.

36. Schneider J, Matsuoka M, Takeuchi M, Zhang J, Horiuchi Y, Anpo M, et al. Understanding TiO2photocatalysis: mechanisms and materials. Chem Rev. 2014;114:9919–86.

37. Gini C. Variabilità e mutabilità. Memorie di metodologica statistica. 1955th edition. Rome: Libreria Eredi Virgilio Veschi; 1912.

38. Golbamaki N, Rasulev B, Cassano A, Marchese Robinson RL, Benfenati E, Leszczynski J, et al. Genotoxicity of metal oxide nanomaterials: review of recent data and discussion of possible mechanisms. Nanoscale. 2015;7: 2154–98. https://doi.org/10.1039/C4NR06670G.

39. Rice Z, Cady NC, Bergkvist M, Lobert PE, Bourgeois D, Pampin R, et al. Terminal phosphate group influence on DNA - TiO2 nanoparticle interactions. MRS Proc. 2009;1236:1236-NaN-15. https://doi.org/10.1557/PROC-1236-SS05-15.

40. Jugan M-L, Barillet S, Simon-Deckers A, Herlin-Boime N, Sauvaigo S, Douki T, et al. Titanium dioxide nanoparticles exhibit genotoxicity and impair DNA repair activity in A549 cells. Nanotoxicology. 2012;6:501–13. https://doi.org/10.3109/17435390.2011.587903.

41. Romoser AA. Cytotoxicological response to engineered nanomaterials: a pathway-driven process. 2012.

42. Trouiller B, Reliene R, Westbrook A, Solaimani P, Schiestl RH. Titanium dioxide nanoparticles induce DNA damage and genetic instability in vivo in mice. Cancer Res. 2009;69:8784–9. https://doi.org/10.1158/0008-5472.CAN-09-2496.

43. Barillet S, Simon-Deckers A, Herlin-Boime N, Mayne-L'Hermite M, Reynaud C, Cassio D, et al. Toxicological consequences of TiO2, SiC nanoparticles and multi-walled carbon nanotubes exposure in several mammalian cell types: an in vitro study. J Nanopart Res. 2010;12:61–73. https://doi.org/10.1007/s11051-009-9694-y.

44. Li K, Zhao X, K. Hammer B, Du S, Chen Y. Nanoparticles Inhibit DNA Replication by Binding to DNA: Modeling and Experimental Validation. ACS Nano. 2013;7(11):9664–74. https://doi.org/10.1021/nn402472k.

45. Mano SS, Kanehira K, Sonezaki S, Taniguchi A. Effect of polyethylene glycol modification of TiO2 nanoparticles on cytotoxicity and gene expressions in human cell lines. Int J Mol Sci. 2012;13:3703–17.

46. Falck GCM, Lindberg HK, Suhonen S, Vippola M, Vanhala E, Catalan J, et al. Genotoxic effects of nanosized and fine TiO2. Hum Exp Toxicol. 2009;28: 339–52. https://doi.org/10.1177/0960327109105163.

47. Magdolenova Z, Bilaničová D, Pojana G, Fjellsbø LM, Hudecova A, Hasplova K, et al. Impact of agglomeration and different dispersions of titanium dioxide nanoparticles on the human related in vitro cytotoxicity and genotoxicity. J Environ Monit. 2012;14:455. https://doi.org/10.1039/c2em10746e.

48. Karlsson HL, Di Bucchianico S, Collins AR, Dusinska M. Can the comet assay be used reliably to detect nanoparticle-induced genotoxicity? Environ Mol Mutagen. 2015;56:82–96. https://doi.org/10.1002/em.21933.

49. EC. Types and uses of nanomaterials, indcluding safety aspects. 2012. http://eur-lex.europa.eu/LexUriServ/LexUriServ.do?uri=SWD:2012:0288:FIN:EN:PDF.

50. SCCS. Opinion on Titanium Dioxide (nano form). 2014.

51. Schröder K, Pohlenz-Michel C, Simetska N, Voss JU, Escher S, Mangersdorf I. Carcinogenicity and Mutagenicity of Nanoparticles – Assessment of Current Knowledge as Basis for Regulation. Hannover; 2014. http://www.umweltbundesamt.de/sites/default/files/medien/378/publikationen/texte_50_2014_carcinogenicity_and_mutagenicity_of_nanoparticles_1.pdf.

52. Marchese Robinson RL, Lynch I, Peijnenburg W, Rumble J, Klaessig F, Marquardt C, et al. How should the completeness and quality of curated nanomaterial data be evaluated? Nanoscale 2016. https://doi.org/10.1039/C5NR08944A.

53. TDMA/TDIC. Industry Comment on behalf of Titanium Dioxide Manufacturer Association/Titanium Dioxide Industry Consortium (TDMA/TDIC) on the CLH Report for Harmonised Classification and Labelling (Comment #99). 2016. https://echa.europa.eu/documents/10162/4fd87a5d-e671-43e4-a3b8-30e51a723107.

54. European Industry. Comments and response to comments on CLH on Titaniuim dioxide: Proposal and justification comments. 2016;1–406. https://echa.europa.eu/documents/10162/13626/clh_comments_titanium_dioxide_en.pdf.

55. Gerloff K, Landesmann B, Worth A, Munn S, Palosaari T, Whelan M. The

Grouping of nanomaterials to read-across hazard endpoints: from data collection to assessment...

31

adverse outcome pathway approach in nanotoxicology. Comput Toxicol. 2017;1:3–11. https://doi.org/10.1016/j.comtox.2016.07.001.

56. Worth A, Aschberger K, Asturiol D, Bessems J, Gerloff K, Graepel R, Joossens E, Lamon L, Palosaari T, Richarz A. Evaluation of the availability and applicability of computational approaches in the safety assessment of nanomaterials. Luxembourg: EUR 28617 EN, Publications Office of the European Union; 2017:JRC106386. http://publications.jrc.ec.europa.eu/repository/handle/JRC106386.

57. ECHA. Guidance for identification and naming of substances under REACH and CLP. 2012.

58. Rajapakse K, Drobne D, Kastelec D. Experimental evidence of false-positive comet test results due to TiO 2 particle – assay interactions experimental evidence of false-positive comet test results due to TiO 2 particle – assay interactions. Nanotoxicology. 2013;7:1043–51.

59. OECD. Test No. 318: Dispersion Stability of Nanomaterials in Simulated Environmental Media. 2017. http://www.oecd-ilibrary.org/environment/test-no-318-dispersion-stability-of-nanomaterials-in-simulated-environmental-media_9789264284142-en.

60. OECD. Test No. 412: Subacute Inhalation Toxicity: 28-Day Study. 2017. http://www.oecd-ilibrary.org/environment/test-no-412-subacute-inhalation-toxicity-28-day-study_9789264070783-en.

61. Mast J, De Temmerman P-J. Protocol(s) for size-distribution analysis of primary NM particles in air, powders, and liquids. 2016. http://www.nanoreg.eu/images/D2.10_Protocol_for_size-distribution_analysis_of_primary_NM_particles_in_air_powders_and_liquids_-approvedpublic_for_website_final09.11.pdf. Accessed 24 Mar 2017.

62. ECHA. How to prepare registration dossiers that cover nanoforms: best practices 2017. https://doi.org/10.2823/128306.

3

The crystal structure of titanium dioxide nanoparticles influences immune activity in vitro and in vivo

Rob J. Vandebriel[1]*[ID], Jolanda P. Vermeulen[1], Laurens B. van Engelen[1], Britt de Jong[1], Lisa M. Verhagen[2], Liset J. de la Fonteyne-Blankestijn[1], Marieke E. Hoonakker[2] and Wim H. de Jong[1]

Abstract

Background: The use of engineered nanoparticles (NP) is widespread and still increasing. There is a great need to assess their safety. Newly engineered NP enter the market in a large variety; therefore safety evaluation should preferably be in a high-throughput fashion. In vitro screening is suitable for this purpose. TiO_2 NP exist in a large variety (crystal structure, coating and size), but information on their relative toxicities is scarce. TiO_2 NP may be inhaled by workers in e.g. paint production and application. In mice, inhalation of TiO_2 NP increases allergic reactions. Dendritic cells (DC) form an important part of the lung immune system, and are essential in adjuvant activity. The present study aimed to establish the effect of a variety of TiO_2 NP on DC maturation in vitro. Two NP of different crystal structure but similar in size, uncoated and from the same supplier, were evaluated for their adjuvant activity in vivo.

Methods: Immature DC were differentiated in vitro from human peripheral blood monocytes. Exposure effects of a series of fourteen TiO_2 NP on cell viability, CD83 and CD86 expression, and IL-12p40 and TNF-α production were measured. BALB/c mice were intranasally sensitized with ovalbumin (OVA) alone, OVA plus anatase TiO_2 NP, OVA plus rutile TiO_2 NP, and OVA plus Carbon Black (CB; positive control). The mice were intranasally challenged with OVA. OVA-specific IgE and IgG1 in serum, cellular inflammation in bronchoalveolar lavage fluid (BALF) and IL-4 and IL-5 production in draining bronchial lymph nodes were evaluated.

Results: All NP dispersions contained NP aggregates. The anatase NP and anatase/rutile mixture NP induced a higher CD83 and CD86 expression and a higher IL-12p40 production in vitro than the rutile NP (including coated rutile NP and a rutile NP of a 10-fold larger primary diameter). OVA-specific serum IgE and IgG1 were increased by anatase NP, rutile NP, and CB, in the order rutile<anatase<CB. The three particles similarly increased IL-4 and IL-5 production by bronchial LN cells and eosinophils and lymphocytes in the BALF. Neutrophils were induced by rutile NP and CB but not by anatase NP.

Conclusions: Our data show that measuring CD83 and CD86 expression and IL-12p40 and TNF-α production in DC in vitro may provide an efficient way to screen NP for potential adjuvant activity; future studies should establish whether this also holds for other NP. Based on antigen-specific IgE and IgG1, anatase NP have higher adjuvant activity than rutile NP, confirming our in vitro data. Other parameters of the allergic response showed a similar response for the two NP crystal structures. From the viewpoint of safe(r) by design products, rutile NP may be preferred over anatase NP, especially when inhalation exposure can be expected during production or application of the product.

Keywords: Titanium dioxide, Anatase, Rutile, Dendritic cell, Maturation, Inhalation, LgE, LgG1, Ovalbumin, Adjuvant

* Correspondence: rob.vandebriel@rivm.nl
[1]Centre for Health Protection, National Institute for Public Health and the Environment (RIVM), PO Box 1, 3720, BA, Bilthoven, The Netherlands
Full list of author information is available at the end of the article

Background

The use of engineered nanoparticles (NP) is widespread and still increasing. Therefore, there is great need to assess their effect on human health. Newly developed NP enter the market frequently and in a large variety, therefore safety evaluation should preferably provide results quickly and in a high-throughput fashion. An in vitro screening assay with demonstrated predictive value is suitable for this purpose. A further advantage of such an approach is that it reduces the use of animals, as animal experiments can be designed using knowledge obtained from in vitro experiments [1]. TiO_2 NP are one of the most frequently used nanomaterials in paints; both production and application may result in inhalation exposure. Following inhalation TiO_2 NP are known to be able to enhance an allergic response (adjuvant activity) [2–5] via the NF-κB pathway [6]. Dendritic cells (DC) form an important part of the lung immune system [7]. DC maturation is an essential step in the adaptive immune response [8] and plays an important role in enhancing an allergic response after inhalation of diesel soot particles [9, 10] and particulate matter [11] and likely also of TiO_2 NP. In fact, TiO_2 NP have been shown to induce DC maturation [12] via the NF-κB pathway [13]. Therefore, in the present study DC maturation is used as in vitro screening assay to determine the activation potency of TiO_2 NP.

A series of TiO_2 NP with different crystal structure, coating, and size were evaluated in the DC maturation assay in order to evaluate their DC activation potency as measure for their safety from the viewpoint of safe(r) by design products, especially when inhalation exposure can be expected during production or application of the product. Two NP of different crystal structure but similar in size, uncoated and from the same supplier, were evaluated for their adjuvant activity in vivo.

Results

Particle characterization

Size of the nanoparticles in dispersion

Table 1 lists the fourteen NP tested including their primary size and their size in dispersion (in 0.05% BSA in H_2O). The mean size of the various NP was between 157 and 212 nm, suggesting that, with the exception of the rutile NP of 200 nm, in suspension all NP were aggregated. The median size (the highest point in the peak of the size distribution) of the various NP was between 84 and 175 nm, and showed more variation between the various NP than the mean size.

Endotoxin content of the nanoparticles

Using the endoLISA kit an endotoxin concentration in the dispersion solution without NP of 52 EU/ml was found, while the endotoxin concentration in the dispersions containing NP ranged between 0 and 84 EU/ml. Multi-group ANOVA indicated no relationship between crystal structure of the NP and their endotoxin concentration ($P = 0.46$).

In vitro study

Exposure effect on viability

WST-1 staining indicated no loss of viability for the highest NP concentration tested (128 μg/ml; Additional file 1: Table S1). Live dead staining was performed to gate

Table 1 List of TiO_2 NP used in this study, including their size in dispersion

Manu-facturer	identification or product #	crystal form [a]	primary size [a] (nm)	SSA [a] (m^2/g)	purity [a] (%)	coating [a]	mean ± SD (nm)	median ± SD (nm)
JRC	NM-102	anatase	20	90	N/A	none	182.6 ± 21.1	86.6 ± 30.8
JRC	NM-103	rutile	20	60	N/A	hydrophobic	157.4 ± 8.9	102.0 ± 49.2
JRC	NM-104	rutile	20	60	N/A	hydrophilic	162.4 ± 5.8	147.4 ± 14.5
Skyspring	7910DL	anatase	10–25	50–150	99.5	none	186.4 ± 14.2	175.4 ± 29.7
Skyspring	7918DL	anat./rut.	10–30	50–100	99.5	none	169.6 ± 7.9	129.4 ± 38.9
Skyspring	7920DL	rutile	10–30	≈50	99.5	none	169.6 ± 25.7	139.8 ± 47.3
Skyspring	7923DL	rutile	20–40	> 40	99	SiO_2	177.2 ± 40.9	84.2 ± 17.8
Skyspring	7925DL	rutile	20–40	> 40	99	Al_2O_3	194.0 ± 15.9	128.8 ± 57.2
Io-Li-Tec	NO-0038-HP	anatase	20	> 120	99.5	none	208.6 ± 22.0	144.6 ± 42.0
Io-Li-Tec	NO-0046-HP	rutile	10–30	≈50	99.5	none	170.6 ± 13.2	139.2 ± 10.6
Io-Li-Tec	NO-0051-HP	rutile	200	8	99.5	none	212.4 ± 22.1	140.2 ± 61.5
Io-Li-Tec	NO-0058-HP	anatase	10–25	50–150	99.5	none	157.4 ± 28.3	121.2 ± 35.5
Io-Li-Tec	NO-0065-HP	rutile	20–40	40	99	silicon oil	161.6 ± 9.5	153.0 ± 2.8
Io-Li-Tec	NO-0066-HP	rutile	20–40	> 40	99	SiO_2	175.8 ± 19.0	157.0 ± 5.7

SSA specific surface area, N/A not available
[a]Information form the manufacturer or, in case of JRC [34], the supplier

viable cells and to evaluate possible NP exposure effects on viability. No clear dose-related effects were seen for any of the NP. For some NP, two or more consecutive doses induced staining levels below 80% of the non-exposed controls (10–30 nm uncoated anatase/rutile mixture, 20–40 nm SiO_2 coated rutile, 20–40 nm Al_2O_3 coated rutile, and 20–40 nm silicon oil coated rutile NP); these staining levels never fell below 50%. Additional file 1: Table S2 shows the results of live dead staining for the highest NP concentration tested.

Exposure effect on surface marker expression

Maturation of DC leads to an increased expression of surface markers, such as CD40, CD80, CD83, CD86 and HLA-DR [8]. In order to determine whether exposure to the different NP leads to DC maturation, the effect on the expression of these markers was measured using flow cytometry. Next to the aforementioned markers, as a control the expression was measured of CD14, a surface marker found on monocytes but not on DC. During culture of DC from monocytes, CD14 expression should disappear. After maturation, CD14 expression was found to be low and not affected by NP exposure. This protocol has consistently shown a clear upregulation by LPS of CD40, CD80, CD83, CD86 and HLA-DR [14].

For all NP tested exposure resulted in a dose-dependent effect on the mean fluorescence index (MFI) of CD83 and CD86, while no exposure effects on the MFI of CD40, CD80 and HLA-DR were seen.

In order to make a comparison between the NP in their capacity to induce DC maturation the MFI of CD83 at the highest NP concentration tested was divided by that of the blank control and the NP were ranked according to these ratios (Additional file 1: Table S3). The results show that anatase and anatase/rutile NP have a higher CD83 inducing capacity than rutile ones. Multi-group ANOVA indicated a statistically significant difference between the crystal structures ($P = 0.00013$).

For CD86 a similar approach was taken as for CD83 (Additional file 1: Table S4). Anatase and anatase/rutile NP have a higher CD86 inducing capacity than rutile ones, except for Skyspring SiO_2 coated rutile NP. Multi-group ANOVA indicated a statistically significant difference between the crystal structures ($P = 0.00697$). The range in CD83 induction was almost twice that of CD86 (4.5 versus 2.4).

Exposure effect on cytokine production

The induction of IL-6, IL-8, IL-10, IL-12p40, IL-12p70 and TNF-α production was measured. The production of IL-10 and IL-12p70 was lower than the detection limit, while IL-8 production did not show a dose-response relationship. IL-6, IL-12p40 and TNF-α showed a dose-response relationship and the NP were ranked,

using the same approach as described above: production at the highest NP concentration tested was divided by that of the blank control, and the NP were ranked according to these ratios.

Ranking the NP according to the ratio of IL-12p40 induction shows that the anatase NP (including the anatase/rutile NP) more strongly induced IL-12p40 production than the rutile NP (Additional file 1: Table S5). Multi Group ANOVA indicated a statistically significant difference between the crystal structures ($P = 0.01256$).

Ranking the NP according to the ratio of TNF-α induction shows that the anatase NP (including the anatase/rutile NP) more strongly induced TNF-α production than the rutile NP, except for Io-Li-Tec uncoated 200 nm NP (Additional file 1: Table S6). Multi Group ANOVA indicated that this difference between the crystal structures was, however, not statistically significant ($P = 0.24924$).

IL-6 induction showed no consistent relation with crystal structure, coating or manufacturer (Additional file 1: Table S7). Multi-group ANOVA indicated no statistically significant difference between the crystal structures ($P = 0.99891$).

Table 2 shows the ranking based on CD83, CD86, and IL-12p40. Using Support Vector Machines on the combined results on CD83, CD86, and IL-12p40, the accuracy of classification of the crystal structure was found to be 100%. Classification of coating or manufacturer did not result in a prediction that was better than a random prediction.

In vivo study
Serum immunoglobulins

IgE In the treatment groups where OVA was administered only during the challenge phase, OVA-specific IgE was 14 ng/ml; NP exposure during the "sensitization" phase did not affect this level (results not shown).

When OVA was administered during both the sensitization and challenge phase, OVA-specific IgE was 4 times higher relative to the animals that received OVA only during the challenge phase. Co-exposure to OVA and anatase TiO_2 NP, or OVA and the positive control Carbon Black (CB) during the sensitization phase increased OVA-specific IgE ($P < 0.01$; Fig. 1a). For rutile TiO_2 NP the increase was small and not statistically significant; OVA-specific IgE was 2 times higher after anatase NP co-exposure compared to rutile NP co-exposure ($P < 0.05$). These results may suggest that anatase NP have adjuvant activity, whereas rutile NP do not.

IgG1 In the treatment groups where OVA was administered only during the challenge phase, OVA-specific IgG1

Table 2 Ranking of TiO$_2$ NPs based on induction of CD83 and CD86 expression, and IL-12p40 production. 1, strongest induction; 14, weakest induction. The ranks for the three parameters were summed and the TiO$_2$ NPs were ranked accordingly

crystal form	primary size (nm)	coating	manufacturer	CD83	CD86	IL-12p40	score
anat./rut.	10–30	none	Skyspring	1	1	3	5
anatase	20	none	JRC	3	2	1	6
anatase	10–25	none	Io-Li-Tec	4	5	2	11
anatase	20	none	Io-Li-Tec	5	4	4	13
anatase	10–25	none	Skyspring	2	**6**	5	13
rutile	20–40	SiO$_2$	Skyspring	6	**3**	9	18
rutile	20–40	Al$_2$O$_3$	Skyspring	8	7	6	21
rutile	10–30	none	Skyspring	7	8	8	23
rutile	200	none	Io-Li-Tec	9	9	7	25
rutile	20	hydrophobic	JRC	12	11	10	33
rutile	10–30	none	Io-Li-Tec	14	10	11	35
rutile	20–40	SiO$_2$	Io-Li-Tec	10	13	13	36
rutile	20	hydrophilic	JRC	11	12	14	37
rutile	20–40	silicon oil	Io-Li-Tec	13	14	12	39

Bold: ranking does not fit the anatase vs. rutile difference in induction

was 74 ng/ml; NP exposure during the "sensitization" phase did not affect this level (results not shown).

When OVA was administered during both the sensitization and challenge phase, OVA-specific IgG1 was 160 times higher relative to the animals that received OVA only during the challenge phase. Co-exposure to OVA and rutile TiO$_2$ NP, OVA and anatase TiO$_2$ NP, or OVA and CB increased OVA-specific IgG1 ($P < 0.05$ for rutile NP; $P < 0.001$ for anatase NP and CB; Fig. 1b). OVA-specific IgG1 was 3 times higher after anatase NP co-exposure compared to rutile NP co-exposure ($P < 0.001$). These results may suggest that both rutile and anatase TiO$_2$ NP have an adjuvant activity and that the adjuvant activity is greater for anatase NP than for rutile NP.

Cytokines produced by bronchial lymph node cells and spleen cells
In the supernatants of the bronchial lymph node (LN) and spleen cell cultures IFN-γ, IL-1β, IL-4, IL-5, IL-17A, MCP-1 and TNF-α were measured.

Bronchial lymph node cells In the treatment groups where OVA was administered only during the challenge phase, production of IL-1β, IL-17 and MCP-1 was found not to be consistently above the detection limit. For the other cytokines, no treatment–related effects were seen.

In the treatments groups where OVA was administered during both the sensitization and challenge phase, production of IL-1β and MCP-1 was found not to be consistently above the detection limit. For IFN-γ, IL-17A and TNF-α, no treatment-related effects were seen. In the supernatants of the OVA-alone animals the IL-4

concentration was 8 pg/ml. Co-exposure to OVA and rutile TiO$_2$ NP, OVA and anatase TiO$_2$ NP, or OVA and CB resulted in a 4-fold increase in IL-4 levels ($P < 0.05$) compared to OVA-alone (Fig. 2a). IL-5 was absent from the supernatants of the OVA-alone animals. In the supernatants of the animals co-exposed to OVA and rutile NP, OVA and anatase NP, or OVA and CB, the IL-5 concentration was 24 pg/ml (Fig. 2b).

Spleen cells For spleen cells no effect of NP treatment was observed.

Cells in the lung lavage

Eosinophils An infiltrate of eosinophils is suggestive of an allergic inflammatory response. For the treatment groups where OVA was administered only during challenge, the lungs of the control animals did not show eosinophils, whereas the animals that were exposed to rutile NP and anatase NP showed a low percentage of eosinophils (Fig. 3a). CB exposed animals showed a higher percentage of eosinophils compared to rutile NP and anatase NP exposed animals ($P < 0.05$). When the effects were expressed as number of eosinophils a similar pattern was found but without statistical significance (Fig. 3b).

The treatment groups that were both sensitized and challenged to OVA showed a considerably higher percentage of eosinophils compared to the groups where OVA was administered only during challenge (Fig. 3c). For these groups the percentage of eosinophils was higher after co-exposure to OVA and rutile NP, and OVA and CB, compared to OVA alone ($P < 0.05$). When

a

IgE

b

IgG1

Fig. 1 a. OVA-specific IgE in serum. **b**. OVA-specific IgG1 in serum. Mice were sensitized with OVA alone, OVA + rutile TiO$_2$ NP, OVA + anatase TiO$_2$ NP, or OVA + Carbon Black (CB), and challenged with OVA. $N = 6$, mean ± SEM is shown. (*), (**), and (***) $P < 0.05$, $P < 0.01$, and $P < 0.001$vs. OVA alone; (+), (++), and (+++) $P < 0.05$, $P < 0.01$, and $P < 0.001$ vs. OVA + rutile NP; (###) $P < 0.001$ vs. OVA + anatase NP

a

br LN IL-4

b

br LN IL-5

Fig. 2 a. IL-4 production by LN cells. **b**. IL-5 production by LN cells. Mice were sensitized with OVA alone, OVA + rutile NP, OVA + anatase NP, or OVA + CB, and challenged with OVA. LN cell preparations were made and incubated with Con A for 24 h. N = 6, mean ± SEM is shown. (*) $P < 0.05$ vs. OVA alone

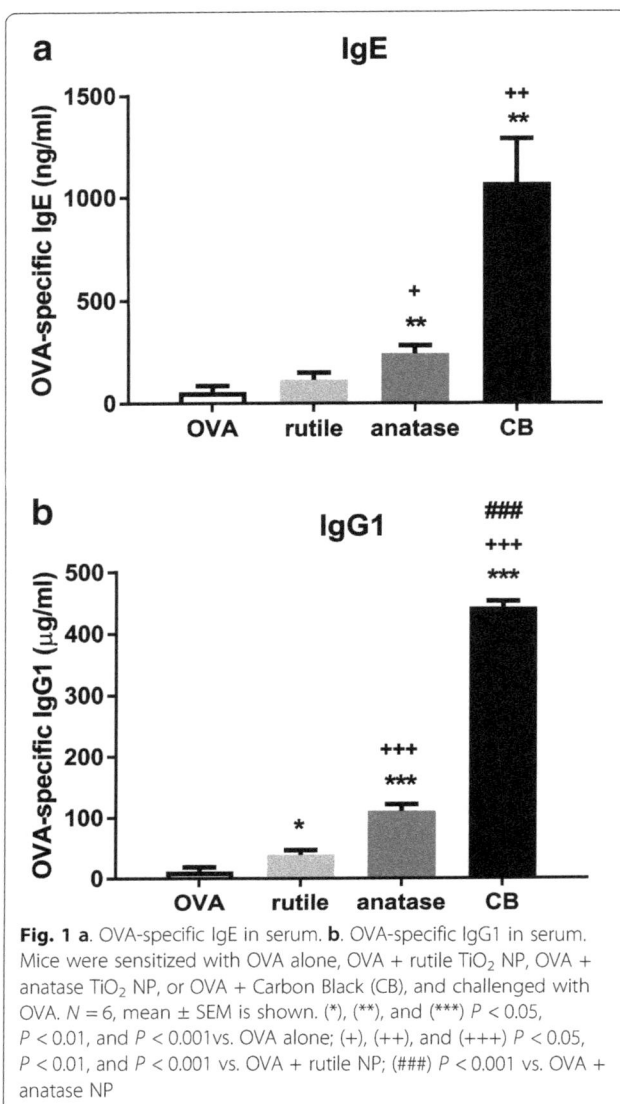

the effects were expressed as number of eosinophils a similar pattern was found but without statistical significance (Fig. 3d).

Lymphocytes An infiltrate of lymphocytes is suggestive of a chronic inflammatory response. For the treatment groups where OVA was administered only during challenge, exposure to anatase NP and CB increased the percentage of lymphocytes in the lungs ($P < 0.01$ and $P < 0.05$, respectively; Fig. 4a). Exposure to anatase NP and CB resulted in a higher percentage of lymphocytes compared to rutile NP ($P < 0.05$). Rutile NP and CB exposure resulted in an increased number of lymphocytes (Fig. 4b).

The treatment groups that were both sensitized and challenged to OVA showed a higher percentage of lymphocytes compared to the groups where OVA was administered only during challenge (Fig. 4c). For these groups the percentage of lymphocytes was higher after co-exposure to OVA and rutile NP, OVA and anatase NP, and OVA and CB, compared to OVA alone ($P < 0.001$, $P < 0.01$, and $P < 0.01$, respectively). Co-exposure to OVA and CB resulted in a higher percentage of lymphocytes compared to co-exposure to OVA and anatase NP ($P < 0.05$). Co-exposure to OVA and rutile NP, and OVA and CB resulted in an increased number of lymphocytes ($P < 0.05$ and $P < 0.01$, respectively; Fig. 4d). Co-exposure to OVA and CB resulted in an increased number of lymphocytes compared to co-exposure to OVA and rutile NP, and OVA and anatase NP ($P < 0.05$ and $P < 0.01$, respectively).

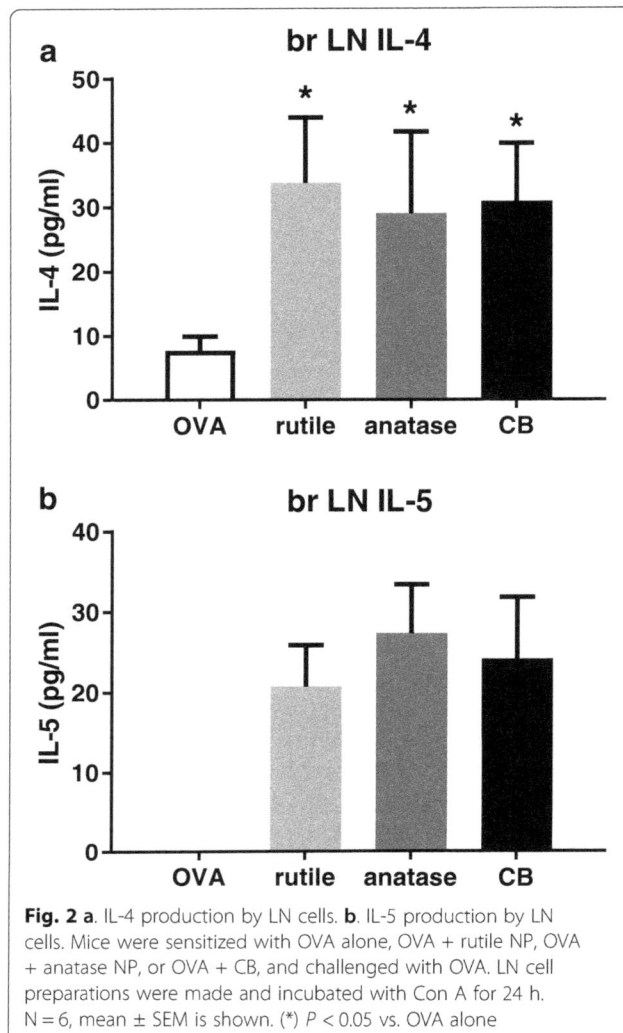

Neutrophils An infiltrate of neutrophils is suggestive of a non-allergic, acute inflammatory response.

For the treatment groups where OVA was administered only during challenge, exposure to anatase NP

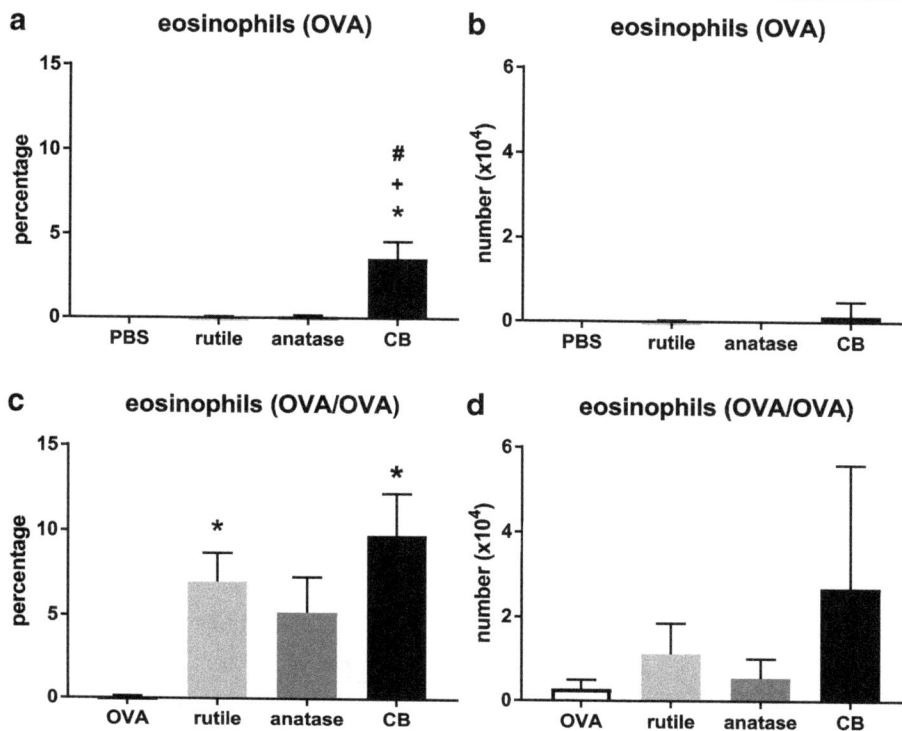

Fig. 3 a. Percentage of eosinophils in the BALF after OVA challenge. **b**. Number of eosinophils in the BALF after OVA challenge. **c**. Percentage of eosinophils in the BALF after OVA sensitization and challenge. **d**. Number of eosinophils in the BALF after OVA sensitization and challenge. A, B. Mice were sensitized with PBS, rutile NP, anatase NP, or CB, and challenged with OVA. C, D. Mice were sensitized with OVA alone, OVA + rutile NP, OVA + anatase NP, or OVA + CB, and challenged with OVA. N = 6, mean ± SEM is shown. In A and B, (*) $P < 0.05$ vs. PBS alone; (+) $P < 0.05$ vs. rutile NP; (#) $P < 0.05$ vs. anatase NP. In C and D, (*) $P < 0.05$ vs. OVA alone

resulted in a higher percentage of neutrophils in the lungs ($P < 0.01$; Fig. 5a). Exposure to CB resulted in a lower percentage of neutrophils compared to anatase NP ($P < 0.05$). Exposure to rutile NP and CB resulted in an increased number of neutrophils ($P < 0.05$ and $P < 0.001$, respectively; Fig. 5b). Exposure to anatase NP resulted in a smaller number of neutrophils compared to rutile NP and CB ($P < 0.01$ and $P < 0.05$, respectively).

The treatment groups that were both sensitized and challenged to OVA showed a rather similar percentage of neutrophils compared to the groups where OVA was administered only during challenge (Fig. 5c). Co-exposure to OVA and anatase NP resulted in a lower percentage of neutrophils compared to OVA alone, and to co-exposure to OVA and rutile NP ($P < 0.01$). Co-exposure to OVA and rutile NP and to OVA and CB resulted in a higher number of neutrophils compared to OVA alone ($P < 0.01$; Fig. 5d). Co-exposure to OVA and anatase NP resulted in a smaller number of neutrophils compared to OVA and rutile NP, and OVA and CB ($P < 0.01$ and $P < 0.05$, respectively).

Macrophages Macrophages are the dominant cell type in the lung lavage and their numbers are in general relatively constant; a decrease in their percentage is often due to an increase in the percentage of neutrophils, lymphocytes and eosinophils. For the treatment groups where OVA was administered only during challenge, exposure to rutile NP resulted in a higher percentage of macrophages in the lungs ($P < 0.05$; Fig. 6a), whereas exposure to CB resulted in a lower percentage ($P < 0.05$). Exposure to anatase NP and CB resulted in a lower percentage of macrophages compared to rutile NP ($P < 0.01$ and $P < 0.05$, respectively). No treatment related effects on the number macrophages was seen (Fig. 6b).

The treatment groups that were both sensitized and challenged to OVA showed a somewhat lower percentage of macrophages compared to the groups where OVA was administered only during challenge (Fig. 6c). The percentage of macrophages was lower after co-exposure to OVA and rutile NP, and to OVA and CB, compared to OVA alone ($P < 0.001$). The percentage of macrophages was higher after co-exposure to OVA and anatase NP compared to co-exposure to OVA and rutile NP and to OVA and CB ($P < 0.05$ and $P < 0.01$, respectively). This is likely due to a higher percentage of neutrophils (in case of rutile NP) and lymphocytes (in case of rutile

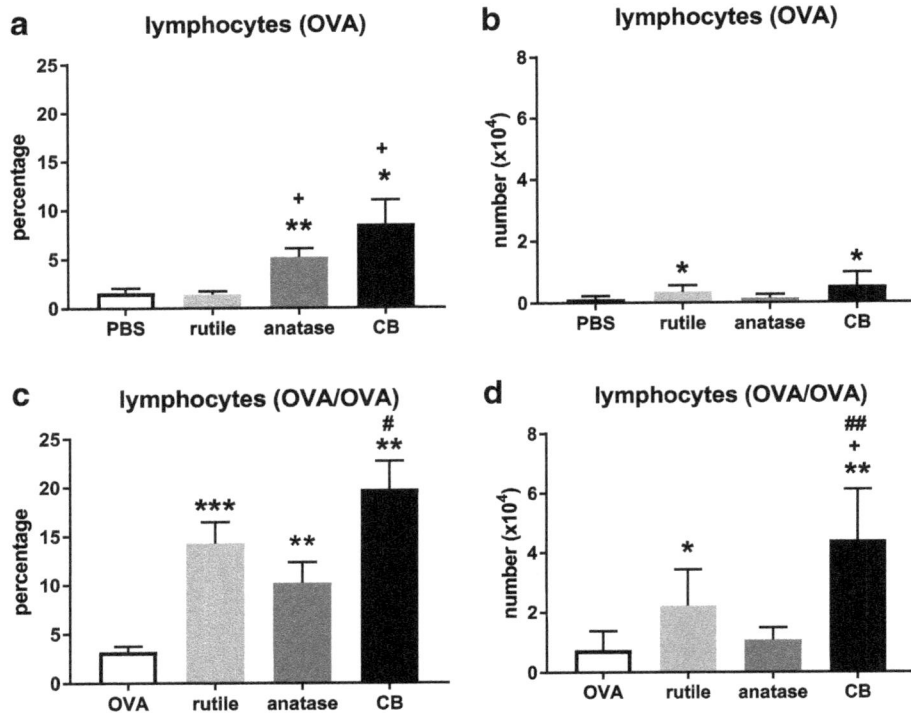

Fig. 4 a. Percentage of lymphocytes in the BALF after OVA challenge. **b**. Number of lymphocytes in the BALF after OVA challenge. **c**. Percentage of lymphocytes in the balf after ova sensitization and challenge. **d**. Number of lymphocytes in the BALF after OVA sensitization and challenge. See legend to Fig. 3. In A and B, (*) and (**) $P < 0.05$ and $P < 0.01$ vs. PBS alone; (+) $P < 0.05$ vs. rutile NP. In C and D, (*), (**) and (**) $P < 0.05$, $P < 0.01$ and $P < 0.01$ vs. OVA alone; (+) $P < 0.05$ vs. OVA + rutile NP; (##) $P < 0.05$ vs. OVA + anatase NP

NP and CB). Due to the small percentage of eosinophils in general, effects on these percentages have a minor influence on the percentage of macrophages. The number of macrophages was increased after co-exposure to OVA and CB compared to OVA alone ($P < 0.05$; Fig. 6d).

Overall, for eosinophils and lymphocytes no clear difference in the response to rutile NP and anatase NP is seen. For neutrophils, the response to rutile NP is higher than to anatase NP.

Discussion

Here we have shown that in vitro anatase and anatase/rutile TiO$_2$ NP induced a higher expression of CD83 and CD86 and a higher production of IL-12p40, than rutile NP, suggesting that DC maturation is induced to a greater extent by anatase and anatase/rutile NP than by rutile NP.

No effect of the size of the primary NP, their coating, and their manufacturer was found. The primary size of the NP is 10–40 nm, with the exception of one product having a primary particle size of 200 nm. NanoSight measurements showed that during cell culture all NP had a rather similar size distribution with a mean size of 160–210 nm. This suggests that, with the exception of the 200 nm particle, all NP showed aggregation and/or

agglomeration. This may be an explanation for the absence of a size effect on the test results. It cannot be ruled out, however, that some of the coatings play a possible role in DC maturation. For instance, SiO$_2$ NP have been shown to induce DC maturation [15, 16].

Different responses to anatase and rutile TiO$_2$ NP have been reported earlier. Anatase NP induced a higher IL-8 production than rutile NP in A549 human lung epithelial cells [17]. Anatase and anatase/rutile NP induced a higher amount of reactive oxygen species (ROS) than rutile NP in a cell-free system [18]. Anatase NP induced stronger glutathione depletion and a greater reduction of superoxide dismutase than rutile NP in PC12 neuronal cells [19]. In this study, only anatase NP showed an increase in malondialdehyde; this molecule is formed by ROS from unsaturated fatty acids. Intranasal instillation of mice with 155 nm anatase NP resulted in higher IL-1β and TNF-α levels in the brain compared to similar treatment with 80 nm rutile NP [20]. In contrast to the previous studies, rutile NP induced higher ROS production than anatase NP in HEL30 keratinocytes [21]. These authors also found that rutile NP initiated cell death by apoptosis through formation of ROS, while anatase NP induced cell death by necrosis. In a co-culture of human blood vessel endothelial cells and DC, anatase NP

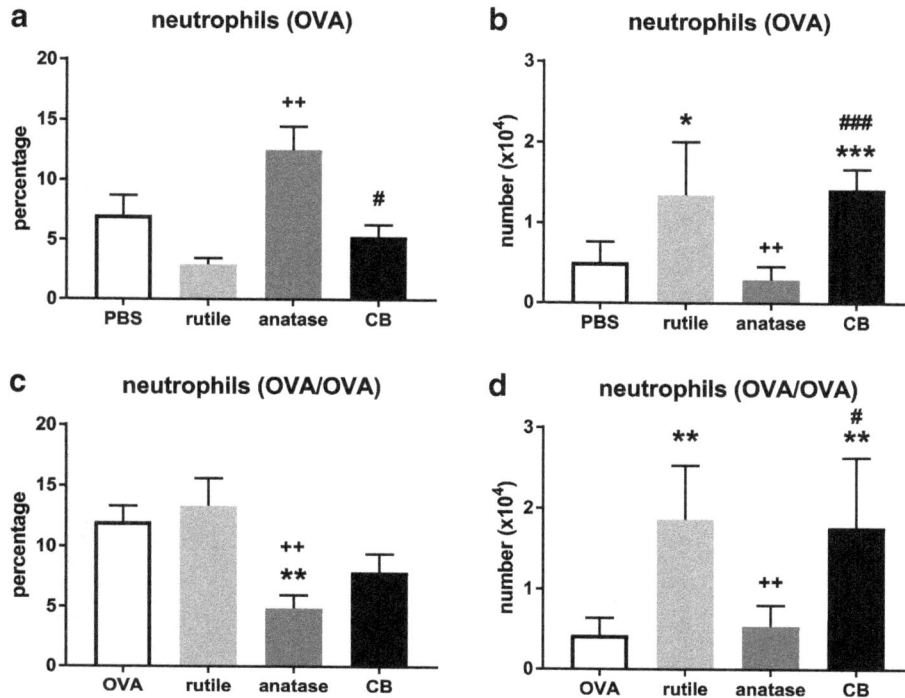

Fig. 5 a. Percentage of neutrophils in the BALF after OVA challenge. **b**. Number of neutrophils in the BALF after OVA challenge. **c**. Percentage of neutrophils in the BALF after OVA sensitization and challenge. **d**. Number of neutrophils in the BALF after OVA sensitization and challenge. See legend to Fig. 3. In A and B, (*) and (***) $P < 0.05$ and $P < 0.001$ vs. PBS alone; (++) $P < 0.01$ vs. rutile NP; (#) and (###) $P < 0.05$ and $P < 0.001$ vs. anatase NP. In C and D, (**) $P < 0.01$ vs. OVA alone; (++) $P < 0.01$ vs. OVA + rutile NP; (#) $P < 0.05$ vs. OVA + anatase NP

induced a higher IL-1β, IL-10 and IFN-γ production than rutile NP [22]. Unlike our study, a similar expression of CD83 and CD86 on DC was found after exposure to anatase and rutile NP. In addition, they observed a similar induction of allogeneic naive CD4$^+$ T-cells by DC that had been exposed to anatase and rutile NP. In conclusion, except for the studies by Braydich-Stolle et al. [21] and Schanen et al. [22], these studies are in line with our study suggesting that anatase and anatase/rutile TiO$_2$ NP have a stronger adjuvant activity than rutile ones.

When comparing the responses between rutile and anatase NP for the various parameters, two markers of the allergic response, IgE and IgG1, are induced more strongly by anatase compared to rutile NP, whereas other markers for this response, IL-4, IL-5, eosinophils and lymphocytes are similarly induced by both NP, and neutrophils are induced more strongly by rutile compared to anatase NP. The conclusion of a stronger adjuvant activity of anatase NP compared to rutile NP should thus be made with some prudence.

The in vitro assay used here is generally accepted to measure effects on DC maturation. Since DC maturation is important in the induction of an adaptive immune response, and DC play an important role in the stimulation by particles of the adaptive immune response in the

respiratory tract [10], the assumption was that stimulation of DC maturation in vitro might be translated to identify adjuvant activity for the immune response in vivo by NP, such as in the mouse ovalbumin allergy model. When inhaled, TiO$_2$ NP can induce or enhance an allergic response (adjuvant activity) when co-administered with the allergen [2–5]. In our study two NP with different crystal structures but otherwise very similar, were selected to be tested in the mouse ovalbumin allergy model. The NP are of similar size (10–30 nm rutile NP, 10–25 nm anatase NP), are both uncoated, and are both from the same producer (Io-Li-Tec). By using the in vitro model prior to the experimental animal study, the number of NP for which testing in vivo was deemed relevant was limited to two.

In the animal study reported here we have shown that co-administration of an allergen (ovalbumin) and TiO$_2$ NP, results, especially for the anatase TiO$_2$ NPs in a marked adjuvant activity; these results are consistent with the in vitro findings using the DC model. Intratracheal instillation of rats of 80% anatase/20% rutile TiO$_2$ NP but not of two rutile NP induced an increase in neutrophils and cytotoxicity in the bronchoalveolar lavage and proliferation of tracheobronchial epithelial cells and lung parenchymal cells [23]. Similar to our study, this study showed stronger effects of anatase NP compared to

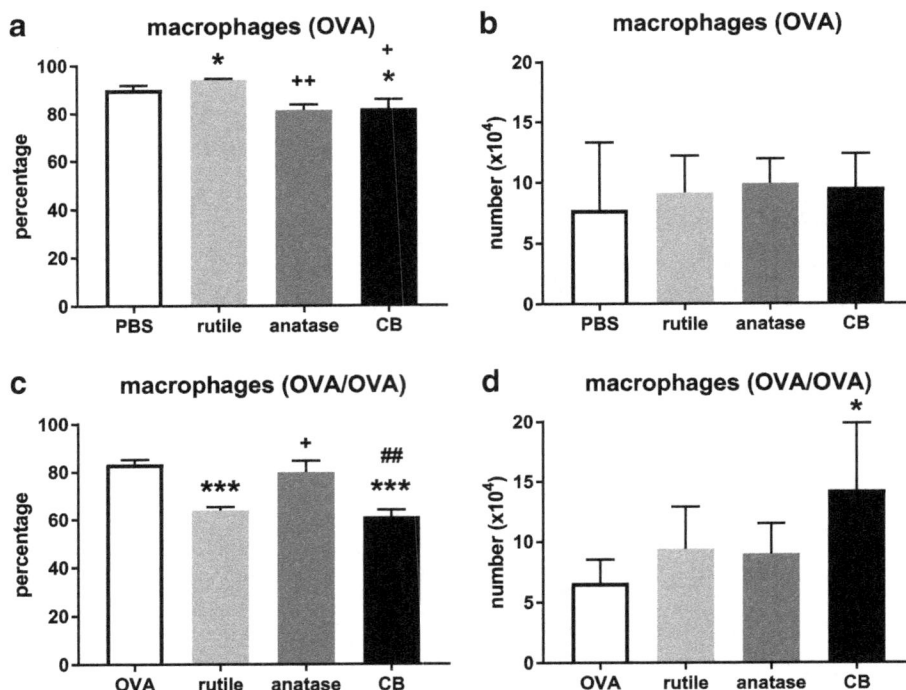

Fig. 6 a. Percentage of macrophages in the BALF after OVA challenge. **b**. Number of macrophages in the BALF after OVA challenge. **c**. Percentage of macrophages in the BALF after OVA sensitization and challenge. **d**. Number of macrophages in the BALF after OVA sensitization and challenge. See legend to Fig. 3. In A and B, (*) $P < 0.05$ vs. PBS alone; (+) and (++) $P < 0.05$ and $P < 0.01$ vs. rutile NP. In C and D, (***) $P < 0.001$ vs. OVA alone; (+) $P < 0.05$ vs. OVA + rutile NP; (##) $P < 0.01$ vs. OVA + anatase NP

rutile NP on the rodent lungs. It should be noted, however, that this study did not involve an allergy model.

A more general question is whether physico-chemical properties of NP can provide information on the degree of oxidative stress, and thus glutathione depletion, DC maturation and allergic reactions. The higher ROS activity induced by anatase NP compared to rutile NP can be explained by their differences in surface chemistry [18]. Anatase is more suitable to adsorb oxygen in the form of $O2^-$ and O^- than rutile TiO_2 [24]. Water is bound by anatase as H^+ and OH^-, and by rutile as H_2O [25, 26]. Both processes (adsorption of $O2^-$ and O^-; binding of H^+ and OH^-) facilitate ROS formation [24]. Glutathione (GSH) is an essential antioxidant that protects against oxidative stress. GSH in the cell decreases from exposure to oxidants [27]. GSH levels in antigen-presenting cells (such as DC) influence the Th1 versus the Th2 response; reduction in GSH levels leads to a decreased Th1 response [28]. The following chain of events may thus be suggested to explain differences for anatase vs. rutile TiO_2 NP: higher adsorption of $O2^-$ and O^-, and stronger binding of H^+ and OH^- on the surface of anatase NP → ROS ⇑ → glutathione depletion ⇑ → Th1 ⇓ → allergic Th2 response ⇑.

Li et al. [29] have shown that in an ovalbumin allergy model the response is determined by the oxidant potential of co-administered particulate matter. Our findings

of a larger response due to co-administration of anatase NP compared to rutile NP are in line with this observation.

Relationships between physico-chemical properties of NP and biological effects have been established for band gap energy levels and cytotoxicity [30] and surface charge and lung fibrosis [31]. In this paper we established a relationship between crystal structure and induction of DC maturation as well as adjuvant activity.

The lower adjuvant activity of rutile TiO_2 NP relative to anatase NP may be a reason to preferably apply rutile NP in order to reduce adjuvant activity during possible respiratory exposure. For a final choice of NP to be used additional NP characteristics should also be considered.

Finally, the in vitro DC maturation assay appears to be predictive for the adjuvant activity in vivo and may therefore be used as in vitro screening assay. However, this requires that first additional NP (multiple anatase and rutile NP, and also NP of other chemical identity such as SiO_2) be compared in vitro and in vivo.

Conclusions

In summary, we have shown that anatase TiO_2 NP more strongly induce DC maturation than rutile NP; moreover, anatase NP show a stronger adjuvant activity in an in vivo allergy model. From the viewpoint of safe(r) by design products, rutile NP may be preferred over anatase NP, especially when inhalation exposure can be expected during production or application of the product The DC maturation assay used is a promising in vitro screen for adjuvant activity of NP.

Methods
In vitro studies
Materials
Fourteen TiO_2 nanoparticles (NP) obtained from various suppliers (Joint Research Centre, Institute for Health and Consumer Protection, European Union; Skyspring Nano Materials Inc., Houston, TX, USA; Ionic Liquids Technologies GmbH, Heilbronn, Germany) were included in the study. They are listed in Table 1.

NP dispersion and size determination
The NP (powder) were pre-wetted by adding a drop of absolute ethanol. The NP were then taken up in dispersion liquid (H_2O + 0.05% BSA) to a concentration of 2.56 mg/mL. These suspensions were sonicated using a 450 W Digital Sonifier (Branson, Danbury, CT, USA) with 10% of the maximum energy for 16 min according to the Nanogenotox protocol [32]. The particle size was determined using Nanoparticle Tracking Analysis (Nanosight, Amesbury, UK), which is based on the Brownian movement of the NP. Each suspension was measured five times, filtered through a 0.45-μm filter and measured again five times. The particle size in the filtered suspensions is shown. It is expressed as median (size, to match the peak in the size distribution), and as an average, both ± SD of the five measurements.

Generation, exposure, and maturation of DC
Human-derived buffy coats were obtained from Sanquin (Amsterdam, the Netherlands). Peripheral blood mononuclear cells were isolated from buffy coats by density centrifugation (Lymphoprep; Axis Shield, Oslo, Norway). The cells were washed, harvested, and resuspended in RPMI-1640 (Gibco, Grand Island, NY, USA) supplemented with 2% heat-inactivated human serum (Harlan, Boxmeer, the Netherlands), 100 μg/mL streptomycin, 100 IU/mL penicillin, and 0.3 mg/mL L-glutamine. They were seeded in culture flasks (Corning, Amsterdam, the Netherlands) and were let to attach for 1 h. The cells were rinsed with warm (37°C) PBS and medium was added (RPMI-1640 supplemented with 10% heat-inactivated Foetal Calf Serum ("FCS"; Hyclone; GE Healthcare, Logan, UT, USA), streptomycin, penicillin, L-glutamine, 500 U/mL GM-CSF and 250 U/mL IL-4. At day 3, fresh cytokines were added. At day 6, the immature DC were harvested. Cell culture conditions were 37 °C in a humidified atmosphere containing 5% CO_2.

The DC were exposed to a concentration range of the TiO_2 NP (0–128 μg/mL) for 48 h. After this, the viability of the cells was measured using the WST-1 assay. Next to staining for viability ("live-dead" staining), the expression of CD14, CD40, CD80, CD83, CD86, and HLA-DR was measured. To this end, the cells were washed twice with PBS and twice with FACS buffer (PBS pH 7.2, 0.5% BSA, 0.5 mM EDTA). To 100 μL of these cells, 100 μL staining mix 1 or staining mix 2 was added (see below). After incubation at 4 °C for 30 min, the cells were spun down, included in FACS buffer, and measured using the FACS Canto (Becton Dickinson Biosciences, Breda, the Netherlands)

Marker	Label	Dilution
Staining mix 1		
CD80	FITC	1:40
CD14	PE	1:25
HLA-DR	Pacific Blue	1:1600
Live-dead	Aqua	1:200
Staining mix 2		
CD83	FITC	1:40
CD40	PE	1:20
CD86	Pacific Blue	1:800
Live-dead	Aqua	1:200

IL-12p40 was measured by ELISA (Becton Dickinson Biosciences) according to the manufacturer's instructions. The other cytokines (IL-6, IL-8, IL-10, IL-12p70 and TNF-α) were measured using a Bio-Plex System (Bio-Rad, Veenendaal, the Netherlands).

Statistics
Each NP was tested at least three times; in Additional file 1: Tables S1-S7 a representative result is shown. To establish the significance of the difference in induction of CD83, CD86, IL-12p40, TNF-α and IL-6 between the groups of particles, a multi-group ANOVA was used for crystal structure, coating, and manufacturer. The analyses were run on a single surface marker or cytokine, versus the three categorical factors of crystal structure, coating and manufacturer, in one analysis. In addition, the accuracy of classification to the crystal structure was established using Support Vector Machines (SVM). Using the radial kernel on scaled data, SVM [33] creates a separating hyperplane. The rank data is the input. The crystal structure is binary, with anatase/rutile taken as anatase.

In vivo study
Animals
Specific pathogen-free (SPF) female BALB/cAnNCrl mice [2], 6–8 weeks of age, were obtained from Charles

River (Sulzfeld, Germany) and randomly assigned to a treatment group. Animals were bred under SPF conditions and barrier maintained during the experiment. Drinking water and conventional feed were provided ad libitum. Husbandry conditions were maintained according to all applicable provisions of the national laws, Experiments on Animals Decree and Experiments on Animals Act. The experiment was approved by an independent ethical committee (the Animal Experiments Committee of the National Institute for Public Health and the Environment) prior to the study.

Animal treatment and euthanasia

Uncoated 10–30 nm rutile TiO_2 NP ("ILT46"; NO-0046-HP, Io-Li-Tec, Germany), uncoated 10–25 nm anatase TiO_2 NP ("ILT58"; NO-0058-HP, Io-Li-Tec, Germany), and Carbon Black ("CB", Printex 90, Degussa, Germany) were tested. They were dissolved in PBS to 6.67 mg/mL. Ovalbumin ("OVA"; Grade VII; Sigma-Aldrich, Zwijndrecht, the Netherlands) was dissolved in PBS to 10 mg/mL. Endotoxin was removed from OVA using a Detoxi-Gel Endotoxin Removing Column (Pierce; Thermo Fisher Scientific, Etten Leur, the Netherlands) according to the manufacturer's instructions. For the OVA-alone group, 1 mL OVA was diluted with 1 mL PBS. To 1 mL of each of the NP suspensions, 1 mL PBS or 1 mL OVA was added. To each of the eight samples (PBS, OVA, ILT46, ILT58, CB, ILT46/OVA, ILT58/OVA, and CB/OVA), 100 µL mouse albumin (Sigma-Aldrich) was added. The samples were sonicated using a Digital Sonifier (Branson) with 10% of the maximum energy for 16 min. Animals were sensitized intranasally under deep isoflurane anaesthesia by adding 20 µL of the sample in each of the two nostrils (40 µL per animal; 0.45% OVA and 120 µg NP) at days 0, 1, and 2. Animals were challenged intranasally under deep isoflurane anaesthesia by adding 20 µL OVA in each of the two nostrils (40 µl per animal; 0.45% OVA) at days 25, 26, and 27.

At day 28, the animals were weighed. They were sacrificed by isoflurane euthanasia. Blood was collected (Greiner MiniCollect tubes) and the serum samples were stored at − 80 °C. The lungs were lavaged with PBS (1 mL per 25 g animal weight). This was repeated twice. Bronchoalveolar lavage (BAL) fluid cells were centrifuged and the cell pellets were resuspended in PBS, counted using a Coulter Counter (Coulter Electronics, Luton, UK), and visually differentiated after Giemsa staining. Bronchial lymph nodes (LN) were excised and cell suspensions were prepared (see below).

Cell culture

The culture medium used was RPMI-1640 supplemented with 10% FCS, 100 µg/mL streptomycin, and 100 IU/mL penicillin. Cell suspensions were made by pressing the LNs through a cell strainer (Falcon, Franklin Lakes, NJ, USA). Cells were counted using a Coulter Counter. LN cell suspensions were cultured at 10^6 cells/mL culture medium with 5 µg/mL Concanavalin A (MP Biomedicals, Irvine, CA, USA) in 96-well tissue culture plates (Nunc, Roskilde, Denmark) for 24 h. Spleen cell suspensions were cultured at 10^6 cells/mL culture medium with 1 mg/mL OVA in 96-well tissue culture plates (Nunc) for 120 h. Culture conditions were 37 °C in a humidified atmosphere containing 5% CO_2.

Serum Ig and cytokine measurements

OVA-specific IgE and OVA-specific IgG1 were measured using an ELISA (Cayman Chemicals, Sanbio, Uden, the Netherlands). A 10-plex panel containing beads for mouse IL-1β, IL-4, IL-5, IL-17A, IFN-γ, MCP-1, and TNF-α (Merck, Darmstadt, Germany) was used.

Statistics

Statistical analysis of animal weights, BALF cell percentages, spleen and LN weights and cellularity, serum IgE and IgG1 levels, and cytokine production was performed using the independent-samples t-test (SPSS Inc., Chicago, IL, USA). Number of animals per group = 6.

Additional file

Additional file 1: Table S1. Effect of exposure to TiO_2 nanoparticles on viability (WST-1). Table S2. Effect of exposure to TiO_2 nanoparticles on viability (live-dead). Table S3. Effect of exposure to TiO_2 nanoparticles on CD83 expression. Table S4. Effect of exposure to TiO_2 nanoparticles on CD86 expression. Table S5. Effect of exposure to TiO_2 nanoparticles on IL-12p40 production. Table S6. Effect of exposure to TiO_2 nanoparticles on TNF-α production. Table S7. Effect of exposure to TiO_2 nanoparticles on IL-6 production. (DOCX 36 kb)

Abbreviations

NP: Nanoparticles; OVA: Ovalbumin

Acknowledgements

Geert van der Horst, Daan Leseman, and Dr. Margriet Park are acknowledged for support, Dr. Tessa Pronk and Dr. Jeroen Pennings for statistics, and Prof Henk van Loveren for critical review of the manuscript.

Funding

The study was supported by the Netherlands Food and Consumer Product Safety Authority, project V090016.

Authors' contributions

RJV and WDJ were involved in conception and design of the study; JPV, LBVE, BDJ, LMH, LJDLFB, and MEH were involved in acquisition of data; RJV, MEH, and WDJ were involved in analysis and interpretation of data. RJV and WDJ drafted the manuscript. All authors have given final approval of the version to be published.

Competing interests

The authors declare that they have no competing interests.

Author details

[1]Centre for Health Protection, National Institute for Public Health and the Environment (RIVM), PO Box 1, 3720, BA, Bilthoven, The Netherlands.
[2]Intravacc, PO Box 450, 3720, AL, Bilthoven, The Netherlands.

References

1. Nel AE, Nasser E, Godwin H, Avery D, Bahadori T, Bergeson L, Beryt E, Bonner JC, Boverhof D, Carter J, Castranova V, Deshazo JR, Hussain SM, Kane AB, Klaessig F, Kuempel E, Lafranconi M, Landsiedel R, Malloy T, Miller MB, Morris J, Moss K, Oberdorster G, Pinkerton K, Pleus RC, Shatkin JA, Thomas R, Tolaymat T, Wang A, Wong J. A multi-stakeholder perspective on the use of alternative test strategies for nanomaterial safety assessment. ACS Nano. 2013;7:6422–33.
2. de Haar C, Hassing I, Bol M, Bleumink R, Pieters R. Ultrafine but not fine particulate matter causes airway inflammation and allergic airway sensitization to co-administered antigen in mice. Clin Exp Allergy. 2006;36: 1469–79.
3. Larsen ST, Roursgaard M, Jensen KA, Nielsen GD. Nano titanium dioxide particles promote allergic sensitization and lung inflammation in mice. Basic Clin Pharmacol Toxicol. 2010;106:114–7.
4. Rossi EM, Pylkkänen L, Koivisto AJ, Nykäsenoja H, Wolff H, Savolainen K, Alenius H. Inhalation exposure to nanosized and fine TiO2 particles inhibits features of allergic asthma in a murine model. Part Fibre Toxicol. 2010;7:35.
5. Jonasson S, Gustafsson A, Koch B, Bucht A. Inhalation exposure of nano-scaled titanium dioxide (TiO2) particles alters the inflammatory responses in asthmatic mice. Inhal Toxicol. 2013;25:179–91.
6. Mishra V, Baranwal V, Mishra RK, Sharma S, Paul B, Pandey AC. Titanium dioxide nanoparticles augment allergic airway inflammation and Socs3 expression via NF-κB pathway in murine model of asthma. Biomaterials. 2016;92:90–102.
7. Lambrecht BN, Hammad H. The role of dendritic and epithelial cells as master regulators of allergic airway inflammation. Lancet. 2010;376:835–43.
8. Banchereau J, Steinman RM. Dendritic cells and the control of immunity. Nature. 1998;392:245–52.
9. Porter M, Karp M, Killedar S, Bauer SM, Guo J, Williams D, Breysse P, Georas SN, Williams MA. Diesel-enriched particulate matter functionally activates human dendritic cells. Am J Respir Cell Mol Biol. 2007;37:706–19.
10. Provoost S, Maes T, Willart MA, Joos GF, Lambrecht BN, Tournoy KG. Diesel exhaust particles stimulate adaptive immunity by acting on pulmonary dendritic cells. J Immunol. 2010;184:426–32.
11. de Haar C, Kool M, Hassing I, Bol M, Lambrecht BN, Pieters R. Lung dendritic cells are stimulated by ultrafine particles and play a key role in particle adjuvant activity. J Allergy Clin Immunol. 2008;121:1246–54.
12. Schanen BC, Das S, Reilly CM, Warren WL, Self WT, Seal S, Drake DR 3rd: Immunomodulation and T helper TH1/TH2 response polarization by CeO2 and TiO2 nanoparticles. PLoS One 2013, 8:e62816.
13. Zhu R, Zhu Y, Zhang M, Xiao Y, Du X, Liu H, Wang S. The induction of maturation on dendritic cells by TiO2 and Fe3O4@TiO2 nanoparticles via NF-κB signaling pathway. Mater Sci Eng C Mater Biol Appl. 2014;39:305–14.
14. Hoefnagel MH, Vermeulen JP, Scheper RJ, Vandebriel RJ. Response of MUTZ-3 dendritic cells to the different components of the Haemophilus influenzae type B conjugate vaccine: towards an in vitro assay for vaccine immunogenicity. Vaccine. 2011;29:5114–21.
15. Winter M, Beer HD, Hornung V, Krämer U, Schins RP, Förster I. Activation of the inflammasome by amorphous silica and TiO2 nanoparticles in murine dendritic cells. Nanotoxicology. 2011;5:326–40.
16. Malachin G, Lubian E, Mancin F, Papini E, Tavano R. Combined action of human commensal bacteria and amorphous silica nanoparticles on the viability and immune responses of dendritic cells. Clin Vaccine Immunol. 2017;24:e00178–17.
17. Sayes CM, Wahi R, Kurian PA, Liu Y, West JL, Ausman KD, Warheit DB, Colvin VL. Correlating nanoscale titania structure with toxicity: a cytotoxicity and inflammatory response study with human dermal fibroblasts and human lung epithelial cells. Toxicol Sci. 2006;92:174–85.
18. Jiang J, Oberdörster G, Elder A, Gelein R, Mercer P, Biswas P. Does nanoparticle activity depend upon size and crystal phase? Nanotoxicology. 2008;2:33–42.
19. Wu J, Sun J, Xue Y. Involvement of JNK and P53 activation in G2/M cell cycle arrest and apoptosis induced by titanium dioxide nanoparticles in neuron cells. Toxicol Lett. 2010;199:269–76.
20. Wang J, Liu Y, Jiao F, Lao F, Li W, Gu Y, Li Y, Ge C, Zhou G, Li B, Zhao Y, Chai Z, Chen C. Time-dependent translocation and potential impairment on central nervous system by intranasally instilled TiO(2) nanoparticles. Toxicology. 2008;254:82–90.
21. Braydich-Stolle LK, Schaeublin NM, Murdock RC, Jiang J, Biswas P, Schlager JJ, Hussain SM. Crystal structure mediates mode of cell death in TiO2 nanotoxicity. J Nanopart Res. 2009;11:1361–74.
22. Schanen BC, Karakoti AS, Seal S, Drake DR 3rd, Warren WL, Self WT. Exposure to titanium dioxide nanomaterials provokes inflammation of an in vitro human immune construct. ACS Nano. 2009;3:2523–32.
23. Warheit DB, Webb TR, Reed KL, Frerichs S, Sayes CM. Pulmonary toxicity study in rats with three forms of ultrafine-TiO2 particles: differential responses related to surface properties. Toxicology. 2007;230:90–104.
24. Sclafani A, Herrmann JM. Comparison of the photoelectronic and photocatalytic activities of various anatase and rutile forms of titania in pure liquid organic phases and in aqueous solutions. J Phys Chem. 1996;100: 13655–61.
25. Selloni A, Vittadini A, Grätzel M. The adsorption of small molecules on the TiO2 anatase (101) surface by first-principles molecular dynamics. Surf Sci. 1998;402–404:219–22.
26. Vittadini A, Selloni A, Rotzinger FP, Grätzel M. Structure and energetics of water adsorbed at TiO2 anatase (101) and (001) surfaces. Phys Rev Lett. 1998;81:2954–7.
27. Rahman I, MacNee W. Oxidative stress and regulation of glutathione in lung inflammation. Eur Respir J. 2000;16:534–54.
28. Peterson JD, Herzenberg LA, Vasquez K, Waltenbaugh C. Glutathione levels in antigen-presenting cells modulate Th1 versus Th2 response patterns. Proc Natl Acad Sci U S A. 1998;95:3071–6.
29. Li N, Wang M, Bramble LA, Schmitz DA, Schauer JJ, Sioutas C, Harkema JR, Nel AE. The adjuvant effect of ambient particulate matter is closely reflected by the particulate oxidant potential. Environ Health Perspect. 2009;117: 1116–23.
30. Zhang H, Ji Z, Xia T, Meng H, Low-Kam C, Liu R, Pokhrel S, Lin S, Wang X, Liao YP, Wang M, Li L, Rallo R, Damoiseaux R, Telesca D, Mädler L, Cohen Y, Zink JI, Nel AE. Use of metal oxide nanoparticle band gap to develop a predictive paradigm for oxidative stress and acute pulmonary inflammation. ACS Nano. 2012;6:4349–68.
31. Li R, Wang X, Ji Z, Sun B, Zhang H, Chang CH, Lin S, Meng H, Liao YP, Wang M, Li Z, Hwang AA, Song TB, Xu R, Yang Y, Zink JI, Nel AE, Xia T. Surface charge and cellular processing of covalently functionalized multiwall carbon nanotubes determine pulmonary toxicity. ACS Nano. 2013;7:2352–68.
32. Jensen KA, Kembouche Y, Christiansen E, Jacobsen NR, Wallin H, Guiot C, Spalla O, Witschger O: Final protocol for producing suitable manufactured nanomaterial exposure media. The generic NANOGENOTOX dispersion protocol. (2011). https://www.anses.fr/en/system/files/nanogenotox_deliverable_5.pdf Accessed 30 Nov 2017.
33. Rifkin R, Mukherjee S, Tamayo P, Ramaswamy S, Yeang C-H, Angelo M, Reich M, Poggio T, Lander ES, Golub TR, Mesirov JP. An analytical method for multiclass molecular cancer classification. SIAM Rev. 2003;45:706–23.
34. European Commission. Joint Research Centre. Institute for Health and Consumer Protection (2014): Titanium Dioxide, NM-100, NM-101, NM-102, NM-103, NM-104, NM-105: Characterisation and Physico-Chemical Properties https://eceuropaeu/jrc/en/publication/eur-scientific-and-technical-research-reports/titanium-dioxide-nm-100-nm-101-nm-102-nm-103-nm-104-nm-105-characterisation-and-physico Accessed 30 Nov, 2017.

4

Radical containing combustion derived particulate matter enhance pulmonary Th17 inflammation via the aryl hydrocarbon receptor

Sridhar Jaligama[1,2], Vivek S. Patel[1,2,3,4], Pingli Wang[5], Asmaa Sallam[1,2], Jeffrey Harding[1,2,3], Matthew Kelley[6], Skylar R. Mancuso[7], Tammy R. Dugas[4] and Stephania A. Cormier[1,2,3,4*]

Abstract

Background: Pollutant particles containing environmentally persistent free radicals (EPFRs) are formed during many combustion processes (e.g. thermal remediation of hazardous wastes, diesel/gasoline combustion, wood smoke, cigarette smoke, etc.). Our previous studies demonstrated that acute exposure to EPFRs results in dendritic cell maturation and Th17-biased pulmonary immune responses. Further, in a mouse model of asthma, these responses were enhanced suggesting exposure to EPFRs as a risk factor for the development and/or exacerbation of asthma. The aryl hydrocarbon receptor (AHR) has been shown to play a role in the differentiation of Th17 cells. In the current study, we determined whether exposure to EPFRs results in Th17 polarization in an AHR dependent manner.

Results: Exposure to EPFRs resulted in Th17 and IL17A dependent pulmonary immune responses including airway neutrophilia. EPFR exposure caused a significant increase in pulmonary Th17 cytokines such as IL6, IL17A, IL22, IL1β, KC, MCP-1, IL31 and IL33. To understand the role of AHR activation in EPFR-induced Th17 inflammation, A549 epithelial cells and mouse bone marrow-derived dendritic cells (BMDCs) were exposed to EPFRs and expression of *Cyp1a1* and *Cyp1b1*, markers for AHR activation, was measured. A significant increase in *Cyp1a1* and *Cyp1b1* gene expression was observed in pulmonary epithelial cells and BMDCs in an oxidative stress and AHR dependent manner. Further, in vivo exposure of mice to EPFRs resulted in oxidative stress and increased *Cyp1a1* and *Cyp1b1* pulmonary gene expression. To further confirm the role of AHR activation in pulmonary Th17 immune responses, mice were exposed to EPFRs in the presence or absence of AHR antagonist. EPFR exposure resulted in a significant increase in pulmonary Th17 cells and neutrophilic inflammation, whereas a significant decrease in the percentage of Th17 cells and neutrophilic inflammation was observed in mice treated with AHR antagonist.

Conclusion: Exposure to EPFRs results in AHR activation and induction of *Cyp1a1* and in vitro this is dependent on oxidative stress. Further, our in vivo studies demonstrated a role for AHR in EPFR-induced pulmonary Th17 responses including neutrophilic inflammation.

Keywords: Free radicals, Particulate matter, Th17, Inflammation, Asthma, Aryl hydrocarbon receptor, Neutrophils

* Correspondence: stephaniacormier@lsu.edu
[1]Department of Pediatrics, University of Tennessee Health Science Center, Memphis, TN 38103, USA
[2]Children's Foundation Research Institute, Le Bonheur Children's Hospital, Memphis, TN 38103, USA
Full list of author information is available at the end of the article

Background

Combustion of hazardous waste and biofuels produces many atmospheric pollutants including reactive trace gases, polycyclic aromatic hydrocarbons, and particulate matter (PM) [1, 2]. It is estimated that about 40–70% PM is attributed to emissions from combustion and thermal remediation sources [3]. Several epidemiological studies have provided substantial evidence that long-term exposure to PM contribute to the development of asthma and aggravate existing asthma symptoms [4–6]. Although several studies including our own studies have demonstrated an association between exposure to PM derived from combustion sources and exacerbation of asthma and respiratory tract infections [7, 8], very limited data exists about the underlying mechanisms of their toxicity and the deteriorating effects leading to the development of respiratory diseases as a result of their complexity and non-uniformity in composition. Recent studies have identified environmentally persistent free radicals (EPFRs) in PM from a variety of combustion sources including thermal remediation of hazardous wastes, diesel/gasoline combustion, wood smoke, cigarette smoke, etc. [9–14]. In the current study, we utilized an EPFR-containing ultrafine pollutant particle system that was created by exposure of PM surrogates (CuO on silica substrate) to 2-monochlorophenol vapors at 230 °C (MCP230) [15, 16]. This procedure has been shown to mimic the formation of EPFRs in the cooling zone of combustion systems. It represents the chlorinated phenol containing surface stabilized semi-quinone type free radical emitted as the effluent from a variety of combustion sources including biomass fuels, fossil fuels, and hazardous materials where chlorinated hydrocarbons and Cu(II)O are typically present [16, 17].

Our previous studies demonstrated that acute exposure of mice to EPFRs resulted in cytotoxicity, pulmonary oxidative stress, and lung dysfunction [8, 15]. Lung dysfunction correlated with increased maturation of dendritic cells and a Th17-biased immunophenotype in the lungs, however the mechanism of these responses was not completely understood. IL17A and Th17 cells have been shown to play an important role in the pathophysiology of airway diseases such as asthma and COPD [18, 19]. Cellular infiltration involving neutrophils and eosinophils is a characteristic feature of chronic inflammatory diseases [20]. Further, exaggerated neutrophilic inflammation and Th17 immune responses are hallmarks of severe asthma and are implicated in the development and promotion of steroid-resistant asthma [18, 21–23]. Th17 effector cytokines such as IL17A recruit neutrophils into the airway [24, 25]. These data warranted the investigation of underlying molecular pathways leading to EPFR-induced IL17A and Th17 responses.

Aryl hydrocarbon receptor (AHR) is a ubiquitous ligand-dependent transcription factor [26]. AHR binds to a wide array of exogenous and endogenous ligands resulting in the induction of xenobiotic metabolizing enzymes. Several researchers have demonstrated induction of cytochrome P450 metabolizing enzymes such as Cyp1A1 as a result of environmental exposure to known AHR ligands such as 2,3,7,8-tetrachlorodibenzo-p-dioxin (TCDD). The levels of AHR and its activity are modulated by exposure to its ligands [27]. Recent studies on AHR have implicated them in induction of various cytokines and chemokines and have demonstrated the role of AHR in regulating the differentiation of Th17 cells and production of Th17 cytokines such as IL17A and IL22 [28]. Depending on the type of ligand, activation of AHR can cause either Th17 or regulatory T cell differentiation leading to exacerbation of inflammation or immunosuppression, respectively [29–31]. The role of AHR in PM-induced pulmonary Th17 inflammation has not been well studied.

In the current study, we determined the mechanism underlying EPFR-induced Th17 inflammation. We demonstrated that Th17 cells are essential for EPFR-induced pulmonary neutrophilic inflammation and cytokine response. Further, we demonstrated that exposure to EPFRs results in AHR activation, as evidenced by increased expression of AHR dependent genes $Cyp1a1$ and $Cyp1b1$, which is dependent on EPFR-induced oxidative stress and cellular uptake of the particles. Inhibition of AHR nuclear translocation and DNA binding abated EPFR-induced pulmonary Th17 immune responses and associated neutrophilic inflammation. Thus, EPFR-induced Th17 inflammatory responses are dependent on AHR activation.

Methods

Animals

Male and female C57BL/6 mice (age 8–10 weeks) were purchased from Harlan (Indianapolis, IN). Male Ahr knockout ($Ahr^{-/-}$; B6.129-$Ahr^{tm1Gonz}$/Nci) mice (age 16 weeks) were obtained from National Cancer Institute (Frederick, MD). The IL17Ra$^{-/-}$ ($Il17ra^{tm1Koll}$) and IL23p19$^{-/-}$ ($Il23a^{tm1Lex}$) on C57BL/6 background were obtained from Amgen Inc. and Taconic, respectively. Both male and female mice (age 8–10 weeks) were used for experiments involving IL17Ra$^{-/-}$ and IL23p19$^{-/-}$ mice. All mice were given free access to rodent chow and water ad libitum and were maintained under controlled conditions with 12 h light/dark cycle, temperature, humidity, and specific pathogen free conditions. All animal protocols were prepared according to the *Guide for the Care and Use of Laboratory Animals*, and were approved by the Institutional Animal Care and Use Committee at the University of Tennessee Health Science Center and Louisiana State University Health Sciences Center. Timepoints were chosen to capture peak antigen presenting cell (hours) and Th cell responses (generally peak within a week after initial antigen stimulation) and reduce animal numbers needed to observe these responses.

Exposure to PM and treatment with AHR antagonist

Radical containing ultrafine PM with mean aerodynamic diameter of approximately 0.2 μm was previously characterized by our colleague Dr. Slawo Lomnicki at the Louisiana State University as described earlier [16]. MCP230 particles were suspended in sterile saline containing 0.02% tween 80 (particle solution) at 1 mg/mL concentration. The resulting suspension was subjected to probe sonication on ice to disperse the particles and maintain a suspension free of particulate aggregates. Mice received 50 μl of the resulting suspension via oropharyngeal aspiration as described earlier [32]. Control mice were administered 50 μl of particle solution (Vehicle). Two hours prior to exposure to vehicle or MCP230, AHR activation was blocked by treating mice with 10 mg/kg dose (i.p.) of CH223191 (1-Methyl-N-[2-methyl-4-[2-(2-methylphenyl) diazenyl] phenyl-1H-pyrazole-5-carboxamide) (Cayman Chemical, Ann Arbor, MI), which was shown to be a selective antagonist of AHR [33, 34]. Here after, CH223191 will be referred as AHR antagonist.

Luciferase assay for AHR activation

A549 cells were transfected with both a DRE-luciferase reporter for AHR activation and a Renilla luciferase reporter (Dual-Luciferase Reporter Assay System, Promega). After 24 h, the cells were exposed to 50 μg/cm^2 particles or 50 nM TCDD with or without 100 μM Trolox, an antioxidant. Four hours after exposure to PM, firefly luciferase activity was measured as increase in luminescence in the presence of luciferin. Renilla luciferase activity, assessed as increase in luminescence in the presence of coelenterazine, was used to normalize the AHR activation data for differences in transfection efficiencies and cell number.

Cyp1a1 and Cyp1b1 expression in vitro

Human lung epithelial cells (A549) were cultured in growth medium consisting of DMEM, 10% heat-inactivated fetal bovine serum (FBS) and 100 U-mg/mL penicillin-streptomycin. Cells were plated at a density of 4×10^4 cells/cm^2 in 6-well plates and incubated for 24 h to achieve ~ 80–85% confluence. Treatment groups included media-only control; vehicle control (2.7% DMSO); antioxidant 10 mM N-tert-Butyl-α-phenylnitrone (PBN); uptake blocker cocktail (2.5 μg/mL Filipin III; 10 μg/mL chlorpromazine; 10 μM Wortmannin); 50 μg/cm^2 MCP50 (non-EPFR-containing particles); 50 μg/cm^2 MCP230; MCP230+PBN; MCP50+uptake blocker cocktail; MCP230+uptake blocker cocktail. Cells receiving both particles and PBN and/or uptake blocker

cocktail were pre-treated with PBN and/or uptake blocker cocktail for one hour before exposure to particles as described previously [35]. Each group was done in triplicate and cells were incubated for 4 h at 37 °C and 5% CO$_2$. At the end of incubation, supernatants were collected and flash frozen in liquid nitrogen. Cells were washed twice with ice-cold PBS, scraped off the plate using a rubber policeman, pelleted and flash frozen in liquid nitrogen and stored at − 80 °C.

Quantitative real time PCR

Total RNA was isolated using RNeasy Plus Mini Kit (Qiagen, Valencia, CA) following manufacturer's instructions and cDNA was synthesized using Superscript III First Strand Synthesis Supermix as per manufacturer's instructions (Life Technologies, Carlsbad, CA). 50 ng of cDNA was mixed with Power SYBR Green PCR Master Mix and qPCR was performed using Roche LightCycler 480, (Applied Biosystems, Foster City, CA). Primers sequences for *Cyp1a1* (Amplicon Length: 148; Forward: GAGGAGCTA GACACAGTGATTG; Reverse: TGTCTCTTGTTGTGCT GTGG); *Cyp1b1* (Amplicon Length: 151; Forward: CAC CAGGTATCCTGATGTGC; Reverse: AGGCACAAAGC TGGAGAAG); *Hprt1* (Amplicon Length: 181; Forward: TGGCGTCGTGATTAGTGATG; Reverse: ACAGAGGG CTACAATGTGATG). *Il17a* expression was determined using TaqMan gene expression assay (Applied Biosystems, Waltham, MA). Data are normalized for *Hprt1* or *Gapdh* and plotted as relative gene expression using ΔΔCt analysis.

Bronchoalveolar lavage fluid (BALF) cellularity

Mice were humanely euthanized, and a small incision was made in the upper region of the trachea and an 18-gauge cannula was inserted into the incision. 1 mL of BALF isolation buffer (PBS containing 0.5% BSA) was slowly instilled and removed from the lungs. Cells were counted and 20,000 cells were spun on to a glass slide using a cytospin. The slides were air dried and subsequently stained with Hema-3 staining kit (Fisher Scientific, Pittsburgh, PA) following supplier's instructions. Differential cell counts were determined based on the morphology and staining of the cells by counting at least 300 cells per slide.

Establishment of mouse model of asthma

A mouse model of asthma using chicken egg white ovalbumin (OVA) (Sigma-Aldrich, St. Louis, MO) was generated. Briefly, a mixture of 20 μg of OVA emulsified in Imject Alum (Pierce, Rockford, IL) was prepared and mice were sensitized by injecting with the mixture i.p. on protocol days 0, and 14. MCP230 (50 μg) was administered to wild type and IL17Ra$^{-/-}$ OVA+MCP230 group mice on protocol day 23. Subsequently, mice were challenged with 1% OVA solution made in saline by inhalation exposure for 20 min on protocol days 24, 25, and 26. Mice were euthanized on protocol day 28; BALF was collected for differential cell count analysis and lungs were collected for performing histopathological assessment.

Lung histopathology and in situ hybridization

Mice were euthanized, lungs were isolated and inflated with zinc-formalin fixative at 25 cm constant water pressure and fixed for 24 h before they were transferred to 70% ethanol. The lungs were then dehydrated, embedded in paraffin and sectioned to 4 μm thick sections and stained with hematoxylin and eosin to visualize the inflammation. In situ hybridization for *Cyp1a1* RNA was performed as described earlier [36] using RNAscope 2.5 HD assay kit (Advanced Cell Diagnostics, Newark, CA) on lung sections of mice exposed to vehicle or MCP230. Representative images of lung sections were acquired using EVOS FL Auto cell imaging system (Life Science Technologies, Grand Island, NY). To quantify inflammation, ten random airway microscopy fields were captured at 10× magnification on the Nikon Eclipse Ci-L (Nikon Corporation, Tokyo, Japan). Area of inflammation was quantified using ImageJ software (National Institutes of Health, Bethesda, MD). Data are represented as the area of inflammation surrounding airway and normalized to the size of the respective airway.

Flow cytometry

Single cell suspension of the lung cells and flow cytometric staining of cells was performed as described earlier [7, 32]. Mice were euthanized; lungs were subjected to retrograde vascular perfusion with Hank's Balanced Salt solution (HBSS) to remove excess red blood cells. The isolated lungs were coarsely dissociated using an Octodissociator (Miltenyi, Germany). The dissociated lungs were incubated with collagenase I (Invitrogen, NY) , and 150 ng/mL DNase I (Sigma Aldrich, MO) for 30 min in HBSS. Following incubation, the lungs were further subjected to dissociation with Octodissociator to reduce the remaining cell clumps to single cell suspension. Cells were strained through a 40 μm cell strainer (BD Biosciences, CA). The resulting cell suspension was treated with RBC lysis buffer to remove any residual blood cells. Cells were incubated for five hours at 37 °C with a stimulatory cocktail containing 5% heat-inactivated fetal bovine serum, 500 ng/mL ionomycin, 5 ng/mL phorbol 12-myristate 13-acetate (PMA) (Sigma-Aldrich), and a protein transport inhibitor (GolgiPlug, BD Biosciences) made in RPMI 1640 media. Cells were stained with a Fixable live/dead dye eFluor 780 (eBiosciences, San Diego, CA) and were subsequently fixed, permeabilized and stained for T cell and intracellular cytokine markers using antibodies eFluor450-CD3

(eBiosciences, CA), PerCP-CD4 (BioLegend, CA), FITC-CD8 (eBiosciences, CA), and PE-IFNγ (eBiosciences, CA), PE-Cy7-IL4 (eBiosciences, CA), APC-IL17A (eBiosciences, CA). A total of 1.2 million cells/sample were analyzed by FACS Canto II (BD Biosciences) and dead cells were excluded from analysis. Flow cytometry data was analyzed using FlowJo Software v.10 (FLOWJO LLC, OR).

Cytokine analysis

Cytokine levels in homogenized lung supernatants were determined using MILLIPLEX MAP Mouse Th17 cytokine magnetic bead panel (Millipore, Billerica, MA) using Luminex 200 system (Luminex Corporation). The following cytokines were assayed: IL1β, IL6, IL17A, IL17E, IL21, IL22, IL31, IL33, keratinocyte-derived chemokine (KC) and monocyte chemotactic protein (MCP-1). Raw data were plotted against a standard curve using a five-parameter logistic regression to derive the concentrations for unknown samples. Data presented exclude numbers beyond the sensitivity of the assay.

Statistics

Data are presented as means ± SEM. Data are analyzed by GraphPad Prism software (Version 6). ANOVA with post hoc analysis was performed to determine the level of difference between experimental groups. $p < 0.05$ was considered as statistically different.

Results

EPFRs induce pulmonary Th17 immune responses

Our previous study demonstrated that acute exposure to EPFRs results in Th17-biased pulmonary inflammation with increased neutrophils [35]. IL23 serves as a survival and maintenance factor for Th17 cells [37, 38] and promotes Th17 differentiation [39, 40]. IL23p19$^{-/-}$ mice are deficient in Th17 cells and, therefore, this mouse model was used to confirm that Th17 cells mediate the increase in lung IL17A and neutrophil recruitment upon MCP230 exposure. We exposed wild type (WT) and IL23p19$^{-/-}$ mice to either vehicle or MCP230 (EPFR). Percent Th17 cells and *Il17a* expression were measured. A schematic for the MCP230 exposure and analysis of Th17 cells, *Il17a* expression and cell differential in BALF at 5 days post-exposure (dpe) is presented in Fig. 1a. In congruence with our previously published results, a significant increase in the percent of pulmonary Th17 cells was observed in WT mice exposed to MCP230 compared to vehicle. On the contrary, MCP230-exposed IL23p19$^{-/-}$ mice failed to show an increase in the percent of pulmonary Th17 cells (Fig. 1b and c; CD3$^+$CD4$^+$ cells double positive for IFNγ and IL4 or IL4 and IL17A were excluded while gating). A significant increase in the expression of *Il17a* was observed in MCP230-exposed WT mice compared to vehicle, but no

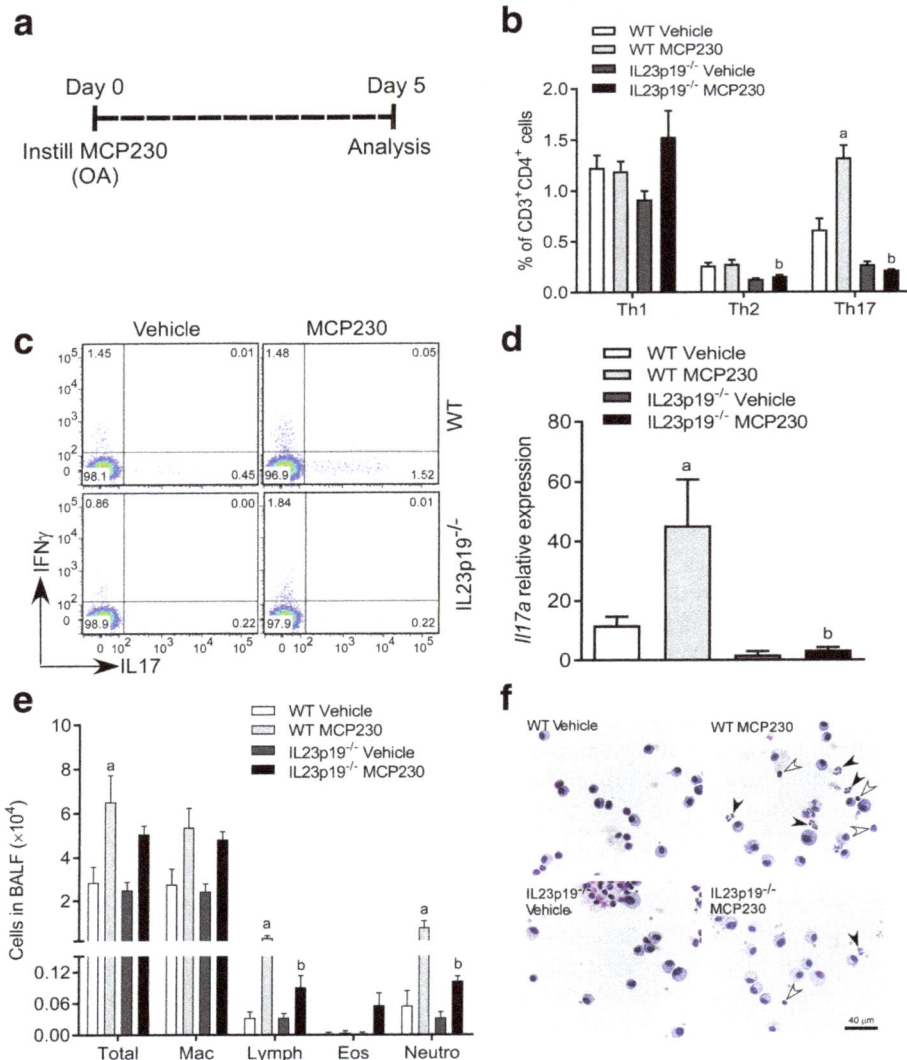

Fig. 1 Exposure to MCP230 induces immune responses in the lung in Th17 dependent manner. (**a**) Schematic of MCP230 exposure protocol. Mice were exposed to MCP230 (50 μg) by oropharyngeal aspiration on day 0 and BAL fluid (BALF) or whole-lungs were collected on day 5 post-exposure. (**b**) T cell subsets were quantified using flow cytometry. Pulmonary T helper cell responses were measured after vehicle or MCP230 exposure in WT and IL23p19$^{-/-}$ mice. PMA/ionomycin-stimulated lung cells were stained with surface (CD3, CD4, and CD8) and intracellular (IFNγ, IL4, and IL17A) antibodies for Th1, Th2, and Th17 cells. (**c**) Representative pseudo color dot plots of CD4$^+$ T cells gated for IFNγ, and IL17A in WT and IL23p19$^{-/-}$ mice. (**d**) The expression of *Il17a* relative to *Gapdh* in whole-lung homogenates of WT and IL23p19$^{-/-}$ mice exposed to vehicle or MCP230 was determined using RT-qPCR. **e** Differential cell count of BALF from vehicle or MCP230-exposed WT or IL23p19$^{-/-}$ mice. **f** Representative photomicrographs of BALF cells collected from WT and IL23p19$^{-/-}$ mice exposed to vehicle or MCP230. Arrowheads represent the neutrophils (black) and lymphocytes (white). Data represent mean ± SEM from 3 to 5 mice. $^a p < 0.05$, compared to WT Vehicle group. $^b p < 0.05$, compared to WT MCP230 group, one-way ANOVA with Tukey's multiple comparisons test

difference was seen in IL23p19$^{-/-}$ mice (Fig. 1d), suggesting that increased *Il17a* expression in MCP230-exposed WT mice is Th17 dependent. Expression of *Il17f* was less than that of *Il17a* and there was no difference between MCP230-exposed WT mice compared to vehicle or to MCP230-exposed IL23p19$^{-/-}$ mice (Additional file 1: Figure S1).

To determine the role of Th17 cells in EPFR-induced pulmonary neutrophilic inflammation, we performed differential cell counts in WT and IL23p19$^{-/-}$ mice exposed to either vehicle or MCP230. In WT mice, exposure to MCP230 significantly increased the numbers of lymphocytes and neutrophils compared to that in vehicle control, whereas these numbers were significantly less in MCP230-exposed IL23p19$^{-/-}$ mice compared to that in MCP230-exposed WT mice (Fig. 1e). Exposure to MCP230 in both WT and IL23p19$^{-/-}$ mice resulted in increases in the total number of leukocytes and macrophages compared to respective vehicle exposed mice. The numbers of total leukocytes and macrophages were comparable between WT and IL23p19$^{-/-}$ mice following exposure to MCP230 (Fig. 1e). Representative images of higher numbers of neutrophils and lymphocytes (black and white arrowheads, respectively) in MCP230-exposed WT mice compared to MCP230-exposed IL23p19$^{-/-}$ mice are shown in Fig. 1f.

EPFRs induce pulmonary neutrophilic inflammation in an IL17A-dependent manner

To demonstrate that MCP230 exacerbates asthma and determine if MCP230-induced pulmonary neutrophilic inflammation is dependent on IL17A, an OVA-induced mouse model of asthma was developed in WT and IL17 receptor alpha knockout (IL17Ra$^{-/-}$) mice. A schematic for the development of the mouse model of asthma, exposure to MCP230, and BALF and histopathology assessment is presented in Fig. 2a. BALF was collected for differential cell counts and pulmonary inflammation

was determined by hematoxylin and eosin staining of lung sections obtained at 5 dpe. A significant increase in the percentage of neutrophils was observed in WT mice exposed to OVA and MCP230 (WT OVA+MCP230) compared to WT OVA mice; however, the percentage of neutrophils was significantly less in IL17Ra$^{-/-}$ OVA +MCP230 mice compared to MCP230-exposed WT mice (Fig. 2b). No difference in the percentage of neutrophils was observed in IL17Ra$^{-/-}$ OVA+MCP230 mice compared to IL17Ra$^{-/-}$ OVA mice. The percentage of eosinophils was significantly decreased in WT OVA +MCP230 mice compared to WT OVA mice (Fig. 2b); and there were no significant changes in the numbers of macrophages and lymphocytes. Total numbers of cells are shown in Additional file 2: Figure S2. Histopathological analysis revealed inflammation in the peribronchiolar/ perivascular areas in lungs of WT OVA+MCP230 mice, while such inflammation was absent or mild in IL17Ra$^{-/-}$ OVA+MCP230 mice (Fig. 2c and d). Together, these results suggest that MCP230-induced pulmonary

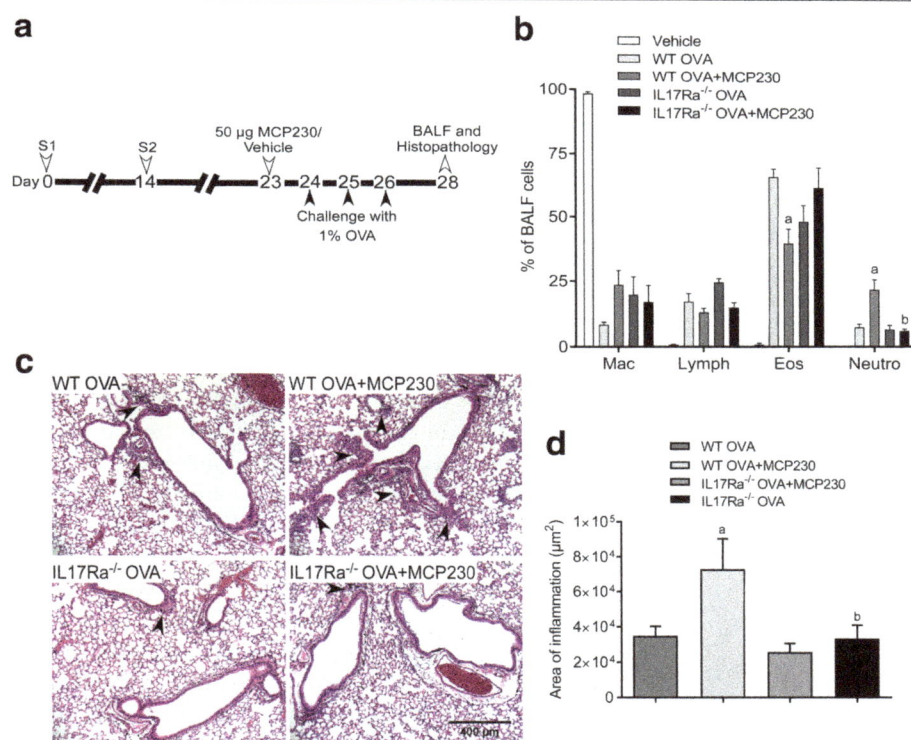

Fig. 2 IL17A mediates MCP230-exacerbated pulmonary neutrophilic inflammation in asthma. **a** Schematic representing the protocol followed to induce inflammation in a mouse model of asthma. WT and IL17Ra$^{-/-}$ mice were sensitized with OVA (Ovalbumin complexed to Imject Alum) on days 0 and 14. Mice were exposed to either vehicle or MCP230 (50 μg) on protocol day 23 and challenged with OVA on days 24, 25, and 26. BALF or lungs were collected on day 28. **b** Differential cell counts of BALF cells at 5 days post-exposure (i.e. day 28) from mice challenged with OVA and exposed to vehicle or MCP230. Data are represented as percentage of total BALF cells. Data represent mean ± SEM from 4 to 5 mice. $^{a}p < 0.05$, compared to WT OVA group. $^{b}p < 0.05$, compared to WT OVA+MCP230 group, one-way ANOVA with Holm-Sidak's multiple comparisons test. **c** Representative photomicrographs of the lungs of WT and IL17Ra$^{-/-}$ mice challenged with OVA and exposed to vehicle or MCP230. Arrowheads point to areas of peribronchiolar and perivascular inflammation. **d** Quantification of area of inflammation (μm^2) surrounding the airways. Data represent mean ± SEM from 4 to 5 mice. $^{a}p < 0.05$, compared to WT OVA group. $^{b}p < 0.05$, compared to WT OVA+MCP230, one-way ANOVA with Tukey's multiple comparisons test

a

b

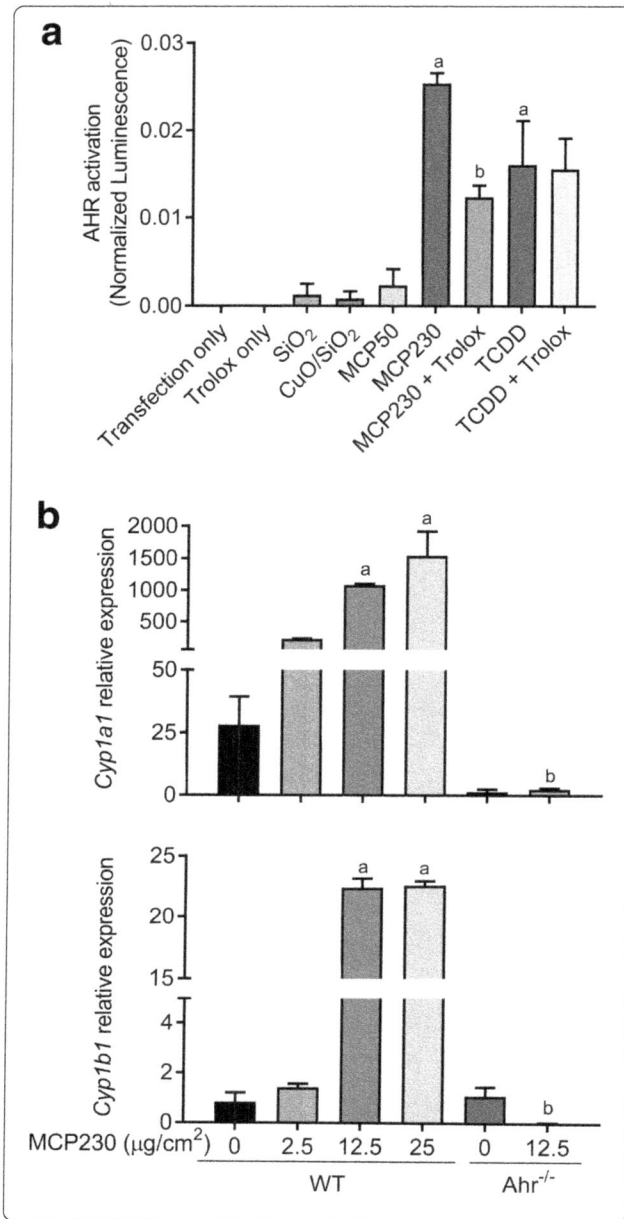

Fig. 3 MCP230 exposure activates aryl hydrocarbon receptor (AHR) and increases the expression of *Cyp1a1*. (**a**) Activation of AHR as measured using a dual AHR luciferase reporter assay in A549 cells. A549 cells were exposed to MCP230 (50 μg/cm²) or TCDD (50 nM) and simultaneously treated with or without trolox (antioxidant; 100 μM) for 4 h. In addition, AHR activation was assessed in cells exposed to non-EPFR-containing particle controls such as SiO₂, CuO/SiO₂, and MCP50 (50 μg/cm²). AHR promoter activity is expressed as normalized luminescence using a Renilla reporter for internal normalization. Data represent mean ± SEM from one of two independent experiments, performed in triplicate. $^a p < 0.05$, compared to MCP50 group. $^b p < 0.05$, compared to MCP230 group, one-way ANOVA with Dunnett's multiple comparisons test. (**b**) Activation of AHR as measured by *Cyp1a1* and *Cyp1b1* expression relative to *Gapdh* using RT-qPCR analysis in the bone marrow-derived dendritic cells (BMDCs). BMDCs from WT and Ahr$^{-/-}$ mice were exposed to various concentrations of MCP230 for 4 h. Data represent mean ± SEM from one of two independent experiments, performed in duplicate. $^a p < 0.05$, compared to WT (0 μg/cm²) group. $^b p < 0.05$, compared to WT (12.5 μg/cm²) group, one-way ANOVA with Tukey's multiple comparisons test

neutrophilic inflammation in WT OVA+MCP230 mice is dependent on IL17A.

Exposure to EPFRs induces activation of AHR

AHR binds to a wide array of exogenous ligands (e.g. air pollutants) resulting in the induction of xenobiotic metabolizing enzymes and cytokines. Depending on the type of ligand, AHR regulates differentiation of Th17 cells and production of Th17 cytokines such as IL17A and IL22 [28]. To understand the role of AHR in MCP230-induced Th17 inflammation, we investigated whether acute exposure to MCP230 activates the AHR pathway. AHR activation was analyzed in vitro using a dual luciferase reporter assay in MCP230-exposed A549 cells. MCP230 exposure caused a significant increase in luciferase activity as measured by luminescence, indicating AHR activation in MCP230-treated cells compared to that of MCP50 (PM containing the organic and particle but lacking the EPFR [16]) treated cells (Fig. 3a). The increase in the luminescence was comparable to the luminescence in TCDD-exposed cells, a known AHR agonist. A significant reduction in AHR activation was observed when MCP230-exposed cells were co-treated with trolox, an antioxidant. However, such reduction was not observed in TCDD exposed cells co-treated with trolox. No significant increase in AHR activation was observed in cells treated with non-EPFR-containing PM (SiO₂, CuO/SiO₂, or MCP50) compared to transfection only group. These observations demonstrate that EPFRs are important for the activation of AHR.

Using in vitro and in vivo studies, we previously demonstrated that MCP230 induces the maturation of DCs and enhances the capacity of DCs to stimulate the proliferation and activation of T cells [35]. Recently, it was reported that AHR activation also induces maturation of DCs [41]. To assess the role of MCP230 to activate AHR in DCs cuing Th17 responses and subsequent neutrophilia, we determined the expression of AHR regulated genes *Cyp1a1* and *Cyp1b1* in bone marrow-derived dendritic cells (BMDCs) isolated from WT and Ahr$^{-/-}$ mice. Treatment of BMDCs derived from WT mice with MCP230 caused a dose-dependent increase in the expression of *Cyp1a1* with significant difference at concentrations 12.5 and 25 µg/cm^2 compared to vehicle treated control cells (Fig. 3b). Also, a significant increase in the expression of *Cyp1b1* was observed with exposure to MCP230 at same concentrations. In contrast, and as expected, treatment of BMDCs isolated from Ahr$^{-/-}$ mice with MCP230 at 12.5 µg/cm^2 did not result in any change in *Cyp1a1* and *Cyp1b1* expression compared to respective vehicle treated control cells (Fig. 3b). Together, these data indicate that exposure to MCP230 induces AHR activation.

EPFRs induce expression of *Cyp1a1* and *Cyp1b1* in vitro in an uptake-dependent and oxidative stress-dependent manner

Previously, we reported that blocking cellular uptake of MCP230 or oxidative stress inhibits the MCP230-induced T cell activation and proliferation [35]. Thus, uptake of MCP230 particles or oxidative stress induced by MCP230 particles is important for its immune-modulating effects. To determine if uptake of MCP230 was necessary for the activation of AHR, we pretreated A549 cells with an uptake blocker cocktail (UB) or anti-oxidant PBN followed by exposure to MCP230 and measured the expression of *Cyp1a1* and *Cyp1b1*. Exposure to MCP230 significantly increased the expression of *Cyp1a1* (> 40-fold) and pretreatment with UB or PBN partially inhibited the effects of MCP230 on *Cyp1a1* expression (Fig. 4a). Expression of *Cyp1b1* was also reduced in cells treated with UB or PBN and exposed to MCP230. Although, exposure to MCP50 caused a significant increase in *Cyp1b1* expression, treatment of cells with UB significantly inhibited the expression of *Cyp1b1* (Fig. 4b). These results indicate that MCP230-induced AHR activation is dependent on both particle uptake and the ability to induce generation of reactive oxygen species (ROS).

Exposure to EPFRs induces *Cyp1a1* and *Cyp1b1* expression in an AHR-dependent manner

To determine if MCP230-induced expression of *Cyp1a1* and *Cyp1b1* was dependent on activation of AHR, we exposed A549 cells to MCP230 in the presence or absence of CH223191, a selective AHR antagonist (AHR anta) that inhibits AHR-dependent transcription even at 10 µmol concentration [34]. FICZ is a high affinity

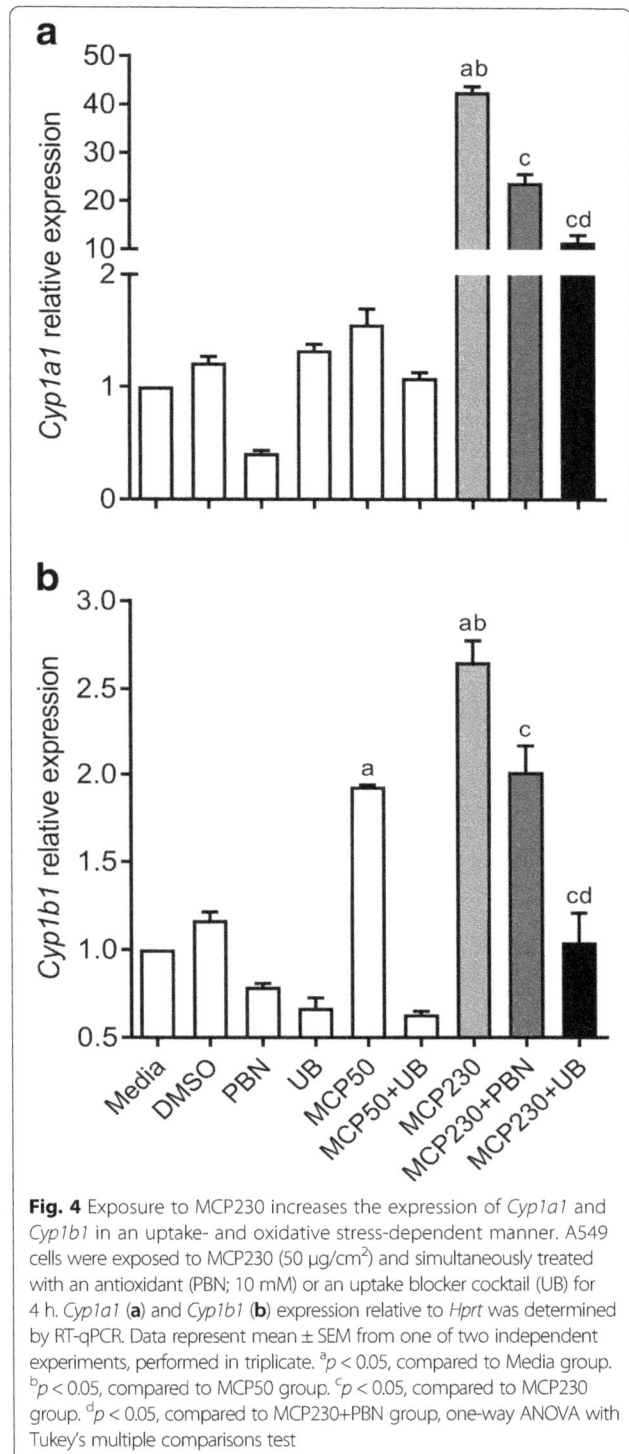

Fig. 4 Exposure to MCP230 increases the expression of *Cyp1a1* and *Cyp1b1* in an uptake- and oxidative stress-dependent manner. A549 cells were exposed to MCP230 (50 µg/cm^2) and simultaneously treated with an antioxidant (PBN; 10 mM) or an uptake blocker cocktail (UB) for 4 h. *Cyp1a1* (**a**) and *Cyp1b1* (**b**) expression relative to *Hprt* was determined by RT-qPCR. Data represent mean ± SEM from one of two independent experiments, performed in triplicate. ^{a}$p < 0.05$, compared to Media group. ^{b}$p < 0.05$, compared to MCP50 group. ^{c}$p < 0.05$, compared to MCP230 group. ^{d}$p < 0.05$, compared to MCP230+PBN group, one-way ANOVA with Tukey's multiple comparisons test

ligand of AHR and it has been shown to enhance Th17 responses and exacerbate immune-mediated diseases in several mouse models [28, 31, 42]. Since the effects of MCP230 are similar to that of FICZ, we switched to using FICZ as a positive control for AHR activation. Exposure to MCP230 and FICZ caused a significant increase in the expression of *Cyp1a1* (Fig. 5a) and *Cyp1b1* (Fig. 5b) compared to media or vehicle (DMSO) controls. Pretreatment of MCP230-exposed cells with AHR antagonist significantly reduced the expression of both *Cyp1a1* and *Cyp1b1* compared to that in cells exposed to MCP230 alone. Similarly, FICZ-induced *Cyp1a1* and *Cyp1b1* expression was also inhibited by AHR antagonist, indicating an AHR dependent expression of these proteins. These results further corroborate the data presented in Figs. 3 and 4 that demonstrate MCP230-induced activation of AHR.

Acute exposure to EPFRs results in transient activation of AHR in vivo

We investigated whether exposure to EPFRs result in transient or persistent activation of AHR in vivo. WT mice were exposed to vehicle or MCP230 (50 µg) via oropharyngeal aspiration, lungs were isolated at 4 and 24 h post-exposure, and expression of *Cyp1a1* and *Cyp1b1* genes was determined. Exposure to MCP230 resulted in a significant increase in the expression of *Cyp1a1* and *Cyp1b1* at 4 h post-exposure compared to vehicle treated controls (Fig. 6a and b). At 24 h post-exposure, the expression of both *Cyp1a1* and *Cyp1b1* were reduced to that of the vehicle treated control (Fig. 6a and b). These data indicate that acute exposure to MCP230 results in transient, but significant, increases in AHR activity in the lungs. To determine if AHR was activated in airway or

immune cells, in situ hybridization for *Cyp1a1* mRNA was performed in the lungs isolated at 4 h post-exposure from mice exposed to vehicle or MCP230. A significant increase in *Cyp1a1* was observed in the lungs of the mice exposed to MCP230 compared to vehicle control. An increase in *Cyp1a1* positive cells was observed in the airway epithelium and in the parenchymal regions in the lungs of MCP230-treated mice (Fig. 6c). The specific cell types in which MCP230 induced *Cyp1a1* were not identified.

Exposure to EPFRs induces Th17 cytokine response in the lung

In a different study in our lab, we observed that AHR activation is increased through to 12 h and returns to baseline by 24 h (data not shown). To determine the effects of MCP230 exposure on immediate immune responses, we measured Th17 associated cytokines in the lungs of MCP230-exposed mice at 12 h post-exposure and 1 dpe. A total of 10 cytokines (IL1β, IL6, IL21, IL17A, IL22, IL17E, KC, MCP-1, IL33 and IL31) were assessed. Acute exposure to MCP230 significantly increased the levels of Th17 polarizing cytokines IL1β and IL6 at 1 dpe, with significantly higher levels of IL6 (approximately 45 fold increase) as early as 12 h postexposure (Table 1). Th17 effector cytokines IL17A and IL22 significantly increased at 1 dpe in the lungs of MCP230-exposed mice, but were not different at 12 h. These results indicate that exposure to MCP230 induces

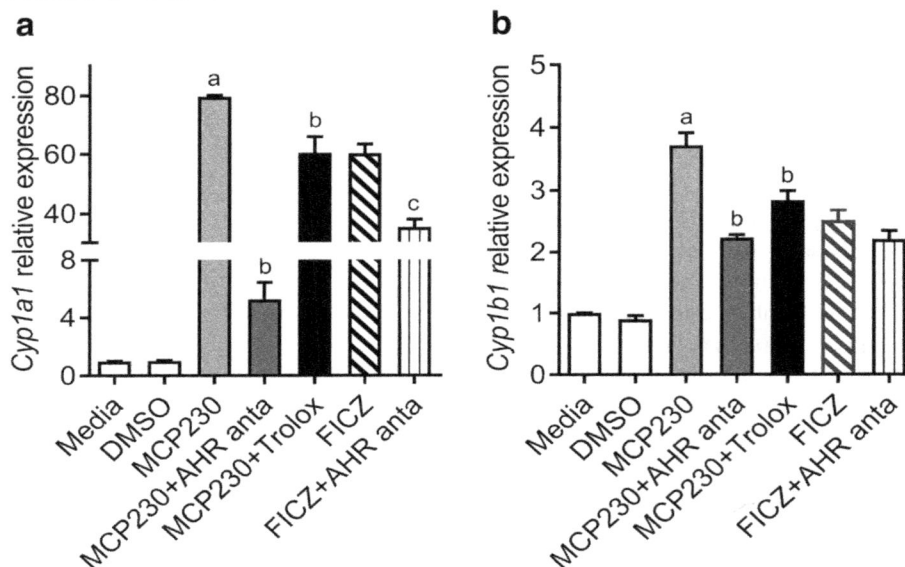

Fig. 5 MCP230-induced expression of *Cyp1a1* and *Cyp1b1* is dependent on AHR activation. A549 cells were treated with MCP230 (50 µg/cm²) or AHR agonist (FICZ; 200 nM) in the presence or absence of AHR antagonist (CH223191; 10 µM) for 4 h. Cell pellets were collected and expression of *Cyp1a1* (**a**) and *Cyp1b1* (**b**) relative to *Hprt* was determined using RT-qPCR analysis. Data represent mean ± SEM from one of two independent experiments, performed in triplicate. [a]$p < 0.05$, compared to Media group. [b]$p < 0.05$, compared to MCP230 group. [c]$p < 0.05$, compared to FICZ group, one-way ANOVA with Tukey's multiple comparisons test

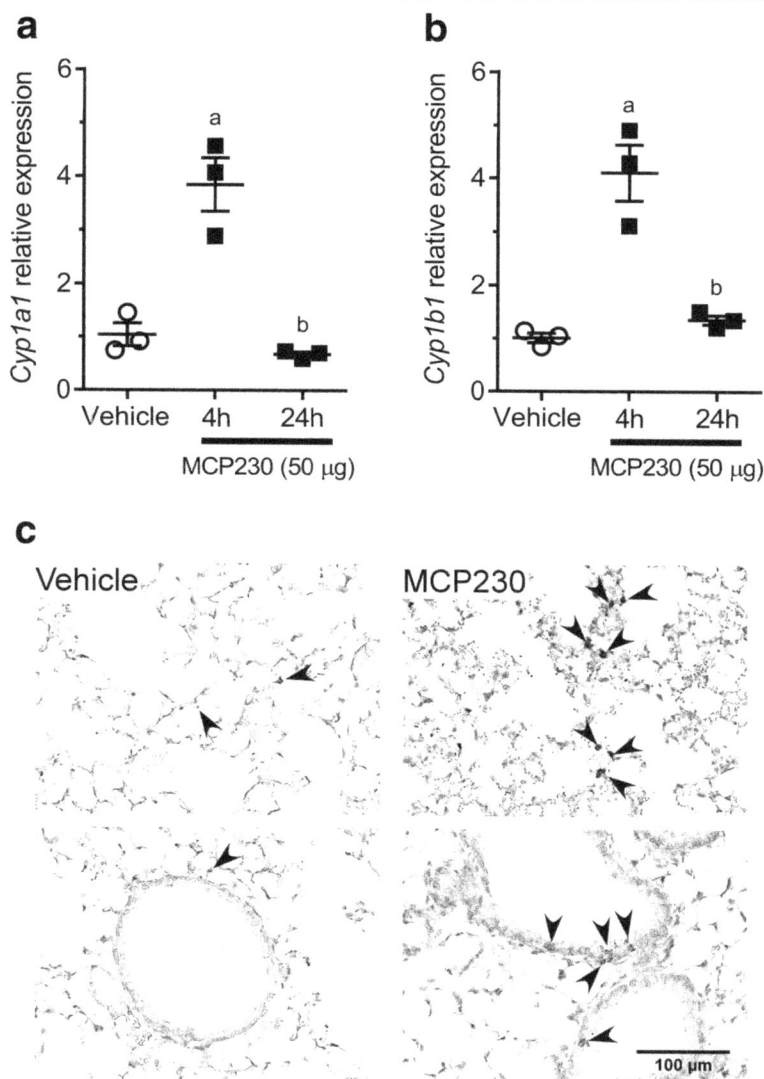

Fig. 6 Acute exposure to MCP230 results in transient activation of AHR and increased expression of *Cyp1a1* and *Cyp1b1* in vivo. (**a**, **b**) WT mice were exposed to vehicle or MCP230 (50 μg) and lungs were isolated at 4 and 24 h post-exposure. Expression of *Cyp1a1* and *Cyp1b1* relative to *Hprt* was measured using RT-qPCR analysis. Data represent mean ± SEM from one of two independent experiments. [a]$p < 0.05$, compared to Vehicle group. [b]$p < 0.05$, compared to 4 h group, one-way ANOVA with Tukey's multiple comparisons test. (**c**) Representative photomicrographs of lungs from WT mice exposed to vehicle or 50 μg MCP230. Lungs were isolated from mice at 4 h post-exposure and stained for *Cyp1a1* RNA using in situ hybridization. Top panel represents expression of *Cyp1a1* in lung parenchyma and bottom panel represents expression of *Cyp1a1* in the airway epithelium. Arrowheads point at cells expressing *Cyp1a1*

a Th17 cell-biased environment in the lungs. We also analyzed the chemokines KC and MCP-1 in the lungs of MCP230-exposed mice. The levels of both KC and MCP-1 were significantly elevated at 1 dpe, with significantly higher levels of MCP-1 as early as 12 h. In addition, we observed an increase in the levels of IL33 at 12 h and 1 dpe. In contrast to the IL33 levels, a reduction in the levels of IL31 was observed, which was significant at 12 h. No significant changes in the levels of IL17E and IL21 were observed in mice exposed to MCP230 compared to vehicle control (Table 1).

EPFR-induced Th17 pulmonary immune response and pulmonary neutrophilic inflammation are dependent on AHR activation

Exposure to MCP230 resulted in a significant increase in the percent of Th17 cells in the lungs of mice as shown in Fig. 1b and previously [35]. Recent reports indicate that AHR activation leads to Th17 cell differentiation thus leading to exacerbation of the inflammatory responses [29–31]. To investigate the role of AHR in the MCP230-induced Th17 response, we inhibited AHR activation in MCP230-exposed mice by treating them with AHR

Table 1 MCP230 exposure results in pulmonary Th17 associated cytokine induction

Cytokines	MCP230	
	12 h	1 d
IL1β	1.446 ± 0.1729	1.691 ± 0.2082[a]
IL6	45.71 ± 8.457[a]	10.61 ± 3.177[a]
IL21	0.7346 ± 0.0256	1.034 ± 0.1367
IL17A	0.6526 ± 0.1302	6.096 ± 1.666[a]
IL22	0.9377 ± 0.0325	1.504 ± 0.158[a]
IL17E	0.7034 ± 0.0941	0.9023 ± 0.0322
KC	5.629 ± 1.54 *p = 0.053*	2.591 ± 0.4729[a]
MCP-1	6.337 ± 1.325[a]	6.825 ± 0.2238[a]
IL33	2.226 ± 0.1384[a]	2.716 ± 0.1907[a]
IL31	0.3472 ± 0.07782[a]	0.4988 ± 0.0489

Levels of Th17 cytokines were determined in the lung homogenates of WT mice exposed to MCP230 at 12 h and 1 day post-exposure. Concentrations (pg/mg of lung protein) of all cytokines were measured using multiplex assay. Data are expressed as means ± SEM of fold change over Vehicle treated controls from 4 to 5 mice. [a]$p < 0.05$ compared to vehicle control, unpaired t test

antagonist (MCP230+AHR anta) and measured pulmonary T cell sub-populations using intracellular cytokine staining. Exposure to MCP230 resulted in a significant increase in Th17 cells (IL17A producing $CD3^+CD4^+$ cells) in the lungs of mice exposed to MCP230 compared to vehicle exposed control mice. Treatment with AHR antagonist significantly reduced the percent of Th17 cells in the lungs of MCP230-exposed mice compared to that in MCP230-exposed mice not treated with AHR antagonist (Fig. 7a and b). There was no significant difference in Th17 numbers between vehicle exposed control group and AHR antagonist treated groups [i.e. Vehicle vs Vehicle+AHR anta ($p = 0.17$) or MCP230 +AHR anta ($p = 0.31$)].

To determine the role of AHR in MCP230-induced neutrophil recruitment, we analyzed the inflammatory cells in airways (BALF) of mice pre-treated with AHR antagonist and exposed to MCP230. The mice were treated with AHR antagonist 2 h prior to MCP230 exposure to inhibit AHR activation (i.e. at 4 h post MCP230 exposure). In accordance with the data presented in Fig. 1, exposure to MCP230 increased the total number of leukocytes in the lungs, with significant increase in the number of neutrophils and lymphocytes compared to that in vehicle control. Pretreatment with AHR antagonist significantly attenuated these high numbers of total leukocytes, including neutrophils and lymphocytes, in MCP230-exposed mice (Fig. 7c). Together, these results suggest that AHR activation is required for MCP230-induced pulmonary Th17 response and recruitment of inflammatory neutrophils in lungs.

Discussion

Several epidemiological studies have demonstrated association between exposure to airborne PM and increased risk to develop asthma and/or acute asthma exacerbations [43–45]. Although an association between elevated levels of PM and respiratory diseases exist, the underlying mechanisms of PM-induced asthma exacerbations are not completely understood. In this study, we utilized an EPFR-containing combustion-derived PM, a common form of PM found in the atmosphere, and present a unique mechanism that mediates the pulmonary immune responses as a result of exposure. The data presented here demonstrate that MCP230, an EPFR-containing PM, results in pulmonary neutrophilia that is dependent on Th17 cells and IL17A. Further, we demonstrate that AHR signaling is important for EPFR-induced Th17 adaptive immune response and pulmonary neutrophilia.

Pulmonary neutrophilic inflammation is a major characteristic of patients with severe asthma. Studies in humans with asthma and animal models of asthma demonstrate that neutrophils play an important role in the pathogenesis of severe asthma [21, 46]. Further, IL17A has been shown to play an important role in the severity of human airway diseases, such as asthma and COPD [47]. Airway inflammation in severe and persistent asthma is associated with IL17A; and Th17 cells play a critical role in the activation and recruitment of neutrophils [23]. Our previous studies have shown that exposure to EPFRs results in maturation of dendritic cells and Th17 biased cell responses that were associated with neutrophilic inflammation [35]. However, the mechanism of EPFR-induced Th17 inflammation and associated neutrophilia was not completely understood. In the current study, MCP230-exposure caused an early immune response in the form of increased Th17 cytokines including neutrophil chemo-attractants. Using IL23p19 knockout ($IL23p19^{-/-}$; mice deficient in Th17 responses) and IL17Ra knockout ($IL17Ra^{-/-}$) mice models, we have confirmed that activation of Th17 cells and IL17A are essential for neutrophilic inflammation in the lungs upon exposure to EPFRs.

AHR binds to a wide array of exogenous and endogenous ligands, activating inflammatory responses in various diseases [27]. AHR is known to play a role in increased differentiation of Th17 cells [30, 31]. Th17 cell differentiation subsequent to ligand-dependent activation of AHR has also been observed in other models of autoimmune diseases [29–31], which may lead to exacerbation of inflammation involving neutrophilia. To understand the role of AHR in MCP230-induced Th17 inflammation, we investigated whether acute exposure to MCP230 activates the AHR pathway. Our results showed that exposure to EPFRs induced activation of AHR (Fig. 3) and was confirmed by increased expression of *Cyp1a1* and *Cyp1b1* in

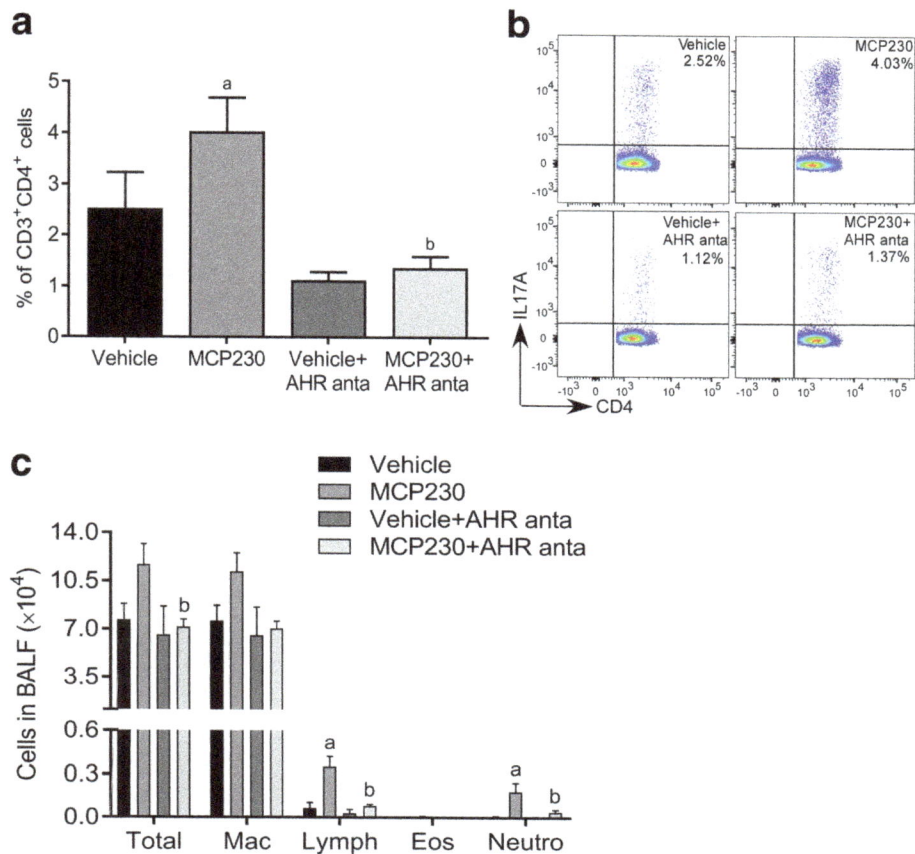

Fig. 7 MCP230-induced pulmonary Th17 immune response is dependent on AHR activation. WT mice were exposed to vehicle or MCP230 (50 μg) that were treated with or without AHR antagonist (CH223191; 10 mg/kg) 2 h prior to the exposure. Lungs or BALF were collected at 5 dpe. (**a, b**) Lungs were used to determine adaptive T cell responses. PMA/ionomycin-stimulated lung cells were stained with surface (CD3 and CD4) and intracellular (IL17A) antibodies. T cell subsets were quantified using flow cytometry. Data are presented as percentage of IL17A+ cells among CD3+CD4+ cells (**a**) and representative flow cytometry pseudo color dot plots of IL17A+CD4+ cells gated on CD3+ T cells (**b**). Data represent mean ± SEM from 4 to 5 mice. $^a p < 0.05$, compared to Vehicle group. $^b p < 0.05$, compared to MCP230 group, one-way ANOVA with Holm-Sidak's multiple comparisons test. (**c**) BALF were used to assess differential cell counts by counting at least 300 cells/sample. Data represent mean ± SEM from one of two independent experiments, 4 to 5 mice. $^a p < 0.05$, compared to Vehicle group. $^b p < 0.05$, compared to MCP230 group, one-way ANOVA with Dunnett's multiple comparisons test

lung cells in vitro (Figs. 3, 4 and 5) and in vivo (Fig. 6). This EPFR-induced *Cyp1a1* and *Cyp1b1* expression was inhibited by an AHR antagonist (Fig. 5). Previously, we reported that EPFR-induced oxidative stress and cellular uptake of MCP230 particles are important for its immune-modulating effects [35]. Oxidative stress is known to promote the polarization of T cell differentiation towards Th2 phenotype [48]; however, the role of oxidative stress in polarizing the T cell differentiation towards Th17 phenotype is not completely understood and in the literature there is conflicting information on the induction of oxidative stress as a result of AHR activation [49, 50]. Interestingly, our data showed that using an antioxidant or an uptake blocker significantly inhibited the EPFR-induced *Cyp1a1* and *Cyp1b1* expression (Fig. 5), suggesting a role of EPFR-induced oxidative stress in AHR activation.

IL17 mediates the influx of neutrophils in the lungs in an OVA-induced mouse model of asthma and inhibiting IL17, using monoclonal antibodies, reduces the bronchial influx of neutrophils [51]. In addition, Th17 cells can induce neutrophilia by directly releasing chemoattractants for neutrophils [25]. We demonstrate that exposure to EPFRs results in increased levels of Th17 inducing cytokines IL1β and IL6 levels at 1 dpe, with significantly high levels of IL6 as early as 12 h post-exposure. IL6 is an important regulator of balance between regulatory T cells and Th17 cells [52]. The levels of IL33 were also higher at 12 h post-exposure and 1 dpe, which can directly stimulate mast cells to produce IL1β and IL6, and enhance the Th17 response [53, 54]. Further, we observed increase in cytokines IL17A and an increase in the levels of neutrophil chemo attractants

KC and MCP-1 in the airways at 1 dpe. Although we observed only a transient activation of AHR, such AHR activation can drive cytokine induction that leads to Th17 biased responses. We observed EPFR-induced immune responses in mice beginning at 12 h post-exposure that persisted until 5 dpe. Further studies are required to understand the role of AHR activation in early immune response and its effects on subsequent adaptive Th17 response.

We present evidence that AHR activation is necessary for EPFR-induced pulmonary immune responses. Treatment with AHR antagonist resulted in suppression of EPFR-induced pulmonary Th17 responses and the associated neutrophilic inflammation. AHR is expressed at high levels in Th17 cells compared to other T cell subsets [28] and we observed a significant reduction of EPFR-induced Th17 cells in mice pre-treated with AHR antagonist.

Conclusions

We demonstrated that EPFRs associated with combustion-derived PM result in pulmonary immune response in the form of early Th17 cytokine expression and subsequent pulmonary neutrophilic inflammation. This EPFR-induced pulmonary neutrophilic inflammation was shown to be dependent on Th17 and IL17A. Our in vitro data demonstrated that EPFR-induced AHR activation is mediated to some extent by the ability of particles to generate oxidative stress and required uptake of EPFRs. Further, we demonstrated that EPFRs induce AHR activation in vivo and inhibition of AHR activation using selective AHR antagonist resulted in inhibition of pulmonary Th17 inflammation and associated neutrophilia. In summary, our data illustrate a unique mechanism by which radical containing particulate matter mediate pulmonary Th17 immune responses through AHR. In addition to Th17 cells, other cells like $\gamma\delta$ T cells [55, 56] and NKT cells [57] can produce IL17A and contribute to inflammation prior to the development of adaptive Th17 responses. Although beyond the scope of this paper, our future studies will investigate the role of AHR activation in these cells. Using $Th17^{-/-}$ mouse model would directly address the importance of Th17 cells in MCP230-exacerbated asthma severity; however, this model was not available when our experiments were performed. While AHR−/− mice were available at the time of these studies, we chose not to use them, because among other physiological issues (e.g. defects in fertility, perinatal growth, liver size and function, closure, spleen size), they have defects in peripheral lymphocytes [58], which would be important in the inflammatory responses to MCP230. Generation of conditional and cell-specific $AHR^{-/-}$ models will be helpful to confirm our results, but beyond the scope of this manuscript.

Additional files

Additional file 1: Figure S1. *Il17f* expression relative to *Gapdh* in whole-lung homogenates of WT and IL23p19$^{-/-}$ mice exposed to vehicle or MCP230 was determined using TaqMan gene expression assay (Applied Biosystems, Waltham, MA). Expression was determined at 5 dpe. Data represent mean ± SEM from 3 to 5 mice. (TIF 148 kb)

Additional file 2: Figure S2. WT and IL17Ra$^{-/-}$ mice were sensitized with OVA (ovalbumin complexed to Imject Alum) on days 0 and 14. Mice were exposed to either vehicle or MCP230 (50 μg) on protocol day 23 and challenged with OVA on days 24, 25, and 26. BAL fluid or lungs were collected on day 28. Differential cell counts of BALF cells at 5 dpe (i.e. day 28) from mice challenged with OVA and exposed to vehicle or MCP230. Data are presented as mean ± SEM of numbers of cells from 4 to 5 mice. (TIF 9277 kb)

Abbreviations
AHR: Aryl hydrocarbon receptor; ANOVA: Analysis of variance; BALF: Bronchoalveolar lavage fluid; BMDC: Bone marrow-derived dendritic Cell; CH223191: 1-methyl-*N*-[2-methyl-4-[2-(2-methylphenyl)diazenyl]phenyl]-1*H*-pyrazole-5-carboxamide); *Cyp1a1*: Cytochrome p450 1a1; *Cyp1b1*: Cytochrome p450 1b1; EPFR: Environmentally persistent free radicals; FICZ: 6-formylindolo[3,2-b]carbazole; IL17A: Interleukin 17A; IL17E: Interleukin 17E; IL1β: Interleukin 1β; IL21: Interleukin 21; IL22: Interleukin 22; IL31: Interleukin 31; IL33: Interleukin 33; IL6: Interleukin 6; KC: Keratinocyte-derived chemokine; MCP-1: Monocyte chemotactic protein-1; MCP230: EPFR-containing PM; OVA: Ovalbumin; PBN: *N*-tert-Butyl-α-phenylnitrone; PM: Particulate matter; SEM: Standard error of means; TCDD: 2,3,7, 8-tetrachlorodibenzo-p-dioxin; Th17: T-helper 17

Acknowledgements
Dr. Slawo Lomnicki and the Louisiana State University Superfund Research Program supplied all particles including MCP230. Authors would like to thank Dr. Farhana Hasan of Louisiana State University for her assistance in synthesis and characterization of MCP50 and MCP230.

Funding
This work was supported by NIEHS Superfund grant to SAC, SL, and TRD (P42ES013648) and NIEHS grant to SAC (R01ES015050).

Authors' contributions
PW, SJ and SAC conceived and designed the study, and drafted the manuscript. PW participated in the design of the study and assisted with real time PCR, and flow cytometry experiments. VSP performed the multiplex and cell differential experiments, and drafted/revised the manuscript. AS assisted with in vitro experiments and real time PCR. JH assisted with isolation of BALF, differential cell counts and histology quantification. SRM assisted with histology quantification. MK and TRD assisted with luciferase assay for AHR activation analysis. All authors have read and approved the manuscript.

Competing interests
The authors declare that they have no competing interests.

Author details
^{1}Department of Pediatrics, University of Tennessee Health Science Center, Memphis, TN 38103, USA. ^{2}Children's Foundation Research Institute, Le

Bonheur Children's Hospital, Memphis, TN 38103, USA. [3]Department of Biological Sciences, Louisiana State University, Baton Rouge, LA 70803, USA. [4]Department of Comparative Biomedical Sciences, Louisiana State University School of Veterinary Medicine, Room 2510, 1909 Freight Dock, Skip Bertman Drive, Baton Rouge, LA 70803, USA. [5]Department of Respiratory and Critical Care Medicine, Second Affiliated Hospital, Zhejiang University School of Medicine, Hangzhou, China. [6]Department of Pharmacology, Toxicology, and Neuroscience, Louisiana State University Health Sciences Center, Shreveport, LA 71103, USA. [7]St. Joseph's Academy, Baton Rouge, LA 70808, USA.

References

1. Syc M, Horak J, Hopan F, Krpec K, Tomsej T, Ocelka T, et al. Effect of fuels and domestic heating appliance types on emission factors of selected organic pollutants. Environ Sci Technol. 2011;45(21):9427–34. https://doi.org/10.1021/es2017945. https://www.ncbi.nlm.nih.gov/pubmed/21932830.

2. Wiedinmyer C, Yokelson RJ, Gullett BK. Global emissions of trace gases, particulate matter, and hazardous air pollutants from open burning of domestic waste. Environ Sci Technol. 2014;48(16):9523–30. https://doi.org/10.1021/es502250z. https://www.ncbi.nlm.nih.gov/pubmed/25019173.

3. Cass G. Comments on sources, atmospheric levels, and characterization of airborne particulate matter. Inhal Toxicol. 1995;7:765–8.

4. Clark NA, Demers PA, Karr CJ, Koehoorn M, Lencar C, Tamburic L, et al. Effect of early life exposure to air pollution on development of childhood asthma. Environ Health Perspect. 2010;118(2):284–90. https://doi.org/10.1289/ehp.0900916. https://www.ncbi.nlm.nih.gov/pubmed/20123607.

5. Gehring U, Wijga AH, Hoek G, Bellander T, Berdel D, Bruske I, et al. Exposure to air pollution and development of asthma and rhinoconjunctivitis throughout childhood and adolescence: a population-based birth cohort study. Lancet Respir Med. 2015;3(12):933–42. https://doi.org/10.1016/S2213-2600(15)00426-9. https://www.ncbi.nlm.nih.gov/pubmed/27057569.

6. Mamessier E, Nieves A, Vervloet D, Magnan A. Diesel exhaust particles enhance T-cell activation in severe asthmatics. Allergy. 2006;61(5):581–8. https://doi.org/10.1111/j.1398-9995.2006.01056.x. https://www.ncbi.nlm.nih.gov/pubmed/16629788.

7. Lee GI, Saravia J, You D, Shrestha B, Jaligama S, Hebert VY, et al. Exposure to combustion generated environmentally persistent free radicals enhances severity of influenza virus infection. Part Fibre Toxicol. 2014;11:57. https://doi.org/10.1186/s12989-014-0057-1. https://www.ncbi.nlm.nih.gov/pubmed/25358535.

8. Balakrishna S, Saravia J, Thevenot P, Ahlert T, Lominiki S, Dellinger B, et al. Environmentally persistent free radicals induce airway hyperresponsiveness in neonatal rat lungs. Part Fibre Toxicol. 2011;8:11. https://doi.org/10.1186/1743-8977-8-11. https://www.ncbi.nlm.nih.gov/pubmed/21388553.

9. dela Cruz AL, Gehling W, Lomnicki S, Cook R, Dellinger B. Detection of environmentally persistent free radicals at a superfund wood treating site. Environ Sci Technol. 2011;45(15):6356–65. https://doi.org/10.1021/es2012947. https://www.ncbi.nlm.nih.gov/pubmed/21732664.

10. dela Cruz AL, Cook RL, Dellinger B, Lomnicki SM, Donnelly KC, Kelley MA, et al. Assessment of environmentally persistent free radicals in soils and sediments from three Superfund sites. Environ Sci Process Impacts. 2014;16(1):44–52. https://doi.org/10.1039/c3em00428g. https://www.ncbi.nlm.nih.gov/pubmed/24244947.

11. Dellinger B, Pryor WA, Cueto R, Squadrito GL, Hegde V, Deutsch WA. Role of free radicals in the toxicity of airborne fine particulate matter. Chem Res Toxicol. 2001;14(10):1371–7. https://www.ncbi.nlm.nih.gov/pubmed/11599928.

12. Valavanidis A, Fiotakis K, Vlahogianni T, Papadimitriou V, Pantikaki V. <I>Corrigendum to</I>: Determination of Selective Quinones and Quinoid Radicals in Airborne Particulate Matter and Vehicular Exhaust Particles. Environ Chem. 2006;3(3):233. https://doi.org/10.1071/EN05089_CO. http://www.publish.csiro.au/paper/EN05089_CO.

13. Valavanidis A, Iliopoulos N, Gotsis G, Fiotakis K. Persistent free radicals, heavy metals and PAHs generated in particulate soot emissions and residue ash from controlled combustion of common types of plastic. J Hazard Mater. 2008;156(1–3):277–84. https://doi.org/10.1016/j.jhazmat.2007.12.019. https://www.ncbi.nlm.nih.gov/pubmed/18249066.

14. Valavanidis A, Vlachogianni T, Fiotakis K. Tobacco smoke: involvement of reactive oxygen species and stable free radicals in mechanisms of oxidative damage, carcinogenesis and synergistic effects with other respirable particles. Int J Environ Res Public Health. 2009;6(2):445–62. https://doi.org/10.3390/ijerph6020445. https://www.ncbi.nlm.nih.gov/pubmed/19440393.

15. Balakrishna S, Lomnicki S, McAvey KM, Cole RB, Dellinger B, Cormier SA. Environmentally persistent free radicals amplify ultrafine particle mediated cellular oxidative stress and cytotoxicity. Part Fibre Toxicol. 2009;6:11. https://doi.org/10.1186/1743-8977-6-11. https://www.ncbi.nlm.nih.gov/pubmed/19374750.

16. Lomnicki S, Truong H, Vejerano E, Dellinger B. Copper oxide-based model of persistent free radical formation on combustion-derived particulate matter. Environ Sci Technol. 2008;42(13):4982–8. https://www.ncbi.nlm.nih.gov/pubmed/18678037.

17. Dellinger B, Lomnicki S, Khachatryan L, Maskos Z, Hall RW, Adounkpe J, et al. Formation and stabilization of persistent free radicals. Proc Combust Inst. 2007;31(1):521–8. https://doi.org/10.1016/jproci200607.172. https://www.ncbi.nlm.nih.gov/pubmed/25598747.

18. Alcorn JF, Crowe CR, Kolls JK. TH17 cells in asthma and COPD. Annu Rev Physiol. 2010;72:495–516. https://doi.org/10.1146/annurev-physiol-021909-135926. https://www.ncbi.nlm.nih.gov/pubmed/20148686.

19. Bullens DM, Decraene A, Seys S, Dupont LJ. IL-17A in human respiratory diseases: innate or adaptive immunity? Clinical implications. Clin Dev Immunol. 2013;2013:840315. https://doi.org/10.1155/2013/840315. https://www.ncbi.nlm.nih.gov/pubmed/23401702.

20. Fahy JV. Eosinophilic and neutrophilic inflammation in asthma: insights from clinical studies. Proc Am Thorac Soc. 2009;6(3):256–9. https://doi.org/10.1513/pats.200808-087RM. https://www.ncbi.nlm.nih.gov/pubmed/19387026.

21. Nakagome K, Matsushita S, Nagata M. Neutrophilic inflammation in severe asthma. Int Arch Allergy Immunol. 2012;158(Suppl 1):96–102. https://doi.org/10.1159/000337801. https://www.ncbi.nlm.nih.gov/pubmed/22627375.

22. Newcomb DC, Peebles RS Jr. Th17-mediated inflammation in asthma. Curr Opin Immunol. 2013;25(6):755–60. https://doi.org/10.1016/j.coi.2013.08.002. https://www.ncbi.nlm.nih.gov/pubmed/24035139.

23. McKinley L, Alcorn JF, Peterson A, Dupont RB, Kapadia S, Logar A, et al. TH17 cells mediate steroid-resistant airway inflammation and airway hyperresponsiveness in mice. J Immunol. 2008;181(6):4089–97. https://www.ncbi.nlm.nih.gov/pubmed/18768865.

24. Ye P, Rodriguez FH, Kanaly S, Stocking KL, Schurr J, Schwarzenberger P, et al. Requirement of interleukin 17 receptor signaling for lung CXC chemokine and granulocyte colony-stimulating factor expression, neutrophil recruitment, and host defense. J Exp Med. 2001;194(4):519–27. https://www.ncbi.nlm.nih.gov/pubmed/11514607.

25. Pelletier M, Maggi L, Micheletti A, Lazzeri E, Tamassia N, Costantini C, et al. Evidence for a cross-talk between human neutrophils and Th17 cells. Blood. 2010;115(2):335–43. https://doi.org/10.1182/blood-2009-04-216085. https://www.ncbi.nlm.nih.gov/pubmed/19890092.

26. Schmidt JV, Bradfield CAA. Receptor signaling pathways. Annu Rev Cell Dev Biol. 1996;12:55–89. https://doi.org/10.1146/annurev.cellbio.12.1.55. https://www.ncbi.nlm.nih.gov/pubmed/8970722.

27. Harper PA, Riddick DS, Okey AB. Regulating the regulator: factors that control levels and activity of the aryl hydrocarbon receptor. Biochem Pharmacol. 2006;72(3):267–79. https://doi.org/10.1016/j.bcp.2006.01.007. https://www.ncbi.nlm.nih.gov/pubmed/16488401.

28. Veldhoen M, Hirota K, Westendorf AM, Buer J, Dumoutier L, Renauld JC, et al. The aryl hydrocarbon receptor links TH17-cell-mediated autoimmunity to environmental toxins. Nature. 2008;453(7191):106–9. https://doi.org/10.1038/nature06881. https://www.ncbi.nlm.nih.gov/pubmed/18362914.

29. Kimura A, Naka T, Nohara K, Fujii-Kuriyama Y, Kishimoto T. Aryl hydrocarbon receptor regulates Stat1 activation and participates in the development of Th17 cells. Proc Natl Acad Sci U S A. 2008;105(28):9721–6. https://doi.org/10.1073/pnas.0804231105. https://www.ncbi.nlm.nih.gov/pubmed/18607004.

30. Mohinta S, Kannan AK, Gowda K, Amin SG, Perdew GH, August A. Differential regulation of Th17 and T regulatory cell differentiation by aryl hydrocarbon receptor dependent xenobiotic response element dependent and independent pathways. Toxicol Sci. 2015;145(2):233–43. https://doi.org/10.1093/toxsci/kfv046. https://www.ncbi.nlm.nih.gov/pubmed/25716673.

31. Quintana FJ, Basso AS, Iglesias AH, Korn T, Farez MF, Bettelli E, et al. Control of T(reg) and T(H)17 cell differentiation by the aryl hydrocarbon receptor. Nature. 2008;453(7191):65–71. https://doi.org/10.1038/nature06880. https://www.ncbi.nlm.nih.gov/pubmed/18362915.

32. Jaligama S, Chen Z, Saravia J, Yadav N, Lomnicki SM, Dugas TR, et al. Exposure to Deepwater Horizon Crude Oil Burnoff Particulate Matter

Induces Pulmonary Inflammation and Alters Adaptive Immune Response. Environ Sci Technol. 2015;49(14):8769–76. https://doi.org/10.1021/acs.est.5b01439. http://www.ncbi.nlm.nih.gov/pubmed/26115348.

33. Kim SH, Henry EC, Kim DK, Kim YH, Shin KJ, Han MS, et al. Novel compound 2-methyl-2H-pyrazole-3-carboxylic acid (2-methyl-4-o-tolylazo-phenyl)-amide (CH-223191) prevents 2,3,7,8-TCDD-induced toxicity by antagonizing the aryl hydrocarbon receptor. Mol Pharmacol. 2006;69(6):1871–8. https://doi.org/10.1124/mol.105.021832. https://www.ncbi.nlm.nih.gov/pubmed/16540597.

34. Zhao B, Degroot DE, Hayashi A, He G, Denison MS. CH223191 is a ligand-selective antagonist of the ah (dioxin) receptor. Toxicol Sci. 2010;117(2):393–403. https://doi.org/10.1093/toxsci/kfq217. https://www.ncbi.nlm.nih.gov/pubmed/20634293.

35. Wang P, Thevenot P, Saravia J, Ahlert T, Cormier SA. Radical-containing particles activate dendritic cells and enhance Th17 inflammation in a mouse model of asthma. Am J Respir Cell Mol Biol. 2011;45(5):977–83. https://doi.org/10.1165/rcmb.2011-0001OC. http://www.ncbi.nlm.nih.gov/pubmed/21493781.

36. Saravia J, You D, Shrestha B, Jaligama S, Siefker D, Lee GI, et al. Respiratory syncytial virus disease is mediated by age-variable IL-33. PLoS Pathog. 2015;11(10):e1005217. https://doi.org/10.1371/journal.ppat.1005217. https://www.ncbi.nlm.nih.gov/pubmed/26473724.

37. Veldhoen M, Hocking RJ, Atkins CJ, Locksley RM, Stockinger B. TGFbeta in the context of an inflammatory cytokine milieu supports de novo differentiation of IL-17-producing T cells. Immunity. 2006;24(2):179–89. https://doi.org/10.1016/j.immuni.2006.01.001. https://www.ncbi.nlm.nih.gov/pubmed/16473830.

38. Stritesky GL, Yeh N, Kaplan MH. IL-23 promotes maintenance but not commitment to the Th17 lineage. J Immunol. 2008;181(9):5948–55. https://www.ncbi.nlm.nih.gov/pubmed/18941183.

39. Chung Y, Chang SH, Martinez GJ, Yang XO, Nurieva R, Kang HS, et al. Critical regulation of early Th17 cell differentiation by interleukin-1 signaling. Immunity. 2009;30(4):576–87. https://doi.org/10.1016/jimmuni200902.007. https://www.ncbi.nlm.nih.gov/pubmed/19362022.

40. Mus AM, Cornelissen F, Asmawidjaja PS, van Hamburg JP, Boon L, Hendriks RW, et al. Interleukin-23 promotes Th17 differentiation by inhibiting T-bet and FoxP3 and is required for elevation of interleukin-22, but not interleukin-21, in autoimmune experimental arthritis. Arthritis Rheum. 2010;62(4):1043–50. https://doi.org/10.1002/art.27336. https://www.ncbi.nlm.nih.gov/pubmed/20131264.

41. Vogel CF, Wu D, Goth SR, Baek J, Lollies A, Domhardt R, et al. Aryl hydrocarbon receptor signaling regulates NF-kappaB RelB activation during dendritic-cell differentiation. Immunol Cell Biol. 2013;91(9):568–75. https://doi.org/10.1038/icb2013.43. https://www.ncbi.nlm.nih.gov/pubmed/23999131.

42. Singh NP, Singh UP, Rouse M, Zhang J, Chatterjee S, Nagarkatti PS, et al. Dietary Indoles Suppress Delayed-Type Hypersensitivity by Inducing a Switch from Proinflammatory Th17 Cells to Anti-Inflammatory Regulatory T Cells through Regulation of MicroRNA. J Immunol. 2016;196(3):1108–22. https://doi.org/10.4049/jimmunol.1501727. https://www.ncbi.nlm.nih.gov/pubmed/26712945.

43. Baldacci S, Maio S, Cerrai S, Sarno G, Baiz N, Simoni M, et al. Allergy and asthma: effects of the exposure to particulate matter and biological allergens. Respir Med. 2015;109(9):1089–104. https://doi.org/10.1016/jrmed201505.017. https://www.ncbi.nlm.nih.gov/pubmed/26073963.

44. Brauer M, Hoek G, Smit HA, de Jongste JC, Gerritsen J, Postma DS, et al. Air pollution and development of asthma, allergy and infections in a birth cohort. Eur Respir J. 2007;29(5):879–88. https://doi.org/10.1183/09031936.00083406. https://www.ncbi.nlm.nih.gov/pubmed/17251230.

45. Brunekreef B, Beelen R, Hoek G, Schouten L, Bausch-Goldbohm S, Fischer P, et al. Effects of long-term exposure to traffic-related air pollution on respiratory and cardiovascular mortality in the Netherlands: the NLCS-AIR study. Res Rep Health Eff Inst. 2009;139:5–71. discussion 3–89. https://www.ncbi.nlm.nih.gov/pubmed/19554969.

46. Jatakanon A, Uasuf C, Maziak W, Lim S, Chung KF, Barnes PJ. Neutrophilic inflammation in severe persistent asthma. Am J Respir Crit Care Med. 1999;160(5 Pt 1):1532–9. https://doi.org/10.1164/ajrccm.160.5.9806170. https://www.ncbi.nlm.nih.gov/pubmed/10556116.

47. Cazzola M, Matera MG. IL-17 in chronic obstructive pulmonary disease. Expert Rev Respir Med. 2012;6(2):135–8. https://doi.org/10.1586/ers.12.7. https://www.ncbi.nlm.nih.gov/pubmed/22455484.

48. King MR, Ismail AS, Davis LS, Karp DR. Oxidative stress promotes polarization of human T cell differentiation toward a T helper 2 phenotype. J Immunol. 2006;176(5):2765–72. https://www.ncbi.nlm.nih.gov/pubmed/16493032.

49. Wu JP, Chang LW, Yao HT, Chang H, Tsai HT, Tsai MH, et al. Involvement of oxidative stress and activation of aryl hydrocarbon receptor in elevation of CYP1A1 expression and activity in lung cells and tissues by arsenic: an in vitro and in vivo study. Toxicol Sci. 2009;107(2):385–93. https://doi.org/10.1093/toxsci/kfn239. https://www.ncbi.nlm.nih.gov/pubmed/19033395.

50. Dalton TP, Puga A, Shertzer HG. Induction of cellular oxidative stress by aryl hydrocarbon receptor activation. Chem Biol Interact. 2002;141(1–2):77–95. https://www.ncbi.nlm.nih.gov/pubmed/12213386.

51. Hellings PW, Kasran A, Liu Z, Vandekerckhove P, Wuyts A, Overbergh L, et al. Interleukin-17 orchestrates the granulocyte influx into airways after allergen inhalation in a mouse model of allergic asthma. Am J Respir Cell Mol Biol. 2003;28(1):42–50. https://doi.org/10.1165/rcmb.4832. https://www.ncbi.nlm.nih.gov/pubmed/12495931.

52. Kimura A, Kishimoto T. IL-6: regulator of Treg/Th17 balance. Eur J Immunol. 2010;40(7):1830–5. https://doi.org/10.1002/eji.201040391. https://www.ncbi.nlm.nih.gov/pubmed/20583029.

53. Cho KA, Suh JW, Sohn JH, Park JW, Lee H, Kang JL, et al. IL-33 induces Th17-mediated airway inflammation via mast cells in ovalbumin-challenged mice. Am J Physiol Lung Cell Mol Physiol. 2012;302(4):L429–40. https://doi.org/10.1152/ajplung00252.2011. https://www.ncbi.nlm.nih.gov/pubmed/22180658.

54. Moulin D, Donze O, Talabot-Ayer D, Mezin F, Palmer G, Gabay C. Interleukin (IL)-33 induces the release of pro-inflammatory mediators by mast cells. Cytokine. 2007;40(3):216–25. https://doi.org/10.1016/j.cyto.2007.09.013. https://www.ncbi.nlm.nih.gov/pubmed/18023358.

55. O'Brien RL, Roark CL, Born WK. IL-17-producing gammadelta T cells. Eur J Immunol. 2009;39(3):662–6. https://doi.org/10.1002/eji.200839120. https://www.ncbi.nlm.nih.gov/pubmed/19283718.

56. Papotto PH, Ribot JC, Silva-Santos B. IL-17+ gammadelta T cells as kick-starters of inflammation. Nat Immunol. 2017;18(6):604–11. https://doi.org/10.1038/ni.3726. https://www.ncbi.nlm.nih.gov/pubmed/28518154.

57. Monteiro M, Almeida CF, Agua-Doce A, Graca L. Induced IL-17-producing invariant NKT cells require activation in presence of TGF-beta and IL-1beta. J Immunol. 2013;190(2):805–11. https://doi.org/10.4049/jimmunol.1201010. https://www.ncbi.nlm.nih.gov/pubmed/23293359.

58. Sauzeau V, Carvajal-Gonzalez JM, Riolobos AS, Sevilla MA, Menacho-Marquez M, Roman AC, et al. Transcriptional factor aryl hydrocarbon receptor (Ahr) controls cardiovascular and respiratory functions by regulating the expression of the Vav3 proto-oncogene. J Biol Chem. 2011;286(4):2896–909. https://doi.org/10.1074/jbc.M110.187534. https://www.ncbi.nlm.nih.gov/pubmed/21115475.

5

Ambient fine particulate matter exposure induces reversible cardiac dysfunction and fibrosis in juvenile and older female mice

Guohua Qin[1], Jin Xia[1], Yingying Zhang[1], Lianghong Guo[2], Rui Chen[3] and Nan Sang[1*]

Abstract

Background: Cardiovascular disease is the leading cause of mortality in the advanced world, and age is an important determinant of cardiac function. The purpose of the study is to determine whether the $PM_{2.5}$-induced cardiac dysfunction is age-dependent and whether the adverse effects can be restored after $PM_{2.5}$ exposure withdrawal.

Methods: Female C57BL/6 mice at different ages (4-week-old, 4-month-old, and 10-month-old) received oropharyngeal aspiration of 3 mg/kg b.w. $PM_{2.5}$ every other day for 4 weeks. Then, 10-month-old and 4-week-old mice were exposed to $PM_{2.5}$ for 4 weeks and withdrawal $PM_{2.5}$ 1 or 2 weeks. Heart rate and systolic blood pressure were measured using a tail-cuff system. Cardiac function was assessed by echocardiography. Left ventricles were processed for histology to assess myocardial fibrosis. ROS generation was detected by photocatalysis using 2′,7′-dichlorodihydrofluorescein diacetate (DCFHDA). The expression of cardiac fibrosis markers (Col1a1, Col3a1) and possible signaling molecules, including NADPH oxidase 4 (NOX-4), transforming growth factor β1 (TGFβ1), and Smad3, were detected by qPCR and/ or Western blot.

Results: $PM_{2.5}$ exposure induced cardiac diastolic dysfunction of mice, elevated the heart rate and blood pressure, developed cardiac systolic dysfunction of 10-month-old mice, and caused fibrosis in both 4-week-old and 10-month-old mice. $PM_{2.5}$ exposure increased the expression of Col1a1, Col3a1, NOX-4, and TGFβ1, activated Smad3, and generated more reactive oxygen species in the myocardium of 4-week-old and 10-month-old mice. The withdrawal from $PM_{2.5}$ exposure restored blood pressure, heart rate, cardiac function, expression of collagens, and malonaldehyde (MDA) levels in hearts of both 10-month-old and 4-week-old mice.

Conclusion: Juvenile and older mice are more sensitive to $PM_{2.5}$ than adults and suffer from cardiac dysfunction. $PM_{2.5}$ exposure reversibly elevated heart rate and blood pressure, induced cardiac systolic dysfunction of older mice, and reversibly induced fibrosis in juvenile and older mice. The mechanism by which $PM_{2.5}$ exposure resulted in cardiac lesions might involve oxidative stress, NADPH oxidase, TGFβ1, and Smad-dependent pathways.

Keywords: Particulate matter, Cardiac, Fibrosis, Reversible, Different age

Background

Air pollution, mostly by fine particulate matter ($PM_{2.5}$), leads to 3.3 million premature deaths per year worldwide, predominantly in Asia [1]. Epidemiological evidence supports a robust association between exposure to $PM_{2.5}$ and cardiovascular diseases morbidity and mortality, such as myocardial infarction, heart failure, heart attacks, stroke, heart rhythm disturbances, and sudden death [2, 3]. However, the physicochemical properties of ambient $PM_{2.5}$ in different regions varies because of a number of factors including local geography, proximity to emission sources, and meteorology. Even in the same region, $PM_{2.5}$ from different seasons appears to have different chemical composition. It has been reported that seasonal variation in the association between $PM_{2.5}$ and cardiovascular hospitalization [4]. Furthermore, $PM_{2.5}$ does not affect all people equally. Several studies have suggested that susceptible individuals are at greater risk for $PM_{2.5}$-associated cardiovascular morbidity and mortality including the elderly, women, and

* Correspondence: sangnan@sxu.edu.cn
[1]College of Environment and Resource, Research Center of Environment and Health, Shanxi University, Taiyuan, Shanxi 030006, People's Republic of China
Full list of author information is available at the end of the article

patients with preexisting coronary artery disease and diabetes [5, 6].

Recent studies have demonstrated that exposure to $PM_{2.5}$ promotes systolic and diastolic dysfunction [7, 8], and exposure to carbon black impairs cardiac function in senescent mice [9]. Furthermore, exposure to diesel exhaust or $PM_{2.5}$ during early life can cause significant cardiovascular dysfunction in adulthood [10, 11]. However, the susceptibility of individuals of different ages to cardiovascular disease caused by $PM_{2.5}$ exposure has not been investigated. We hypothesized that $PM_{2.5}$ exposure may induce different effects in different life phases, such as juvenile, adult, and older subpopulations.

The specific molecular mechanisms of $PM_{2.5}$-induced cardiotoxicity effects are still under active investigation. Numerous investigations have elucidated potential biological mechanisms, whereby exposure to $PM_{2.5}$ may modulate disease susceptibility, including the progression of atherosclerosis, inflammation, thrombosis, systemic vascular dysfunction, and epigenetic changes [12]. Cardiac fibrosis is a common phenotype found in several cardiac diseases, including myocardial infarction and heart failure. It is characterized by the adverse accumulation of collagen and other extracellular matrix proteins. In addition to the loss of contractile capacity, inhalation of $PM_{2.5}$ is associated with adverse ventricular remodeling and worsening of cardiac fibrosis [7, 11]. Transforming growth factor $\beta1$ (TGF$\beta1$), a critical regulator of fibroblast phenotype and function, acts through Smad-dependent or independent pathways [13]. However, the mechanisms underlying the cardiac fibrosis effects of $PM_{2.5}$ are unclear.

Several previous studies of seasonal patterns of cardiovascular disease (CVD) indicated a peak of CVD in winter months [4, 14, 15]. We found seasonal variation in associations between collagen expression and $PM_{2.5}$ exposure in H9C2 cells in our pilot experiment. The strongest effect on collagen expression was observed after treatment with $PM_{2.5}$ from winter (Additional file 1: Figure S1). Accordingly, winter $PM_{2.5}$ was used for in vivo experiments in mice in the present study. The dose of $PM_{2.5}$ used in the present study was based on the following reasoning. As reported, respiratory volume of one mouse for 2 days reaches 0.259 m^3 [16]. According to the Chinese ambient air quality secondary standards (GB3095–2012) of $PM_{2.5}$ (75 μg/m^3), the amount of $PM_{2.5}$ inhalation for each mouse over 2 days is 19.425 μg. Therefore, $PM_{2.5}$ exposure concentration for mouse (about 20 g b.w.) every 2 days should be 0.97 mg/kg (b.w.). The dose used in the present study was about 3 fold of secondary standards or more than 3.6 fold when considering the deposition fraction [17]. However, the $PM_{2.5}$ concentration could exceed 300 μg/m^3 during the polluted periods

in Beijing [18] or other cities in China (http://113.108.142.147:20035/emcpublish/). The average concentration of $PM_{2.5}$ in northern China with non-haze weather was 161 μg/m^3 [19], and the level with haze weather reached 692 μg/m^3 [20].

Therefore, the purpose of this study was: (1) to determine whether the $PM_{2.5}$-induced cardiac dysfunction is age-dependent; (2) to examine whether the above-mentioned effects could be restored after $PM_{2.5}$ exposure withdrawal; (3) to determine the potential mechanism of susceptibility to $PM_{2.5}$ exposure.

Results

Exposure to $PM_{2.5}$ elevates heart rate and systolic blood pressure of 10-month-old mice

For the heart rate of 4-week-old mice, 4 weeks of $PM_{2.5}$ exposure caused a significant increase compared with pre-exposure but a non-significant increase compared with age-matched control group (Fig. 1a). The systolic blood pressure of 4-week-old mice was not affected by $PM_{2.5}$ during 4 weeks of exposure (Fig. 1b). Neither heart rate nor the systolic blood pressure of 4-month-old mice was changed after $PM_{2.5}$ exposure within the 4 weeks observation period. For 10-month-old mice, 2 weeks of $PM_{2.5}$ exposure caused a significant increase in the heart rate compared with pre-exposure or age-matched control group (Fig. 1a). The heart rate of 10-month-old mice was significantly higher than 4-month-old mice after $PM_{2.5}$ exposure (Fig. 1a). The systolic blood pressure of 10-month-old mice was elevated after 4 weeks of exposure compared with age-matched control group (Fig. 1b). The systolic blood pressure of 10-month-old mice was significantly higher than both 4-week-old and 4-month-old mice after $PM_{2.5}$ exposure (Fig. 1b). Interestingly, the heart rate of 10-month-old mice decreased to base level after withdrawal from $PM_{2.5}$ exposure for 2 weeks (Fig. 1c). The systolic blood pressure of 10-month-old mice was almost completely restored after withdrawal from $PM_{2.5}$ exposure for only 1 week (Fig. 1d).

Exposure to $PM_{2.5}$ induces cardiac dysfunction in mice

The data obtained from echocardiography are presented in Fig. 2. The ratio of peak early diastolic flow velocities and peak early motion wave values (E/E') was significantly changed in mice at different ages after $PM_{2.5}$ exposure (Fig. 2a). The E/E' of 10-month-old mice and 4-week-old mice was restored after withdrawal from $PM_{2.5}$ exposure for 2 weeks (Fig. 2c, e). $PM_{2.5}$ exposure caused a significant decrease in the ejection fraction (EF) of 10-month-old mice compared to age-matched control group. (Fig. 2b). The EF of 10-month-old mice was significantly lower than both 4-week-old and 4-month-old mice after $PM_{2.5}$ exposure (Fig. 2b). The EF of

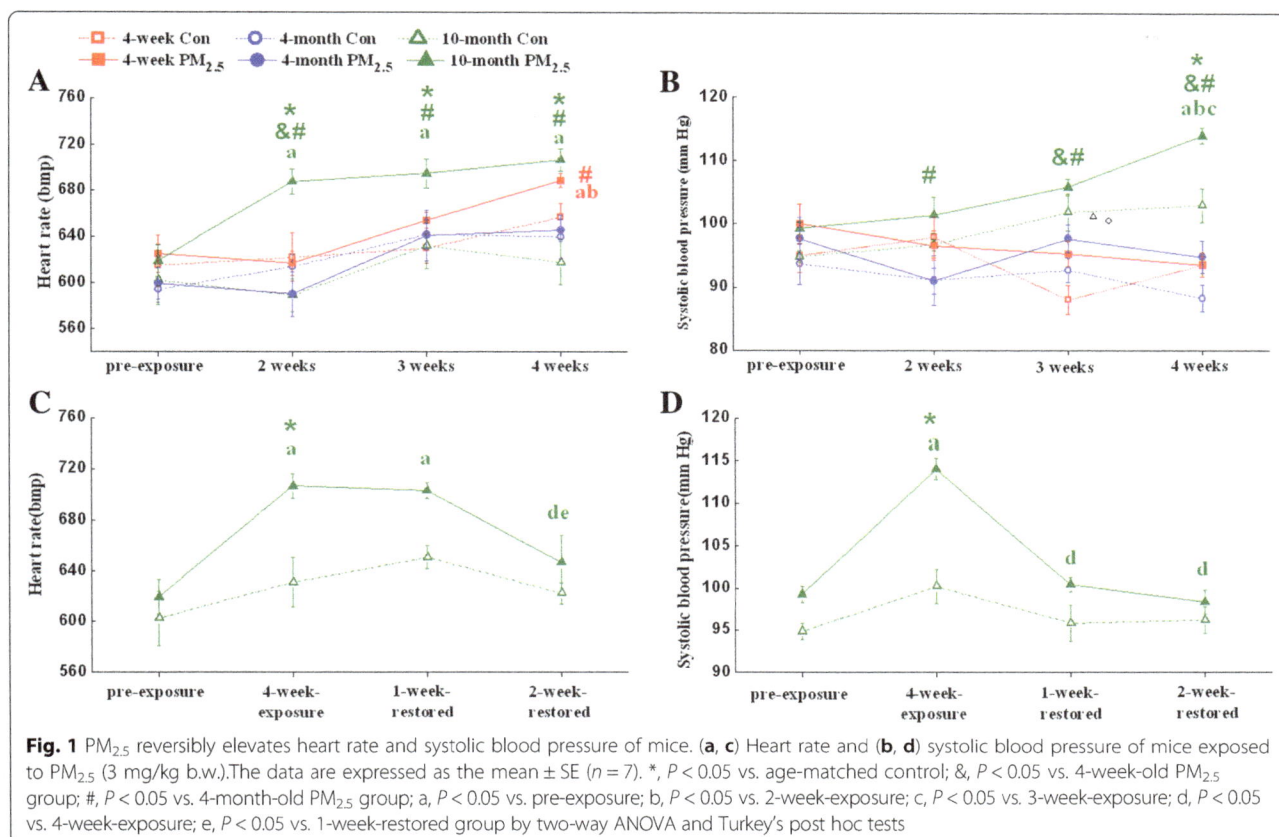

Fig. 1 PM$_{2.5}$ reversibly elevates heart rate and systolic blood pressure of mice. (**a**, **c**) Heart rate and (**b**, **d**) systolic blood pressure of mice exposed to PM$_{2.5}$ (3 mg/kg b.w.).The data are expressed as the mean ± SE ($n = 7$). *, $P < 0.05$ vs. age-matched control; &, $P < 0.05$ vs. 4-week-old PM$_{2.5}$ group; #, $P < 0.05$ vs. 4-month-old PM$_{2.5}$ group; a, $P < 0.05$ vs. pre-exposure; b, $P < 0.05$ vs. 2-week-exposure; c, $P < 0.05$ vs. 3-week-exposure; d, $P < 0.05$ vs. 4-week-exposure; e, $P < 0.05$ vs. 1-week-restored group by two-way ANOVA and Turkey's post hoc tests

10-month-old mice was restored after withdrawal from PM$_{2.5}$ exposure for 1 week (Fig. 2d).

Exposure to PM$_{2.5}$ induces cardiac fibrosis in 4-week-old and 10-month-old mice

Histological examination of PM$_{2.5}$-exposed mouse hearts stained with Masson's trichrome revealed increased collagen deposition/myocardial fibrosis (Fig. 3). The hearts from PM$_{2.5}$-exposed 4-week-old and 10-month-old mice showed interstitial fibrosis distributed diffusely across the left ventricular free wall (Fig. 3a). Quantification of the fibrotic area demonstrated that fibrosis was significantly greater in the PM$_{2.5}$-exposed 4-week-old and 10-month-old mice than the corresponding control mice (Fig. 3b). The fibrotic area in hearts from 10-month-old mice was significantly greater than in hearts form 4-month-old mice after PM$_{2.5}$ exposure (Fig. 3b). The fibrosis area reduced in 10-month-old mice after withdrawal from exposure to PM$_{2.5}$ for 2 weeks (Fig. 3A, e-f; C). The fibrosis area was reduced in 4-week-old mice after withdrawal from exposure to PM$_{2.5}$ for 2 weeks (Fig. 3A, i-j; D).

Exposure to PM$_{2.5}$ induces cardiac fibrosis marker expression in 4-week-old and 10-month-old mice

PM$_{2.5}$ exposure of 4-week-old and 10-month-old mice led to increased transcription of Col1a1 and Col3a1, the major structural collagen in the myocardium, suggesting that PM$_{2.5}$ exposure alters gene expression consistent with a profibrotic phenotype (Fig. 4a, b). Western blot analyses confirmed increased protein expression of Col1a1 and Col3a1 in PM$_{2.5}$-exposed 10-month-old mice and Col1a1 in PM$_{2.5}$-exposed 4-week-old (Fig. 4c, d). Furthermore, consistent with above results regarding cardiac dysfunction and collagen deposition, the expression of Col1a1 and Col3a1 of 10-month-old and 4-week-old mice were restored after withdrawal from exposure to PM$_{2.5}$ for one or 2 weeks (Fig. 4c-f).

PM$_{2.5}$ induces ROS in hearts of 4-week-old and 10-month-old mice

The generation of ROS induced by PM$_{2.5}$ was detected by photocatalysis using an ROS-sensitive probe – 2',7'-dichlorodihydrofluorescein diacetate (DCFHDA, Invitrogen). The ROS levels in the hearts of 4-week-old and 10-month-old mice exposed to PM$_{2.5}$ were significantly increased compared to those of the corresponding control mice and 4-month-old mice after PM$_{2.5}$ exposure (Fig. 5).

PM$_{2.5}$ induces inflammation and oxidative damage in hearts and lungs of 4-week-old and 10-month-old mice

In order to indicate whether the occurrence of oxidative damage is a consequence of the local oxidative stress of

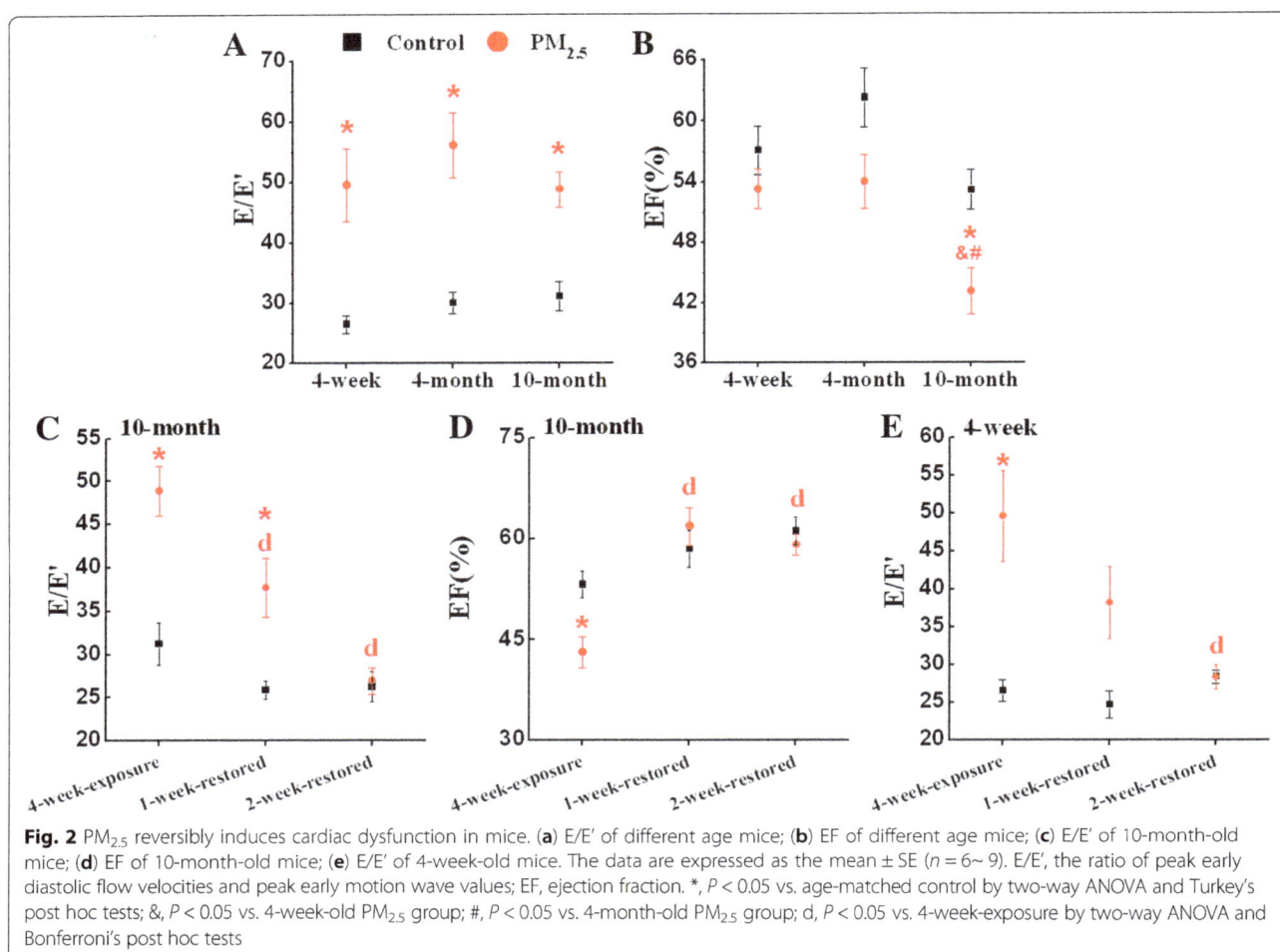

Fig. 2 PM$_{2.5}$ reversibly induces cardiac dysfunction in mice. (**a**) E/E' of different age mice; (**b**) EF of different age mice; (**c**) E/E' of 10-month-old mice; (**d**) EF of 10-month-old mice; (**e**) E/E' of 4-week-old mice. The data are expressed as the mean ± SE (n = 6~9). E/E', the ratio of peak early diastolic flow velocities and peak early motion wave values; EF, ejection fraction. *, P < 0.05 vs. age-matched control by two-way ANOVA and Turkey's post hoc tests; &, P < 0.05 vs. 4-week-old PM$_{2.5}$ group; #, P < 0.05 vs. 4-month-old PM$_{2.5}$ group; d, P < 0.05 vs. 4-week-exposure by two-way ANOVA and Bonferroni's post hoc tests

lungs, we detected the mRNA levels of TGFβ1 and interleukin 6 (IL-6), and MDA levels in hearts and lungs. The mRNA levels of TGFβ1 were significantly increased in both lungs and hearts of 4-week-old and 10-month-old mice after PM$_{2.5}$ exposure (Fig. 6a, b). The highest expression of TGFβ1 mRNA was observed in hearts of 10-month-old mice after PM$_{2.5}$ exposure (Fig. 6b). The mRNA levels of IL-6 were significantly increased in lungs of all exposed groups mice and in hearts of 4-week-old and 10-month-old mice after PM$_{2.5}$ exposure (Fig. 6c, d).

The MDA levels in the hearts and lungs of 4-week-old and 10-month-old mice exposed to PM$_{2.5}$ were significantly higher than in aged-matched controls (Fig. 7a, b). The MDA levels in hearts and lungs of 10-month-old mice decreased to base level after withdrawal from exposure to PM$_{2.5}$ for 1 week (Fig. 7c-d). The MDA levels of 4-week-old mice did not change compared to corresponding controls after withdrawal from exposure to PM$_{2.5}$ for one or 2 weeks (Fig. 7e-f).

PM$_{2.5}$-induced cardiac fibrosis is associated with NOX4-ROS-TGFβ1-Smad signaling

Western blotting was used to detect the protein expression of possible signaling molecules involved in PM$_{2.5}$-induced cardiac fibrosis. NOX-4 and TGFβ1 protein levels were significantly increased in the hearts of 4-week-old and 10-month-old mice after PM$_{2.5}$ exposure (Fig. 8a-c). After exposure for 4 weeks, PM$_{2.5}$ treatment activated Smad3 in the hearts of 4-week-old and 10-month-old mice (Fig. 8a & d). No significant differences in the protein levels of NOX-4 or TGFβ1 or in the phosphorylation of Smad3 were observed in the hearts of 4-month-old mice compared with the control group (Fig. 8).

Discussion

The results of our present study provide evidence that PM$_{2.5}$ aspiration induced cardiac dysfunction and fibrosis in 4-week-old and 10-month-old mice, and the adverse effects could be resolved after PM$_{2.5}$ exposure withdrawal. Cardiovascular disease is the leading cause

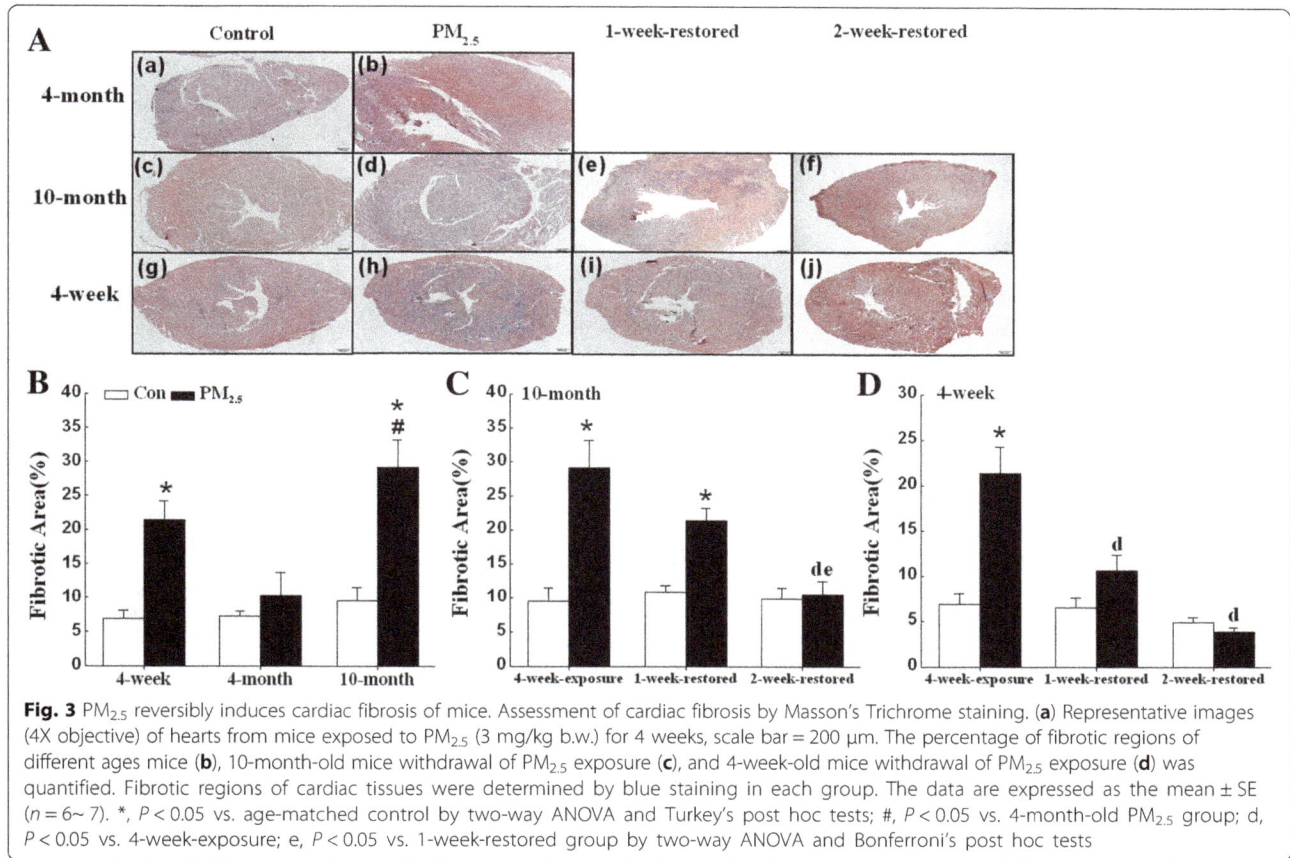

Fig. 3 PM$_{2.5}$ reversibly induces cardiac fibrosis of mice. Assessment of cardiac fibrosis by Masson's Trichrome staining. (**a**) Representative images (4X objective) of hearts from mice exposed to PM$_{2.5}$ (3 mg/kg b.w.) for 4 weeks, scale bar = 200 μm. The percentage of fibrotic regions of different ages mice (**b**), 10-month-old mice withdrawal of PM$_{2.5}$ exposure (**c**), and 4-week-old mice withdrawal of PM$_{2.5}$ exposure (**d**) was quantified. Fibrotic regions of cardiac tissues were determined by blue staining in each group. The data are expressed as the mean ± SE ($n = 6 \sim 7$). *, $P < 0.05$ vs. age-matched control by two-way ANOVA and Turkey's post hoc tests; #, $P < 0.05$ vs. 4-month-old PM$_{2.5}$ group; d, $P < 0.05$ vs. 4-week-exposure; e, $P < 0.05$ vs. 1-week-restored group by two-way ANOVA and Bonferroni's post hoc tests

of mortality in the advanced world, and age is an important determinant of cardiac function. The morbidity and mortality rates associated with PM$_{2.5}$-induced cardiovascular disease are significantly higher in the elderly than in adults. Based on preliminary epidemiologic evidence, infants less than 2 years old and adults over 65 years old are the most susceptible subpopulations to PM [21]. Numerous findings support the association between PM exposure and electrocardiogram abnormalities in elderly subjects [22]. Several epidemiological studies have demonstrated associations between acute and chronic PM$_{2.5}$ exposure and the elevation of heart rate and blood pressure, especially among elderly or susceptible individuals [5, 23, 24]. However, the effects of childhood air pollution exposure on cardiovascular risk in human populations are not well defined.

Most studies on the cardiac effects of PM are performed in susceptible models, such as hypertensive [25, 26], ligation of coronary arteries [27], and gene deficient animals [28, 29]. In the present study, 4-week-old, 4-month-old, and 10-month-old mice were employed as juvenile, adult, and older subpopulations, respectively. It is reported that during the juvenile stages, the valve, left atrial size, left ventricular end-diastolic dimension, aortic root, and ascending aorta dimensions show linear growth and, during the adult stages, the dimensions plateau [30]. There is evidence for atrial hypertrophy and dilatation, and LV wall thickness increases with age in older mice. Other age-dependent cellular changes reported in aging rodents include fibroblast proliferation, collagen accumulation, and interstitial fibrosis in both the atria and the ventricles [31]. Our data revealed that subchronic exposure to PM$_{2.5}$ significantly increased the heart rate and systolic blood pressure in older mice. Furthermore, the PM$_{2.5}$ effects on heart rate and blood pressure of 10-month-old mice were reversible. This finding is consistent with previous studies showing that chronic inhalation exposure to concentrated ambient particulate matter increased heart rate and blood pressure in C57BL/6 mice [7, 32]. Ying et al. reported that chronic exposure to concentrated ambient particulate matter (CAP) significantly increased blood pressure of spontaneously hypertensive rats, and withdrawal from CAP exposure restored blood pressure [26]. In combination, these data provide strong evidence that exposure to PM$_{2.5}$ may have significant effects on elderly because they are more susceptible to cardiovascular disease.

Wold and colleagues reported that a 9-month inhalation exposure to CAP resulted in systolic and diastolic dysfunction [7]. In utero and early life exposure to diesel

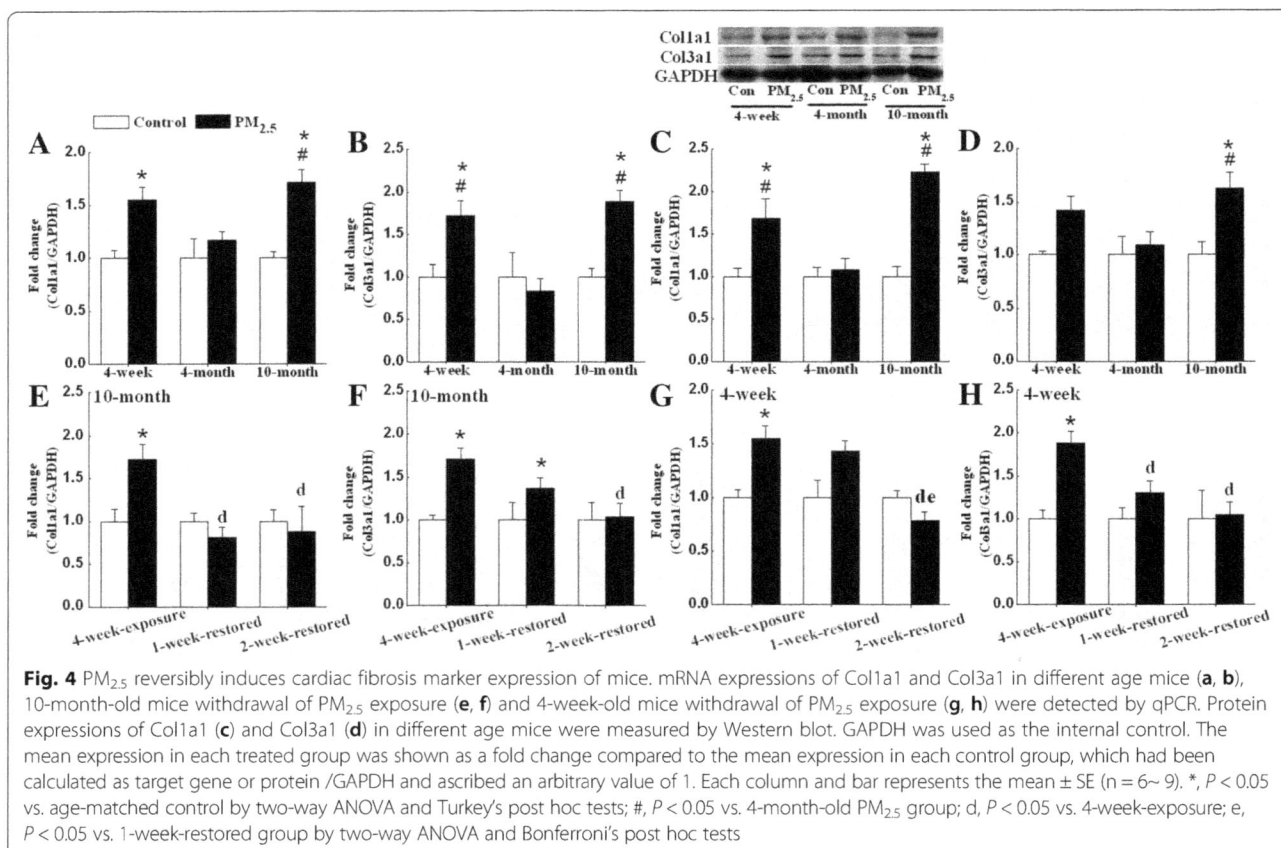

Fig. 4 PM$_{2.5}$ reversibly induces cardiac fibrosis marker expression of mice. mRNA expressions of Col1a1 and Col3a1 in different age mice (**a**, **b**), 10-month-old mice withdrawal of PM$_{2.5}$ exposure (**e**, **f**) and 4-week-old mice withdrawal of PM$_{2.5}$ exposure (**g**, **h**) were detected by qPCR. Protein expressions of Col1a1 (**c**) and Col3a1 (**d**) in different age mice were measured by Western blot. GAPDH was used as the internal control. The mean expression in each treated group was shown as a fold change compared to the mean expression in each control group, which had been calculated as target gene or protein /GAPDH and ascribed an arbitrary value of 1. Each column and bar represents the mean ± SE (n = 6~ 9). *, $P < 0.05$ vs. age-matched control by two-way ANOVA and Turkey's post hoc tests; #, $P < 0.05$ vs. 4-month-old PM$_{2.5}$ group; d, $P < 0.05$ vs. 4-week-exposure; e, $P < 0.05$ vs. 1-week-restored group by two-way ANOVA and Bonferroni's post hoc tests

exhaust or PM$_{2.5}$ induces adult cardiac dysfunction [10, 11]. In the present study, the hearts of PM$_{2.5}$-exposed mice of different ages displayed a phenotype of diastolic dysfunction, indicated by the index of E/E' ratios. The E/E' ratio is a reliable index for detecting diastolic dysfunction [33]. EF is a basic parameter that assess systolic functions of the heart. Decreases in EF suggest that subchronic exposure to PM$_{2.5}$ induced systolic dysfunctions only in 10-month-old mice. Furthermore, PM$_{2.5}$-induced cardiac dysfunction of 10-month-old and 4-week-old mice could be restored after PM$_{2.5}$ withdrawal. It is in accordance with previous study that withdrawal from CAP exposure restored cardiac function in spontaneously hypertensive rats [26]. Some pharmacological agents/genetic modification could reduce PM$_{2.5}$-induced hypertension in rats [8, 34]. It indicated that PM$_{2.5}$-induced cardiac dysfunction is reversible.

We found that 10-month-old and 4-week-old mice developed more fibrosis following PM$_{2.5}$-exposure. The impairment in heart function observed in 4-week-old and 10-month-old mice correlated with increases of collagen deposition. The increases in fibrillar collagen in the heart interstitium contribute to tissue stiffness, and increases in collagen deposition may contribute to

impaired heart function. We observed PM$_{2.5}$-induced fibrosis changes in 4-week-old and 10-month-old mice accompanied by increases in the gene expression of major structural collagen types (Col1a1 and Col3a1) in the myocardium. Other studies have documented similar results with exposure to concentrated ambient PM [7, 35] and carbon black [9].

The heart rate, blood pressure, cardiac functional and structural changes, and molecular marker data showed that older mice are the most susceptible group to PM$_{2.5}$. Similar results were observed with secondhand smoke or lipopolysaccharide (LPS) treatment. Secondhand smoke or LPS induce more cardiac dysfunction, fibrosis, inflammation, and oxidative stress in aged mice than in young mice [36, 37]. Aging-associated cardiac abnormalities are manifested as diastolic cardiac dysfunction, cardiac hypertrophy, and fibrosis, as well as impaired contractile function [38, 39]. The negative effects of PM$_{2.5}$ on older mice might accelerate the development of aging. Furthermore, our data showed that 4-week-old mice were more susceptible than 4-month-old mice. PM$_{2.5}$ exposure induced cardiac fibrosis, elevated Col1a1 and Col3a1 expression in 4-week-old mice, but not in 4-month-old mice. One possible reason for the difference in susceptibility to PM$_{2.5}$ of mice is their

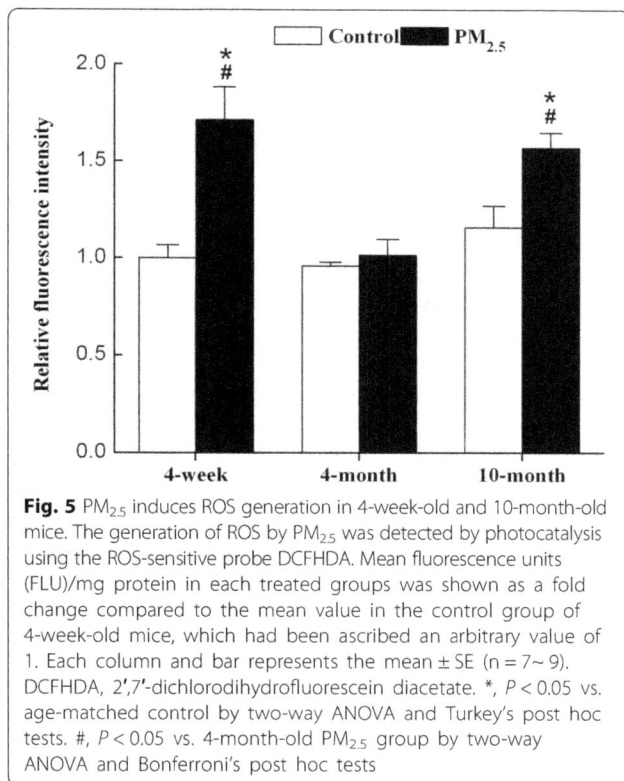

Fig. 5 $PM_{2.5}$ induces ROS generation in 4-week-old and 10-month-old mice. The generation of ROS by $PM_{2.5}$ was detected by photocatalysis using the ROS-sensitive probe DCFHDA. Mean fluorescence units (FLU)/mg protein in each treated groups was shown as a fold change compared to the mean value in the control group of 4-week-old mice, which had been ascribed an arbitrary value of 1. Each column and bar represents the mean ± SE (n = 7~ 9). DCFHDA, 2',7'-dichlorodihydrofluorescein diacetate. *, $P < 0.05$ vs. age-matched control by two-way ANOVA and Turkey's post hoc tests. #, $P < 0.05$ vs. 4-month-old $PM_{2.5}$ group by two-way ANOVA and Bonferroni's post hoc tests

differences in estrogen levels. It is well established that the incidence of cardiovascular disease is reduced in females prior to menopause, which may be due to estrogen levels [40]. Estrogen protects cardiomyocytes against angiotensin II-induced sensitization of hypertension [41]. In the present study, we observed that $PM_{2.5}$ elevated non-significantly the estradiol 2 (E2) levels of 4-week-old and 4-month-old mice. The E2 levels of 10-month-old mice were lower than 4-month-old mice in $PM_{2.5}$ groups (Additional file 2: Figure S2). It still needs further research to study whether male mice display different age-dependent responses from female mice. Another possible mechanism of $PM_{2.5}$-induced cardiac functional changes might involve the role of ROS. Oxidative stress is increased in human heart failure and animal models of cardiac hypertrophy and fibrosis [42]. The heart consists of various types of cells, such as cardiomyocytes and nonmyocytes, including fibroblasts, endothelial cells, smooth muscle cells, and immune system–related cells [43]. ROS could be produced in cardiomyocytes or endothelial cells [44]. Our recent study has shown that $PM_{2.5}$ dose-dependently induced ROS production in H9C2 cells [45]. In the present study, $PM_{2.5}$ induced ROS generation in hearts and lungs of 4-week-old and 10-month-old mice. These observations indicated that ROS and oxidative stress might play important roles in $PM_{2.5}$-induced cardiac fibrosis.

Different potential mechanisms for PM-associated cardiovascular disease have been hypothesized as either activated by direct effects of pollutants on the cardiovascular system, or by indirect effects due to pulmonary oxidative stress and inflammatory responses [46]. In the present study, we observed the elevation of TGFβ1 and IL-6 mRNA expression and MDA levels in lungs and hearts of 4-week-old and 10-month-old mice. Although this does not exclude the possibility of direct particle translocation, it is possible that $PM_{2.5}$ triggers the release of soluble inflammatory mediators from the lungs and subsequently causes cardiac inflammation through systemic inflammatory responses. Similarly, it is reported that extra-pulmonary effects due to carbon nanoparticles inhalation are dominated by indirect effects (particle-cell interactions in the lung) rather than direct effects (translocated carbon nanoparticles) [47].

ROS generation has been detected in rat ventricular myocytes exposed to diesel exhaust, and it is likely mediated through NADPH oxidase-dependent pathways [48]. NADPH oxidases are multisubunit enzymes that are largely distributed within heart cells [49]. NOX-4 is essential for the differentiation of human cardiac fibroblasts into myofibroblasts [42]. A similar phenomenon was observed in the present study by the examination of NOX-4 expression and direct measurement of intracellular ROS as DCFHDA-fluorescence in mice. Following activation, membrane-bound NADPH oxidase initiates single-electron transfers to molecular oxygen, resulting in the formation of ROS [50]. Our data showed that NOX-4 expression was increased in 4-week-old and 10-month-old mice after $PM_{2.5}$ exposure. The increase in NOX-4 expression was accompanied by the elevation of TGFβ1 protein expression. ROS stimulates the release and activation of cytokines, such as TGFβ1 [51]. TGF-β1 is expressed and released by many cell types, including cardiomyocytes, cardiac fibroblasts, and immune cells [52]. Cardiac tissue fibrosis in mice hearts is associated with an increased expression of the profibrotic marker TGF-β1 in cardiac macrophages [53]. TGFβ1 is upregulated in various experimental models of cardiac hypertrophy [54], and functional blockade of TGFβ1 prevents cardiac interstitial fibrosis induced by pressure overload in rats [55]. However, TGFβ1 upregulates the expression of NADPH oxidase and induces further ROS generation [42]. Hu and colleagues suggested positive feedback between TGFβ1, NADPH oxidase-mediated ROS generation, and LOX-1 [56]. Among numerous fibrotic signals, TGFβ1 is reported to be a key fibrogenic mediator. Smad2 and Smad3 are well-documented downstream mediators of TGFβ1-induced fibrosis, and activations of Smad2 and Smad3 are known to stimulate matrix-component synthesis, such as collagens [13]. TGF-β1 activates Smad-mediated signaling pathways on binding to TGF-β receptors on cardiomyocytes and cardiac fibroblasts [57]. In our study, Smad3 was activated in both 4-week-old and 10-month-old mice after PM$_{2.5}$ exposure. This finding implied that PM$_{2.5}$ induced cardiac fibrosis might involve the TGFβ1-Smad pathway.

Many studies have documented that Zn and Mn can enter systemic circulation and lead to lung fibrosis and cardiovascular disease [58–60]. In our latest study, we found that PM$_{2.5}$-bound metals could reach and deposit in the heart with a developmental window-dependent property. The content of Zn increased significantly in hearts of 4-week-old and 10-month-old mice. The contents of Mn and Cd increased significantly in hearts of 10-month-old mice [61]. It is speculated that heavy metals, such as Zn, Mn, and Cd, might be responsible for PM$_{2.5}$ induced cardiac toxicity. However, further experiments are needed to confirm the hypothesis.

There are several limitations to our study. The first limitation is the exposure method. Although oropharyngeal aspiration has been commonly used for experimental PM exposure [62–64]. Because it delivers a bolus high dose of particles to the lung, rather than repeated inhalation at lower doses, it may produce different effects in the lungs and hearts compare with exposure by inhalation. An additional limitation pertains to the low sensitivity of the tail-cuff method used to assay heart rate and blood pressure in this study. It is reported that

tail-cuff readings are on average 39 mmHg lower than telemetric measurements for systolic blood pressure [65]. We exerted considerable care in the measurements with careful training of the mice. The data of each animal were measured as the mean of at least 5 successful measurements.

Conclusion

In this report, we provide evidence that PM$_{2.5}$ exposure induced cardiac dysfunction in mice at all ages tested, elevated heart rate and blood pressure in 10-month-old mice, and caused cardiac fibrosis in 10-month-old and 4-week-old mice. In combination, these data provide strong evidence that exposure to PM$_{2.5}$ has significant effects on juveniles and the elderly because they are more susceptible to cardiovascular disease. Furthermore, all the above adverse effects in 10-month-old and 4-week-old mice could be restored after withdrawal PM$_{2.5}$ exposure for 2 weeks. The mechanisms by which PM$_{2.5}$ exposure resulted in cardiac lesions might involve the generation of oxidative stress and inflammation in lungs and the activation of TGFβ1-Smad pathway.

Methods
Collection of PM$_{2.5}$ samples
Sampling was performed between 2012 and 2013 in Taiyuan, Northern China. The PM$_{2.5}$ samples were

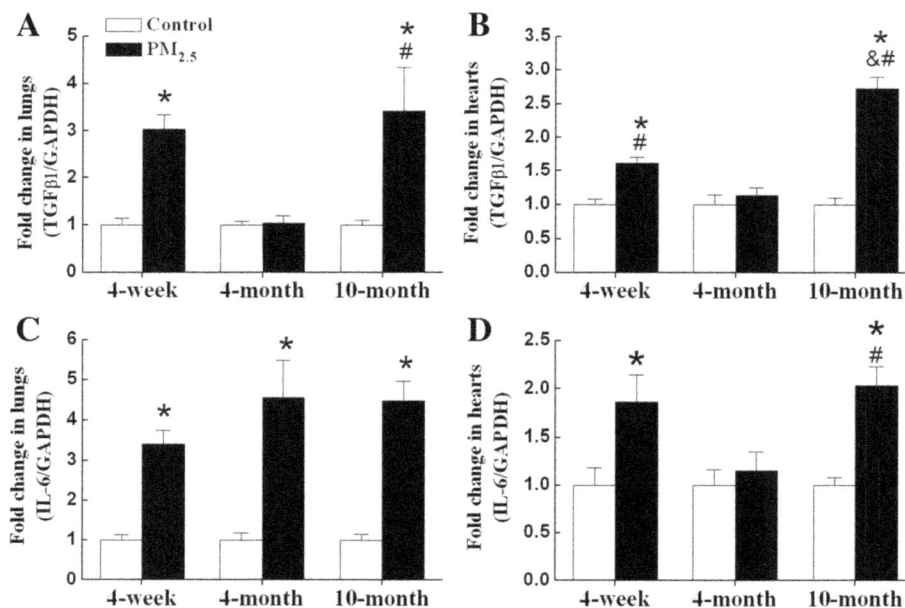

Fig. 6 PM$_{2.5}$ induces mRNA expression of TGFβ1 and IL-6 in lungs and hearts of mice. mRNA expression of TGFβ1 and IL-6 in lungs (**a**, **c**) and hearts (**b**, **d**) were detected by qPCR. GAPDH was used as the internal control. The mean expression in each treated group was shown as a fold change compared to the mean expression in each control group, which had been calculated as target gene /GAPDH and ascribed an arbitrary value of 1. Each column and bar represents the mean ± SE (n = 6–9). TGFβ1, transforming growth factor β1; IL-6, interleukin-6. *$P < 0.05$ vs. age-matched control by two-way ANOVA and Turkey's post hoc tests; & $P < 0.05$ vs. 4-week-old PM$_{2.5}$ group; # $P < 0.05$ vs. 4-month-old PM$_{2.5}$ group by two-way ANOVA and Bonferroni's post hoc tests

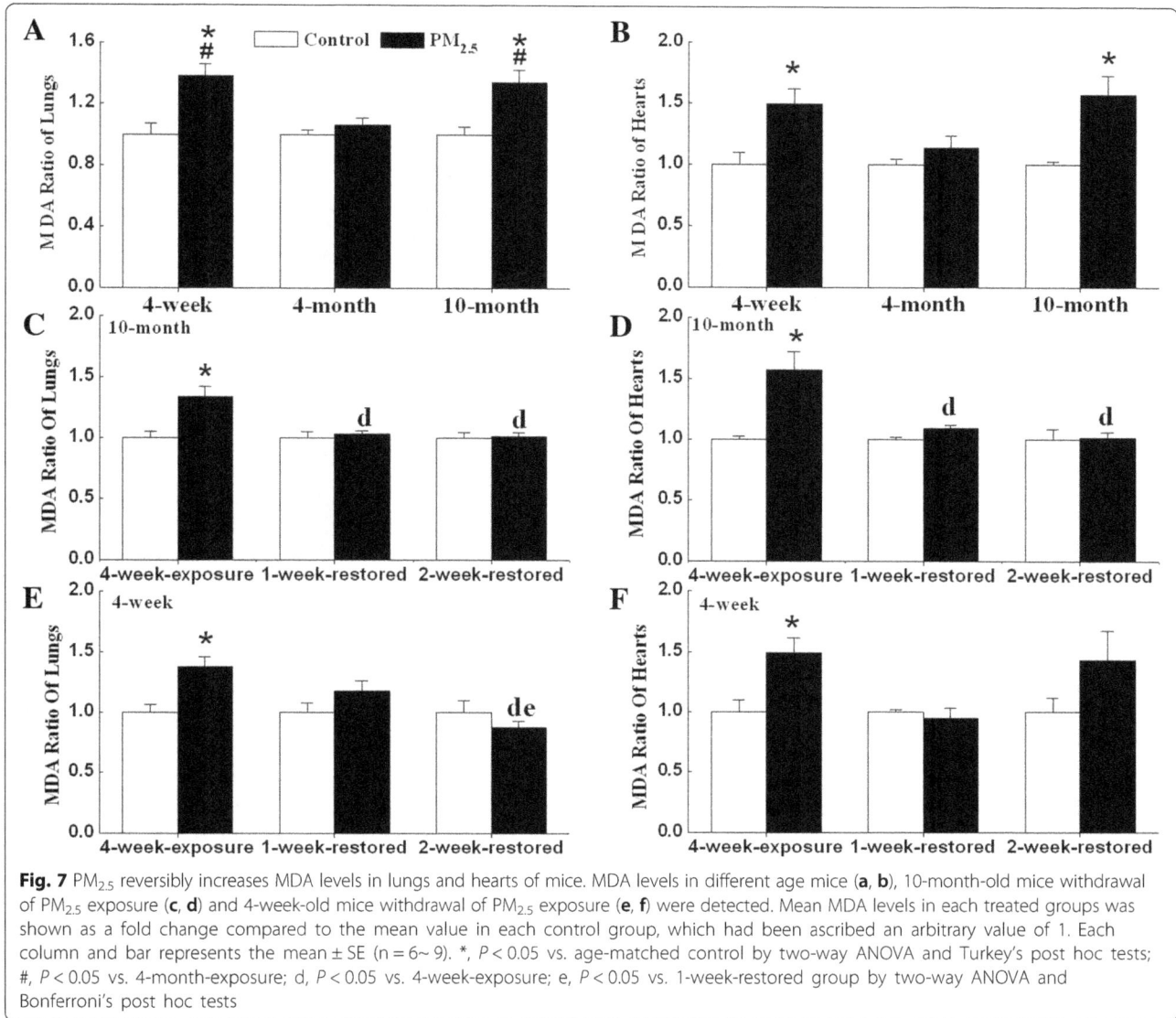

Fig. 7 $PM_{2.5}$ reversibly increases MDA levels in lungs and hearts of mice. MDA levels in different age mice (**a, b**), 10-month-old mice withdrawal of $PM_{2.5}$ exposure (**c, d**) and 4-week-old mice withdrawal of $PM_{2.5}$ exposure (**e, f**) were detected. Mean MDA levels in each treated groups was shown as a fold change compared to the mean value in each control group, which had been ascribed an arbitrary value of 1. Each column and bar represents the mean ± SE (n = 6~ 9). *, $P < 0.05$ vs. age-matched control by two-way ANOVA and Turkey's post hoc tests; #, $P < 0.05$ vs. 4-month-exposure; d, $P < 0.05$ vs. 4-week-exposure; e, $P < 0.05$ vs. 1-week-restored group by two-way ANOVA and Bonferroni's post hoc tests

collected onto quartz filters (Φ90 mm, Munktell, Falun, Dalarna, Sweden) with PM middle-volume air samplers (TH-150CIII, Wuhan, China). Details of sample collection and components analysis of $PM_{2.5}$ have been previously described [66] and provided in Additional file 3: Table S1-Table S4 in Supporting information.

Animals and exposure

Female C57BL/6 mice were purchased from the Junke Biological Engineering Co., LTD (Nanjing, China). Animals were housed in individual stainless steel cages under standard conditions (24 ± 2 °C and 50 ± 5% humidity) with a 12 h light–dark cycle in SPF conditions. The protocol of animal procedures was conducted in accordance with the National Institutes of Health Guide for the Care and Use of Laboratory Animals and was

approved by the Institutional Animal Care and Use Committee of Shanxi University.

In *study-1*, C57BL/6 mice at 4 weeks, 4 months and 10 months were randomized into two subgroups. The mice received oropharyngeal aspiration of 0.9% saline (control groups) or 3 mg/kg. b.w. $PM_{2.5}$ suspension (3 mg/ml, $PM_{2.5}$ groups) 15–30 μl depend on the body weight of each animal every other day for 4 weeks. When not being treated, the mice had free access to standard food and water. Mice were sacrificed 24 h after the final exposure.

In *study-2*, C57BL/6 mice at 4-week-old or 10-month-old were received oropharyngeal aspiration of 0.9% saline (controls) or 3 mg/kg. b.w. $PM_{2.5}$ suspension ($PM_{2.5}$ groups) every other day for 4 weeks. Mice were sacrificed 24 h, 1 week, or 2 weeks after the final exposure, respectively. The hearts and lungs were removed, and all

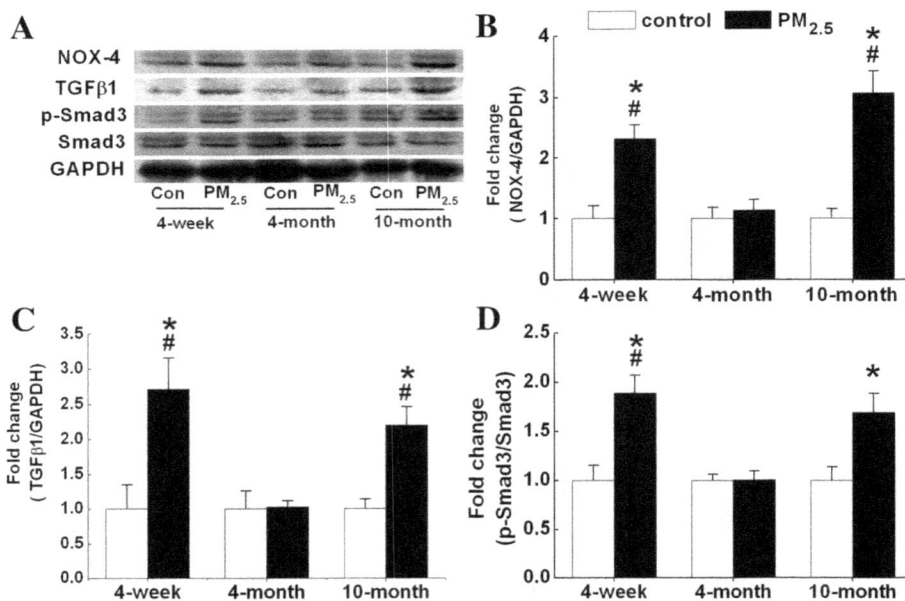

Fig. 8 PM$_{2.5}$-induced cardiac fibrosis is associated with NOX4-TGFβ1-Smad signaling. Protein levels were measured by Western blot. (**a**), Representative Western blot results of each protein. The protein levels of NOX-4 (**b**), TGFβ1 (**c**), and ratio of p-Smad3 and Smad 3 (**d**). Each column and bar represents the mean ± SE ($n = 3 \sim 6$). The mean expression in each treated group was shown as a fold change compared to the mean expression in each control group, which had been calculated as target protein /GAPDH and ascribed an arbitrary value of 1. NOX-4, NADPH oxidase 4; TGFβ1, transforming growth factor β1. *, $P < 0.05$ vs. age-matched control by two-way ANOVA and Turkey's post hoc tests; #, $P < 0.05$ vs. 4-month-exposure by two-way ANOVA and Bonferroni's post hoc tests

samples were fixed or quick frozen in liquid nitrogen and stored at − 80 °C.

Heart rate and blood pressure assay

Heart rate and blood pressure were measured using a standard tail-cuff system (BP-2010A System, Softron). The blood pressure and heart rate data of each mice were measured as the mean of at least 5 successful measurements.

Echocardiographic assessment

Heart function and structure were assessed by echocardiography using a Vevo 770™ ultrasound system (VisualSonics, Toronto, Ontario, Canada), which included a 21-MHz transducer. Mice were anesthetized with 2% isoflurane administered via a nose cone, were shaved from the chest, and were placed in the supine position on a hotplate. Echocardiography and off-line data analysis was performed by a single observer. The observer was blinded as to the age and group of mice being analyzed. Two-dimensional (2D) and M-mode echocardiography images were obtained from the parasternal region and viewed to measure left ventricular end-diastolic dimension (LVEDD), left ventricular end-systolic dimension (LVESD), posterior wall thickness in diastole (LVPWd), left ventricular end diastolic volume (LVEDV), and left ventricular end systolic volume (LVESV). Left

ventricle filling parameters were assessed from the ends of mitral leaflets in apical quadrilocular image, and peak early (E) and after (A) diastolic flow velocities were measured. Tissue Doppler assessment was conducted on apical quadrilocular image. Peak early motion (E') and peak after motion (A') wave values were measured. Ejection fraction (EF), fractional shortening (FS), E/A ratio, E'/A' ratio, and E/E' ratio were obtained using defined calculations. Each parameter was measured in at least 3 cycles, and mean figures were utilized. All measurements were performed offline using the Vevo 770™ system software (VisualSonics, Toronto, Ontario, Canada).

Histological analysis by Masson's trichrome staining

The cardiac tissue from mice of each group was rapidly removed, washed several times with 0.1 μM phosphate buffered saline (PBS, pH 7.4), fixed in 10% formalin for 24 h at room temperature, dehydrated by graded ethanol, and embedded in paraffin. Sections (5–6 μm-thick) were deparaffinized with xylene, stained with Masson's trichrome staining, and observed by microscopy. Quantitative planimetric analyses were performed on three successive sections per slide, and at least 7 sections from 3 consecutive slides per mouse were examined. Each image was digitized using a digital camera and analyzed under a research microscope (Olympus, Japan) using Image-Pro Plus software (version 5.0). The left ventricular cross-section collagen accumulation was quantified by the ratio of blue area to total myocardium area. All analyses were performed by an investigator blinded to the group assignments.

ROS detection

Fresh hearts were used to prepare a 10% (*w/v*) PBS homogenate. After centrifuging at 1000 g for 10 min at 4 °C, the supernatant was collected and used to evaluate reactive oxygen species (ROS) and protein content. In 96-well plates, 190 µL of the supernatant and 10 µL of 1 mM DCFHDA were added to each well. After incubating at 37 °C for 30 min in the dark, the fluorescence was read at 485 nm for excitation and 530 nm for emission with a fluorescent plate reader (Varioskan Flash, Thermo Scientific, America). The results were calculated as the fluorescence units (FLU)/mg protein. The value of the 4-week-old mice in control group was set to 1.

Oxidative stress analysis

The heart or lung tissues were homogenized and centrifuged, and the supernatants were collected for biomarker and protein concentration determination. The level of the lipid peroxidation product malondialdehyde (MDA) was measured using commercial kits (Nanjing Jiancheng Bioengineering Institute, Nanjing, China).

Quantitative real-time PCR

Total RNA was isolated using TRIzol Reagent (TaKaRa, Dalian, China) according to the manufacturer's instructions. Total RNA was then treated with DNase I (TaKaRa, Dalian, China), and cDNA was synthesized using a First Strand cDNA Synthesis kit (TaKaRa, Dalian, China) The cDNA product was stored at − 80 °C until used.

Real-time quantitative PCR (qPCR) was performed using an IQ5 Real-Time PCR System (Bio-Rad, USA) and SYBR Green qPCR Master Mix kit (Takara, Dalian, China). The primers are listed in Additional file 3: Table S5. The cycling conditions were as follows: 3 min at 95 ° C, 40 cycles of 20 s at 94 °C, 20 s at 55–60 °C, and 20 s at 72 °C. The threshold cycle (Ct) values for the experimental samples were plotted onto the dilution series standard curve. The target quantities were calculated from separate standard curves generated for each experiment. The relative expression values were then determined by dividing the quantities of the target sequence of interest with the quantity obtained for GAPDH as an internal reference gene. The qPCR was repeated three times for each gene.

Western blot analysis

Proteins were extracted in ice-cold lysis buffer (1% Nonidet P-40, 1 mM EDTA, 125 mM sodium fluoride, 0.5 mM sodium vanadate, 2.5 µg/mL of aprotinin, 5 µg/mL of pepstatin, 50 µg/mL of leupeptin, 25 µM PMSF, and 25 µg/mL of trypsin inhibitor). The protein concentration was determined according to the Bradford method using BSA as the standard protein [67]. Sodium dodecyl sulfate–polyacrylamide gel electrophoresis was performed on 50 µg protein samples using 12% resolving/4% stacking Tris-HCl gels. Electrophoresis proteins were transferred to nitrocellulose membranes using Bio-Rad Mini Trans-Blot Electrophoretic Transfer Cell Instruments. Membranes were blocked in 3% BSA solution for 1 h at room temperature and incubated overnight at 4 °C with antibodies to targeted proteins (anti-GAPDH antibody, CST; anti-Col1a1 antibody, Bioss; anti-Col3a1 antibody, Bioss; anti-TGFβ1 antibody, Proteintech; anti- NADPH oxidase 4 (NOX-4)antibody, BBI; anti-Smad 3 antibody, BBI; and anti-P-Smad 3 antibody, BBI). After washing, the membranes were incubated with fluorescently labeled secondary antibody (1,5000) (IRDye 800CW goat anti-rabbit IgG (H + L), LI-COR), scanned, and detected with the LI-COR Odyssey Infrared Fluorescent System.

Statistical analysis

All data are expressed as the means ± standard error of the mean (SE). Comparison between groups in Fig. 1a and b was conducted using two-way repeated analysis of variance (ANOVA) followed by Tukey's post-test within each x-axis time-point across all groups or Tukey's post-test within each treatment group across x-axis time-points. Two-way non-repeated ANOVA followed by Tukey's post-test within each group across the x-axis time-points or Bonferroni's post-test within each x-axis time-point across the control and $PM_{2.5}$ groups were used to compare between groups in others figures. Differences for all tests were considered significant when $P < 0.05$.

Additional files

Additional file 1: Figure S1. $PM_{2.5}$ induces collagen mRNA (A) and protein (B) expression in H9C2 cells. (A) mRNA expressions of Col1a1 and Col3a1 in H9C2 cells were detected by qPCR. (B) The protein levels of Col1a1 and Col3a1 were detected by Western blot. GAPDH was used as the internal control. The mean expression in four seasons $PM_{2.5}$ treated group was shown as a fold change compared to the mean expression of control group, which had been calculated as target gene or protein /GAPDH and ascribed an arbitrary value of 1. Each column and bar represents the mean ± SE (n=3). Significantly different from control by one-way ANOVA with Tukey's post-test. * P<0.05 vs. control group; a P<0.05 vs. spring $PM_{2.5}$ group; b P<0.05 vs. summer $PM_{2.5}$ group; c P<0.05 vs. autumn $PM_{2.5}$ group. (TIF 440 kb)

Additional file 2: Figure S2. Estrogen levels in plasma of different age mice. Each column and bar represents the mean ± SE (n=6). # P<0.05 vs. 4-week-exposure by two-way ANOVA and Bonferroni's post hoc tests. (TIF 106 kb)

Additional file 3: Table S1. Contents of inorganic ion in $PM_{2.5}$ samples from different seasons (unit: µg/m³). **Table S2.** Element contents in $PM_{2.5}$

samples from different seasons (unit: ng/m^3). **Table S3.** Contents of polycyclic aromatic hydrocarbons (PAHs) in PM$_{2.5}$ samples from different seasons (unit: ng/m^3). **Table S4.** Carbon contents in PM$_{2.5}$ samples from different seasons (unit: μg/m^3). **Table S5.** Sequences of primers used in real-time PCR. (DOCX 35 kb)

Abbreviations
ANOVA: Analysis of variance; bpm: Beats per minute; cDNA: Complimentary deoxyribonucleic acid; Col1a1: Collagen I; Col3a1: Collagen III; DCFHDA: 2',7 dichlorodihydro fluorescein diacetate; DMEM: Dulbecco's modified eagle's medium; E/E': Ratio of peak early diastolic flow velocities and peak early motion wave values; EF: Ejection fraction; GAPDH: Glyceraldehye 3-phosphatede hydrogenase; IL-6: Interleukin 6; LPS: Lipopolysaccharide; LV: Left ventricle; mRNA: Messenger ribonucleic acid; NOX-4: NADPH oxidase subunit 4; PM: Particulate matter; PM$_{2.5}$: Particulate matter with a diameter of 2.5 μm or less; qRT-PCR: Quantitative real time polymerase chain reaction; ROS: Reactive oxygen species; TGFβ1: Transforming growth factor β1

Acknowledgements
The authors thank Hao Li for the heart function assessment and data analysis using ultrasound (from Fuwai Hospital, National Center for Cardiovascular Diseases, China).

Funding
This research was supported by the National Natural Science Foundation of China(21777091, 91543203, 21377076, 91543206, 11435002, 21222701), Research Project for Young Sanjin Scholarship of Shanxi, Program for the Outstanding Innovative Teams of Higher Learning Institutions of Shanxi, State Key Laboratory of Environmental Chemistry and Ecotoxicology, Research Center for Eco-Environmental Sciences, Chinese Academy of Sciences (KF2016–17), Research Project Supported by Shanxi Scholarship Council of China (015–006).

Authors' contributions
GQ, contributed to generating hypothesis and experimental design, conducted experiments, interpreted data, wrote the manuscript and is the primary author of the manuscript; JX, performed heart rate and blood pressure assay, H9C2 cell culture, ROS assay, qRT-PCR and Western experiments, contributed to preparation of figures; YZ, performed PM$_{2.5}$ collection and animal exposure; LG, contributed to supervising the entire project; RC, contributed to manuscript preparation. NS, contributed to supervising the entire project and was responsible for overall coordination of the project. All authors read and approved the final manuscript.

Competing interests
The authors declare that they have no competing interests.

Author details
[1]College of Environment and Resource, Research Center of Environment and Health, Shanxi University, Taiyuan, Shanxi 030006, People's Republic of China. [2]State Key Laboratory of Environmental Chemistry and Ecotoxicology, Research Center for Eco-Environmental Sciences, Chinese Academy of Sciences, Beijing 100085, People's Republic of China. [3]CAS Key Laboratory for Biomedical Effects of Nanomaterials and Nanosafety& CAS Center for Excellence in Nanoscience, Beijing Key Laboratory of Ambient Particles Health Effects and PreventionTechniques, National Center for Nanoscience & Technology of China, Beijing 100190, People's Republic of China.

References
1. Lelieveld J, Evans JS, Fnais M, Giannadaki D, Pozzer A. The contribution of outdoor air pollution sources to premature mortality on a global scale. Nature. 2015;525:367–71.
2. Brook RD, Franklin B, Cascio W, Hong Y, Howard G, Lipsett M, Luepker R, Mittleman M, Samet J, Smith SC. Air pollution and cardiovascular disease: a statement for healthcare professionals from the expert panel on population and prevention science of the american heart association. Circulation. 2004; 109:2655–71.
3. Shah AS, Langrish JP, Nair H, Mcallister DA, Hunter AL, Donaldson K, Newby DE, Mills NL. Global association of air pollution and heart failure: a systematic review and meta-analysis. Lancet. 2013;382:1039.
4. Bell ML, Ebisu K, Peng RD, Walker J, Samet JM, Zeger SL, Dominici F. Seasonal and regional short-term effects of fine particles on hospital admissions in 202 us counties, 1999–2005. Am J Epidemiol. 2008;168:1301–10.
5. Brook RD, Rajagopalan S, Pope CA, Brook JR, Bhatnagar A, Diezroux AV, Holguin F, Hong Y, Luepker RV, Mittleman MA. Particulate matter air pollution and cardiovascular disease. Circulation. 2010;121:2331–78.
6. Lee BJ, Kim B, Lee K. Air pollution exposure and cardiovascular disease. Toxicol Res. 2014;30:71.
7. Wold LE, Ying Z, Hutchinson KR, Velten M, Gorr MW, Velten C, Youtz DJ, Wang A, Lucchesi PA, Sun Q. Cardiovascular remodeling in response to long-term exposure to fine particulate matter air pollution. Circ Heart Failure. 2012;5:452.
8. Ying Z, Yue PX, Zhong M, Sun Q, Mikolaj M, Wang A, Brook RD, Chen LC, Rajagopalan S. Air pollution and cardiac remodeling: a role for rhoa/rho-kinase. Am J Physiol Heart Circ Physiol. 2009;296:H1540.
9. Tankersley CG, Champion HC, Takimoto E, Gabrielson K, Bedja D, Misra V, Elhaddad H, Rabold R, Mitzner W. Exposure to inhaled particulate matter impairs cardiac function in senescent mice. Ajp Regul Integr Comp Physiol. 2008;295:R252–63.
10. Gorr MW, Velten M, Nelin TD, Youtz DJ, Sun Q, Wold LE. Early life exposure to air pollution induces adult cardiac dysfunction. Am J Physiol Heart Circ Physiol. 2014;307:1353–60.
11. Weldy CS, Liu Y, Chang YC, Medvedev IO, Fox JR, Larson TV, Chien WM, Chin MT. In utero and early life exposure to diesel exhaust air pollution increases adult susceptibility to heart failure in mice. Part Fibre Toxicol. 2013;10:59.
12. Newby DE, Mannucci PM, Tell GS, Baccarelli AA, Brook RD, Donaldson K, Forastiere F, Franchini M, Franco OH, Graham I. Expert position paper on air pollution and cardiovascular disease. Eur Heart J. 2015;36:83.
13. Biernacka A, Dobaczewski M, Frangogiannis NG. Tgf-β signaling in fibrosis. Growth Factors. 2011;29:196–202.
14. Fares A. Winter cardiovascular diseases phenomenon. N Am J Med Sci. 2013;5:266–79.
15. Hsu WH, Hwang SA, Kinney PL, Lin S. Seasonal and temperature modifications of the association between fine particulate air pollution and cardiovascular hospitalization in New York state. Sci Total Environ. 2017;578: 626–32.
16. Gurkan OU, O'Donnell C, Brower R, Ruckdeschel E, Becker PM. Differential effects of mechanical ventilatory strategy on lung injury and systemic organ inflammation in mice. Am J Physiol Lung Cell Mol Physiol. 2003;285:710–8.
17. Yin W, Hou J, Xu T, Cheng J, Wang X, Jiao S, Wang L, Huang C, Zhang Y, Yuan J. Association of individual-level concentrations and human respiratory tract deposited doses of fine particulate matter with alternation in blood pressure. Environ Pollut. 2017;230:621.
18. Guo S, Hu M, Zamora ML, Peng J, Shang D, Zheng J, Du Z, Wu Z, Shao M, Zeng L. Elucidating severe urban haze formation in China. Proc Natl Acad Sci U S A. 2014;111:17373.
19. Li RJ, Kou XJ, Geng H, Dong C, Cai ZW. Pollution characteristics of ambient pm 2.5 -bound pahs and npahs in a typical winter time period in Taiyuan. Chin Chem Lett. 2014;25:663–6.
20. Cao LX, Geng H, Yao CT, Zhao L, Duan PL, Xuan YY, Li H. Investigation of chemical compositions of atmospheric fine particles during a wintertime haze episode in Taiyuan city. China Environ Sci. 2014;34:837–43.
21. 3Rd PCA. Epidemiology of fine particulate air pollution and human health: biologic mechanisms and who's at risk? Environ Health Perspect. 2000;108: 713–23.
22. Gold DR, Litonjua AA, Zanobetti A, Coull BA, Schwartz J, Maccallum G, Verrier RL, Nearing BD, Canner MJ, Suh H. Air pollution and st-segment depression in elderly subjects. Environ Health Perspect. 2005;113:883–7.

23. Liang R, Zhang B, Zhao X, Ruan Y, Lian H, Fan Z. Effect of exposure to pm2. 5 on blood pressure: a systematic review and meta-analysis. J Hypertens. 2014;32:2130–41.

24. Wu S, Deng F, Huang J, Wang H, Shima M, Wang X, Qin Y, Zheng C, Wei H, Hao Y. Blood pressure changes and chemical constituents of particulate air pollution: results from the healthy volunteer natural relocation (hvnr) study. Environ Health Perspect. 2013;121:66–72.

25. Kamal AS, Rohr AC, Mukherjee B, Morishita M, Keeler GJ, Harkema JR, Wagner JG. Pm2.5-induced changes in cardiac function of hypertensive rats depend on wind direction and specific sources in Steubenville, Ohio. Inhal Toxicol. 2011;23:417–30.

26. Ying Z, Xie X, Bai Y, Chen M, Wang X, Zhang X, Morishita M, Sun Q, Rajagopalan S. Exposure to concentrated ambient particulate matter induces reversible increase of heart weight in spontaneously hypertensive rats. Part Fibre Toxicol. 2015;12:15.

27. Liu Y, Wei-Ming C, Medvedev IO, Weldy CS, Luchtel DL, Rosenfeld ME, Chin MT. Inhalation of diesel exhaust does not exacerbate cardiac hypertrophy or heart failure in two mouse models of cardiac hypertrophy. Part Fibre Toxicol. 2013;10:49.

28. Carter JD, Madamanchi NR, Stouffer GA, Runge MS, Cascio WE, Tong H. Ultrafine particulate matter exposure impairs vasorelaxant response in superoxide dismutase 2-deficient murine aortic rings. J Toxicol Environ Health A. 2017;81:1–10.

29. Pei Y, Jiang R, Zou Y, Yu W, Zhang S, Wang G, Zhao J, Song W. Effects of fine particulate matter (pm2.5) on systemic oxidative stress and cardiac function in apoe−/− mice. Int J Environ Res Public Health. 2016;13:484.

30. Jr HR, Cm A, Sa W, Bj G, Pr K, Dw B, Ke Y. Mouse heart valve structure and function: echocardiographic and morphometric analyses from the fetus through the aged adult. Am J Physiol. 2008;294:2480–8.

31. Keller KM, Howlett SE. Sex differences in the biology and pathology of the aging heart. Can J Cardiol. 2016;32:1065–73.

32. Ying Z, Xu X, Bai Y, Zhong J, Chen M, Liang Y, Zhao J, Liu D, Morishita M, Sun Q. Long-term exposure to concentrated ambient pm2.5 increases mouse blood pressure through abnormal activation of the sympathetic nervous system: a role for hypothalamic inflammation. Environ Health Perspect. 2014;122:79.

33. Kasner M, Westermann D, Steendijk P, Gaub R, Wilkenshoff U, Weitmann K, Hoffmann W, Poller W, Schultheiss HP, Pauschinger M. Utility of doppler echocardiography and tissue doppler imaging in the estimation of diastolic function in heart failure with normal ejection fraction: a comparative doppler-conductance catheterization study. Circulation. 2007;116:637–47.

34. Lu X, Ye Z, Zheng S, Ren H, Zeng J, Wang X, Jose PA, Chen K, Zeng C. Long-term exposure of fine particulate matter causes hypertension by impaired renal d1 receptor-mediated sodium excretion via upregulation of g-protein-coupled receptor kinase type 4 expression in sprague-dawley rats. Journal of the American Heart Association Cardiovascular & Cerebrovascular Disease. 2018;7. https://doi.org/10.1161/JAHA.117.007185.

35. Sancini G, Farina F, Battaglia C, Cifola I, Mangano E, Mantecca P, Camatini M, Palestini P. Health risk assessment for air pollutants: alterations in lung and cardiac gene expression in mice exposed to Milano winter fine particulate matter (pm2.5). PLoS One. 2014;9:e109685.

36. Jia-Ping W, Dennis Jine-Yuan H, Wei-Wen K, Chien-Kuo H, Peiying P, Yu-Lan Y, Chien-Chung L, V Vijaya P, Cecilia Hsuan D, Chih-Yang H. Secondhand smoke exposure reduced the compensatory effects of igf-i growth signaling in the aging rat hearts. Int J Med Sci. 2015;12:708–18.

37. Li F, Lang F, Zhang H, Xu L, Wang Y, Hao E. Role of tfeb mediated autophagy, oxidative stress, inflammation, and cell death in endotoxin induced myocardial toxicity of young and aged mice. Oxidative Med Cell Longev. 2016;2016:5380319. https://doi.org/10.1155/2016/5380319.

38. Hua Y, Zhang Y, Ceylanisik AF, Wold LE, Nunn JM, Ren J. Chronic akt activation accentuates aging-induced cardiac hypertrophy and myocardial contractile dysfunction: role of autophagy. Basic Res Cardiol. 2011;106:1173–91.

39. Yang X, Sreejayan N, Ren J. Views from within and beyond: narratives of cardiac contractile dysfunction under senescence. Endocrine. 2005;26:127–37.

40. Vitale C, Mendelsohn ME, Rosano GM. Gender differences in the cardiovascular effect of sex hormones. Fundam Clin Pharmacol. 2009;6:675–85.

41. Xue B, Zhang Z, Beltz TG, Guo F, Hay M, Johnson AK. Estrogen regulation of the brain renin-angiotensin system in protection against angiotensin ii-induced sensitization of hypertension. Am J Physiol Heart Circ Physiol. 2014; 307:H191.

42. Cucoranu I, Clempus R, Dikalova A, Phelan PJ, Ariyan S, Dikalov S, Dan S. Nad(p)h oxidase 4 mediates transforming growth factor-β1–induced differentiation of cardiac fibroblasts into myofibroblasts. Circ Res. 2005;97:900–7.

43. Tirziu D, Giordano FJ, Simons M. Cell communications in the heart. Circulation. 2010;122:928–37.

44. Zhang M, Shah AM. Ros signalling between endothelial cells and cardiac cells. Cardiovasc Res. 2014;102:249–57.

45. Zhang Y, Ji X, Ku T, Li G, Sang N. Heavy metals bound to fine particulate matter from northern China induce season-dependent health risks: a study based on myocardial toxicity. Environ Pollut. 2016;216:380.

46. Fiordelisi A, Piscitelli P, Trimarco B, Coscioni E, Iaccarino G, Sorriento D. The mechanisms of air pollution and particulate matter in cardiovascular diseases. Heart Fail Rev. 2017;22:1–11.

47. Ganguly K, Ettehadieh D, Upadhyay S, Takenaka S, Adler T, Karg E, Krombach F, Kreyling WG, Schulz H, Schmid O. Early pulmonary response is critical for extra-pulmonary carbon nanoparticle mediated effects: comparison of inhalation versus intra-arterial infusion exposures in mice. Part Fibre Toxicol. 2017;14:19.

48. Zuo L, Youtz DJ, Wold LE. Particulate matter exposure exacerbates high glucose-induced cardiomyocyte dysfunction through ros generation. PLoS One. 2011;6:e23116.

49. Cave AC, Brewer AC, Narayanapanicker A, Ray R, Grieve DJ, Walker S, Shah AM. Nadph oxidases in cardiovascular health and disease. Antioxid Redox Signal. 2006;8:691.

50. Privratsky JR, Wold LE, Sowers JR, Quinn MT, Ren J. At1 blockade prevents glucose-induced cardiac dysfunction in ventricular myocytes: role of the at1 receptor and nadph oxidase. Hypertension. 2003;42:206–12.

51. Li PF, Dietz R, Von HR. Superoxide induces apoptosis in cardiomyocytes, but proliferation and expression of transforming growth factor-beta1 in cardiac fibroblasts. FEBS Lett. 1999;448:206–10.

52. Kamo T, Akazawa H, Komuro I. Cardiac nonmyocytes in the hub of cardiac hypertrophy. Circ Res. 2015;117:89.

53. Shen JZ, Morgan J, Tesch GH, Rickard AJ, Chrissobolis S, Drummond GR, Fuller PJ, Young MJ. Cardiac tissue injury and remodeling is dependent upon mr regulation of activation pathways in cardiac tissue macrophages. Endocrinology. 2016;157:3213–23.

54. Rosenkranz S. Tgf-beta1 and angiotensin networking in cardiac remodeling. Cardiovasc Res. 2004;63:423.

55. Kuwahara F, Kai H, Tokuda K, Kai M, Takeshita A, Egashira K, Imaizumi T. Transforming growth factor-β function blocking prevents myocardial fibrosis and diastolic dysfunction in pressure-overloaded rats. Circulation. 2002;106:130–5.

56. Hu C, Dandapat A, Sun L, Khan JA, Liu Y, Hermonat PL, Mehta JL. Regulation of tgfbeta1-mediated collagen formation by lox-1: studies based on forced overexpression of tgfbeta1 in wild-type and lox-1 knock-out mouse cardiac fibroblasts. J Biol Chem. 2008;283:10226–31.

57. Dobaczewski M, Chen W, Frangogiannis NG. Transforming growth factor (tgf)-β signaling in cardiac remodeling. J Mol Cell Cardiol. 2011;51:600–6.

58. Kodavanti UP, Schladweiler MC, Gilmour PS, Wallenborn JG, Mandavilli BS, Ledbetter AD, Christiani DC, Runge MS, Karoly ED, Costa DL. The role of particulate matter-associated zinc in cardiac injury in rats. Environ Health Perspect. 2008;116:13–20.

59. Lu X, Zhu Y, Bai R, Li S, Teng X. The effect of manganese-induced toxicity on the cytokine mrna expression of chicken spleen lymphocytes in vitro. Res Vet Sci. 2015;101:165–7.

60. Shao JJ, Yao HD, Zhang ZW, Li S, Xu SW. The disruption of mitochondrial metabolism and ion homeostasis in chicken hearts exposed to manganese. Toxicol Lett. 2012;214:99–108.

61. Ku T, Zhang Y, Ji X, Li G, Sang N. Pm2.5-bound metal metabolic distribution and coupled lipid abnormality at different developmental windows. Environ Pollut. 2017;228:354.

62. Cuevas AK, Niu J, Zhong M, Liberda EN, Ghio A, Qu Q, Chen LC. Metal rich particulate matter impairs acetylcholine-mediated vasorelaxation of microvessels in mice. Part Fibre Toxicol. 2015;12:14.

63. Kim YH, Tong H, Daniels M, Boykin E, Krantz QT, Mcgee J, Hays M, Kovalcik K, Dye JA, Gilmour MI. Cardiopulmonary toxicity of peat wildfire particulate matter and the predictive utility of precision cut lung slices. Part Fibre Toxicol. 2014;11:29.

64. Miller MR, Mclean SG, Duffin R, Lawal AO, Araujo JA, Shaw CA, Mills NL, Donaldson K, Newby DE, Hadoke PW. Diesel exhaust particulate increases the size and complexity of lesions in atherosclerotic mice. Part Fibre Toxicol. 2013;10:61.

65. Fink GD. Does tail-cuff plethysmography provide a reliable estimate of central blood pressure in mice? J Am Heart Assoc. 2017;6:e006554.

66. Chen M, Li B, Sang N. Particulate matter (pm2.5) exposure season-dependently induces neuronal apoptosis and synaptic injuries. J Environ Sci. 2017;54:336–45.

67. Bradford MM. A rapid and sensitive method for the quantitation of microgram quantities of protein utilizing the principle of protein-dye binding. Anal Biochem. 1976;72:248–54.

6

Pro-inflammatory adjuvant properties of pigment-grade titanium dioxide particles are augmented by a genotype that potentiates interleukin 1β processing

Sebastian Riedle[1,2,3], Laetitia C. Pele[4], Don E. Otter[1,5], Rachel E. Hewitt[4,6], Harjinder Singh[2], Nicole C. Roy[1,2†] and Jonathan J. Powell[4,6*†]

Abstract

Background: Pigment-grade titanium dioxide (TiO_2) particles are an additive to some foods (E171 on ingredients lists), toothpastes, and pharma–/nutraceuticals and are absorbed, to some extent, in the human intestinal tract. TiO_2 can act as a modest adjuvant in the secretion of the pro-inflammatory cytokine interleukin 1β (IL-1β) when triggered by common intestinal bacterial fragments, such as lipopolysaccharide (LPS) and/or peptidoglycan.
Given the variance in human genotypes, which includes variance in genes related to IL-1β secretion, we investigated whether TiO_2 particles might, in fact, be more potent pro-inflammatory adjuvants in cells that are genetically susceptible to IL-1β-related inflammation.

Methods: We studied bone marrow-derived macrophages from mice with a mutation in the nucleotide-binding oligomerisation domain-containing 2 gene ($Nod2^{m/m}$), which exhibit heightened secretion of IL-1β in response to the peptidoglycan fragment muramyl dipeptide (MDP). To ensure relevance to human exposure, TiO_2 was food-grade anatase (119 ± 45 nm mean diameter ± standard deviation). We used a short 'pulse and chase' format: pulsing with LPS and chasing with TiO_2 +/− MDP or peptidoglycan.

Results: IL-1β secretion was not stimulated in LPS-pulsed bone marrow-derived macrophages, or by chasing with MDP, and only very modestly so by chasing with peptidoglycan. In all cases, however, IL-1β secretion was augmented by chasing with TiO_2 in a dose-dependent fashion (5–100 μg/mL). When co-administered with MDP or peptidoglycan, IL-1β secretion was further enhanced for the $Nod2^{m/m}$ genotype. Tumour necrosis factor α was triggered by LPS priming, and more so for the $Nod2^{m/m}$ genotype. This was enhanced by chasing with TiO_2, MDP, or peptidoglycan, but there was no additive effect between the bacterial fragments and TiO_2.

Conclusion: Here, the doses of TiO_2 that augmented bacterial fragment-induced IL-1β secretion were relatively high. In vivo, however, selected intestinal cells appear to be loaded with TiO_2, so such high concentrations may be 'exposure-relevant' for localised regions of the intestine where both TiO_2 and bacterial fragment uptake occurs. Moreover, this effect is enhanced in cells from $Nod2^{m/m}$ mice indicating that genotype can dictate inflammatory signalling in response to (nano)particle exposure. In vivo studies are now merited.

Keywords: Nano, Particle, TiO_2, E171, NOD2, IL-1β, TNF-α, Muramyl dipeptide, Peptidoglycan

* Correspondence: jonathan.powell@mrc-ewl.cam.ac.uk
†Equal contributors
[4]Biomineral Research Group, MRC Human Nutrition Research, Elsie Widdowson Laboratory, 120 Fulbourn Road, Cambridge CB1 9NL, UK
[6]Department of Veterinary Medicine, Biomineral Research Group, University of Cambridge, Madingley Road, Cambridge CB3 0ES, UK
Full list of author information is available at the end of the article

Background

Potential toxicological effects following exposure to titanium dioxide (TiO_2) are of current interest [1, 2]. TiO_2 is a mineral pigment which, when used in a particulate form, is valued for its properties as a whitening or brightening agent, and is included in some processed foods (E171 on ingredients lists), toothpastes, capsules and tablets. From these sources, the average daily intake of pigment-grade TiO_2 for an adult in the UK is about 10^{12} particles/day [3, 4], nominally ~0.04 mg/kg/day for a 70 kg adult. These findings are supported by a recent Dutch study with mean long term intakes of pigment-grade TiO_2 ranging from 0.06 mg/kg/day in elderly subjects to 0.17 mg/kg/day for 7–69-year-olds [5]. In 2–6 year old children, however, it was higher at 0.67 mg/kg/day [5].

It is well established that particles of TiO_2, likely derived from sources of the Western lifestyle described above, accumulate in certain cells, such as macrophages in Peyer's patches of the human small intestine [6–10]. Whether they have any deleterious impact in this environment remains a matter of speculation, but, if they do, both cell accumulation and host factors are likely to be important [4]. Indeed, it has been often noted that the accumulation of these particles occurs where the earliest signs of Crohn's disease have been reported [11]. With respect to cell accumulation and stimulation, the pristine particle is probably of limited relevance. The intestinal lumen is a 'soup' of proteins, bacterial fragments, ions, small organic molecules etc. and these will modify the surface of the particles through adsorptive interactions. Consistent with this, there are several reports of how TiO_2 particles act as an adjuvant for cellular responses to the bacterial-derived molecule lipopolysaccharide (LPS), either through formation of 'conjugates' or by co-incubation [12–15].

More recently it has been shown that pigment-grade TiO_2 is a modest trigger of the NLR family pyrin domain-containing 3 (NLRP3) inflammasome and that this activity may contribute to intestinal inflammatory properties of the particle in murine models [16]. The inflammasome regulates the activation of caspase-1 which, in turn, determines cleavage of inactive pro-interleukin 1β (pro-IL-1β) to form mature pro-inflammatory interleukin 1β (IL-1β). If such a pro-inflammatory effect from oral TiO_2 exposure translates significantly from murine models to humans, it must be occurring in a small minority of the population because most children and adults do not have intestinal disease. In this respect some variants of human genotype could be important. Indeed, it is well recognised that inflammatory bowel diseases are complex polygenic disorders [17]. Certain mutations in the nucleotide-binding oligomerisation domain-containing 2 (*NOD2*) gene, for example, are associated with an increased risk of the inflammatory

bowel disease, Crohn's disease [18, 19]. Maeda et al. have shown that in mice at least one form of *Nod2* mutation potentiates IL-1β processing and enhances risk of intestinal inflammation [20]. These mice carry a known Crohn's disease-associated 'knockin' mutation in the *Nod2* locus but also carry a duplication of the 3′ end of the wild-type (WT) *Nod2* locus [21], and herein are designated as *Nod2*$^{m/m}$ mice. Specifically, development of a modest pro-inflammatory phenotype in these animals is reportedly triggered by a bacterial peptidoglycan moiety, muramyl dipeptide (MDP), in an IL-1β-dependent fashion [20]. Since bacterial peptidoglycan is taken up by Peyer's patch phagocytes [22, 23] it raises the possibility that TiO_2 could act as an adjuvant for the pro-inflammatory effects of peptidoglycan, and especially so where the genotype potentiates IL-1β processing. Hence, using bone marrow-derived macrophages (BMDMs) from WT and *Nod2*$^{m/m}$ mice, we have tested these possibilities using an assay of short 'pulse and chase' format, to determine if and how TiO_2 could amplify IL-1β secretion at the cellular level.

Methods

Study design

The macrophage-stimulatory effects of dietary TiO_2 were investigated, either alone or in combination with microbial-associated molecular patterns (MAMPs), using cells from WT and *Nod2*$^{m/m}$ mice. MAMP concentrations were fixed whereas a range of TiO_2 concentrations was investigated. LPS pre-stimulation of cells was employed as this MAMP is abundant in the intestinal lumen and can prime cells for an inflammasome-driven response (IL-1β secretion), as described in the Introduction. Parameters assessed were overall cell viability, particle uptake, and secretion of the pro-inflammatory cytokines IL-1β and tumour necrosis factor alpha (TNF-α).

TiO_2 particles

Food- and pharmaceutical-grade TiO_2 particles with anatase crystal structure and a purity of not less than 99% were obtained from Sensient Colors (St. Louis, USA). According to the manufacturer, the TiO_2 particles had an average particle size of 300 nm and a maximum particle size of 1.0 μm, which had been determined using a sediograph instrument. We undertook further analysis of the powder, initially with transmission electron microscopy. A 1 mg/mL suspension of TiO_2 powder in distilled water (Life Technologies, Auckland, New Zealand) with 0.5% bovine serum albumin (BSA; Life Technologies) as a dispersant was prepared. A drop of the TiO_2 particle suspension was placed on a 200-mesh carbon-coated copper grid, and excessive liquid was absorbed with filter paper. The particles were analysed with a Philips CM10 transmission electron microscope at 80 kV. The image analysis software iTEM (Olympus Soft Imaging Solutions, Münster, Germany) was used to record the images digitally and subsequently measure the diameter of the particles.

In addition, particle size under cell culture conditions was determined with nanoparticle tracking analysis, which is a method to analyse dispersed particles based on their Brownian motion, similar to analysis with dynamic light scattering [24]. A 100 µg/mL TiO$_2$ particle suspension was prepared in tissue culture medium (TCM) consisting of RPMI 1640 medium (Sigma-Aldrich, Gillingham, UK) with 10% foetal bovine serum (FBS; PAA Laboratories, Yeovil, UK) and 1% penicillin-streptomycin antibiotics (Sigma-Aldrich). The suspension was sonicated for 10 min to facilitate distribution of the TiO$_2$ particles in the medium. The motion of the particles in suspension was digitally recorded with a NanoSight NS500 instrument (NanoSight, Amesbury, UK). Three TiO$_2$ suspensions were analysed independently. The particle sizes were calculated from the recorded videos with nanoparticle tracking analysis software (Nanosight).

Animals

For the cell culture experiments, bone marrow was obtained from 10 to 18 week old female C57BL/6 WT and $Nod2^{m/m}$ mice. The original WT breeding pairs were purchased from the Jackson Laboratory (Bar Harbor, USA) and bred at the AgResearch Small Animal Colony (Hamilton, New Zealand). Breeding pairs for $Nod2^{m/m}$ mice on a C57BL/6 background were kindly provided by Lars Eckmann [20], and backcrossed with WT mice for 10 generations at the AgResearch Small Animal Colony. The mice were kept under conventional conditions at all times [25].

Harvest of BMDMs and cell culture

For the bone marrow collection, the mice were euthanised with CO$_2$ asphyxiation and cervical dislocation. Femurs and tibias were collected, sterilised in 70% ethanol for 10 s, and the bone marrow flushed out with cold RPMI 1640 medium (Life Technologies). Single cell suspensions were prepared by passing the cells repeatedly through a 19G needle (BD Biosciences, Singapore) and a 70 µm cell strainer (BD Labware, Franklin Lakes, USA). Bone marrow cells were re-suspended in TCM consisting of RPMI 1640 medium (Life Technologies) with 10% FBS (Life Technologies), 1% penicillin-streptomycin antibiotics (Life Technologies), and 10 µg/mL macrophage colony-stimulating factor (eBioscience, San Diego, USA). The cells were transferred to non-tissue culture treated 24-well plates (BD Labware) at a concentration of 1 × 10^6 cells/well in 1 mL TCM and cultured at 37 °C in 7% CO$_2$/93% air. Half of the TCM was replaced every 3 days

with fresh TCM throughout the culture period. Bone marrow cells were fully differentiated into BMDMs on day 7 and used for experiments between day 8 and day 10.

Stimulation of BMDMs with TiO$_2$ particles +/– peptidoglycan or MDP

As previously noted, a short 'pulse (LPS) and chase (TiO$_2$ +/– peptidoglycan or MDP)' format was used to dissect out the point in the pathway that the particles might act as pro-inflammatory adjuvants of MAMPs. To that effect, harvested murine BMDMs from each genotype, +/– LPS pre-stimulation, were exposed to a range of TiO$_2$ particle concentrations +/– peptidoglycan or MDP, as detailed below.

To activate the cells, especially for pro-IL-1β induction, BMDMs were first primed in culture with 1 mL TCM containing 10 ng/mL LPS from *Escherichia coli* O111:B4 (Sigma-Aldrich, Auckland, New Zealand) for 3 h at 37 °C in 7% CO$_2$/93% air. Unprimed BMDMs were cultured under identical conditions but without LPS. All cells were then washed in TCM before the TiO$_2$ suspensions were added. A 1 mg/mL TiO$_2$ stock suspension was first prepared in distilled water and autoclaved. This stock suspension was used to prepare TiO$_2$ suspensions in the TCM with final concentrations from 5 µg/mL to 100 µg/mL. Similar concentrations have been used in previous studies that examined cytokine secretion by phagocytic cells after TiO$_2$ exposure [13, 26–28]. The TiO$_2$ suspensions were sonicated in a water bath for 10 min before 1 mL of the respective TiO$_2$ suspension was added to the cells. When the BMDMs were co-stimulated with MAMPs, either synthetic MDP or peptidoglycan from *Bacillus subtilis* (both from Sigma-Aldrich) was added to the respective TiO$_2$ suspensions in TCM, both at a final concentration of 10 µg/mL. The BMDMs were incubated with TiO$_2$ particles in TCM with or without the co-stimulants for 3 h at 37 °C in 7% CO$_2$/93% air.

Flow cytometry analysis of BMDMs

Only LPS pre-stimulated BMDMs were used for flow cytometry analysis. After incubation with particle suspensions with or without the other MAMPs, the cells were collected for analysis with flow cytometry. Briefly, cells were washed with TCM, incubated for 30 min with cold phosphate-buffered saline (PBS; Life Technologies) on ice, and collected by vigorous pipetting. The BMDMs were re-suspended in 150 µL PBS containing 5% FBS, 2% ethylenediaminetetraacetic acid (Life Technologies), and 1% sodium azide (BDH Laboratory Supplies, Poole, UK). The cells were first incubated for 15 min on ice with 1 µg/mL anti-mouse CD16/32 blocking antibody (clone 93; BioLegend, San Diego, USA) and then stained for 15 min on ice with 1 µg/mL anti-mouse phycoerythrin-labelled F4/80 antibody (clone BM8; BioLegend), a specific marker for murine macrophages. In addition, 0.8 μg/mL propidium iodide (PI; Life Technologies) was added to each sample immediately before analysis for viability assessment. The cells were analysed with a FACS Calibur flow cytometer (BD Biosciences, San Jose, USA), and at least 12,000 events per sample were acquired with the CellQuest Pro software (BD Biosciences). Data analysis was performed with FlowJo (Tree Star, Ashland, USA). For details on the gating strategy see Additional file 1. The percentage of viable cells in relation to the total number of detected events was assessed with PI staining. Cells that did not show PI staining (PI$^-$) were considered to be viable cells. BMDMs were identified among the PI$^-$ cells based on the expression of F4/80, i.e. viable cells that expressed F4/80 (PI$^-$F4/80$^+$) were classified as viable BMDMs. The percentages of PI$^-$F4/80$^+$ cells in relation to the total number of viable cells are shown in Additional file 2. Uptake of TiO$_2$ particles by BMDMs was assessed with the median side scatter (SSC) intensity of the PI$^-$F4/80$^+$ cell populations. According to previous studies, an increase in SSC intensity indicated TiO$_2$ particle uptake [12, 29, 30].

Validation of SSC analysis by flow cytometry as a measure of TiO$_2$ cellular uptake

To confirm that increases in SSC intensity did indeed indicate TiO$_2$ particle uptake, we undertook correlative studies with conventional flow cytometry and imaging cytometry which allows visualisation of TiO$_2$ uptake by individual cells [31]. This technique was not available in the laboratory that undertook the above work and is impractical for a very large number of samples, so only the lower concentration range was investigated and correlated to ensure true discrimination from background.

To quantify TiO$_2$ cellular uptake (i.e. association and localisation) by peripheral myeloid cell populations, fresh leukocyte cones were purchased from the National Blood Service (Cambridge, UK). Peripheral blood mononuclear cells (PBMCs) were isolated by density centrifugation using the separating medium Lymphoprep (Axis Shield Diagnostics, Dundee, UK) and frozen until use. PBMCs from 3 leucocyte cones were thawed and rested for 2 h prior to incubation at 1×10^6 cells/mL with 0 μg/mL, 5 μg/mL, or 10 μg/mL TiO$_2$ and incubated for 24 h in RPMI 1640 medium (Sigma-Aldrich, Gillingham, UK) supplemented with 10% FBS (Sigma-Aldrich).

After incubation, cells were washed with ice cold PBS (Sigma-Aldrich) containing 1% BSA (Sigma-Aldrich) and stained for the human monocyte/myeloid cell markers CD14 Alexa Fluor 488 or CD11c fluorescein isothiocyante (both from BD Biosciences), respectively. Single

stain compensation tubes and unstained PBMC tubes, with and without TiO$_2$, were also prepared at this time from PBMC samples for the generation of compensation matrices. After staining, PBMCs were washed with ice cold PBS containing 1% BSA, re-suspended in a small volume of PBS containing 2% paraformaldehyde (Sigma-Aldrich) solution, and placed on ice in the dark until acquisition.

Imaging cytometry analysis was undertaken using an ImageStreamX Mark I platform (Amnis-Merck-Millipore, Seattle, USA), equipped with 405 nm and 488 nm lasers for excitation, a 785 nm laser for a scatter signal with standard filter sets, multi magnification (20×/40×/60×) and extended depth of field. INSPIRE software (Amnis) was used for acquisition and IDEAS software (Amnis) for analysis. The machine passed all tests and was fully calibrated prior to acquisition of samples. Before acquisition, cells were filtered through 35 μm cell strainers (BD Labware). A minimum of 10,000 events per sample were acquired. Compensation matrices were generated by running single stained cells (i.e. single cell surface marker) and analysed using IDEAS software. For analysis, TiO$_2$ positive cells were identified and quantified using a spot count analysis of dark spots appearing within the cells based on bright-field images of CD14 positive (CD14$^+$) cells. Briefly, cells were first plotted as area versus aspect ratio of the bright-field images and a single cell gate drawn, followed by a focused gate. CD14$^+$ cells were then gated based on fluorescence intensity. A custom dark spot count mask was generated to quantify CD14$^+$ cells, with cells positive for 2 or more darks pots gated as dark spot positive.

Conventional flow cytometry analysis was performed using a CyAn ADP 9 colour analyser (Beckman Coulter, Brea, USA) equipped with 405 nm, 488 nm and 642 nm solid-state lasers and 11 detectors in standard configuration. Summit software was used for acquisition and analysis (Beckman Coulter, USA). At least 500,000 events were acquired on the flow cytometer using a lowered SSC setting on a logarithmic scale. Samples were filtered through 35 μm cell strainers (BD Labware) directly prior to acquisition. For data analysis, events were first plotted as forward versus side scatter using SSC on a logarithmic scale, and a large gate was drawn excluding debris. Cells were then further gated for CD11c positivity based on fluorescence intensity for the mean fluorescence intensity (MFI) of the SSC signal of CD11c$^+$ myeloid cells.

Stimulation of PBMCs with monosodium urate crystals or silica nanoparticles

We confirmed that other exemplar inflammasome-activating particles to which humans are exposed, namely monosodium urate (MSU) crystals and silica nanoparticles (SNPs) [32, 33], promote IL-1β processing in our short 'pulse and chase' format. Isolated PBMCs ($n = 4$) were thawed and rested overnight. Cells (1.10^6 cells/mL) were then subjected to LPS pre-stimulation (10 ng/mL, *Escherichia coli* O111:B4; Sigma-Aldrich) to induce the production of pro-IL-1β or with TCM as a negative control. Following 3 h, cells were washed and then challenged with 100 μg/mL MSU crystals (Caltag Medsystems, Buckingham, UK) or 100 μg/mL SNPs (InvivoGen, San Diego, USA) for a further 3 h. Following this, cells were washed and replenished with fresh TCM for a further 21 h (3 + 21 h). Supernatants were collected at the 3 h and 3 + 21 h time points for IL-1β analyses.

Cytokine detection in cell supernatants

Cell supernatants were collected at the time points indicated and stored at −20 °C until required for cytokine analysis. IL-1β (TiO_2 and exemplar inflammasome-activating particles) and TNF-α (TiO_2 only) were investigated with enzyme-linked immunosorbent assay (ELISA) using DuoSet ELISA kits (R&D Systems, Minneapolis, USA) according to the manufacturer's instructions. The cytokine concentrations were generally determined with a FlexStation 3 microplate scanner (Molecular Devices, Sunnyvale, USA) and Soft Max Pro software (Molecular Devices).

Statistical analysis

All statistical comparisons were carried out using R (R Development Core Team, Vienna, Austria). For analysis of the flow cytometry results, the groups according to genotype (WT or $Nod2^{m/m}$ BMDMs) were compared with two-way analysis of variance (ANOVA) using co-stimulation condition and TiO_2 exposure as the two factors. For analysis of the cytokine secretion results without co-stimulation, the groups according to genotype (WT or $Nod2^{m/m}$ BMDMs) were compared with one-way ANOVA using TiO_2 exposure as the single factor. For analysis of the cytokine secretion results with co-stimulation, the groups according to co-stimulation condition (MDP or peptidoglycan) were compared with two-way ANOVA using genotype and TiO_2 exposure as the two factors. In instances where two-way ANOVA results showed a significant interaction effect or the one-way ANOVA results indicated a significant difference between groups, pairwise group comparisons were performed with Tukey's post-hoc test. Figures depict group means ± standard deviation (SD). Finally, paired T tests were used to compare supernatant levels of IL-1β for cells exposed to MSU crystals or SNPs versus non-particle-exposed control cells. Group means ± standard error of the mean (SEM) are depicted in the corresponding figure.

Results

TiO$_2$ particle characterisation

Several images of TiO_2 particles were obtained with transmission electron microscopy and a representative image is shown in Fig. 1. The diameters of individual particles were measured with image analysis software. The average primary particle size was 119 nm with a SD of 45 nm, and the observed particle sizes ranged from 50 nm to 350 nm with a maximum frequency at 100 nm (Fig. 2a). Approximately 54% of the particles had a diameter between 125 nm and 200 nm, and about 40% had a diameter of 100 nm or less.

TiO_2 particles were suspended in TCM for the subsequent cell culture experiments, so the particle sizes in TCM were also investigated, using nanoparticle tracking analysis. According to this method, the average particle size was 160 nm, and the sizes ranged between 20 nm and 450 nm (Fig. 2b). Approximately 20% of the particles had a diameter of less than 100 nm. The slight increase in particle sizes versus electron microscopy measures probably results from the differing environments as, in solution, particles have a hydration shell and are liable to adsorb TCM molecules. However, the possibility of a small degree of agglomeration in this environment cannot be precluded.

Cellular effects of TiO$_2$ particles

As intended with our short 'pulse and chase' style assay, BMDMs of both genotypes that were not primed with LPS (i.e. sham-pulsed) did not secrete meaningful amounts of IL-1β when chased for 3 h with TiO_2 from

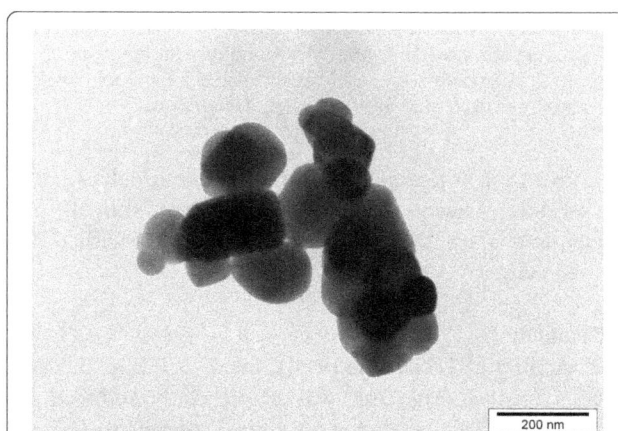

Fig. 1 Transmission electron microscopy image of TiO_2 particles. Food- and pharmaceutical-grade anatase TiO_2 particles were suspended in distilled water with 0.5% BSA at a concentration of 1 mg/mL. The particle suspension was analysed with transmission electron microscopy at 80 kV. A representative image is shown; scale bar = 200 nm

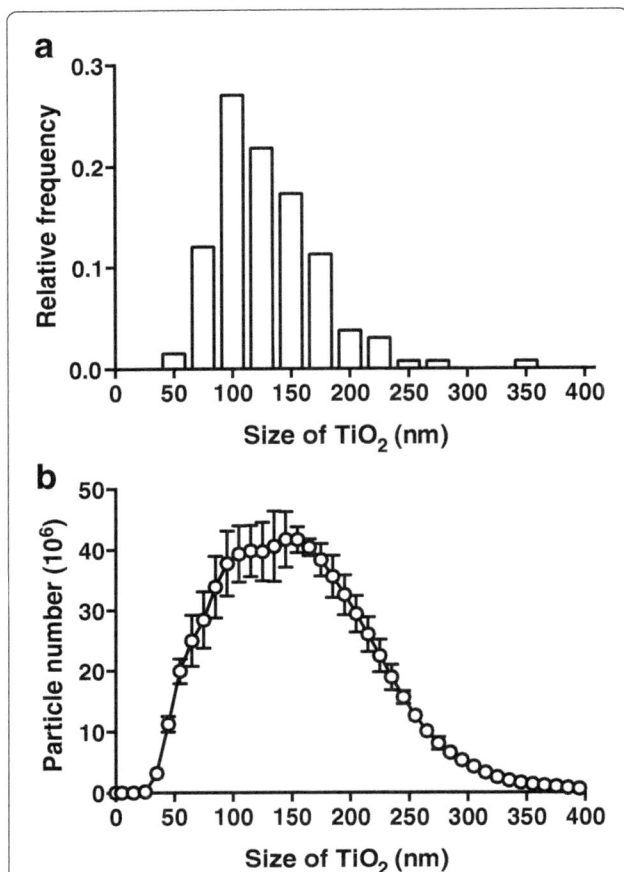

Fig. 2 Size determination of TiO$_2$ particles. **a** Food- and pharmaceutical-grade anatase TiO$_2$ particles were suspended in distilled water with 0.5% BSA at a concentration of 1 mg/mL. The particle suspension was analysed with transmission electron microscopy at 80 kV. TiO$_2$ particle diameters were measured with image analysis software. The distribution of the particle diameters, grouped in sizes of 25 nm, is shown as a relative frequency histogram, $n = 133$. **b** Food- and pharmaceutical-grade anatase TiO$_2$ particles were suspended in RPMI 1640 medium with 10% FBS and 1% penicillin-streptomycin at a concentration of 1 mg/mL. TiO$_2$ particle sizes were determined with nanoparticle tracking analysis, and the size distribution of the particles is plotted as a line graph. Data represent mean ± SD from three independent experiments

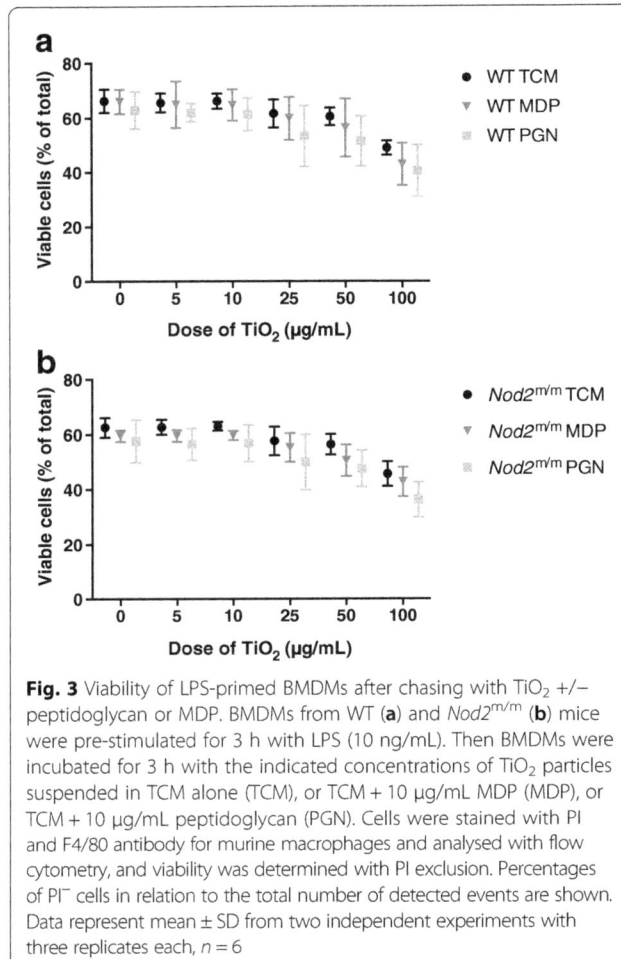

Fig. 3 Viability of LPS-primed BMDMs after chasing with TiO$_2$ +/−peptidoglycan or MDP. BMDMs from WT (**a**) and $Nod2^{m/m}$ (**b**) mice were pre-stimulated for 3 h with LPS (10 ng/mL). Then BMDMs were incubated for 3 h with the indicated concentrations of TiO$_2$ particles suspended in TCM alone (TCM), or TCM + 10 μg/mL MDP (MDP), or TCM + 10 μg/mL peptidoglycan (PGN). Cells were stained with PI and F4/80 antibody for murine macrophages and analysed with flow cytometry, and viability was determined with PI exclusion. Percentages of PI$^-$ cells in relation to the total number of detected events are shown. Data represent mean ± SD from two independent experiments with three replicates each, $n = 6$

0 μg/mL to 100 μg/mL +/− MDP or peptidoglycan (IL-1β secretion always <5 pg/mL; data not shown). All subsequent data therefore refer to results with LPS-primed cells.

Cell viability

The viability of LPS-pulsed cells, from WT (Fig. 3a) and $Nod2^{m/m}$ mice (Fig. 3b), was significantly reduced by chasing with TiO$_2$ particles, in a dose-responsive fashion ($p < 0.001$ for trend, Fig. 3a and b). Addition of peptidoglycan or MDP during the chase phase marginally, but significantly, decreased cell viability further ($p < 0.001$ for trend), although there was no interaction effect with TiO$_2$ exposure (Fig. 3a and b).

Particle uptake

Particle uptake was assessed by flow cytometric SSC intensities for LPS-pulsed viable (PI$^-$) F4/80$^+$ WT (Fig. 4a) and $Nod2^{m/m}$ BMDMs (Fig. 4b). During the chase phase, SSC intensities of WT and $Nod2^{m/m}$ BMDMs increased with increasing TiO$_2$ concentrations ($p < 0.001$ for trend) but were unaffected by the presence of peptidoglycan or MDP (Fig. 4a and b). To confirm that such increases in SSC intensities did result from TiO$_2$ uptake, as anticipated and as previously reported [12, 29, 30], we compared this form of analysis with imaging cytometry which allows visualisation of particle uptake [31]. Using PBMCs, and the lower end of the exposure range (where error would be greatest), increases in SSC intensity of myeloid-gated cells correlated positively and closely with observed TiO$_2$ uptake ($r = 0.84$, $p < 0.01$; Fig. 5).

IL-1β secretion

In LPS-pulsed BMDMs chased with TCM alone (i.e. zero dose TiO$_2$ in Fig. 6a), there was no secretion of mature IL-1β, consistent with the role of LPS in stimulating pro-IL-1β but not triggering the inflammasome [34, 35].

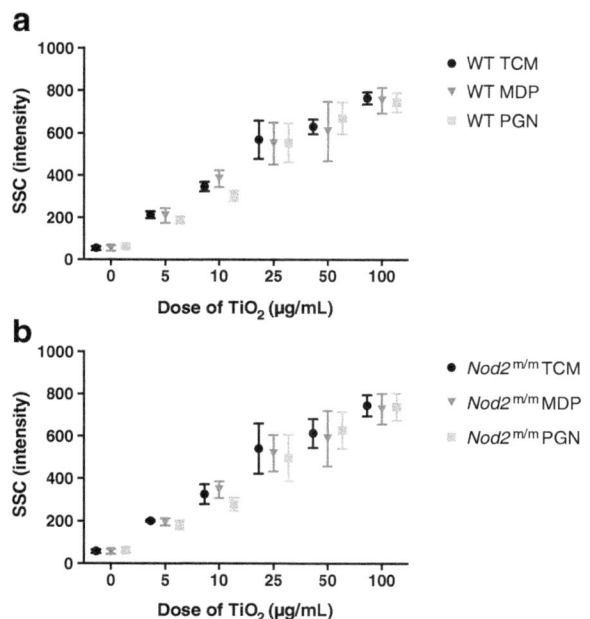

Fig. 4 Particle uptake by LPS-primed BMDMs after chasing with TiO$_2$ +/− peptidoglycan or MDP. BMDMs from WT (**a**) and Nod2$^{m/m}$ (**b**) mice were pre-stimulated for 3 h with LPS (10 ng/mL). Then BMDMs were incubated for 3 h with the indicated concentrations of TiO$_2$ particles suspended in TCM alone (TCM), TCM + 10 μg/mL MDP (MDP), or TCM + 10 μg/mL peptidoglycan (PGN). Cells were stained with PI and F4/80 antibody for murine macrophages and analysed with flow cytometry, and median SSC intensities of PI$^-$F4/80$^+$ cells were recorded. Data represent mean ± SD from two independent experiments with three replicates each, n = 6

Again as anticipated, chasing LPS-primed BMDMs with TiO$_2$ led to mature IL-1β secretion in a dose-dependent fashion ($p < 0.001$; Fig. 6a) as these particles are a modest activator of the inflammasome [16, 28]. Pairwise group comparison with Tukey's post-hoc test indicated significant IL-1β stimulation with TiO$_2$ doses in TCM of ≥50 μg/mL (p between <0.01 and <0.001; Fig. 6a).

Similarly, chasing LPS-primed BMDMs with TiO$_2$ + peptidoglycan or MDP increased IL-1β secretion in a dose-dependent fashion, for cells of both genotypes ($p < 0.001$, Fig. 6b). However, genotype significantly influenced the extent of the IL-1β response ($p < 0.01$ for + MDP and $p < 0.001$ for + peptidoglycan). Furthermore, an interaction effect between genotype and TiO$_2$ exposure was observed for peptidoglycan ($p < 0.001$), but not for MDP. Pairwise comparisons between groups with Tukey's post-hoc test, when chasing with TiO$_2$ + peptidoglycan, showed that the amount of IL-1β released by WT and Nod2$^{m/m}$ BMDMs differed significantly when the cells were similarly exposed to ≥10 μg/mL TiO$_2$ (p between <0.05 and <0.001; Fig. 6b).

TNF-α secretion

LPS priming led to marked secretion of TNF-α even when chased with TCM alone (Fig. 7a) because, unlike IL-1β [36], there is no requirement for a second signal to enable protein formation and secretion of this cytokine. Chasing LPS-primed BMDMs with TiO$_2$ led to further TNF-α secretion in a dose-dependent fashion ($p < 0.001$; Fig. 7a) and, again, Tukey's post-hoc test indicated significant TNF-α stimulation with TiO$_2$ doses in TCM of ≥50 μg/mL (p between <0.05 and <0.001; Fig. 7a).

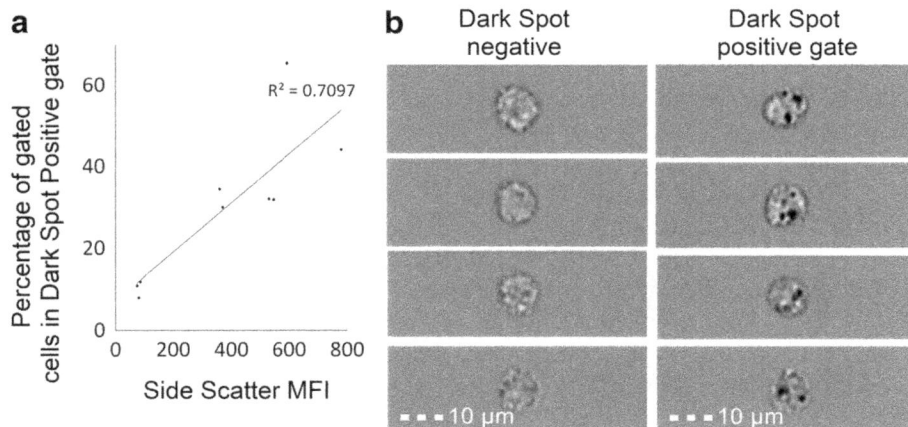

Fig. 5 Correlation of SSC intensity and dark spots in bright-field images by flow and imaging cytometry. PBMCs from human blood were incubated for 24 h with 0 μg/mL, 5 μg/mL, or 10 μg/mL TiO$_2$ particles in TCM and stained with either CD11c or CD14 antibodies for human monocytes/myeloid cells and analysed with conventional flow or imaging cytometry, respectively. **a** Correlation between increases in SSC MFI of CD11c$^+$ myeloid cells identified using conventional flow cytometry and the percentages of CD14$^+$ cells bearing dark spots in bright-field measured by imaging cytometry; Pearson correlation $p < 0.01$, $r = 0.8424$. **b** Representative images of cells designated 'dark spot negative' or 'dark spot positive' by imaging cytometry; scale bar = 10 μm

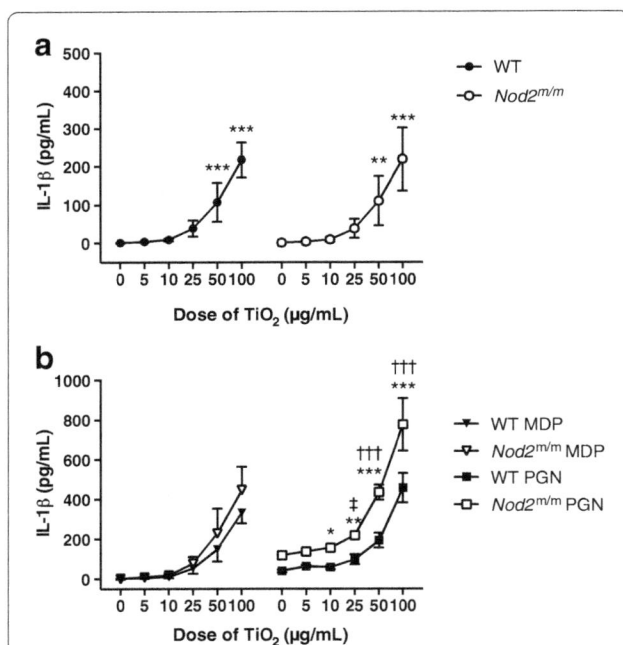

Fig. 6 IL-1β secretion by LPS-primed BMDMs after chasing with TiO₂ +/− peptidoglycan or MDP. BMDMs from WT and Nod2^{m/m} mice were pre-stimulated for 3 h with LPS (10 ng/mL). Then BMDMs were incubated for 3 h with the indicated concentrations of TiO₂ particles suspended in TCM alone (**a**) or suspended in TCM + 10 μg/mL MDP (MDP) or TCM + 10 μg/mL peptidoglycan (PGN) (**b**). Supernatant concentrations of IL-1β were analysed by ELISA. Data represent mean ± SD from two independent experiments with three replicates each, n = 6. **a** Results were analysed with one-way ANOVA and Tukey's post-hoc test; **p < 0.01, ***p < 0.001 compared to respective WT or Nod2^{m/m} cells incubated without TiO₂. **b** Results were analysed with two-way ANOVA and Tukey's post-hoc test; *p < 0.05, **p < 0.01, ***p < 0.001 for Nod2^{m/m} cells compared to WT cells cultured with the same TiO₂ concentration, †††p < 0.001 for WT and Nod2^{m/m} cells compared to respective WT or Nod2^{m/m} cells incubated without TiO₂, ‡p < 0.05 for Nod2^{m/m} cells compared to Nod2^{m/m} cells incubated without TiO₂

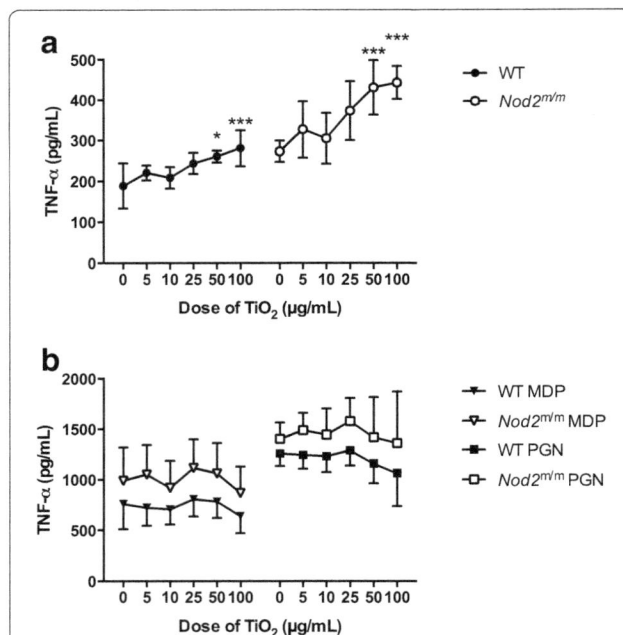

Fig. 7 TNF-α secretion by LPS-primed BMDMs after chasing with TiO₂ +/− peptidoglycan or MDP. BMDMs from WT and Nod2^{m/m} mice were pre-stimulated for 3 h with LPS (10 ng/mL). Then BMDMs were incubated for 3 h with the indicated concentrations of TiO₂ particles suspended in TCM alone (**a**) or suspended in TCM + 10 μg/mL MDP (MDP) or TCM + 10 μg/mL peptidoglycan (PGN) (**b**). Supernatant concentrations of TNF-α were analysed by ELISA. Data represent mean ± SD from two independent experiments with three replicates each, n = 6. **a** Results were analysed with one-way ANOVA and Tukey's post-hoc test; *p < 0.05, ***p < 0.001 compared to respective WT or Nod2^{m/m} cells incubated without TiO₂

exposure (e.g. over 24 h) can lead to false positives [35]. SNPs and MSU crystals are considered exemplar particulate stimulants of the inflammasome, and we confirmed that, with similar short exposures as for our TiO₂ particles (3 h) and LPS priming, IL-1β secretion was enhanced compared to non-particle-exposed cells (Fig. 8).

Discussion
Relevance and context of our findings
The distal intestinal tract is bathed in high concentrations of MAMPs such as LPS and peptidoglycan (and their fragments) due to the continuous turnover of the microbiome. Since ingested particles, such as pigment-grade TiO₂, are taken up by intestinal cells from this distal environment it is important to consider interactions of these components (i.e. MAMPs + particles) when looking at potential cellular effects. In this work we have further considered the impact of genotype, namely one that imparts greater potential for an inflammatory phenotype (Nod2^{m/m}) than the WT version. We confirm that (a) primed cells from Nod2^{m/m} mice secrete higher concentrations of pro-inflammatory cytokines,

In contrast to IL-1β, the secretion of TNF-α by LPS-primed BMDMs that were chased with MDP or peptidoglycan was not affected by additional TiO₂ exposure regardless of dose (i.e. the MAMPs rather than the particles dominated the scene for TNF-α secretion; Fig. 7b).

Although in all cases the genotype had a significant influence (p < 0.001) on TNF-α secretion, being greater for cells from Nod2^{m/m} than WT mice, there was no interaction effect between genotype and TiO₂ exposure (Fig. 7a and b).

Specificity of TiO₂ effect
Activation of the inflammasome is by no means specific to TiO₂ particles although Pele et al. have shown that correct design of in vitro experiments is critical. Notably, cell gorging of particles through extended particle

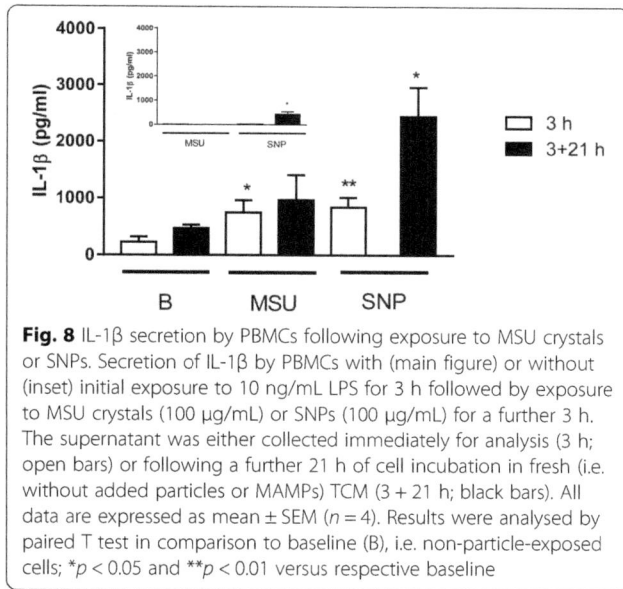

Fig. 8 IL-1β secretion by PBMCs following exposure to MSU crystals or SNPs. Secretion of IL-1β by PBMCs with (main figure) or without (inset) initial exposure to 10 ng/mL LPS for 3 h followed by exposure to MSU crystals (100 μg/mL) or SNPs (100 μg/mL) for a further 3 h. The supernatant was either collected immediately for analysis (3 h; open bars) or following a further 21 h of cell incubation in fresh (i.e. without added particles or MAMPs) TCM (3 + 21 h; black bars). All data are expressed as mean ± SEM (n = 4). Results were analysed by paired T test in comparison to baseline (B), i.e. non-particle-exposed cells; *p < 0.05 and **p < 0.01 versus respective baseline

namely IL-1β and TNF-α, in response to MDP-containing MAMPs than cells from WT mice [20] and (b) TiO₂ particles are mediators of inflammasome activation [12, 16, 28, 33]. Additionally, we show for the first time that, in primed cells exposed to peptidoglycan, the concentration of TiO₂ that is required to trigger the inflammasome and induce IL-1β secretion is lower for cells from $Nod2^{m/m}$ mice than it is from WT mice. This may have important implications as discussed below.

It is established that at least some ingested TiO₂ particles are taken up by intestinal cells, especially by macrophages of large lymphoid follicles of the ileum termed Peyer's patches [6–10]. Recent data suggest that cells of the large bowel can also scavenge particles of pigment-grade TiO₂ and that oral administration of this pigment can lead to pre-cancerous lesions of the colon, termed aberrant crypt foci, in about a third of WT animals but not in controls without TiO₂ exposure [37]. In that work, intestinal mucosal levels of TNF-α and IL-1β were modestly increased for animals fed TiO₂ versus controls [37]. Whilst our data support these findings from a cell culture perspective they also show that particle dose is critical as a determinant of the cytokine response. The precise pathway of TiO₂ uptake by intestinal cells is still not understood, but it is likely that particles in the lumen have their surfaces 'decorated' by soluble molecules of the intestinal lumen so that conjugates (with MAMPs for example), rather than pristine particles, are seen by intestinal cells. Moreover, it is not clear how basal macrophages of the human Peyer's patches become loaded with particles such as TiO₂ as, following M cell uptake, particles should be scavenged by phagocytes that are more apical than the observed basal tissue-fixed macrophages [38]. However, despite the pathway not

being fully elucidated, the important point is that macrophages of the Peyer's patches *do* accumulate TiO₂ particles in humans [9, 39]. If, as we show here, certain genotypes require a lesser cell dose of particles to respond in a pro-inflammatory fashion compared to other genotypes then, in vivo, the initiation of a cascade of inflammation may be host-dependent as well as dose-dependent.

Specificity of the IL-1β adjuvant effect to TiO₂ nanoparticles

The 'role' of the TiO₂ particles in the work presented here involves boosting the pro-inflammatory effects of MAMPs via particle-activation of the inflammasome. Many materials activate the inflammasome, including other (nano)particles, and some of these will be more potent than pigment-grade TiO₂ given the modest efficacy of the latter. For example, MSU crystals and silica particles are activators of the inflammasome (as exemplified here (Fig. 8) and [28, 32, 33]) and have direct relevance in terms of human exposure. MSU crystals may precipitate ectopically and are the cause of joint inflammation in patients with gout, whilst silica exposure to the lungs is well established as an occupational hazard that leads to silicosis in miners. However, in terms of an adjuvant effect on MAMP-primed cells, TiO₂ deserves particular scrutiny because (a) humans are widely exposed to it orally [3, 5], (b) MAMPs are ubiquitous at high concentrations in the intestinal lumen which is unlike anywhere else in the body, and (c) pigment-grade TiO₂ is one of two major particle types that accumulates in intestinal (Peyer's patch) macrophages [7, 9, 39]. The second major particle type, namely aluminosilicate which is mostly in the kaolinite form [7], has not been obviously linked to inflammasome activation although this merits further careful assessment as prolonged macrophage exposure to kaolinite leads to modest IL-1β secretion even in the absence of MAMPS [40].

Interestingly, Winkler et al. have shown that food-grade silica induced production of pro-IL-1β and secretion of mature IL-1β when dendritic cells were exposed to these particles [41]. In other words, silica particles have the capacity to both prime IL-1β formation in the precursor (pro-) form and to induce cleavage to a mature form via inflammasome activation. Although, unlike TiO₂, this silica has not been demonstrated to accumulate in human intestinal immune cells [7], further studies are merited as there is significant oral exposure and perhaps intestinal cells other than those that have been so far characterised for particle accumulation in the intestine are impacted.

In summary for this section, pigment-grade TiO₂ is especially relevant as a potential inflammasome adjuvant in intestinal tissue because of human exposure, accumulation, *and* activity. However, other particles, such as aluminosilicates and silica, should not be ignored as there is certainly exposure and accumulation for the former and exposure and potential for activity for the latter.

IL-1β secretion is not a simple consequence of TiO₂-induced cell death

Non-biological particles in a size range that enables phagocytosis, which includes pigment-grade TiO₂, are readily engulfed by macrophages and accumulate in lysosomes [7, 9, 42]. This in turn leads to lysosomal membrane disruption which is a trigger for two concomitant events. The first is cathepsin-dependent IL-1β release which requires inflammasome activation, and the second is cell death which again is cathepsin-dependent but is independent of the inflammasome [42]. Hence, as expected, both events were observed in this study in a dose-dependent fashion when cells were exposed to TiO₂. In vivo, cell death can lead to pro-IL-1β leakage into the extracellular environment and its activation through 'alternative' pathways, such as cathepsin C-neutrophil proteases. However, this does not occur in 'clean' cell culture media in vitro [42]. Moreover, a short 'pulse and chase' routine protects against such longer term complications. It is therefore anticipated that our observed IL-1β-inducing effect of TiO₂ in LPS-primed macrophages is independent of the concomitantly observed cell death. Regardless of mechanism, it does not alter the potential relevance of these findings to the in vivo situation where, as noted, pigment-grade TiO₂ accumulates in selective intestinal cells of humans.

In vivo relevance for health and disease

Notwithstanding the above, and as discussed earlier, TiO₂ is only a modest activator of the inflammasome, so whether realistic oral exposure to TiO₂ leads to interactions with MAMPs and whether intestinal cell loading of both materials is sufficient to trigger inflammation merits closer attention in a relevant genetically susceptible model. In particular, such work should focus on (a) the Peyer's patches as sites of cellular TiO₂ accumulation with the potential for early inflammatory processes [11] and (b) the colon, given the association of large bowel cancer with early inflammation and potential exacerbation of disease by TiO₂ [43].

In addition, our specific interest concerns inflammatory bowel disease, especially Crohn's disease, and the potential for TiO₂ as an adjuvant for pro-inflammatory responses in recipient Peyer's patch cells [7, 38, 39]. Although the murine model used here does not accurately mimic Crohn's type mutations for *NOD2* because of the duplication of the 3′-end of the WT *Nod2* locus [21], it does, nonetheless, have a heightened susceptibility to

inflammation in response to certain MAMPs, precisely as has been proposed for Crohn's disease [44]. Further work with patient samples is therefore merited to scrutinise the potential for a TiO₂ adjuvant effect on MAMPs in terms of IL-1β secretion.

Conclusions

In summary, in this study we have shown that dietary TiO₂ particles have an impact on the production of the pro-inflammatory cytokines IL-1β and TNF-α by LPS pre-stimulated murine macrophages in vitro, and that TiO₂ particles can act as IL-1β-inducing adjuvants for bacterial MAMPs that contain MDP moieties. We also demonstrated that the impact of this adjuvant effect is genotype-dependent. Primed macrophages from $Nod2^{m/m}$ mice showed an elevated IL-1β response to incubation with TiO₂ particles and peptidoglycan compared to cells from WT mice. Further work will need to consider if any human genotypes (sub-populations) are at greater inflammatory risk than the background population from TiO₂ exposure.

Abbreviations
ANOVA: Analysis of variance; BMDM: Bone marrow-derived macrophage; BSA: Bovine serum albumin; FBS: Foetal bovine serum; IL-1β: Interleukin 1β; LPS: Lipopolysaccharide; MAMP: Microbial-associated molecular pattern; MDP: Muramyl dipeptide; MFI: Mean fluorescence intensity; MSU: Monosodium urate; NLRP3: NLR family pyrin domain-containing 3; NOD2: Nucleotide-binding oligomerisation domain-containing 2; $Nod2^{m/m}$: Homozygous *Nod2* gene mutation (as described); PBMC: Peripheral blood mononuclear cell; PBS: Phosphate-buffered saline; PGN: Peptidoglycan; PI: Propidium iodide; pro-IL-1β: pro-interleukin 1β; SD: Standard deviation; SEM: Standard error of the mean; SNP: Silica nanoparticle; SSC: Side scatter; TCM: Tissue culture medium; TiO₂: Titanium dioxide; TNF: Tumour necrosis factor; WT: Wild-type

Acknowledgements
The authors would like to thank Doug Hopcroft from the Manawatu Microscopy and Imaging Centre (Massey University, Palmerston North, New Zealand) for assistance with electron microscopy. The authors gratefully acknowledge the technical support provided by Drs Nuno Faria and Carolin Haas (Biomineral Research Group, MRC Human Nutrition Research, Cambridge, UK) for nanoparticle tracking analysis and the support for animal-related work and BMDMs preparation from Genevieve Sheriff (nee Baildon) and Ric Broadhurst (Campus Services, AgResearch, Hamilton, New Zealand), and Leigh Ryan and Dr. Wayne Young (Food Nutrition & Health Team, Food & Bio-based Products Group, AgResearch, Palmerston North, New Zealand). The authors are grateful for advice on statistical analysis from Dr. John Koolaard and Catherine Lloyd-West (Campus Services, AgResearch, Palmerston North, New Zealand) and comments on the manuscript from Drs Matthew Barnett and Wayne Young (Food Nutrition & Health Team, Food & Bio-based Products Group, AgResearch, Palmerston North, New Zealand). The authors thank Dr. Sabine Kuhn (Institut für Klinische Chemie und Pathobiochemie, Klinikum rechts der Isar, Technische Universität München, Munich, Germany) for her kind assistance with designing the figures and three anonymous reviewers for their constructive feedback which helped to improve the manuscript.

Funding

The research was mainly supported by the Riddet Institute through its Centre of Research Excellence funding which has been awarded to the Riddet Institute by the New Zealand government. Additional funding was provided by AgResearch, MRC Elsie Widdowson Laboratory (formerly MRC Human Nutrition Research, Grant number U105960399) and Nutrigenomics New Zealand, a collaboration between AgResearch, Plant & Food Research, and The University of Auckland (primarily supported by funding from the Ministry for Science & Innovation contract C11X1009). SR was supported by doctoral scholarships from Massey University and AgResearch. The funding bodies had no influence on the research or preparation of this manuscript.

Authors' contributions

LCP and JJP developed the research hypothesis. LCP and SR designed the study with contributions from DEO, HS, NCR, and JJP. SR performed the experiments, analysed the results, and, together with LCP, designed the figures (except Figs. 5 and 8). REH and LCP provided the data and associated analyses for Figs. 5 and 8, respectively, and wrote the corresponding methods and results sections. All authors contributed to the interpretation of the results. SR and JJP wrote the manuscript with contributions from all authors. All authors read and approved the final manuscript.

Competing interests

The authors declare that they have no competing interests.

Author details

[1]Food Nutrition & Health Team, Food & Bio-based Products Group, AgResearch, Grasslands Research Centre, Tennent Drive, Private Bag 11008, Palmerston North 4442, New Zealand. [2]Riddet Institute, Massey University, Private Bag 11222, Palmerston North 4442, New Zealand. [3]Present address: Conreso GmbH, Neuhauser Str. 47, 80331, München, Germany. [4]Biomineral Research Group, MRC Human Nutrition Research, Elsie Widdowson Laboratory, 120 Fulbourn Road, Cambridge CB1 9NL, UK. [5]Present address: Center for Dairy Research, University of Wisconsin-Madison, 1605 Linden Drive, Madison, WI 53706-1565, USA. [6]Department of Veterinary Medicine, Biomineral Research Group, University of Cambridge, Madingley Road, Cambridge CB3 0ES, UK.

References

1.	Shi H, Magaye R, Castranova V, Zhao J. Titanium dioxide nanoparticles: a review of current toxicological data. Part Fibre Toxicol. 2013;10:15.
2.	Kreyling WG, Holzwarth U, Schleh C, Kozempel J, Wenk A, Haberl N, et al. Quantitative biokinetics of titanium dioxide nanoparticles after oral application in rats: part 2. Nanotoxicology. 2017;11:443–53.
3.	Lomer MCE, Hutchinson C, Volkert S, Greenfield SM, Catterall A, Thompson RPH, et al. Dietary sources of inorganic microparticles and their intake in healthy subjects and patients with Crohn's disease. Brit J Nutr. 2004;92:947–55.
4.	Powell JJ, Faria N, Thomas-McKay E, Pele LC. Origin and fate of dietary nanoparticles and microparticles in the gastrointestinal tract. J Autoimmun. 2010;34:J226–J33.
5.	Rompelberg C, Heringa MB, van Donkersgoed G, Drijvers J, Roos A, Westenbrink S, et al. Oral intake of added titanium dioxide and its nanofraction from food products, food supplements and toothpaste by the Dutch population. Nanotoxicology. 2016;10:1404–14.
6.	Hummel TZ, Kindermann A, Stokkers PCF, Benninga MA, ten Kate FJW. Exogenous pigment in Peyer's patches of children suspected for inflammatory bowel disease. J Pediatr Gastr Nutr. 2014;58:477–80.
7.	Powell JJ, Ainley CC, Harvey RSJ, Mason IM, Kendall MD, Sankey EA, et al. Characterisation of inorganic microparticles in pigment cells of human gut associated lymphoid tissue. Gut. 1996;38:390–5.
8.	Shepherd NA, Crocker PR, Smith AP, Levison DA. Exogenous pigment in Peyer's patches. Hum Pathol. 1987;18:50–4.
9.	Thoree V, Skepper J, Deere H, Pele LC, Thompson RPH, Powell JJ. Phenotype of exogenous microparticle-containing pigment cells of the human Peyer's patch in inflamed and normal ileum. Inflamm Res. 2008;57:374–8.
10.	Urbanski SJ, Arsenault AL, Green FH, Haber G. Pigment resembling atmospheric dust in Peyer's patches. Mod Pathol. 1989;2:222–6.
11.	Fujimura Y, Kamoi R, Iida M. Pathogenesis of aphthoid ulcers in Crohn's disease: correlative findings by magnifying colonoscopy, electron microscopy, and immunohistochemistry. Gut. 1996;38:724–32.
12.	Ashwood P, Thompson RPH, Powell JJ. Fine particles that adsorb lipopolysaccharide *via* bridging calcium cations may mimic bacterial pathogenicity towards cells. Exp Biol Med. 2007;232:107–17.
13.	Butler M, Boyle JJ, Powell JJ, Playford RJ, Ghosh S. Dietary microparticles implicated in Crohn's disease can impair macrophage phagocytic activity and act as adjuvants in the presence of bacterial stimuli. Inflamm Res. 2007;56:353–61.
14.	Evans SM, Ashwood P, Warley A, Berisha F, Thompson RPH, Powell JJ. The role of dietary microparticles and calcium in apoptosis and interleukin-1β release of intestinal macrophages. Gastroenterology. 2002;123:1543–53.
15.	Powell JJ, Harvey RSJ, Ashwood P, Wolstencroft R, Gershwin ME, Thompson RPH. Immune potentiation of ultrafine dietary particles in normal subjects and patients with inflammatory bowel disease. J Autoimmun. 2000;14:99–105.
16.	Ruiz PA, Morón B, Becker HM, Lang S, Atrott K, Spalinger MR, et al. Titanium dioxide nanoparticles exacerbate DSS-induced colitis: role of the NLRP3 inflammasome. Gut. 2017;66:1216–24.
17.	Khor B, Gardet A, Xavier RJ. Genetics and pathogenesis of inflammatory bowel disease. Nature. 2011;474:307–17.
18.	Hugot JP, Chamaillard M, Zouali H, Lesage S, Cézard JP, Belaiche J, et al. Association of NOD2 leucine-rich repeat variants with susceptibility to Crohn's disease. Nature. 2001;411:599–603.
19.	Ogura Y, Bonen DK, Inohara N, Nicolae DL, Chen FF, Ramos R, et al. A frameshift mutation in *NOD2* associated with susceptibility to Crohn's disease. Nature. 2001;411:603–6.
20.	Maeda S, Hsu LC, Liu HJ, Bankston LA, Iimura M, Kagnoff MF, et al. *Nod2* mutation in Crohn's disease potentiates NF-κB activity and IL-1β processing. Science. 2005;307:734–8.
21.	Maeda S. Corrections and clarifications: *Nod2* mutation in Crohn's disease potentiates NF-κB activity and IL-1β processing [Maeda S et al. (2005) Science 307(5710): 734-738]. Science. 2011;333:288.
22.	Powell JJ, Thomas-McKay E, Thoree V, Robertson J, Hewitt RE, Skepper JN, et al. An endogenous nanomineral chaperones luminal antigen and peptidoglycan to intestinal immune cells. Nat Nanotechnol. 2015;10:361–9.
23.	Klasen IS, Melief MJ, van Halteren AG, Schouten WR, van Blankenstein M, Hoke G, et al. The presence of peptidoglycan-polysaccharide complexes in the bowel wall and the cellular responses to these complexes in Crohn's disease. Clin Immunol Immunopathol. 1994;71:303–8.
24.	Filipe V, Hawe A, Jiskoot W. Critical evaluation of nanoparticle tracking analysis (NTA) by NanoSight for the measurement of nanoparticles and protein aggregates. Pharm Res. 2010;27:796–810.
25.	Roy N, Barnett M, Knoch B, Dommels Y, McNabb W. Nutrigenomics applied to an animal model of inflammatory bowel diseases: transcriptomic analysis of the effects of eicosapentaenoic acid- and arachidonic acid-enriched diets. Mutat Res. 2007;622:103–16.
26.	Morishige T, Yoshioka Y, Tanabe A, Yao X, Tsunoda S, Tsutsumi Y, et al. Titanium dioxide induces different levels of IL-1β production dependent on its particle characteristics through caspase-1 activation mediated by reactive oxygen species and cathepsin B. Biochem Biophys Res Commun. 2010;392:160–5.
27.	Palomäki J, Karisola P, Pylkkänen L, Savolainen K, Alenius H. Engineered nanomaterials cause cytotoxicity and activation on mouse antigen presenting cells. Toxicology. 2010;267:125–31.
28.	Winter M, Beer HD, Hornung V, Kärmer U, Schins RPF, Förster I. Activation of the inflammasome by amorphous silica and TiO₂ nanoparticles in murine dendritic cells. Nanotoxicology. 2011;5:326–40.
29.	Suzuki H, Toyooka T, Ibuki Y. Simple and easy method to evaluate uptake potential of nanoparticles in mammalian cells using a flow cytometric light scatter analysis. Environ Sci Technol. 2007;41:3018–24.
30.	Zucker RM, Massaro EJ, Sanders KM, Degn LL, Boyes WK. Detection of TiO₂ nanoparticles in cells by flow cytometry. Cytometry A. 2010;77:677–85.
31.	Hewitt RE, Vis B, Pele LC, Faria N, Powell JJ. Imaging flow cytometry assays for quantifying pigment grade titanium dioxide particle internalization and interactions with immune cells in whole blood. Cytometry A. 2017;91A:1009–20.
32.	Martinon F, Pétrilli V, Mayor A, Tardivel A, Tschopp J. Gout-associated uric acid crystals activate the NALP3 inflammasome. Nature. 2006;440:237–41.
33.	Yazdi AS, Guarda G, Riteau N, Drexler SK, Tardivel A, Couillin I, et al. Nanoparticles activate the NLR pyrin domain containing 3 (Nlrp3)

inflammasome and cause pulmonary inflammation through release of IL-1α and IL-1β. Proc Natl Acad Sci U S A. 2010;107:19449–54.

34. Latz E, Xiao TS, Stutz A. Activation and regulation of the inflammasomes. Nat Rev Immunol. 2013;13:397–411.

35. Pele L, Haas CT, Hewitt R, Faria N, Brown A, Powell J. Artefactual nanoparticle activation of the inflammasome platform: *in vitro* evidence with a nano-formed calcium phosphate. Nanomedicine (Lond). 2015;10:1379–90.

36. Dinarello CA. Immunological and inflammatory functions of the interleukin-1 family. Annu Rev Immunol. 2009;27:519–50.

37. Urrutia-Ortega IM, Garduno-Balderas LG, Delgado-Buenrostro NL, Freyre-Fonseca V, Flores-Flores JO, Gonzalez-Robles A, et al. Food-grade titanium dioxide exposure exacerbates tumor formation in colitis associated cancer model. Food Chem Toxicol. 2016;93:20–31.

38. Powell JJ, Thoree V, Pele LC. Dietary microparticles and their impact on tolerance and immune responsiveness of the gastrointestinal tract. Br J Nutr. 2007;98(Suppl 1):S59–63.

39. Lomer MCE, Thompson RPH, Powell JJ. Fine and ultrafine particles of the diet: influence on the mucosal immune response and association with Crohn's disease. Proc Nutr Soc. 2002;61:123–30.

40. Kato T, Toyooka T, Ibuki Y, Masuda S, Watanabe M, Totsuka Y. Effect of physicochemical character differences on the genotoxic potency of kaolin. Genes Environ. 2017;39:12.

41. Winkler HC, Kornprobst J, Wick P, von Moos LM, Trantakis I, Schraner EM, et al. MyD88-dependent pro-interleukin-1β induction in dendritic cells exposed to food-grade synthetic amorphous silica. Part Fibre Toxicol. 2017;14:21.

42. Orlowski GM, Sharma S, Colbert JD, Bogyo M, Robertson SA, Kataoka H, et al. Frontline science: multiple cathepsins promote inflammasome-independent, particle-induced cell death during NLRP3-dependent IL-1β activation. J Leukoc Biol. 2017;102:7–17.

43. Bettini S, Boutet-Robinet E, Cartier C, Comera C, Gaultier E, Dupuy J, et al. Food-grade TiO$_2$ impairs intestinal and systemic immune homeostasis, initiates preneoplastic lesions and promotes aberrant crypt development in the rat colon. Sci Rep. 2017;7:40373.

44. de Souza HSP, Fiocchi C, Iliopoulos D. The IBD interactome: an integrated view of aetiology, pathogenesis and therapy. Nat Rev Gastroenterol Hepatol. 2017; doi:10.1038/nrgastro.2017.110.

7

Genotoxic and epigenotoxic effects in mice exposed to concentrated ambient fine particulate matter (PM$_{2.5}$)

Antonio Anax Falcão de Oliveira[1†], Tiago Franco de Oliveira[1,5†], Michelle Francini Dias[1], Marisa Helena Gennari Medeiros[2], Paolo Di Mascio[2], Mariana Veras[3], Miriam Lemos[3], Tania Marcourakis[1], Paulo Hilário Nascimento Saldiva[3,4] and Ana Paula Melo Loureiro[1*] ⓘ

Abstract

Background: The Metropolitan Area of São Paulo has a unique composition of atmospheric pollutants, and positive correlations between exposure and the risk of diseases and mortality have been observed. Here we assessed the effects of ambient fine particulate matter (PM$_{2.5}$) on genotoxic and global DNA methylation and hydroxymethylation changes, as well as the activities of antioxidant enzymes, in tissues of AJ mice exposed whole body to ambient air enriched in PM$_{2.5}$, which was concentrated in a chamber near an avenue of intense traffic in São Paulo City, Brazil.

Results: Mice exposed to concentrated ambient PM$_{2.5}$ (1 h daily, 3 months) were compared to in situ ambient air exposed mice as the study control. The concentrated PM$_{2.5}$ exposed group presented increased levels of the oxidized nucleoside 8-oxo-7,8-dihydro-2'-deoxyguanosine in lung and kidney DNA and increased levels of the etheno adducts 1,N^6-etheno-2'-deoxyadenosine and 1,N^2-etheno-2'-deoxyguanosine in kidney and liver DNA, respectively. Apart from the genotoxic effects, the exposure to PM$_{2.5}$ led to decreased levels of the epigenetic mark 5-hydroxymethylcytosine (5-hmC) in lung and liver DNA. Changes in lung, liver, and erythrocyte antioxidant enzyme activities were also observed. Decreased glutathione reductase and increased superoxide dismutase (SOD) activities were observed in the lungs, while the liver presented increased glutathione S-transferase and decreased SOD activities. An increase in SOD activity was also observed in erythrocytes. These changes are consistent with the induction of local and systemic oxidative stress.

Conclusions: Mice exposed daily to PM$_{2.5}$ at a concentration that mimics 24-h exposure to the mean concentration found in ambient air presented, after 3 months, increased levels of DNA lesions related to the occurrence of oxidative stress in the lungs, liver, and kidney, in parallel to decreased global levels of 5-hmC in lung and liver DNA. Genetic and epigenetic alterations induced by pollutants may affect the genes committed to cell cycle control, apoptosis, and cell differentiation, increasing the chance of cancer development, which merits further investigation.

Keywords: Particulate matter, Oxidative stress, DNA adducts, DNA methylation

* Correspondence: apmlou@usp.br
†Antonio Anax Falcão de Oliveira and Tiago Franco de Oliveira contributed equally to this work.
[1]Departamento de Análises Clínicas e Toxicológicas, Faculdade de Ciências Farmacêuticas, Universidade de São Paulo, Av. Prof. Lineu Prestes 580, Bloco 13 B, São Paulo CEP 05508-000, Brazil
Full list of author information is available at the end of the article

Background

Epidemiologic studies conducted mostly in the United States and Europe have shown that cardiovascular diseases, respiratory diseases, and cancer of different tissues (e.g., lung, breast, skin, hematopoietic, bladder, kidney, larynx, and thyroid) are empirically associated with exposure to air pollution [1–12]. Nonetheless, the balance between polluting activities and public policies to control air pollution dictates specific air pollutant compositions in each region, whose effects on disease risk, particularly cancer, are far from being completely understood [9].

The atmospheric chemical composition of the Metropolitan Area of São Paulo is characterized by emissions of approximately 2000 industries with high pollution potential and a fleet of approximately 7 million vehicles, which are the main sources of air pollutants in a region inhabiting approximately 21 million individuals [12, 13]. Automotive fuels in use are gasohol (gasoline containing 20–25% ethanol), hydrated ethanol (95% ethanol), compressed natural gas, and diesel containing 5% biodiesel [12], creating a unique composition of atmospheric pollutants with increased levels of formaldehyde, acetaldehyde, and ethanol compared to those found in other countries [14, 15]. Policies to reduce pollutant emissions by vehicles and industries in São Paulo State have been implemented since the 1980s and a diminishing tendency of regulated air pollutants (CO, hydrocarbons, nitrogen oxides, PM_{10}, and sulfur oxides) has been observed, except for ozone, even with the increase in vehicular fleet and fuel consumption [12]. However, the current levels in São Paulo are far from the recommended limits of the WHO [16], and high positive correlations between air pollution exposure and risk of cardiovascular disease, cancer, and mortality have been observed, as also shown in developed countries [7, 17–19].

The particulate matter (PM) fraction of air pollution includes solid and liquid particles of aerodynamic diameters ranging from 5 nm to 100 μm, originating from fuel combustion, biomass burning, and nucleation events based on vapor condensation (sulfuric acid, nitric acid, organic matter) in the atmosphere [9, 12, 18]. Coarse PM, with a 2.5 to 10 μm aerodynamic diameter (PM_{10}), are retained in the upper airways, while fine and ultrafine PM, with aerodynamic diameters in the 0.1–2.5 μm ($PM_{2.5}$) range and smaller than 0.1 μm ($PM_{0.1}$), respectively, can penetrate into the terminal portion of bronchi and alveoli [4, 7, 18], where they can elicit inflammatory reactions that increase the risk of diseases [2, 20, 21]. In addition to the lung absorption of particle compounds, airway mucociliary clearance results in gastrointestinal tract exposure to swallowed particles, which may trigger systemic effects [22]. Fine particles are important carriers of organic and inorganic chemicals, such as polycyclic aromatic hydrocarbons (PAHs), nitro-PAHs, aldehydes, ketones, carboxylic acids, quinolines, metals, and water-soluble ions, which may lead to harmful effects, such as inflammation, oxidative stress, mutations and cancer [10, 23–25]. Carcinogenic PAHs, such as benzo[a]pyrene, can be metabolized to reactive intermediates able to damage biomolecules, including the DNA [26, 27]. Diverse types of genome damage (chromosomal aberrations, DNA strand breaks, sister chromatid exchange, DNA adducts, micronuclei) and mutations have been shown as consequences of exposure to benzo[a]pyrene [26, 27]. The increase in the generation of reactive oxygen species (ROS) induced by PAHs may also contribute to the observed effects [28]. Based on strong evidence from epidemiological and experimental studies, the International Agency for Research on Cancer (IARC), in 2013, classified outdoor air pollution and airborne particulate matter as carcinogenic to humans (Group 1) [10].

Among the useful biomarkers for the assessment of chemical carcinogenesis pathways, DNA adducts and oxidized nucleobases or nucleosides provide information on early events triggered by exposure, such as the bioactivation of xenobiotics and oxidative stress, while DNA methylation changes depict early biological effects that may evolve to cancer [5]. Accordingly, the levels of the oxidized base 8-oxo-7,8-dihydro-guanine (8-oxoGua) or the deoxyribonucleoside 8-oxo-7,8-dihydro-2′-deoxyguanosine (8-oxodGuo, Fig. 1) are consistently increased in the mononuclear blood cells and urine of subjects exposed to ambient air pollution [5]. Regarding cancer risk, lung 8-oxodGuo levels were correlated with the induction of lung tumors in mice exposed to diesel exhaust particles (DEPs) [29], while in humans the urinary excretion of 8-oxodGuo was associated with the risk of lung cancer [30] and the incidence of colorectal cancer and benign adenoma [31].

In addition to direct DNA oxidation, oxidative stress may induce the formation of mutagenic exocyclic DNA adducts, such as propano, etheno, and malonaldehyde adducts, via reactive carbonyls resulting from lipid peroxidation [32]. The potential role of these lesions as biomarkers of oxidative stress and in cancer etiology has been determined since their quantification in vivo became feasible by using highly sensitive and selective methods [33–43]. Interestingly, the etheno adducts 1,N^2-etheno-2′-deoxyguanosine (1,N^2-εdGuo, Fig. 1) and 1,N^6-etheno-2′-deoxyadenosine (1,N^6-εdAdo, Fig. 1) were the most increased (3- to 4-fold) DNA lesions among others investigated (DNA oxidation and deamination products) in spleen, liver and kidney DNA samples from the nitric oxide overproduction SJL mouse model of inflammation [37]. Despite their potential use as biomarkers in the pathophysiology of inflammation [36, 37], the assessment of these etheno adducts under conditions of PM exposure has only been addressed by a few studies focusing on the effects of wood smoke and ambient PM resulting from wood stoves [44, 45]. Regardless of the inflammatory response [20, 21, 46–48], there are no studies on the effects of urban air PM exposure on the tissue levels of DNA etheno adducts.

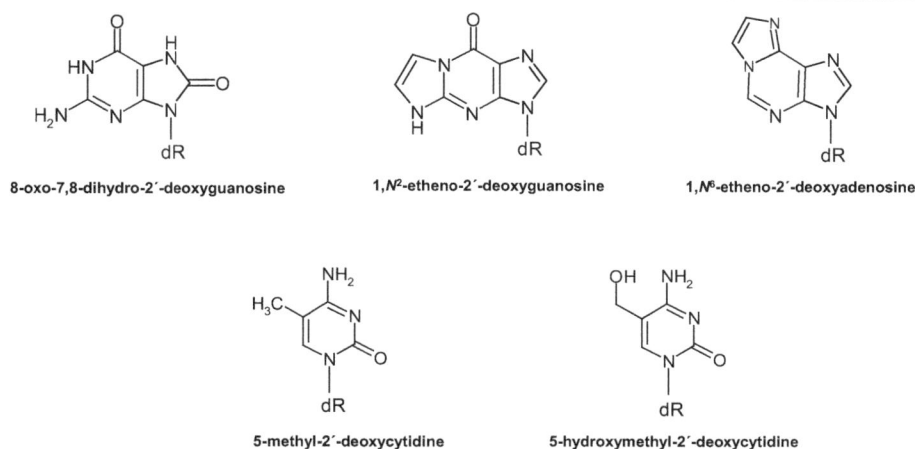

Fig. 1 Chemical structures of the DNA lesions and epigenetic marks quantified in the present study. dR = 2'-deoxyribose

Current research has uncovered epigenetic changes associated with PM exposure, which may play a role in cardiovascular disease and cancer development [47, 49–52]. The current best characterized epigenetic mark is DNA 5-methylcytosine (5-mC, Fig. 1), maintained by DNA methyltransferases (DNMTs) at approximately 4% of the cytosine levels in adult human DNA, with important roles in development, genomic imprinting, silencing of transposable elements, and regulation of gene expression [50, 53–56]. While DNMTs catalyze the C-5 methylation of cytosine bases pertaining to CpGs sequences, the Ten-Eleven-Translocation (TET) methylcytosine hydroxylases are involved in the oxidation of 5-mC to 5-hydroxymethylcytosine (5-hmC, Fig. 1), which is considered the first step in the demethylation process [57].

Studies on global DNA methylation in the whole blood of humans have been associated with a hypomethylation effect of PM exposure [47, 49, 51, 58–62], whereas the outcomes of PM exposure on the global DNA methylation of other target tissues have been studied in mice sperm, rat lung, human placenta, and human buccal cells [63–67]. Increased levels of 5-hmC were detected in blood samples from humans exposed to ambient PM_{10} [68], but human bronchial epithelial cells (HBECs) exposed to DEPs (5 mg/ cm^2, 24 h) in vitro presented decreased 5-hmC levels [69]. Additionally, the increase in human exposure to $PM_{2.5}$ or PM_{10} was associated with a decrease of 5-hmC levels in buccal cells [65].

To better understand the toxicity pathways of fine particulate matter, considering that studies focusing on the genotoxic and epigenotoxic effects of ambient air pollution in South America are scarce [5, 8], we used HPLC-ESI-MS/MS methods to evaluate the effects of ambient $PM_{2.5}$ on genotoxic (8-oxodGuo, $1,N^2$-εdGuo and $1,N^6$-εdAdo lesions) and global DNA 5-mC and 5-hmC changes in different tissues (lung, liver and kidney) of AJ mice. The

animals were exposed whole body to ambient air enriched in $PM_{2.5}$ and compared to in situ ambient air exposed mice as the study control. The fine particulate matter was concentrated in a chamber placed near an avenue of intense traffic in São Paulo City, Brazil.

Methods
Chemicals and enzymes
All the chemicals employed here were of the highest purity grade commercially available. Chromatography grade acetonitrile and methanol, isopropyl alcohol, chloroform, hydrochloric acid, ethanol, magnesium chloride, and tris(hydroxymethyl)-aminomethane were obtained from Carlo Erba Reagents (Milan, Italy). Sodium hydroxide, potassium phosphate, and ammonium acetate were acquired from Merck (Darmstadt, Germany). DNA extraction solutions were obtained from QIAGEN (Valencia, CA). DNase I was acquired from Bio Basic Inc. (Ontario, Canada). $[^{15}N_5]$-2'-deoxyguanosine and $[^{15}N_5]$-2'-deoxyadenosine were provided by Cambridge Isotope Laboratories (Andover, MA). All the other reagents were obtained from Sigma-Aldrich Co. (St. Louis, MO). The catalogue numbers of the reagents are described in Additional file 1: Table S1. Water was purified in a Milli-Q system (Millipore, Bedford, MA).

Adduct standards
$1,N^2$-Etheno-2'-deoxyguanosine ($1,N^2$-εdGuo) and the isotopic standards $[^{15}N_5]1,N^2$-εdGuo, $[^{15}N_5]1,N^6$-εdAdo and $[^{15}N_5]8$-oxodGuo were prepared as described [35, 70]. Their identities were confirmed by their spectral properties, as follows. $1,N^2$-εdGuo: UV, $\lambda_{max} = 285$ nm, $\varepsilon = 16,785$ M^{-1} cm^{-1} [71], pH 7.0; positive ESI-MS: m/z 292 [M + H]$^+$, m/z 176 [M − 2'-deoxyribose + H]$^+$. $[^{15}N_5]1,N^2$-εdGuo: positive ESI-MS: m/z 297 [M + H]$^+$, m/z 181 [M − 2'-deoxyribose + H]$^+$. $[^{15}N_5]1,N^6$-εdAdo: UV, $\lambda_{max} = 260$ nm,

$\varepsilon = 10,300$ M^{-1} cm^{-1} [72], pH 7.0; positive ESI-MS: m/z 281 [M + H]$^+$, m/z 165 [M − 2′-deoxyribose + H]$^+$. [^{15}N$_5$]8-oxodGuo: UV, λ_{max} = 294 nm, ε = 9700 M^{-1} cm^{-1} [73] in water; positive ESI-MS: m/z 289 [M + H]$^+$, m/z 173 [M − 2′-deoxyribose + H]$^+$.

5-mC standard

5-methyl-2′-deoxycytidine (5-mC) standard was obtained by HPLC purification from a solution of commercial dCyd (1 mg/mL). Its spectral properties are as follows: UV in H$_2$O, λ_{max} 277 nm, ε = 8500 M^{-1} cm^{-1} [74]; positive ESI-MS: m/z 242 [M + H]$^+$, m/z 126 [M − 2′-deoxyribose + H]$^+$. The standard was used for quantification of 5-mC and 5-hmC, but the retention time of 5-hmC was defined using a sample of calf thymus DNA presenting a main peak with m/z 258 [M + H]$^+$ → m/z 142 [M - 2′-deoxyribose + H]$^+$.

Experimental groups

Four week old male AJ mice, specific pathogen free, were obtained from the Breeding Center of Laboratory Animals of Fundação Oswaldo Cruz (FIOCRUZ), Rio de Janeiro, Brazil, and were treated accordingly to the Ethics Committee of the Faculty of Medicine, University of São Paulo (protocol n 1310/09). The animals were submitted to a controlled exposure system in a Harvard Ambient Fine-Particle Concentrator designed to concentrate PM$_{2.5}$ up to 30 times. It works separating particles from gases by particle inertia using virtual impaction [75]. It has two chambers, one receiving the air concentrated with particles and the other receiving the ambient air. Two experimental groups were considered, eight animals each: one group breathed concentrated PM$_{2.5}$ and the other group breathed ambient air. They were exposed 1 h/day in the afternoon, 5 days/week, along 3 months (September to November). Between exposures, animals were maintained in plastic cages, at a controlled temperature, in a 12-h light-dark cycle; they also received clean air (HEPA air), food (CR-1 Nuvilab, Colombo, PR, Brazil) and water ad libitum. Immediately after the last exposure, they were anesthetized by i.p. injection of xylazine and ketamine (87.5 mg/kg ketamine and 12.5 mg/kg xylazine). Blood samples were collected, centrifuged (2000 g), and the red blood cells separated for antioxidant enzyme activity assessment. Animals were euthanized by exsanguination. Lung, liver, and kidney were immediately collected, frozen in liquid nitrogen and kept under -80 °C until processing.

Site of exposure

The exposure site was the same described by Akinaga and colleagues [76], located in an area of the Medical School of University of São Paulo, 20 m from the roadside and 150 m from a busy traffic crossroad. The Cerqueira César monitoring station of the São Paulo State Environmental Agency (CETESB, São Paulo, Brazil) is located 160 m from the exposure site. The region is impacted mainly by the emissions of light duty gasohol / hydrated ethanol and heavy duty diesel vehicles.

Exposure chambers

Animals were maintained in special cages that allowed homogeneous distribution of air. Both experimental groups were exposed at the same time and conditions of temperature and pressure. Animals in the 30 times concentrator chamber were exposed daily to PM$_{2.5}$ (5 days/week, 3 months), constantly monitored by a nephelometer. The calculated PM$_{2.5}$ concentration (mean ± SD) for the entire period of exposure was 682 ± 532 μg/m^3. Twice a week, samples of the PM$_{2.5}$ were collected onto polycarbonate filters for elemental analysis [77]. For determination of specific polycyclic aromatic hydrocarbons in PM$_{2.5}$, we used a Hi-vol particle sampler to collect these particles on quartz filters. Analyses of these filters were conducted according to Magalhães and coworkers [78].

Antioxidant enzyme activities

Enzymatic activities of glutathione peroxidase (GPx), glutathione reductase (GR), glutathione S-transferase (GST), and superoxide dismutase (SOD) were determined by spectrophotometric method in lung, liver, kidney, and erythrocytes. Catalase activity (CAT) was evaluated only in erythrocytes. GPx activity was performed using the procedure described by Flohé and Günzler [79]. Tert-butyl hydroperoxide was used as substrate and the formation of oxidized glutathione (GSSG) was indirectly monitored spectrophotometrically through NADPH consumption at 340 nm during 5 min. GR activity was assayed according to Carlberg and Mannervik [80]. The reduction of GSSG to GSH was measured through NADPH consumption and monitored spectrophotometrically at 37 °C for 10 min at 340 nm. GST activity assay was conducted measuring the conjugation of 1-chloro-2,4-dinitrobenzene (CDNB) with reduced glutathione, according to Habig [81]. The formation of the complex was monitored spectrophotometrically at 25 °C for 5 min at 340 nm. Superoxide dismutase (SOD) activity was measured based on McCord & Fridovich, and Flohé & Ötting methods that use the system hypoxanthine-xanthine as a superoxide anion donor [82, 83]. The O$_2$$^{\bullet-}$ production is coupled to the reduction of ferricytochrome C, which is followed spectrophotometrically, allowing for quantitative measurement. SOD in samples converts superoxide free radical to H$_2$O$_2$ and O$_2$, therefore slowing the rate of ferricytochrome C reduction. During the assay, the absorbance was detected in a spectrophotometer at 550 nm, 25 °C. SOD, GPx, GR and GST assays were performed in spectrophotometer Power Wave × 340 (Bio-Tek Instruments INC, software KC4 v3.0). Catalase activity was evaluated measuring the consumption of hydrogen peroxide (H$_2$O$_2$) [84]. The decrease in absorbance was monitored at 25 °C for 30 s at 240 nm in a spectrophotometer (Biochrom Libra S12). All enzyme activities in lung, liver and kidney are expressed as U/μg of protein. The enzyme activities conducted in erythrocytes were corrected by hemoglobin content and expressed as U/g of hemoglobin. Protein and hemoglobin contents were determined by Bradford and Doles® reagents, respectively. All enzymatic assays were conducted in triplicate.

DNA extraction
DNA samples from lung, liver, and kidney were extracted using a QIAGEN kit according to manufacturer's instructions for 1 g of animal tissue, maintaining the correct proportions. Briefly, tissue samples (with average weight of 1.0 g) were homogenized with 10 mL of the cell lysis solution (QIAGEN, Cat. No. 158908) plus 0.5 mM deferoxamine. The obtained homogenates were added to 150 μL of 20 mg/mL proteinase K solution. The samples were homogenized and remained at room temperature overnight. After this period, 40 μL of ribonuclease A (15 mg/mL) were added and kept 2 h at room temperature. The proteins were precipitated by adding 5 mL of protein precipitation solution (QIAGEN, Cat. No. 158912) and centrifuged at 2000 g for 10 min. The supernatants were transferred to tubes containing 10 mL of cold isopropanol. The precipitated DNA was collected into tubes containing 4 mL of 10 mM Tris buffer, 1 mM deferoxamine, pH 7.0, and extracted three times with 4 mL of a chloroform solution containing 4% of isoamyl alcohol. The DNA was again precipitated by adding 8 mL of absolute ethanol and 0.4 mL of a 5 M NaCl solution, and washed twice with 3 mL of 70% ethanol. After air drying, the samples were suspended in 200 μL of 0.1 mM deferoxamine solution and stored at -20 °C. The DNA concentration was determined by measuring the absorbance at 260 nm and its purity was established based on the 260/280 nm absorbance ratio.

DNA enzymatic hydrolysis
For analyses of etheno adducts in liver, aliquots containing 150 μg of DNA were transferred to a final volume of 200 μL of deionized water. 7.5 μL of 200 mM Tris/MgCl$_2$ buffer (pH 7.4), 1.4 μL of the internal standard solution containing [^{15}N$_5$]1,N^6-εdAdo and [^{15}N$_5$]1,N^2-εdGuo (250 fmol/μL), and 6 μL (15 units) of deoxyribonuclease I (Bio Basic Inc., Ontario, Canada) were added. The samples were incubated at 37 °C, 90 rpm for 1 h. Then, 6 μL (0.006 units) of phosphodiesterase I from *Crotalus atrox* (Sigma Aldrich, St. Louis, MO, USA) and 7.5 μL (15 units) of alkaline phosphatase from bovine intestinal mucosa (Sigma Aldrich, St. Louis, USA) were added, incubating again at 37 °C, 90 rpm for 1 h. Finally, samples were centrifuged at 14,000 g for 10 min. Aliquots of 10 μL were withdrawn for quantification of deoxynucleosides (dAdo,

dGuo) by HPLC/PDA. The residual volume of sample was submitted to solid phase extraction, as described below.

Analyses of etheno adducts in kidney and lung were performed using 100 μg of DNA, maintaining the correct proportions of enzymes and the other reagents.

The same procedure was used for quantification of 8-oxodGuo in liver, lung and kidney, using 80 μg of DNA and 1000 fmol of the internal standard [^{15}N$_5$]8-oxodGuo in the injection volume.

Samples containing 12 μg DNA and 3000 fmol of [^{15}N$_5$]1,N^6-εdAdo were also hydrolyzed for analyses of 5-mC and 5-hmC, using the same procedure adjusted to a final volume of 60 μL. The hydrolyzed samples were, then, added to 140 μL of acetonitrile, vortexed for 20 s, centrifuged at 9300 g for 10 min, and aliquots of 20 μL were injected into the HPLC-ESI-MS/MS system described below.

Solid phase extraction
Samples for the analyses of etheno adducts were pre-purified by solid phase extraction, using SPE-C18 cartridges (30 mg/mL, 33 μm, 1 mL, Strata-X, Phenomenex, Torrance, CA, Cat. No. 8B-S100-TAK). This step was not performed for quantification of 8-oxodGuo. The cartridges were loaded in the following sequence: 100% methanol, deionized water, hydrolyzed DNA sample, deionized water, 10% methanol, 15% methanol, and 100% methanol. The last elution fraction containing the adducts of interest was collected. Samples were then vacuum dried and resuspended in 83.1 μL of MiliQ water immediately prior to the HPLC-ESI-MS/MS analysis, to obtain 200 fmol of internal standards in 50 μL of each sample.

Quantification of DNA lesions, 5-mC and 5-hmC
The levels of 1,N^6-εdAdo, 1,N^2-εdGuo, 8-oxodGuo, 5-mC and 5-hmC in DNA samples were assessed by HPLC-ESI-MS/MS. The analytical system consisted of an Agilent 1200 series HPLC (Wilmington, DE, USA) equipped with a binary pump (Agilent 1200 G1312B), an isocratic pump (Agilent 1200 G1310A), a column oven (Agilent 1200 G1316B), a diode array detector (Agilent 1200 DAD G1315C), and an auto sampler (G1367C Agilent 1200) interfaced with a Linear Quadrupole Ion Trap mass spectrometer, Model 4000 QTRAP (Applied Biosystems/MDS Sciex Instruments, Foster City). The ESI-MS/MS parameters were set in the positive ion mode as described in Additional file 1: Table S2.

Analyses were carried out with multiple reaction monitoring (MRM) by using the following fragmentations: m/z 276 [M + H]$^+$ → m/z 160 [M - 2′-deoxyribose + H]$^+$ and m/z 281 [M + H]$^+$ → m/z 165 [M - 2′-deoxyribose + H]$^+$ for detection of 1,N^6-εdAdo and respective internal standard [^{15}N$_5$]1,N^6-εdAdo; m/z 292 [M + H]$^+$ → m/z 176 [M - 2′-deoxyribose + H]$^+$ and m/z 297 [M + H]$^+$ → m/z 181

$[M - 2'$-deoxyribose $+ H]^+$ for detection of $1,N^2$-εdGuo and respective internal standard $[^{15}N_5]1,N^2$-εdGuo; m/z 284 $[M + H]^+ \rightarrow m/z$ 168 $[M - 2'$-deoxyribose $+ H]^+$ and m/z 289 $[M + H]^+ \rightarrow m/z$ 173 $[M - 2'$-deoxyribose $+ H]^+$ for detection of 8-oxodGuo and respective internal standard $[^{15}N_5]$8-oxodGuo; m/z 242 $[M + H]^+ \rightarrow m/z$ 126 $[M - 2'$-deoxyribose $+ H]^+$ for detection of 5-mC; m/z 258 $[M + H]^+ \rightarrow m/z$ 142 $[M - 2'$-deoxyribose $+ H]^+$ for detection of 5-hmC; m/z 228 $[M + H]^+ \rightarrow m/z$ 112 $[M - 2'$-deoxyribose $+ H]^+$ for detection of dCyd.

The calibration curves were constructed at the intervals of 367 to 5875 fmol of 8-oxodGuo, with a fixed amount of $[^{15}N_5]$8-oxodGuo (1000 fmol); 1 to 40 fmol of $1,N^6$-εdAdo and $1,N^2$-εdGuo, with fixed amounts of $[^{15}N_5]1,N^6$-εdAdo and $[^{15}N_5]1,N^2$-εdGuo (200 fmol); and 150 to 1500 pmol of dCyd, 5 to 500 fmol of 5-mC for quantification of 5-hmC, and 5 to 80 pmol of 5-mC for quantification of 5-mC, with a fixed amount of $[^{15}N_5]1,N^6$-εdAdo (300 fmol). Data were acquired and processed using Analyst software 1.4 (Applied Biosystems/MDS Sciex). The molar fractions 8-oxodGuo/dGuo, $1,N^6$-εdAdo/dAdo, $1,N^2$-εdGuo/dGuo, 5-mC/(5-mC + 5-hmC + dCyd), 5-hmC/(5-mC + 5-hmC + dCyd) present in each DNA sample were determined. The following chromatography conditions were used for the analyses. All solvents used were previously filtered and degassed.

8-oxodGuo analysis: A 50×2.0 mm i.d., 2.5 µm, Luna C18(2)-HST column (Phenomenex, Torrance, CA) with a C18(2) security guard cartridge, 4.0×3.0 mm i.d. (Phenomenex, Torrance, CA) was eluted with a gradient of 0.1% formic acid (solvent A) and methanol containing 0.1% formic acid (solvent B) at a flow rate of 150 µL/min and 25 °C, as follows: from 0 to 25 min, 0–15% of solvent B; 25 to 28 min, 15–80% of solvent B; 28 to 31 min, 80% of solvent B; 31 to 33 min, 80–0% of solvent B; 33 to 46 min, 0% of solvent B. The first 16 min of eluent was directed to waste and the 16–32 min fraction was diverted to a second column (150×2.0 mm i.d., 3.0 µm, Luna C18(2)) connected to the ESI source and conditioned by a third isocratic pump with a solution of 15% methanol in water containing 0.1% formic acid (150 µL/min) (Additional file 1: Figure S1). The lesion 8-oxodGuo eluted from the second column at approximately 36 min.

Etheno adducts analyses: A 150×2.0 mm i.d., 3.0 µm, Luna C18(2) column (Phenomenex, Torrance, CA) with a C18(2) security guard cartridge, 4.0×3.0 mm i.d. (Phenomenex, Torrance, CA) was eluted with a gradient of 5 mM ammonium acetate, pH 6.6 (solvent A) and acetonitrile (solvent B) at a flow rate of 130 µL/min and 25 °C, as follows: from 0 to 10 min, 0% of solvent B; 10 to 39 min, 0–20% of solvent B; 39 to 41 min, 20–75% of solvent B; 41 to 46 min, 75% of solvent B; 46 to 47 min, 75–0% of solvent B; 47 to 60 min, 0% of solvent B. The first 15 min of eluent was directed to waste and the 15–18 min fraction was diverted to the ESI source.

5-mC and 5-hmC analyses: A 150×4.6 mm i.d., 5 µm, *Syncronis* HILIC(2) column (Thermo Scientific, USA), with a HILIC security guard cartridge, 4.0×3.0 mm i.d. (Thermo Scientific, USA), was eluted with a gradient of acetonitrile (solvent A) and 5 mM ammonium acetate, pH 8.2 (solvent B) at a flow rate of 300 µL/min and 35 °C, as follows: from 0 to 35 min, 0–40% of solvent B; 35 to 36 min, 40–0% of solvent B; 36 to 56 min, 0% of solvent B. The first 16 min of eluent was directed to waste and the 16–27 min fraction was diverted to the ESI source.

Method validation for 8-oxodGuo quantification in DNA samples

Method accuracy and precision were determined by adding varying amounts of 8-oxodGuo (367, 734, 1469, and 2204 fmol) and a fixed amount of $[^{15}N_5]$8-oxodGuo (1000 fmol) to 100 µg of calf thymus DNA and carrying out the enzymatic hydrolysis and analysis. Samples were processed in quadruplicate in two different days. The limit of quantitation (LOQ) was estimated from the lowest amount of 8-oxodGuo injected on column, with S/N = 10.

Method validation for $1,N^6$-εdAdo and $1,N^2$-εdGuo quantification in DNA samples

Varying amounts of $1,N^6$-εdAdo (1, 5, 10, and 20 fmol in the injection volume) and $1,N^2$-εdGuo (1, 5, 10, and 20 fmol in the injection volume) and fixed amounts of $[^{15}N_5]1,N^6$-εdAdo and $[^{15}N_5]1,N^2$-εdGuo (200 fmol in the injection volume) were added to 100 µg of calf thymus DNA and the analyses were carried out. Samples were processed in quadruplicate in two different days for method accuracy and precision assessment. Recovery was calculated by adding the internal standards $[^{15}N_5]1,N^6$-εdAdo and $[^{15}N_5]1,N^2$-εdGuo (200 fmol) to 100 µg of calf thymus DNA before and after solid phase extraction, carrying out the analyses as described above. The DNA used for recovery calculation was contaminated with 7.5 fmol of $1,N^6$-εdAdo and 20 fmol of $1,N^2$-εdGuo in the beginning of the process. The limit of detection (LOD) was estimated from the lowest amount of adducts added to the calf thymus DNA sample.

Normal 2'-deoxynucleosides quantification in DNA samples used for analyses of 8-oxodGuo, $1,N^6$-εdAdo and $1,N^2$-εdGuo

The quantification of normal 2'-deoxynucleosides was carried out with a Shimadzu (Kyoto, Japan) HPLC system equipped with two LC-20AT pumps, a photo diode array detector (PDA-20AV), an auto-injector (Proeminence SIL-20 AC), and a column oven (CTO-10AS/VP) controlled by a CBM-20A communication module and the software LC-Solution. Elution system was as follows: a 250 mm × 4.6 mm i.d., 5 µm,

Luna C18(2) column (Phenomenex, Torrance, CA) attached to a C18(2) guard column (4,0 × 3.0 mm i.d., 4 μm, Phenomenex, Torrance, CA), eluted with a gradient of 0.1% formic acid and CH_3OH (from 0 to 25 min, 0 to 18% CH_3OH; from 25 to 27 min, 18 to 0% CH_3OH; from 27 to 37 min, 0% CH_3OH) at a flow rate of 1 mL/min and 30 °C. The PDA detector was set at 260 nm. Calibration curves were constructed at intervals of 0.05–1 nmol for dGuo and dAdo.

Statistics

Data were expressed as average ± SEM or average ± SD, as indicated in the text and tables. Means between the two groups (ambient air and $PM_{2.5}$) were compared using t test for 8-oxodGuo, $1,N^2$-εdGuo, $1,N^6$-εdAdo, 5-mC and antioxidant enzymes activities, or Mann-Whitney test for 5-hmC. Results were considered statistically significant when P value was less than 0.05. Normality of the samples was checked by the Kolmogorov-Smirnov test and homogeneity of variances with the Levene test. The statistical analyses were conducted using GraphPad Prism version 6 for Windows (GraphPad Software, San Diego California USA).

Results

Exposure assessment

The elemental characterization of $PM_{2.5}$ is depicted in Table 1. Table 2 presents the mean concentrations of specific polycyclic aromatic hydrocarbons detected in $PM_{2.5}$ collected near the site of exposure.

Antioxidant enzyme activities

Mice exposed to concentrated $PM_{2.5}$ presented changes in lung, liver, and erythrocyte antioxidant enzyme activities, as shown in Table 3. Statistically significant decreased GR and statistically significant increased SOD activities were observed in the lungs, while the liver presented statistically significant increased GST and statistically significant decreased SOD activities. A statistically significant increase in SOD activity was also observed in erythrocytes.

Genotoxic effects of $PM_{2.5}$ in the lungs, liver, and kidneys

The genotoxic effects of $PM_{2.5}$ were assessed by the quantification of 8-oxodGuo and the etheno adducts $1,N^2$-εdGuo and $1,N^6$-εdAdo in lung, liver, and kidney DNA samples. The levels of each lesion in each organ of mice exposed to $PM_{2.5}$ concentrated 30 times compared to those exposed to ambient air are shown in Table 4.

Table 1 Elements (ng/m^3) detected in $PM_{2.5}$ (μg/m^3)

	Minimum	Q1	Median	Q3	Maximum	Mean	SD	SEM
$PM_{2.5}$	65.2	222	574	1047	2094	682	532	95.5
Na	0.00	10.68	432.95	613.42	3774.50	525.64	711.31	125.74
Mg	0.00	0.00	44.13	302.58	6061.46	363.25	1059.70	187.33
Al	289.82	1130.75	1785.09	4219.14	65,846.50	5610.86	11,559.93	2043.53
Si	93.81	827.61	1840.58	4954.59	83,737.34	6489.89	14,685.73	2596.10
P	0.00	39.55	219.26	512.15	8645.44	584.46	1492.15	263.78
S	573.18	2935.17	7074.47	12,747.56	27,164.33	9374.97	8051.74	1423.36
Cl	0.00	75.99	433.59	932.43	4994.57	772.92	1038.12	183.52
K	62.70	778.64	1488.44	3005.62	35,421.57	3458.71	6403.12	1131.92
Ca	44.18	447.99	1233.81	2473.66	40,539.07	3267.85	7148.36	1263.66
Ti	8.70	54.86	151.17	564.01	6261.38	641.99	1429.13	252.64
V	0.00	0.73	6.43	14.18	71.68	11.50	16.50	2.92
Cr	0.00	0.00	0.00	13.09	198.64	14.21	35.27	6.23
Mn	6.21	47.19	90.59	121.04	1432.81	157.48	255.25	45.12
Fe	5.74	1094.30	2042.59	4479.96	65,800.18	5304.88	11,441.17	2022.53
Ni	0.00	0.00	2.96	6.74	81.34	7.99	15.40	2.72
Cu	0.00	23.14	54.24	102.69	868.51	99.66	155.25	27.44
Zn	0.00	146.45	300.87	509.58	3411.48	500.06	703.91	124.43
Se	0.00	0.00	0.00	0.16	10.27	1.24	2.69	0.48
Br	0.00	10.55	15.17	45.03	223.70	36.15	45.36	8.02
Rh	0.00	0.00	0.00	80.53	391.62	51.97	91.40	16.42
Pb	0.00	9.68	31.84	36.13	207.06	37.88	45.23	10.66

Table 2 Polycyclic aromatic hydrocarbons in $PM_{2.5}$ collected at the site of exposure

	Filters (n)	Mean ± SEM (range) ng/m^3
Pyrene	6	1.66 ± 0.42 (3.6–9.0)
Benz[e]acephenantrylene	6	6.81 ± 1.88 (2.44–13.97)
Benzo[k]fluoranthene	8	1.42 ± 0.37 (0.44–3.17)
Benzo[a]pyrene	7	0.72 ± 0.14 (0.27–1.083)

The levels of 8-oxodGuo were increased in the lung and kidney DNA of mice exposed to concentrated $PM_{2.5}$, while 1,N^2-εdGuo was preferentially formed in the liver DNA of mice exposed to concentrated $PM_{2.5}$. A significant increase in 1,N^6-εdAdo was observed in the kidneys of mice exposed to concentrated $PM_{2.5}$. Representative chromatograms are shown in Fig. 2a and b.

Effects of $PM_{2.5}$ on global 5-mC and 5-hmC in lung, liver, and kidney DNA

Epigenetic effects of $PM_{2.5}$ were evaluated by quantification of 5-mC and 5-hmC in lung, liver, and kidney DNA samples. The levels obtained for each organ from mice exposed to $PM_{2.5}$ concentrated 30 times compared to those of mice exposed to ambient air are shown in Table 4. While exposure to concentrated $PM_{2.5}$ did not lead to statistically significant changes in global 5-mC levels, the lung and liver samples of AJ mice exposed to concentrated $PM_{2.5}$ presented lower levels of 5-hmC. An inverse correlation between 5-hmC and 8-oxodGuo was observed in the lung DNA (Fig. 3a). The ratios 5-mC/5-hmC in the lung DNA also differed significantly between the ambient air and

Table 3 Enzymatic activities of glutathione peroxidase (GPx), glutathione reductase (GR), glutathione S-transferase (GST), superoxide dismutase (SOD), and catalase (CAT) in lung, liver, kidney (U/μg protein), and erythrocytes (U/g hemoglobin)

	Ambient Air Average ± SEM (U/μg protein or U/g hemoglobin)	$PM_{2.5}$ Average ± SEM (U/μg protein or U/g hemoglobin)	Number	P value
Lung				
GPx	2.832 ± 0.083	2.967 ± 0.114	4	NS
GR	1.454 ± 0.047	1.142 ± 0.074	4	0.02
GST	12.96 ± 0.600	12.96 ± 0.480	4	NS
SOD	133,436 ± 5858	190,269 ± 13,951	4	0.02
Liver				
GPx	9.900 ± 0.110	10.11 ± 0.150	5	NS
GR	1.390 ± 0.040	1.350 ± 0.060	5	NS
GST	31.82 ± 1.040	35.25 ± 0.700	5	0.02
SOD	296,609 ± 37,767	142,425 ± 21,046	5	<0.01
Kidney				
GPx	6.540 ± 0.090	6.170 ± 0.230	5	NS
GR	3.110 ± 0.080	2.910 ± 0.140	5	NS
GST	13.37 ± 0.240	13.020 ± 0.570	5	NS
SOD	114,203 ± 7149	109,789 ± 17,576	5	NS
Erythrocytes				
GPx	2175 ± 72.00	2292 ± 63.00	6	NS
GR	103.8 ± 4.500	97.98 ± 3.070	5	NS
GST	168.0 ± 7.900	173.8 ± 3.800	4	NS
SOD	151,304 ± 14,350	216,638 ± 4807	4	<0.01
CAT	110,883 ± 5300	113,442 ± 3196	6	NS

NS Not Significant

Table 4 Levels of DNA lesions, 5-mC and 5-hmC in samples from AJ mice exposed to ambient air and to $PM_{2.5}$ concentrated 30 times

	Ambient Air Average ± SEM	$PM_{2.5}$ Average ± SEM	Number	P value
Lung				
8-oxodGuo/10^8 dGuo	2124 ± 56.96	2466 ± 93.10	6	0.01
1,N^2-εdGuo/10^8 dGuo	ND	ND	–	–
1,N^6-εdAdo/10^8 dAdo	1.41 ± 0.23	1.44 ± 0.13	7	NS
5-mC (%)	3.53 ± 0.18	3.84 ± 0.21	8	NS
5-hmC (%)	0.044 ± 0.006	0.029 ± 0.001	8	<0.01
Liver				
8-oxodGuo/10^8 dGuo	2848 ± 183.5	2949 ± 223.8	6; 5	NS
1,N^2-εdGuo/10^8 dGuo	7.79 ± 2.49	24.94 ± 5.21	4	0.02
1,N^6-εdAdo/10^8 dAdo	2.82 ± 0.30	2.18 ± 0.25	6	NS
5-mC (%)	4.68 ± 0.11	4.36 ± 0.38	8; 6	NS
5-hmC (%)	0.060 ± 0.004	0.051 ± 0.002	8; 6	0.04
Kidney				
8-oxodGuo/10^8 dGuo	1854 ± 87.13	2363 ± 157.0	6	0.02
1,N^2-εdGuo/10^8 dGuo	ND	ND	–	–
1,N^6-εdAdo/10^8 dAdo	1.09 ± 0.15	1.52 ± 0.12	7	0.04
5-mC (%)	4.84 ± 0.24	4.20 ± 0.37	8	NS
5-hmC (%)	0.048 ± 0.003	0.048 ± 0.003	8	NS

NS Not Significant, *ND* Not Detected

$PM_{2.5}$ groups (Fig. 3b). A representative chromatogram is shown in Fig. 2c.

Method validation for 8-oxodGuo quantification in DNA samples

For 8-oxodGuo quantification, the system illustrated in Additional file 1: Figure S1 was used. A typical calibration curve in the 367–5875 fmol range, with a fixed amount of the internal standard [$^{15}N_5$]8-oxodGuo (1000 fmol), is presented in Additional file 1: Figure S2. The MS response was linear in the range measured. The method accuracy and precision are presented in Table 5. Good agreement was observed between added and detected amounts of 8-oxodGuo (86–104% accuracy). The intra-day precision was determined by calculating the coefficient of variation (%) for each concentration. The inter-day precision calculated for DNA aliquots supplemented with 367 fmol of 8-oxodGuo was 16.97%. The LOQ (S/N = 10) was 25 fmol for the standard on-column injection.

Method validation for 1,N^6-εdAdo and 1,N^2-εdGuo quantification in DNA samples

The calibration curves presented in Additional file 1: Figure S2 show that the MS response was linear in the 1–40 fmol range. Good agreement was also observed between added and detected amounts of 1,N^6-εdAdo and 1,N^2-εdGuo (93–101% accuracy for 1,N^2-εdGuo, and 100–118% accuracy for 1,N^6-εdAdo) (Table 5). Intra-day precision was determined by calculating the coefficient of variation (%) for each concentration. The inter-day precision calculated for DNA aliquots supplemented with 10 fmol of 1,N^2-εdGuo and 1 fmol of 1,N^6-εdAdo was 14.01 and 16.66%, respectively. The limits of on-column quantification (S/N = 10) were 0.3 fmol for 1,N^6-εdAdo and 1 fmol for 1,N^2-εdGuo.

Discussion

A complex mixture of gases, vapors and particles of varying size and chemical composition is found in urban air, resultant from diverse polluting human activities [6, 17]. To study the effects of specific components of this complex mixture, taking into account the dynamics of pollutants in real ambient air, a feasible approach is to selectively concentrate the desired component over a background of real pollution [75]. Using this approach, we found here that mice exposed to $PM_{2.5}$ from a busy traffic crossroad in São Paulo City presented altered antioxidant system activity in lung, liver, and erythrocytes, concomitantly to increased levels of lung and kidney 8-oxodGuo, kidney 1,N^6-εdAdo, and liver 1,N^2-εdGuo, as well as decreased levels of lung and liver 5-hmC.

In the present study, mice exposed to ambient air enriched in $PM_{2.5}$ ($682 ± 532$ μg/m^3) for 1 h daily for 3 months (from infancy to adulthood) were compared to a

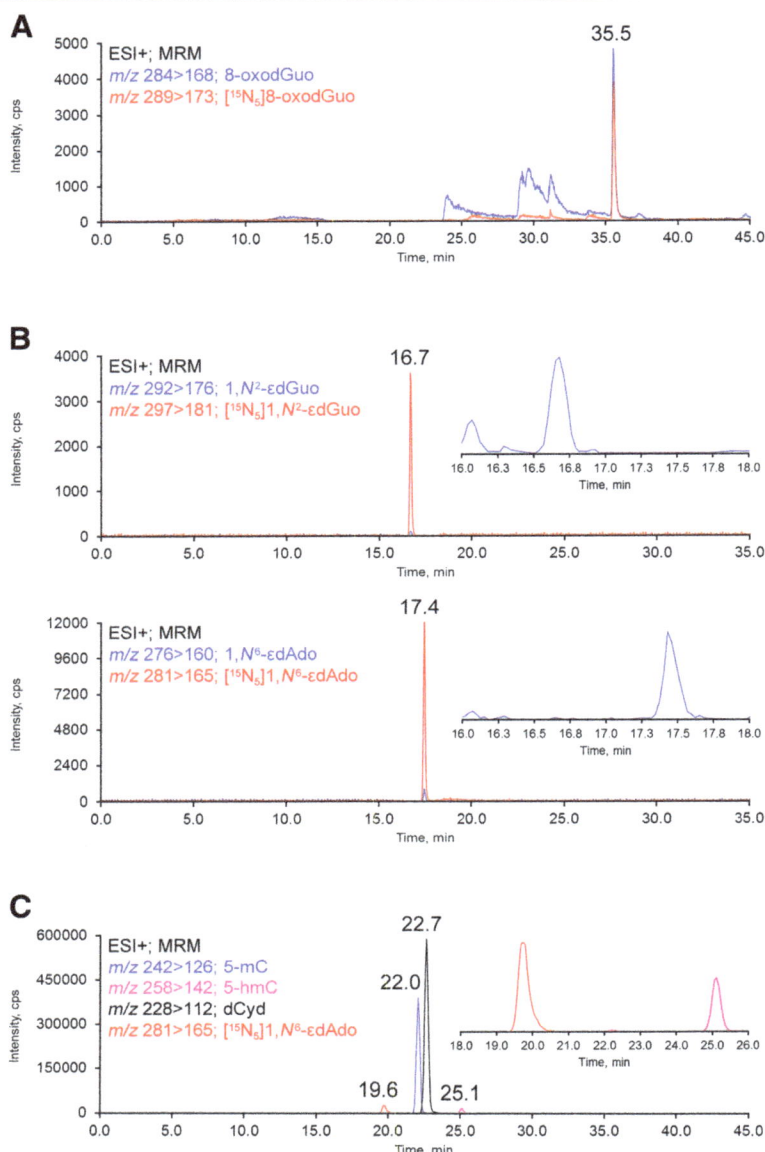

Fig. 2 Representative chromatograms of DNA samples obtained by HPLC-ESI-MS/MS showing **a** 8-oxo-7,8-dihydro-2′-deoxyguanosine (8-oxodGuo); **b** 1,N^2-etheno-2′-deoxyguanosine (1,N^2-εdGuo) and 1,N^6-etheno-2′-deoxyadenosine (1,N^6-εdAdo); **c** 5-methyl-2′-deoxycytidine (5-mC), 5-hydroxymethyl-2′-deoxycytidine (5-hmC), and 2′-deoxycytidine (dCyd). The analyses were performed with multiple reaction monitoring (MRM) by using the fragmentations specified in the images for each analyte. The internal standards are represented by the red traces

control group exposed to ambient air, and both groups were treated inside the chambers of a Harvard Ambient Fine-Particle Concentrator located near the crossroad. The total intake dose (ID) of 70.2 µg (1.08 µg per day of exposure) was estimated according to Alexander et al. [85], with the inhalability of the particles determined according to Menache et al. [86] [ID = C × f × VT × I (d50%, 6g) × t, where C is the $PM_{2.5}$ concentration (600 µg/m³), f is the breathing frequency (250 inhalations/min), VT is the tidal volume (0.15 mL), I is the inhalability (d50%, 6g = 80%), and t is the duration of exposure

(3900 min = 65 days, 5 days per week, 1 h per day)]. If mice were exposed to 20 µg/m³ $PM_{2.5}$ for 24 h, then the estimated intake dose of particles would be 0.864 µg/day (56.16 µg after 65 days). Thus, we can assume that the adopted exposure protocol mimics a 24 h exposure to concentrations of ambient fine particulate matter found in São Paulo City.

The air pollutants data obtained from the Cerqueira César monitoring station of the São Paulo State Environmental Agency (CETESB, São Paulo, Brazil) for the exposure period of the present study (September 1 to

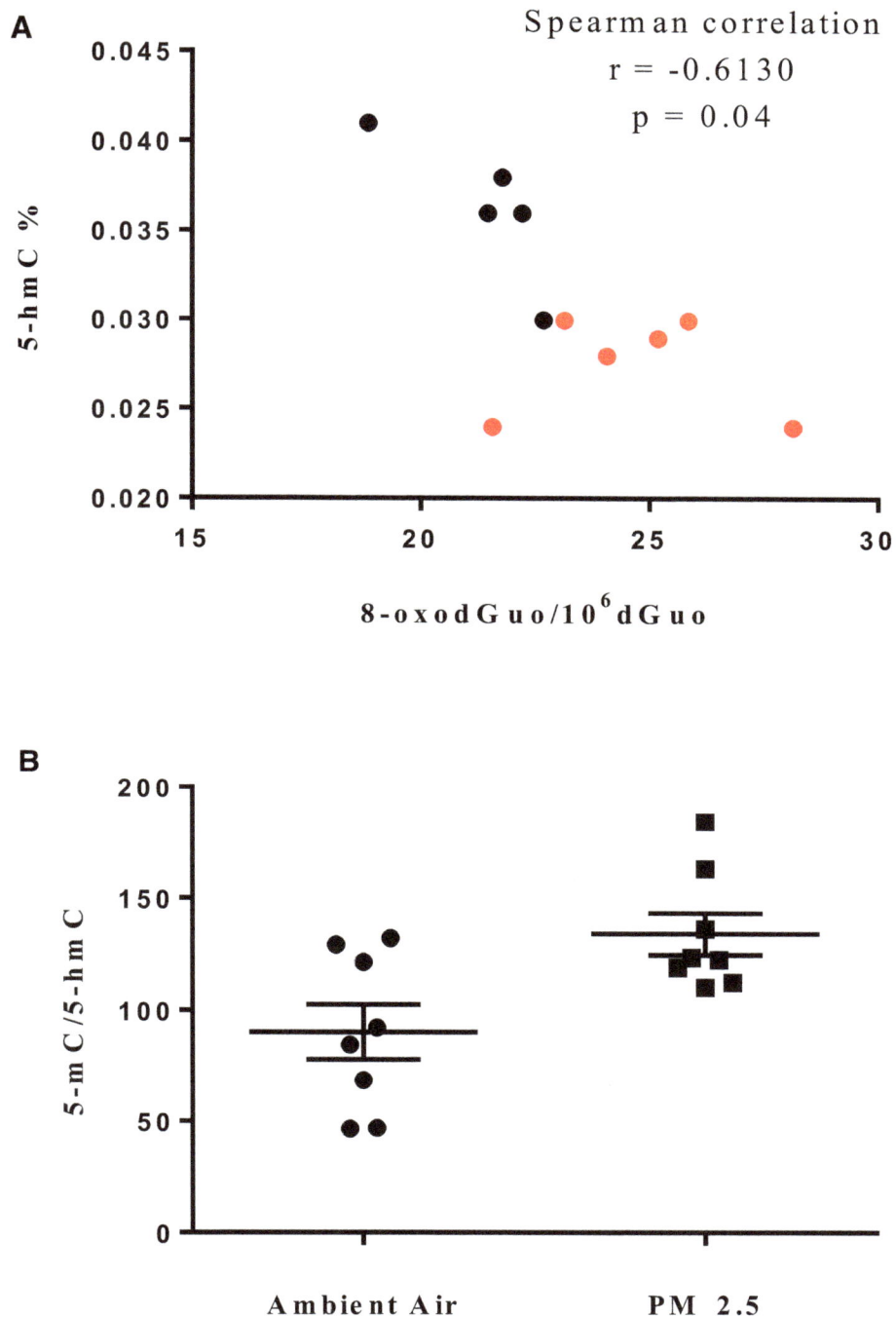

Fig. 3 a Spearman correlation between 5-hmC and 8-oxodGuo in mice lung DNA ($N = 11$, five samples from ambient air are shown in black, and six samples from concentrated $PM_{2.5}$ are shown in red); **b** Ratios between 5-mC and 5-hmC in mice lung DNA (Mean ± SEM, unpaired t test, $p = 0.01$)

November 30, 2010) showed that the ambient air PM_{10} and $PM_{2.5}$ average (± SD) concentrations were 31.61 ± 22.16 $\mu g/m^3$ and 20.36 ± 11.82 $\mu g/m^3$, respectively [87]. The 2008–2010 triennium average (± SD) PM_{10} and $PM_{2.5}$ concentrations in the Cerqueira César monitoring station were 30.86 ± 5.86 $\mu g/m^3$ and 17.73 ±

1.69 $\mu g/m^3$, respectively [87]. Previous characterization of $PM_{2.5}$ collected in the vicinity of the site of exposure showed that approximately 67% of the $PM_{2.5}$ mass was traffic related [76, 88]. Elemental analysis of $PM_{2.5}$ collected inside the concentrated $PM_{2.5}$ exposure chamber also reinforces that vehicular traffic was the major

Table 5 Method accuracy and coefficient of variation (CV) for quantification of 8-oxodGuo, 1,N^2-εdGuo and 1,N^6-εdAdo in DNA

Basal level Average ± SD (fmol)	Added fmol	Detected Average ± SD (fmol)	Detected(−)Basal Average (fmol)	Accuracy %	CV %
8-oxodGuo					
373.00 ± 2.71	0	372.79 ± 50,60	–	–	13.57
373.98 ± 4.86	367	755.41 ± 107,92	381	103.93	14.29
374.84 ± 5.19	734	1069.57 ± 108,51	695	94.65	10.14
357.94 ± 15.05	1469	1671.67 ± 44,27	1314	89.43	2.65
371.07 ± 2.43	2204	2272.01 ± 40,20	1901	86.25	1.77
1,N^2-εdGuo					
0.54 ± 0.01	0	0.54 ± 0.09	–	–	16.88
0.54 ± 0.01	1	1.47 ± 0.16	0.93	93.39	11.17
0.55 ± 0.01	5	5.30 ± 0.72	4.76	95.11	13.50
0.53 ± 0.01	10	10.60 ± 0.39	10.06	100.63	3.67
0.54 ± 0.01	20	20.20 ± 0.93	19.66	98.29	4.60
1,N^6-εdAdo					
2.08 ± 0.10	0	2.29 ± 0.39	–	–	17.05
2.05 ± 0.04	1	3.06 ± 0.47	1.01	100.89	15.31
1.99 ± 0.06	5	7.87 ± 1.66	5.88	117.60	21.10
2.03 ± 0.07	10	12.43 ± 1.25	10.41	104.06	10.06
1.97 ± 0.03	20	22.42 ± 3.89	20.46	102.29	17.34

source of $PM_{2.5}$ in the present study (Table 1), as indicated by the presence of Ca, Mg, Zn, and Pb, which are mainly derived from the combustion of gasoline and oil additives; Zn, Pb, Cd and V, which are derived from diesel tailpipe emissions; and Sb, Fe, Ba, Cu and Al, which are derived from break wear [89]. Polycyclic aromatic hydrocarbons were also detected in $PM_{2.5}$ collected at the site of exposure (Table 2).

The metal content and organic components of $PM_{2.5}$ are important factors for the induction of DNA damage [90, 91]. By direct or indirect mechanisms, both groups of components may induce ROS formation, which, if not equilibrated by cell antioxidant systems, subsequently leads to an increased rate of generation of oxidatively damaged biomolecules [90–96]. A major DNA damage used as a marker of oxidative stress is 8-oxodGuo, a mutagenic lesion formed by the mono electronic oxidation of guanine, or by hydroxyl radical or singlet oxygen attack of guanine in DNA [97].

As reviewed by Møller and coworkers [98], there are few reports on the assessment of oxidatively damaged DNA in the lungs of animals exposed to air pollution particles, with little evidence for associations [98]. Typically, positive associations have been found after rodent exposure to high DEPs concentrations or doses (3 to 80 mg/m^3, exposure by inhalation for few hours or 1 to 12 months; 0.1 to 4 mg by intratracheal instillation, analysis after a few hours or days) [98, 99]. The long-term inhalation of light-duty diesel engine exhaust (DEPs

3.5 mg/m^3, 17 h/day, 3 days/week, for 1 to 12 months) led to the induction of 8-oxodGuo in rat lungs at a rate that was higher during the first 3 months of exposure, despite the continuous linear increase in the lung burden of deposited particles along the 12 months [100]. However, the short-term inhalation of a NIST standard reference material 1650 DEP (5 or 20 mg/m^3, 1.5 h/day, 4 days) did not change the levels of 8-oxodGuo in mouse lungs, which were increased only after a single 1.5 h exposure to 80 mg/m^3 DEP [101]. Contrary to wild-type mice, repair-deficient $Ogg1^{-/-}$ mice exposed by inhalation to the NIST standard reference material 2975 DEP (20 mg/m^3, 1.5 h/day, 4 days) presented increased lung levels of 8-oxodGuo [98]. Indeed, when the mice were exposed to DEP obtained from a diesel engine (0.05, 0.1 and 0.2 mg) for 10 weeks by weekly intratracheal administration, lung 8-oxodGuo levels were increased (for DEP 0.1 and 0.2 mg) and correlated with lung tumor incidence (for DEP 0.05 and 0.1 mg) [29].

Here, we showed that mice exposed for 3 months to ambient $PM_{2.5}$ at a concentration that leads to the estimated total intake dose of 70.2 μg had increased levels of 8-oxodGuo in the lung tissue (Table 4). This is the first time that such an increase has been experimentally demonstrated for an estimated lung burden of particles close to what would be expected after 24 h/day exposure along 3 months to the average $PM_{2.5}$ concentration found in the local ambient air.

Reported basal levels of 8-oxodGuo in rodent lung tissue, based on HPLC analyses, range from 180 to $450/10^8$ dGuo [44, 101–104], $1340 – 2120/10^8$ dGuo [100], or approximately $3000/10^8$ dGuo [29, 105], with the lowest values obtained from DNA extraction methods by using sodium iodide. The mean 8-oxodGuo level found here in the lung of mice exposed to ambient air was $2124/10^8$ dGuo. The level increased to $2466/10^8$ dGuo in the animals exposed to ambient air enriched in $PM_{2.5}$ (Table 4).

An inter-laboratory assessment of 8-oxodGuo in DNA extracted from standard samples of pig liver and distributed by the European Standards Committee on Oxidative DNA Damage (ESCODD) to different research groups revealed a great discrepancy in the levels detected between laboratories, ranging from 223 to $44,100/10^8$ dGuo, with a median level of $1047/10^8$ dGuo [106]. In the present study, the mean 8-oxodGuo levels found in ambient air exposed mice lung, kidney, and liver DNA were, respectively, 2.0, 1.8, and 2.7 times higher than the median basal level obtained by ESCODD. Considering the limitations of 8-oxodGuo analyses, the DNA samples were extracted and stored by using solutions containing deferoxamine for protection against artifactual oxidation, and the hydrolysis procedure was performed by using 80 μg of DNA from each sample to minimize the contribution of spurious oxidation to the final result, as suggested by Helbock and coworkers [107].

It has been shown that human exposure to each 10 μg $PM_{2.5}/m^3$ could result in an 11% increase in the levels of 8-oxodGuo in lymphocyte DNA [92]. Increased levels of urinary or serum 8-oxodGuo in humans were also associated with $PM_{2.5}$ mass, its organic and/or elemental constituents, or the duration of exposure [91, 108–110]. Additionally, children exposed to high levels of a complex mixture of air pollutants in Mexico City presented higher levels of 8-oxodGuo in nasal biopsies from the posterior inferior turbinate compared to those of controls [111].

Consistent with an expected increased rate of generation of superoxide radical ($O_2^{\bullet-}$) in the lung tissue of mice exposed to the concentrated ambient $PM_{2.5}$, lung SOD activity was increased in these animals (Table 3). In a previous study, mice intranasally instilled with a suspension of Residual Oil Fly Ashes (0.2 mg/kg), a surrogate for ambient air PM in many studies, and euthanized 1 or 3 h after exposure, presented increased lung oxygen consumption, NADPH oxidase activity, mitochondrial state 3 respiration, nitric oxide production, phospholipid oxidation, and carbonyl content [112]. Lung SOD activity was also increased in the reported model as a response to the amplified generation of $O_2^{\bullet-}$ by different sources (NADPH oxidase, mitochondria), favoring $O_2^{\bullet-}$ dismutation to H_2O_2 [103]. Catalase, glutathione peroxidases (GPx) and peroxiredoxins (Prxs) reduce H_2O_2 to water, decreasing the chance of its reduction to the highly reactive hydroxyl radical ($^{\bullet}OH$) by transition metals (Fe^{2+}, Cu^+), and preventing the occurrence of oxidative damage [113–115]. While catalase directly decomposes H_2O_2 to H_2O and O_2, the thiol peroxidases GPx and Prxs reduce H_2O_2 to H_2O via simultaneous oxidation of glutathione (GSH) and thioredoxin (Trx). Oxidized glutathione and thioredoxin (GSSG e $TrxS_2$) are reduced by the NADPH-consuming enzymes glutathione reductase (GR) and thioredoxin reductase [113, 115, 116]. Here, the animals exposed to concentrated ambient $PM_{2.5}$ had decreased GR activity in the lung (Table 3), which may unbalance an important defense system against the excess H_2O_2 from $O_2^{\bullet-}$ dismutation, enabling the increased generation of oxidative damage, as observed for 8-oxodGuo. The erythrocytes of the animals exposed to concentrated ambient $PM_{2.5}$ also presented increased SOD activity. This finding is consistent with the knowledge that particles deposited in the lungs not only provoke lung inflammation but also induce a systemic inflammatory response, with the activation of NADPH oxidase in the systemic circulation leading to augmented $O_2^{\bullet-}$ generation [117].

Exposure to concentrated $PM_{2.5}$ also led to increased levels of DNA lesions in internal organs, such as the liver (augmented $1,N^2$-εdGuo) and kidneys (augmented 8-oxodGuo and $1,N^6$-εdAdo). As the animals were exposed whole body to the pollutants, the different routes of absorption (pulmonary, gastrointestinal, and dermal) may contribute to these effects. The lesions $1,N^2$-εdGuo and $1,N^6$-εdAdo are formed by reactive carbonyls resulting from lipid peroxidation [32] and were demonstrated to play a role in the pathophysiology of inflammation [36, 37]. Rats exposed orally to carbon black (0.64 mg/kg b.w.) presented increased levels of 8-oxodGuo, $1,N^6$-εdAdo, and $1,N^2$-εdGuo in the liver, with the highest effect observed for $1,N^2$-εdGuo [44]. However, only $1,N^2$-εdGuo levels were increased in the livers of the animals exposed orally to PM (0.64 mg/kg b.w.) collected from a wood stove-rich area [44]. Thus, different profiles of DNA lesions may be induced in response to the exposure of different tissues to different pollutants. A more comprehensive approach quantifying a large panel of lesions will likely reveal yet unknown effects. The differences in these profiles may be influenced by the time the sample was collected, and the inflammatory condition, pollutant biotransformation, and repair capacity of the target tissues [44]. Decreased SOD and increased GST activities were observed in the livers of mice exposed to concentrated $PM_{2.5}$ in the present study, showing a shift of the detoxification system towards the conjugation of reactive electrophiles with glutathione, consistent with the observed increased levels of $1,N^2$-εdGuo. The present study is the first to show the induction of etheno adducts in the liver and kidneys of mice exposed to ambient $PM_{2.5}$.

The levels of $1,N^6$-εdAdo detected in the present study fall within the range obtained in studies employing ultra-sensitive immunoaffinity/^{32}P-postlabeling and are lower than those described by other groups employing HPLC-ESI-MS/MS (Table 6). Similarly, the $1,N^2$-εdGuo levels quantified in the present study are consistent with the lowest levels reported by Garcia [118] and Angeli [119] by using HPLC-ESI-MS/MS (Table 6).

In addition to the genotoxic effect of PM, another important consequence of the exposure is the induction of epigenetic changes, which may affect gene expression without altering the nucleotide sequence in DNA [120–122]. Approximately 70% of the CpG dinucleotides in DNA are methylated, whereas non methylated CpGs are primarily found in "CpG islands". The dense methylation of promoter regions is associated with gene silencing [123–128].

Here, we observed that $PM_{2.5}$ exposure led to decreased global levels of 5-hmC in lung (34% decrease) and liver (16% decrease) DNA, without affecting the global levels of 5-mC (Table 4). This observation points to global 5-hmC as a more sensitive biomarker. Oxidative stress is a possible contributing factor to the decreased 5-hmC levels. The effect of oxidative stress decreasing the global levels of 5-hmC and modulating the genomic hydroxymethylation profile was demonstrated by Delatte and coworkers [129] in SY5Y human neuroblastoma cell line exposed to buthionine sulfoximine, and in colon epithelia of mice depleted for $GPx1$ and $GPx2$, both situations leading to increased levels of peroxides. We observed a significant inverse correlation between 5-hmC and 8-oxodGuo in mice lung DNA (Fig. 3a). Additionally, several lines of evidence indicate changes in DNA methylation and

hydroxymethylation as key events favoring cancer development due to benzo[a]pyrene exposure [27, 130–133]. Benzo[a]pyrene was one of the PAHs present in the $PM_{2.5}$ collected at the site of exposure (Table 2). Diminished 5-hmC levels were also observed in human bronchial epithelial cells (HBECs) exposed to DEPs (5 mg/cm^2, 24 h) in vitro [69] and in buccal cells of humans exposed to increased concentrations of $PM_{2.5}$ or PM_{10} [65].

As 5-hmC is a first step in the DNA demethylation pathway catalyzed by TET [57], the decrease in its levels may represent decreased TET activity or increased 5-hmC removal from DNA. Previous studies have suggested that the loss of TET activity may lead to the hypermethylation of gene promoter regions, with the consequent deregulation of gene transcription and cell differentiation [128]. Here we observed that the 5-mC/5-hmC ratio increased in lung DNA of the $PM_{2.5}$ exposed mice (Fig. 3b). Differentiated cells in stratified epithelia of several human and mouse organs presented higher levels of 5-hmC than the stem/progenitor cells and cancer cells [134]. The loss of 5-hmC was suggested to be an early event in carcinogenesis [134].

Ding and coworkers [66] evaluated for the first time the effects of traffic-related air pollution on DNA methylation in rat lung. The authors found, using multiple linear regression, that exposure to $PM_{2.5}$, PM_{10} and NO_2 was associated with changes in DNA methylation (decreased methylation of LINE1 and $iNOS$ promoter, and increased promoter methylation of APC and $p16^{CDKN2A}$) [66]. However, the different exposure localities chosen for the control and exposed groups prevented them from ruling out "the effects from the stress induced by other factors" [66]. In the present study, we focused on the effects of $PM_{2.5}$

Table 6 Levels of $1,N^2$-εdGuo and $1,N^6$-εdAdo in DNA from biological samples in different studies

Species/Model	Tissue	Method	Level	References
$1,N^2$-εdGuo				
Human cell line IMR-90	Lung	LC-ESI-MS/MS	$0.2–1.8/10^7$ dGuo	[118]
Human cell line SW480	Colon adenocarcinoma	LC-ESI-MS/MS	$0.5–2/10^7$ dGuo	[119]
Human cell line A549	Lung	LC-ESI-MS/MS	$1.5–5/10^6$ dGuo	[45]
Rat	Liver	LC-ESI-MS/MS	$1–3.25/10^6$ dGuo	[44]
Rat	Lung	LC-ESI-MS/MS	$1.5–2.5/10^6$ dGuo	[44]
$1,N^6$-εdAdo				
Human	Lung	^{32}P-postlabeling	$2.4–146/10^9$ dAdo	[139]
Human cell line A549	Lung	LC-ESI-MS/MS	$0.1–0.45/10^6$ dGuo	[45]
Human	White Blood Cells	^{32}P-postlabeling	$0.08–24.07/10^8$ dAdo	[140]
Human	White Blood Cells	^{32}P-postlabeling	$138–1017/10^9$ dAdo	[141]
Human	White Blood Cells	^{32}P-postlabeling	$0.03–90.15/10^7$ dAdo	[142]
Rat	Liver	LC-ESI-MS/MS	$0.75–2/10^6$ dGuo	[44]
Rat	Liver	LC-ESI-MS/MS	$2.1–6.9/10^8$ tdn	[143]
Rat	Lung	LC-ESI-MS/MS	$0.5–1.25/10^6$ dGuo	[44]

tdn total deoxynucleosides

concentrated from the ambient air, compared to the ambient air exposed group submitted, in the same place and at the same time, to equal conditions of manipulation and stress, except the concentration of $PM_{2.5}$. This is the first assessment of the levels of DNA lesions, 5-mC, 5-hmC, and oxidative stress in different tissues of mice in such an experimental condition, allowing direct evidence of the effects of $PM_{2.5}$ as it occurs in the environment. However, some short-comings of using the ambient air exposed group as the control must be addressed. The endpoints quantified in this group are not the basal levels that could be present in an unexposed control group. Studies using a clean air site or HEPA filtration in situ to prevent any exposure of the control group to PM would improve the sensitivity for detection of differences between groups.

The assessment of the total levels of 5-mC and 5-hmC in DNA is usually a first step in approaches to understand the effects of different agents on the epigenome, as pointed out by Bakulski and Fallin [52]. Although the total 5-mC and 5-hmC levels in DNA do not give information about the genes affected, this type of analysis provides useful data for the direction of greater resolution studies. For example, (1) detecting changes using the whole DNA denotes a broad effect, which probably encompasses different genes; (2) if the investigated agents affect the epigenetic machinery (e.g., TETs, DNMTs, pathways required to recycle the co-substrates of these enzymes, etc.), changes of the total 5-mC and/or 5-hmC levels are expected [69, 121, 133, 135–137]; (3) a broad effect is more likely to replicate in different animal species, compared to specific changes in genes that depend on different factors, including host development and genetics [121, 129, 133]. On the other hand, if no change is observed in the total levels of 5-mC or 5-hmC, biologically important changes across the genome cannot be excluded. The gain and loss of 5-mC or 5-hmC in different genomic locations may be counter-balanced, resulting in no net change of the global levels, which must be interpreted with caution [135].

Jiang and coworkers [133] assessed the DNA methylation profiles of immortalized human bronchial epithelial cells and murine skin exposed to benzo[a]pyrene in vitro and in vivo, respectively. It was evident the broad effect of benzo[a]pyrene modulating the DNA methylation in both systems (2414 differentially methylated regions in the exposed murine skin; 105,958 and 20,577 differentially methylated sites in two exposed human cell lines). A total of 153 genes with altered promoter methylation (hypermethylation or hypomethylation) were found in the exposed murine skin, 45 of them (29%) occurred in the exposed human cells. In contrast, 10,447 genes with altered promoter methylation were detected in the exposed human cells [133]. Delatte and coworkers [129] provided the opportunity to compare differentially hydroxymethylated genes induced by oxidative stress in SY5Y human neuroblastoma cell line and in colon

epithelia of mice. The global levels of 5-hmC were decreased in both systems under oxidative stress, but the genes and pathways altered, although involved in the oxidative stress response, differed between the systems [129]. Studies comparing the specific agent-induced changes in DNA methylation and hydroxymethylation profiles in tissues of animal models, human cells and human tissues would allow a better understanding of the applicability of such detailed information obtained in an animal model.

LINE1 and Alu repeat elements have been used as surrogate assays for quantifying total 5-mC in the majority of the studies on associations between ambient PM exposure and global DNA methylation alterations [47, 49, 58, 59, 61, 62, 66, 67]. Other methods used for quantification of 5-mC and/or 5-hmC in studies of PM exposure were ELISA [68, 69], indirect assays [63], HPLC-UV [51], HPLC-ESI-MS/MS [64, 65]. LINE1 and Alu assays do not distinguish between 5-mC and 5-hmC, and limit the assessment of methylation levels to specific cytosines in bisulfite converted DNA, quantified by pyrosequencing after polymerase chain reaction [135]. Conversely, HPLC based methods allow the direct quantification of the total levels of DNA bases, including 5-mC and 5-hmC separately, and are then considered the "gold standard" for this purpose [135]. A community-wide benchmarking study compared several methods for DNA methylation analysis [136]. Among the six global DNA methylation assays included in the study (HPLC-MS, ELISA, bisulfite pyrosequencing of four repetitive elements), HPLC-MS data most accurately reflected the expected differences between samples [136].

Using HPLC based methods, De Prins and coworkers [51] found that increased exposure to NO_2, PM_{10}, $PM_{2.5}$ and O_3 was associated with decreased total 5-mC levels in human blood DNA; Janssen and coworkers [64] observed that total 5-mC levels in human placenta were inversely associated with $PM_{2.5}$ exposure; and Nys and coworkers [65] were the first to show an association between increased human exposure to $PM_{2.5}$ and PM_{10} and decreased 5-mC and 5-hmC total levels in human buccal cell DNA. So far, to the best of our knowledge, this study is the first to quantify 5-mC and 5-hmC by HPLC-ESI-MS/MS in different tissues (lung, liver and kidney) of mice selectively exposed to ambient $PM_{2.5}$. Our observations encourage further investigation of the effects of $PM_{2.5}$ exposure on the profiles of the genomic methylation and hydroxymethylation of target tissues to obtain a better understanding of the deregulated molecular pathways that may culminate in disease (e.g., cancer, metabolic disorders, cardiovascular disease) development [138].

Conclusions

Mice exposed daily, for 3 months, to $PM_{2.5}$ at a concentration that mimics 24-h exposure to the mean concentration found in ambient air, presented altered antioxidant system activity in lung, liver, and erythrocytes, increased levels of DNA lesions related to oxidative stress in lung, liver, and kidney, and decreased global levels of 5-hmC in lung and liver DNA. This is the first direct demonstration of the occurrence of these effects due to exposure to $PM_{2.5}$ as it occurs in the environment. Genetic and epigenetic alterations induced by pollutants may affect the genes committed to cell cycle control, apoptosis, and cell differentiation, increasing the chance of cancer development, which merits further investigation.

Additional file

Additional file 1: Table S1. Reagents used in the study. Table S2. Parameters used in the ESI-MS/MS equipment for detection of the lesions and epigenetic marks in DNA. Figure S1. System of two columns used for 8-oxo-7,8-dihydro-2′-deoxyguanosine (8-oxodGuo) analyses. A) Configuration used in the first 16 min and from 32 to 46 min of the chromatography; B) Configuration used in the interval 16 – 32 min, allowing further separation and peak narrowing in column B prior to elution to the ESI source of the mass spectrometer. Figure S2. Calibration curves obtained by HPLC-ESI-MS/MS for quantification of 8-oxo-7,8-dihydro-2′-deoxyguanosine (8-oxodGuo), 1,N^2-etheno-2′-deoxyguanosine (1,N^2-εdGuo), 1,N^6-etheno-2′-deoxyadenosine (1,N^6-εdAdo), 2′-deoxycytidine (dCyd), 5-methyl-2′-deoxycytidine (5-mC), and 5-hydroxymethyl-2′-deoxycytidine (5-mC, lower range). (DOCX 738 kb)

Abbreviations

1,N^2-εdGuo: 1,N^2-etheno-2′-deoxyguanosine; 1,N^6-εdAdo: 1,N^6-etheno-2′-deoxyadenosine; 5-hmC: 5-hydroxymethylcytosine; 5-mC: 5-methylcytosine; 8-oxodGuo: 8-oxo-7,8-dihydro-2′-deoxyguanosine; 8-oxoGua: 8-oxo-7,8-dihydro-guanine; APC: Adenomatous polyposis coli; CAT: Catalase; CDNB: 1-chloro-2,4-dinitrobenzene; CETESB: São Paulo State Environmental Agency; dAdo: 2′-deoxyadenosine; dCyd: 2′-deoxycytidine; DEP: Diesel exhaust particles; dGuo: 2′-deoxyguanosine; DNMT: DNA methyltransferase; ESCODD: European Standards Committee on Oxidative DNA Damage; ESI: Electrospray ionization; GPx: Glutathione peroxidase; GR: Glutathione reductase; GSH: Reduced glutathione; GSSG: Oxidized glutathione; GST: Glutathione S-transferase; HBECs: Human bronchial epithelial cells; HPLC: High performance liquid chromatography; IARC: International Agency for Research on Cancer; iNOS: Inducible nitric oxide synthase; LINE1: Long interspersed nucleotide element; LOD: Limit of detection; LOQ: Limit of quantitation; m/z: mass-to-charge ratio; MRM: Multiple reaction monitoring; MS: Mass spectrometry; NADPH: Nicotinamide adenine dinucleotide phosphate; NIST: National Institute of Standards and Technology; Ogg1: 8-oxoguanine DNA glycosylase; PAH: Polycyclic aromatic hydrocarbon; PDA: Photodiode array detector; PM: Particulate matter; Prxs: Peroxiredoxins; ROS: Reactive oxygen species; S/N: Signal-to-noise ratio; SD: Standard deviation; SEM: Standard error of the mean; SOD: Superoxide dismutase; TET: Ten-eleven-translocation; Trx: Thioredoxin

Acknowledgements
Prof. Mary Rosa Rodrigues de Marchi, Departamento de Química Analítica, Instituto de Química, Universidade Estadual Paulista (UNESP) for performing the PAHs analysis. MSc Rosana Astolfo and Prof. Maria de Fátima Andrade Lapat - Laboratório de Análises de Processos Atmosféricos, Instituto de Astronomia, Geofísica e Ciências Atmosféricas, Universidade de São Paulo (USP) for the $PM_{2.5}$ elemental analysis.

Funding
FAPESP (Fundação de Amparo à Pesquisa do Estado de São Paulo, Proc. 2012/22190-3 and 2012/08616-8), CNPq (Proc. 454214/2014-6), CAPES, PRPUSP (Pró-Reitoria de Pesquisa da Universidade de São Paulo), INCT INAIRA (MCT/CNPq/FNDCT/CAPES/FAPEMIG/FAPERJ/FAPESP; Proc. 573813/2008-6), INCT Redoxoma (FAPESP/CNPq/CAPES; Proc. 573530/2008-4), NAP Redoxoma (PRPUSP; Proc. 2011.1.9352.1.8) and CEPID Redoxoma (FAPESP; Proc. 2013/07937-8). T. F. Oliveira and A. A. F. Oliveira received scholarships from FAPESP (Proc. 2012/21636-8, 2011/09891-0, 2012/08617-4) and CAPES (Coordenação de Aperfeiçoamento de Pessoal de Nível Superior). M. H. G. Medeiros, P. Di Mascio, T. Marcourakis, P. H. N. Saldiva, and A. P. M. Loureiro received fellowships from CNPq.

Authors' contributions
AAFO and TFO conducted experiments, performed data analyses and interpretation, drafted the manuscript, and prepared the figures and tables. MD, ML and MMV performed experiments and data analyses. MHGM, PDM and TM performed data interpretation. PHNS designed the study and performed data interpretation. APML designed the study, performed data interpretation, and wrote the manuscript. All authors read and approved the final manuscript.

Competing interests
The authors declare that they have no competing interests.

Author details
[1]Departamento de Análises Clínicas e Toxicológicas, Faculdade de Ciências Farmacêuticas, Universidade de São Paulo, Av. Prof. Lineu Prestes 580, Bloco 13 B, São Paulo CEP 05508-000, Brazil. [2]Departamento de Bioquímica, Instituto de Química, Universidade de São Paulo, Av. Prof. Lineu Prestes 748, São Paulo CEP 05508-000, Brazil. [3]Laboratório de Poluição Atmosférica Experimental – LIM05, Hospital das Clínicas, Faculdade de Medicina, Universidade de São Paulo, Av. Dr. Arnaldo 455, São Paulo CEP 01246903, Brazil. [4]Instituto de Estudos Avançados, Universidade de São Paulo, R. do Anfiteatro, 513, São Paulo CEP 05508060, Brazil. [5]Present address: Departamento de Farmacociências, Universidade Federal de Ciências da Saúde de Porto Alegre, Rua Sarmento Leite 245, Porto Alegre, Rio Grande do Sul CEP 90050-170, Brazil.

References
1. Kok TM, Hogervorst JG, Briedé JJ, Van Herwijnen MH, Maas LM, Moonen EJ, et al. Genotoxicity and physicochemical characteristics of traffic-related ambient particulate matter. Environ Mol Mutagen. 2005;46:71–80.
2. Pope CA III, Dockery DW. 2006 critical review: health effects of fine particulate air pollution: lines that connect. J Air Waste Manage Assoc. 2006;56:709–42.
3. Meng Z, Zhang Q. Damage effects of dust storm PM2.5 on DNA in alveolar macrophages and lung cells of rats. Food Chem Toxicol. 2007;45:1368–74.
4. Møller P, Folkmann JK, Forchhammer L, Bräuner EV, Danielsen PH, Risom L, et al. Air pollution, oxidative damage to DNA, and carcinogenesis. Cancer Lett. 2008;266:84–97.
5. Demetriou CA, Raaschou-Nielsen O, Loft S, Møller P, Vermeulen R, Palli D, et al. Biomarkers of ambient air pollution and lung cancer: a systematic review. Occup Environ Med. 2012;69:619–27.
6. Benbrahim-Tallaa L, Baan RA, Grosse Y, Lauby-Secretan B, El Ghissassi F, Bouvard V, et al. Carcinogenicity of diesel-engine and gasoline-engine exhausts and some nitroarènes. Lancet Oncol. 2012;13:663–4.
7. Yanagi Y, de Assunção JV, Barrozo LV. The impact of atmospheric particulate matter on cancer incidence and mortality in the city of São Paulo, Brazil. Cad Saúde Pública. 2012;28:1737–48.
8. DeMarini DM. Genotoxicity biomarkers associated with exposure to traffic and near-road atmospheres: a review. Mutagenesis. 2013;28:485–505.
9. Fajersztajn L, Veras M, Barrozo LV, Saldiva P. Air pollution: a potentially modifiable risk factor for lung cancer. Nat Rev Cancer. 2013;13:674–8.
10. IARC. IARC Monographs on the Evaluation of Carcinogenic Risks to Humans: Outdoor Air Pollution, vol. 109. Lyon: IARC; 2016. p. 448.
11. Raaschou-Nielsen O, Andersen ZJ, Beelen R, Samoli E, Stafoggia M, Weinmayr G, et al. Air pollution and lung cancer incidence in 17 European cohorts: prospective analyses from the European study of cohorts for air pollution effects (ESCAPE). Lancet Oncol. 2013;14:813–22.
12. Carvalho VSB, Freitas ED, Martins LD, Martins JA, Mazzoli CR, de Fátima Andrade M. Air quality status and trends over the metropolitan area of Sao

Paulo, Brazil as a result of emission control policies. Environ Sci Pol. 2015;47: 68–79.

13. CETESB - Companhia Ambiental do Estado de São Paulo. Qualidade do Ar no Estado de São Paulo 2013. 2013. http://cetesb.sp.gov.br/ar/qualar/. Accessed 29 Oct 2017.

14. Anderson LG. Ethanol fuel use in Brazil: air quality impacts. Energy Environ Sci. 2009;2:1015.

15. Nogueira T, de Souza KF, Fornaro A, Andrade M de F, de Carvalho LRF. On-road emissions of carbonyls from vehicles powered by biofuel blends in traffic tunnels in the metropolitan area of Sao Paulo, Brazil. Atmos Environ. 2015;108:88–97.

16. World Health Organization. WHO Air quality guidelines for particulate matter, ozone, nitrogen dioxide and sulfur dioxide. Global Update 2005. Summary of Risk Assessment. 2005. http://apps.who.int/iris/bitstream/10665/69477/1/WHO_SDE_PHE_OEH_06.02_eng.pdf. Accessed 12 Mar 2018.

17. Brook RD, Rajagopalan S, Pope CA, Brook JR, Bhatnagar A, Diez-Roux AV, et al. Particulate matter air pollution and cardiovascular disease: an update to the scientific statement from the american heart association. Circulation. 2010;121:2331–78.

18. Martins LD, Martins JA, Freitas ED, Mazzoli CR, Gonçalves FLT, Ynoue RY, et al. Potential health impact of ultrafine particles under clean and polluted urban atmospheric conditions: a model-based study. Air Qual Atmos Health. 2010;3:29–39.

19. Samet JM. Some current challenges in research on air pollution and health. Salud Públ Méx. 2014;56:379–85.

20. Dybdahl M, Risom L, Bornholdt J, Autrup H, Loft S, Wallin H. Inflammatory and genotoxic effects of diesel particles in vitro and in vivo. Mutat Res Genet Toxicol Environ Mutagen. 2004;562:119–31.

21. Riva DR, Magalhães CB, Lopes AA, Lanças T, Mauad T, Malm O, et al. Low dose of fine particulate matter (PM2.5) can induce acute oxidative stress, inflammation and pulmonary impairment in healthy mice. Inhal Toxicol. 2011;23:257–67.

22. Møller P, Folkmann JK, Danielsen PH, Jantzen K, Loft S. Oxidative stress generated damage to DNA by gastrointestinal exposure to insoluble particles. Curr Mol Med. 2012;12:732–45.

23. De Martinis BS, Kado NY, Carvalho LRF, Okamoto RA, Gundel LA. Genotoxicity of fractionated organic material in airborne particles from São Paulo, Brazil. Mutat Res. 1999;446:83–94.

24. Karlsson HL, Nygren J, Möller L. Genotoxicity of airborne particulate matter: the role of cell-particle interaction and of substances with adduct-forming and oxidizing capacity. Mutat Res Genet Toxicol Environ Mutagen. 2004;565:1–10.

25. Bell ML, Dominici F, Ebisu K, Zeger SL, Samet JM. Spatial and temporal variation in PM2.5 chemical composition in the United States for health effects studies. Environ Health Perspect. 2007;115:989–95.

26. DeMarini DM, Landi S, Tian D, Hanley NM, Li X, Hu F, et al. Lung tumor KRAS and TP53 mutations in nonsmokers reflect exposure to PAH-rich coal combustion emissions. Cancer Res. 2001;61:6679–81.

27. Chappell G, Pogribny IP, Guyton KZ, Rusyn I. Epigenetic alterations induced by genotoxic occupational and environmental chemical carcinogens: a systematic literature review. Mutat Res. 2016;768:27–45.

28. Ke S, Liu Q, Yao Y, Zhang X, Sui G. An in vitro cytotoxicities comparison of 16 priority polycyclic aromatic hydrocarbons in human pulmonary alveolar epithelial cells HPAEpiC. Toxicol Lett. 2018;290:10–8.

29. Ichinose T, Yajima Y, Nagashima M, Takenoshita S, Nagamachi Y, Sagai M. Lung carcinogenesis and formation of 8-hydroxy-deoxyguanosine in mice by diesel exhaust particles. Carcinogenesis. 1997;18:185–92.

30. Loft S, Svoboda P, Kawai K, Kasai H, Sørensen M, Tjønneland A, et al. Association between 8-oxo-7,8-dihydroguanine excretion and risk of lung cancer in a prospective study. Free Radic Biol Med. 2012;52:167–72 Elsevier Inc.

31. Obtulowicz T, Swoboda M, Speina E, Gackowski D, Rozalski R, Siomek A, et al. Oxidative stress and 8-oxoguanine repair are enhanced in colon adenoma and carcinoma patients. Mutagenesis. 2010;25:463–71.

32. Marnett LJ, Plastaras JP. Endogenous DNA damage and mutation. Trends Genet. 2001;17:214–21.

33. Bartsch H, Nair J. New DNA-based biomarkers for oxidative stress and cancer chemoprevention studies. Eur J Cancer. 2000;36:1229–34.

34. Doerge DR, Churchwell MI, Fang JL, Beland FA. Quantification of etheno-DNA adducts using liquid chromatography, on-line sample processing, and electrospray tandem mass spectrometry. Chem Res Toxicol. 2000;13:1254–9.

35. Loureiro APM, Marques SA, Garcia CCM, Di Mascio P, Medeiros MHG. Development of an on-line liquid chromatography-electrospray tandem

36. mass spectrometry assay to quantitatively determine 1,N2-etheno-2'-deoxyguanosine in DNA. Chem Res Toxicol. 2002;15:1302–8.

36. Nair U, Bartsch H, Nair J. Lipid peroxidation-induced DNA damage in cancer-prone inflammatory diseases: a review of published adduct types and levels in humans. Free Radic Biol Med. 2007;43:1109–20.

37. Pang B, Zhou X, Yu H, Dong M, Taghizadeh K, Wishnok JS, et al. Lipid peroxidation dominates the chemistry of DNA adduct formation in a mouse model of inflammation. Carcinogenesis. 2007;28:1807–13.

38. Medeiros MHG. Exocyclic DNA adducts as biomarkers of lipid oxidation and predictors of disease. Challenges in developing sensitive and specific methods for clinical studies. Chem Res Toxicol. 2009;22:419–25.

39. Garcia CCM, Freitas FP, Di Mascio P, Medeiros MHG. Ultrasensitive simultaneous quantification of 1,N2 -Etheno-2'-deoxyguanosine and 1,N2 -Propano-2'-deoxyguanosine in DNA by an online liquid chromatography electrospray tandem mass spectrometry assay. Chem Res Toxicol. 2010;23:1851.

40. Chen HJ, Lin WP. Quantitative analysis of multiple exocyclic DNA adducts in human salivary dna by stable isotope dilution nanoflow liquid chromatography - nanospray ionization tandem mass spectrometry. Anal Chem. 2011;83:8543–51.

41. Garcia CCM, Freitas FP, Sanchez AB, Di Mascio P, Medeiros MHG. Elevated α-methyl-γ-hydroxy-1,N2-propano-2'-deoxyguanosine levels in urinary samples from individuals exposed to urban air pollution. Chem Res Toxicol. 2013;26: 1602–4.

42. Cui S, Li H, Wang S, Jiang X, Zhang S, Zhang R, et al. Ultrasensitive UPLC-MS-MS method for the quantitation of etheno-DNA adducts in human urine. Int J Environ Res Public Health. 2014;11:10902–14.

43. Monien BH, Schumacher F, Herrmann K, Glatt H, Turesky RJ, Chesne C. Simultaneous detection of multiple DNA adducts in human lung samples by isotope-dilution UPLC-MS/MS. Anal Chem. 2015;87:641–8.

44. Danielsen PH, Loft S, Jacobsen NR, Jensen KA, Autrup H, Ravanat JL, et al. Oxidative stress, inflammation, and DNA damage in rats after intratracheal instillation or oral exposure to ambient air and wood smoke particulate matter. Toxicol Sci. 2010;118:574–85.

45. Danielsen PH, Moller P, Jensen KA, Sharma AK, Wallin H, Bossi R, et al. Oxidative stress, DNA damage, and inflammation induced by ambient air and wood smoke particulate matter in human A549 and THP-1 cell lines. Chem Res Toxicol. 2011;24:168–84.

46. Knaapen AM, Güngör N, Schins RPF, Borm PJA, Van Schooten FJ. Neutrophils and respiratory tract DNA damage and mutagenesis: a review. Mutagenesis. 2006;21:225–36.

47. Bellavia A, Urch B, Speck M, Brook RD, Scott JA, Albetti B, et al. DNA hypomethylation, ambient particulate matter, and increased blood pressure: findings from controlled human exposure experiments. J Am Heart Assoc. 2013;2:1–11.

48. Chen W-L, Lin C-Y, Yan Y-H, Cheng KT, Cheng T-J. Alterations in rat pulmonary phosphatidylcholines after chronic exposure to ambient fine particulate matter. Mol Biosyst. 2014;10:3163–9.

49. Baccarelli A, Wright RO, Bollati V, Tarantini L, Litonjua AA, Suh HH, et al. Rapid DNA methylation changes after exposure to traffic particles. Am J Respir Crit Care Med. 2009;179:572–8.

50. Feil R, Fraga MF. Epigenetics and the environment: emerging patterns and implications. Nat Rev Genet. 2012;13:97–109.

51. De Prins S, Koppen G, Jacobs G, Dons E, Van de Mieroop E, Nelen V, et al. Influence of ambient air pollution on global DNA methylation in healthy adults: a seasonal follow-up. Environ Int. 2013;59:418–24.

52. Bakulski KM, Fallin MD. Epigenetic epidemiology: promises for public health research. Environ Mol Mutagen. 2014;55:171–83.

53. Robertson KD, Wolffe AP. DNA methylation in health and disease. Nat Rev Genet. 2000;1:11–9.

54. Bender J. Dna methylation and epigenetics. Annu Rev Plant Biol. 2004;55:41–68.

55. Magaña AA, Wrobel K, Caudillo YA, Zaina S, Lund G, Wrobel K. High-performance liquid chromatography determination of 5-methyl-2'-deoxycytidine, 2'-deoxycytidine, and other deoxynucleosides and nucleosides in DNA digests. Anal Biochem. 2008;374:378–85.

56. Smith ZD, Meissner A. DNA methylation: roles in mammalian development. Nat Rev Genet. 2013;14:204–20.

57. Branco MR, Ficz G, Reik W. Uncovering the role of 5-hydroxymethylcytosine in the epigenome. Nat Rev Genet. 2012;13:7–13.

58. Tarantini L, Bonzini M, Apostoli P, Pegoraro V, Bollati V, Marinelli B, et al. Effects of particulate matter on genomic DNA methylation content and iNOS promoter methylation. Environ Health Perspect. 2009;117:217–22.

59. Madrigano J, Baccarelli A, Mittleman MA, Wright RO, Sparrow D, Vokonas PS,

et al. Prolonged exposure to particulate pollution, genes associated with glutathione pathways, and DNA methylation in a cohort of older men. Environ Health Perspect. 2011;119:977–82.

60. Guo L, Byun H-M, Zhong J, Motta V, Barupal J, Zheng Y, et al. Effects of short-term exposure to inhalable particulate matter on DNA methylation of tandem repeats. Environ Mol Mutagen. 2014;55:322–35.

61. Chen R, Meng X, Zhao A, Wang C, Yang C, Li H, et al. DNA hypomethylation and its mediation in the effects of fine particulate air pollution on cardiovascular biomarkers: a randomized crossover trial. Environ Int. 2016;94:614–9.

62. Alvarado-Cruz I, Sánchez-Guerra M, Hernández-Cadena L, Vizcaya-Ruiz A, Mugica V, Pelallo-Martínez NA, et al. Increased methylation of repetitive elements and DNA repair genes is associated with higher DNA oxidation in children in an urbanized, industrial environment. Mutat Res. 2017;813:27–36.

63. Yauk C, Polyzos A, Rowan-Carroll A, Somers CM, Godschalk RW, Van Schooten FJ, et al. Germ-line mutations, DNA damage, and global hypermethylation in mice exposed to particulate air pollution in an urban/industrial location. Proc Natl Acad Sci. 2008;105:605–10.

64. Janssen BG, Godderis L, Pieters N, Poels K, Kiciński M, Cuypers A, et al. Placental DNA hypomethylation in association with particulate air pollution in early life. Part Fibre Toxicol. 2013;10:22.

65. Nys S, Duca R, Nawrot T, Hoet P, Meerbeek BV, Landuyt KLV, et al. Temporal variability of global DNA methylation and hydroxymethylation in buccal cells of healthy adults: association with air pollution. Environ Int. 2018;111:301–8.

66. Ding R, Jin Y, Liu X, Zhu Z, Zhang Y, Wang T, et al. Characteristics of DNA methylation changes induced by traffic-related air pollution. Mutat Res. 2016;796:46–53.

67. Cai J, Zhao Y, Liu P, Xia B, Zhu Q, Wang X, et al. Exposure to particulate air pollution during early pregnancy is associated with placental DNA methylation. Sci Total Environ. 2017;607–608:1103–8.

68. Sanchez-Guerra M, Zheng Y, Osorio-Yanez C, Zhong J, Chervona Y, Wang S, et al. Effects of particulate matter exposure on blood 5-hydroxymethylation: results from the Beijing truck driver air pollution study. Epigenetics. 2015;10:633–42.

69. Somineni HK, Zhang X, Biagini Myers JM, Kovacic MB, Ulm A, Jurcak N, et al. Ten-eleven translocation 1 (TET1) methylation is associated with childhood asthma and traffic-related air pollution. J Allergy Clin Immunol. 2016;137:797–805.e5.

70. Mangal D, Vudathala D, Park J-H, Lee SH, Penning TM, Blair IA. Analysis of 7,8-Dihydro-8-oxo-2'-deoxyguanosine in cellular DNA during oxidative stress. Chem Res Toxicol. 2009;22:788–97.

71. Loureiro APM, Di Mascio P, Gomes OF, Medeiros MHG. trans,trans-2,4-Decadienal-induced 1,N2-Etheno-2'-deoxyguanosine adduct formation. Chem Res Toxicol. 2000;13:601–9.

72. Hillestrøm PR, Weimann A, Poulsen HE. Quantification of urinary etheno-DNA adducts by column-switching LC/APCI-MS/MS. J Am Soc Mass Spectrom. 2006;17:605–10.

73. Hofer T, Seo AY, Prudencio M, Leeuwenburgh C. A method to determine RNA and DNA oxidation simultaneously by HPLC-ECD: greater RNA than DNA oxidation in rat liver after doxorubicin administration. Biol Chem. 2006; 387:103–11.

74. Sandhu J, Kaur B, Armstrong C, Talbot CJ, Steward WP, Farmer PB, et al. Determination of 5-methyl-2'-deoxycytidine in genomic DNA using high performance liquid chromatography-ultraviolet detection. J Chromatogr B Anal Technol Biomed Life Sci. 2009;877:1957–61.

75. Kim S, Sioutas C, Chang MC, Gong H. Factors affecting the stability of the performance of ambient fine-particle concentrators. Inhal Toxicol. 2000; 12(Suppl 4):281–98.

76. Akinaga LMY, Lichtenfels AJ, Carvalho-Oliveira R, Caldini EG, Dolhnikoff M, Silva LFF, et al. Effects of chronic exposure to air pollution from Sao Paulo city on coronary of Swiss mice, from birth to adulthood. Toxicol Pathol. 2009;37:306–14.

77. Veras MM, Damaceno-Rodrigues NR, Guimarães Silva RM, Scoriza JN, Saldiva PHN, Caldini EG, et al. Chronic exposure to fine particulate matter emitted by traffic affects reproductive and fetal outcomes in mice. Environ Res. 2009;109:536–43.

78. Magalhães D, Bruns RE, de CVasconcellos P. Hidrocarbonetos policíclicos aromáticos como traçadores da queima de cana-de-açúcar: uma abordagem estatística. Quim Nova. 2007;30:577–81.

79. Flohé L, Günzler WA. Assays of glutathione peroxidase. Methods Enzymol. 1984;105:114–21.

80. Carlberg I, Mannervik B. Purification and characterization of the flavoenzyme glutathione reductase from rat liver. J Biol Chem. 1975;250:5475–80.

81. Habig WH, Pabst MJ, Fleischner G, Gatmaitan Z, Arias IM, Jakoby WB. The identity of glutathione S-transferase B with ligandin, a major binding protein of liver. Proc Natl Acad Sci U S A. 1974;71:3879–82.

82. McCord JM, Fridovich I. The utility of superoxide dismutase in studying free radical reactions. I. Radicals generated by the interaction of sulfite, dimethyl sulfoxide, and oxygen. J Biol Chem. 1969;244:6056–63.

83. Flohé L, Otting F. Superoxide dismutase assays. Methods Enzymol. 1984;105: 93–104.

84. Aebi H. Catalase in vitro. Methods Enzymol. 1984;105:121–6.

85. Alexander DJ, Collins CJ, Coombs DW, Gilkison IS, Hardy CJ, Healey G, et al. Association of inhalation toxicologists (AIT) working party recommendation for standard delivered dose calculation and expression in non-clinical aerosol inhalation toxicology studies with pharmaceuticals. Inhal Toxicol. 2008;20(13):1179–89.

86. Ménache MG, Miller FJ, Raabe OG. Particle inhalability curves for humans and small laboratory animals. Ann Occup Hyg. 1995;39(3):317–28.

87. CETESB - Companhia Ambiental do Estado de São Paulo. Qualar – Sistema de Informações da Qualidade do Ar (2010). http://cetesb.sp.gov.br/ar/qualar/. Accessed 29 Oct 2017.

88. Mauad T, Rivero DHRF, De Oliveira RC, Lichtenfels AJDFC, Guimarães ET, De Andre PA, et al. Chronic exposure to ambient levels of urban particles affects mouse lung development. Am J Respir Crit Care Med. 2008;178:721–8.

89. Schauer JJ, Lough GC, Shafer MM, Christensen WF, Arndt MF, DeMinter JT, et al. Characterization of metals emitted from motor vehicles. Res Rep Health Eff Inst. 2006;133:77–88.

90. Gutiérrez-Castillo ME, Roubicek DA, Cebrián-García ME, De Vizcaya-Ruíz A, Sordo-Cedeño M, Ostrosky-Wegman P. Effect of chemical composition on the induction of DNA damage by urban airborne particulate matter. Environ Mol Mutagen. 2006;47:199–211.

91. Huang HB, Lai CH, Chen GW, Lin YY, Jaakkola JJK, Liou SH, et al. Traffic-related air pollution and DNA damage: a longitudinal study in Taiwanese traffic conductors. PLoS One. 2012;7:1–8.

92. Sørensen M, Autrup H, Hertel O, Wallin H, Knudsen LE, Loft S. Personal exposure to PM2. 5 and biomarkers of DNA damage. Cancer Epidemiol Biomark Prev. 2003;12:191–6.

93. Rossner P, Topinka J, Hovorka J, Milcova A, Schmuczerova J, Krouzek J, et al. An acellular assay to assess the genotoxicity of complex mixtures of organic pollutants bound on size segregated aerosol. Part II: oxidative damage to DNA. Toxicol Lett. 2010;198:312–6.

94. Hou L, Zhang X, Zheng Y, Wang S, Dou C, Guo L, et al. Altered methylation in tandem repeat element and elemental component levels in inhalable air particles. Environ Mol Mutagen. 2014;55:256–65.

95. Hellack B, Quass U, Beuck H, Wick G, Kuttler W, Schins RPF, et al. Elemental composition and radical formation potency of PM10 at an urban background station in Germany in relation to origin of air masses. Atmos Environ. 2015;105:1–6.

96. Valavanidis A, Fiotakis K, Bakeas E, Vlahogianni T. Electron paramagnetic resonance study of the generation of reactive oxygen species catalysed by transition metals and quinoid redox cycling by inhalable ambient particulate matter. Redox Rep. 2005;10:37–51.

97. Cadet J, Loft S, Olinski R, Evans MD, Bialkowski K, Richard Wagner J, et al. Biologically relevant oxidants and terminology, classification and nomenclature of oxidatively generated damage to nucleobases and 2-deoxyribose in nucleic acids. Free Radic Res. 2012;46:367–81.

98. Møller P, Danielsen PH, Karottki DG, Jantzen K, Roursgaard M, Klingberg H, et al. Oxidative stress and inflammation generated DNA damage by exposure to air pollution particles. Mutat Res Rev Mutat Res. 2014;762:133–66.

99. Risom L, Møller P, Loft S. Oxidative stress-induced DNA damage by particulate air pollution. Mutat Res Mol Mech Mutagen. 2005;592:119–37.

100. Iwai K, Adachi S, Takahashi M, Moller L, Udagawa T, Mizuno S, et al. Early oxidative DNA damages and late development of lung cancer in diesel exhaust-exposed rats. Environ Res. 2000;84:255–64.

101. Risom L, Dybdahl M, Bornholdt J, Vogel U, Wallin H, Møller P, et al. Oxidative DNA damage and defence gene expression in the mouse lung after short-term exposure to diesel exhaust particles by inhalation. Carcinogenesis. 2003;24:1847–52.

102. Risom L, Dybdahl M, Møller P, Wallin H, Haug T, Vogel U, et al. Repeated inhalations of diesel exhaust particles and oxidatively damaged DNA in young oxoguanine DNA glycosylase (OGG1) deficient mice. Free Radic Res. 2007;41:172–81.

103. Tsurudome Y, Hirano T, Yamato H, Tanaka I, Sagai M, Hirano H, et al. Changes in levels of 8-hydroxyguanine in DNA, its repair and OGG1 mRNA in rat lungs after intratracheal administration of diesel exhaust particles. Carcinogenesis. 1999;20:1573–6.

104. Marie-Desvergne C, Maître A, Bouchard M, Ravanat JL, Viau C. Evaluation of DNA adducts, DNA and RNA oxidative lesions, and 3-

hydroxybenzo(a)pyrene as biomarkers of DNA damage in lung following intravenous injection of the parent compound in rats. Chem Res Toxicol. 2010;23:1207–14.

105. Schmerold I, Niedermu H. Levels of 8-hydroxy-2'-deoxyguanosine in cellular DNA from 12 tissues of young and old Sprague Dawley rats. Exp Gerontol. 2001;36:1375–86.

106. ESCODD (European Standards Committee on Oxidative DNA Damage). Comparative analysis of baseline 8-oxo-7,8-dihydroguanine in mammalian cell DNA, by different methods in different laboratories: an approach to consensus. Carcinogenesis. 2002;23:2129–33.

107. Helbock HJ, Beckman KB, Shigenaga MK, Walter PB, Woodall AA, Yeo HC, et al. DNA oxidation matters: the HPLC-electrochemical detection assay of 8-oxo-deoxyguanosine and 8-oxo-guanine. Proc Natl Acad Sci. 1998;95:288–93.

108. Kim JY, Mukherjee S, Ngo L, Christiani DC. Urinary 8-hydroxy-2'-deoxyguanosine as a biomarker of oxidative DNA damage in workers exposed to fine particulates. Environ Health Perspect. 2004;112:666–71.

109. Wei Y, Han I, Shao M, Hu M, Zhang JJ, Tang X. PM 2.5 constituents and oxidative DNA damage in humans. Environ Sci Technol. 2009;43:4757–62.

110. Tan C, Lu S, Wang Y, Zhu Y, Shi T, Lin M, et al. Long-term exposure to nigh air pollution induces cumulative DNA damages in traffic policemen. Sci Total Environ. 2017;593–594:330–6.

111. Calderón-Garcidueñas L, Wen-Wang L, Zhang YJ, Rodriguez-Alcaraz A, Osnaya N, Villarreal-Calderón A, et al. 8-hydroxy-2'-deoxyguanosine, a major mutagenic oxidative DNA lesion, and DNA strand breaks in nasal respiratory epithelium of children exposed to urban pollution. Environ Health Perspect. 1999;107:469–74.

112. Magnani ND, Marchini T, Tasat DR, Alvarez S, Evelson PA. Lung oxidative metabolism after exposure to ambient particles. Biochem Biophys Res Commun. 2011;412:667–72.

113. Halliwell B, Gutteridge JMC. Free radicals in biology and medicine. 4th ed. New York: Oxford University Press; 2007.

114. Bartosz G. Reactive oxygen species: destroyers or messengers? Biochem Pharmacol. 2009;77:1303–15.

115. Forman HJ, Ursini F, Maiorino M. An overview of mechanisms of redox signaling. J Mol Cell Cardiol. 2014;73:2–9.

116. Lee S, Kim SM, Lee RT. Thioredoxin and thioredoxin target proteins: from molecular mechanisms to functional significance. Antioxid Redox Signal. 2013;18:1165–207.

117. Kampfrath T, Maiseyeu A, Ying Z, Shah Z, Deiuliis JA, Xu X, et al. Chronic fine particulate matter exposure induces systemic vascular dysfunction via NADPH oxidase and TLR4 pathways. Circ Res. 2011;108:716–26.

118. Garcia CCM, Angeli JPF, Freitas FP, Gomes OF, de Oliveira TF, Loureiro APM, et al. [13C2]-acetaldehyde promotes unequivocal formation of 1,N2-propano-2'-deoxyguanosine in human cells. J Am Chem Soc. 2011;133:9140–3.

119. Angeli JPF, Garcia CCM, Sena F, Freitas FP, Miyamoto S, Medeiros MHG, et al. Lipid hydroperoxide-induced and hemoglobin-enhanced oxidative damage to colon cancer cells. Free Radic Biol Med. 2011;51:503–15.

120. Herceg Z, Vaissière T. Epigenetic mechanisms and cancer: an interface between the environment and the genome. Epigenetics. 2011;6:804–19.

121. Ji H, Khurana Hershey GK. Genetic and epigenetic influence on the response to environmental particulate matter. J Allergy Clin Immunol. 2012;129:33–41.

122. Silveyra P, Floros J. Air pollution and epigenetics: effects on SP-A and innate host defence in the lung. Swiss Med Wkly. 2012;142:w13579.

123. Irizarry RA, Ladd-Acosta C, Wen B, Wu Z, Montano C, Onyango P, et al. The human colon cancer methylome shows similar hypo- and hypermethylation at conserved tissue-specific CpG island shores. Nat Genet. 2009;41:178–86.

124. Doi A, Park I-H, Wen B, Murakami P, Aryee MJ, Irizarry R, et al. Differential methylation of tissue- and cancer-specific CpG island shores distinguishes human induced pluripotent stem cells, embryonic stem cells and fibroblasts. Nat Genet. 2009;41:1350–3.

125. Sharma S, Kelly TK, Jones PA. Epigenetics in cancer. Carcinogenesis. 2010;31:27–36.

126. Brenet F, Moh M, Funk P, Feierstein E, Viale AJ, Socci ND, et al. DNA methylation of the first exon is tightly linked to transcriptional silencing. PLoS One. 2011;6:e14524 Papavasiliou N, editor.

127. Dahl C, Grønbæk K, Guldberg P. Advances in DNA methylation: 5-hydroxymethylcytosine revisited. Clin Chim Acta. 2011;412:831–6.

128. Williams K, Christensen J, Helin K. DNA methylation: TET proteins-guardians of CpG islands? EMBO Rep. 2011;13:28–35.

129. Delatte B, Jeschke J, Defrance M, Bachman M, Creppe C, Calonne E, et al. Genome-wide hydroxymethylcytosine pattern changes in response to oxidative stress. Sci Rep. 2015;5:12714.

130. Damiani LA, Yingling CM, Leng S, Romo PE, Nakamura J, Belinsky SA. Carcinogen-induced gene promoter hypermethylation is mediated by DNMT1 and causal for transformation of immortalized bronchial epithelial cells. Cancer Res. 2008;68:9005–14.

131. Teneng I, Montoya-Durango DE, Quertermous JL, Lacy ME, Ramos KS. Reactivation of L1 retrotransposon by benzo(a)pyrene involves complex genetic and epigenetic regulation. Epigenetics. 2011;6:355–67.

132. Xia B, Yang L-Q, Huang H-Y, Pang L, Yang X-F, Yi Y-J, et al. Repression of biotin-related proteins by benzo[a]pyrene-induced epigenetic modifications in human bronchial epithelial cells. Int J Toxicol. 2016;35:336–43.

133. Jiang C-L, He S-W, Zhang Y-D, Duan H-X, Huang T, Huang Y-C, et al. Air pollution and DNA methylation alterations in lung cancer: a systematic and comparative study. Oncotarget. 2017;8:1369–91.

134. Haffner MC, Chaux A, Meeker AK, Esopi DM, Gerber J, Pellakuru LG, et al. Global 5-hydroxymethylcytosine content is signi cantly reduced in tissue stem/progenitor cell compartments and in human cancers. Oncotarget. 2011;2:627–37.

135. Lisanti S, Omar WA, Tomaszewski B, De Prins S, Jacobs G, Koppen G, et al. Comparison of methods for quantification of global DNA methylation in human cells and tissues. Plos One. 2013;8:e79044.

136. Bock C, Halbritter F, Carmona FJ, Tierling S, Datlinger P, Assenov Y, et al. Quantitative comparison of DNA methylation assays for biomarker development and clinical applications. Nat Biotechnol. 2016;34:726–40.

137. Tammen SA, Dolnikowski GG, Ausman LM, Liu Z, Sauer J, Friso S, et al. Aging and alcohol interact to Alter hepatic DNA Hydroxymethylation. Alcohol Clin Exp Res. 2014;38:2178–85.

138. Jin Z, Liu Y. DNA methylation in human diseases. Gene Dis. 2018;5:1–8.

139. Godshalk R, Nair J, van Schooten FJ, Risch A, Drings P, Kayser K, et al. Comparison of multiple DNA adduct types in tumor adjacent human lung tissue: effect of cigarette smoking. Carcinogenesis. 2002;23:2081–6.

140. Dechakhamphu S, Pinlaor S, Sitthithaworn P, Nair J, Bartsch H, Yongvanit P. Lipid peroxidation and etheno DNA adducts in white blood cells of liver fluke-infected patients: protection by plasma alpha-tocopherol and praziquantel. Cancer Epidemiol Biomark Prev. 2010;19:310–8.

141. Arab K, Pedersen M, Nair J, Meerang M, Knudsen LE, Bartsch H. Typical signature of DNA damage in white blood cells: a pilot study on etheno adducts in Danish mother-newborn child pairs. Carcinogenesis. 2009;30:282–5.

142. Nair J, Vaca CE, Velic I, Mutanen M, Valsta LM, Bartsch H. High dietary omega-6 polyunsaturated fatty acids drastically increase the formation of etheno-DNA base adducts in white blood cells of female subjects. Cancer Epidemiol Biomark Prev. 1997;6:597–601.

143. Churchwell MI, Beland FA, Doerge DR. Quantification of multiple DNA adducts formed through oxidative stress using liquid chromatography and electrospray tandem mass spectrometry. Chem Res Toxicol. 2002;15:1295–301.

Developmental basis for intestinal barrier against the toxicity of graphene oxide

Mingxia Ren[1], Li Zhao[1], Xuecheng Ding[2], Natalia Krasteva[3], Qi Rui[2]* and Dayong Wang[1]* ⓘ

Abstract

Background: Intestinal barrier is crucial for animals against translocation of engineered nanomaterials (ENMs) into secondary targeted organs. However, the molecular mechanisms for the role of intestinal barrier against ENMs toxicity are still largely unclear. The intestine of *Caenorhabditis elegans* is a powerful in vivo experimental system for the study on intestinal function. In this study, we investigated the molecular basis for intestinal barrier against toxicity and translocation of graphene oxide (GO) using *C. elegans* as a model animal.

Results: Based on the genetic screen of genes required for the control of intestinal development at different aspects using intestine-specific RNA interference (RNAi) technique, we identified four genes (*erm-1*, *pkc-3*, *hmp-2* and *act-5*) required for the function of intestinal barrier against GO toxicity. Under normal conditions, mutation of any of these genes altered the intestinal permeability. With the focus on PKC-3, an atypical protein kinase C, we identified an intestinal signaling cascade of PKC-3-SEC-8-WTS-1, which implies that PKC-3 might regulate intestinal permeability and GO toxicity by affecting the function of SEC-8-mediated exocyst complex and the role of WTS-1 in maintaining integrity of apical intestinal membrane. ISP-1 and SOD-3, two proteins required for the control of oxidative stress, were also identified as downstream targets for PKC-3, and functioned in parallel with WTS-1 in the regulation of GO toxicity.

Conclusions: Using *C. elegans* as an in vivo assay system, we found that several developmental genes required for the control of intestinal development regulated both the intestinal permeability and the GO toxicity. With the focus on PKC-3, we raised two intestinal signaling cascades, PKC-3-SEC-8-WTS-1 and PKC-3-ISP-1/SOD-3. Our results will strengthen our understanding the molecular basis for developmental machinery of intestinal barrier against GO toxicity and translocation in animals.

Keywords: Graphene oxide, Intestinal barrier, Intestinal permeability, Molecular basis, PKC-3, *Caenorhabditis elegans*

Background

Graphene and its derivatives are two-dimensional carbon engineered nanomaterials (ENMs) with a single layer of sp^2-bonded carbon atoms. They have the properties of chemical stability, high coefficient of thermal conduction, amphipathicity, large surface area, and ease of functionalization [1]. Graphene oxide (GO) is one of the important graphene derivatives. Due to its unique physical and chemical properties, GO is potentially applied in the fields of drug delivery, biosensor, and environmental remediation [2–5]. Considering the potential of increasing production and various applications [2], a large amount of GO would be released into the environment. In the recent years, the cytotoxicity of GO in inducing oxidative stress, cell division inhibition, apoptosis, or mutagenicity has been observed in different human cell lines [6–10]. Additionally, at least pulmonary and reproductive toxicities could be detected in mammals [11, 12]. The GO distribution assay has further demonstrated the potential of GO translocation into different targeted organs, such as lung, liver, and kidney, in mammals [11, 13].

Caenorhabditis elegans is a widely used non-mammalian animal model for toxicity assessment and toxicological study of various toxicants, including the ENMs [14–17]. Besides properties of short life-cycle and lifespan,

* Correspondence: ruiqi@njau.edu.cn; dayongw@seu.edu.cn
[2]College of Life Sciences, Nanjing Agricultural University, Nanjing 210095, China
[1]Key Laboratory of Environmental Medicine Engineering in Ministry of Education, Medical School, Southeast University, Nanjing 210009, China
Full list of author information is available at the end of the article

transparent body, self-fertilization, and ease of culture [18], *C. elegans* has been shown to be very sensitive to environmental toxicants [14, 19, 20], and frequently used in toxicological study of different ENMs, including the GO [21–27]. In *C. elegans*, GO exposure could cause toxic effects on the functions of both primary targeted organs (such as the intestine) and secondary targeted organs (such as the neurons and the reproductive organs) [22, 28–33]. During the control of ENMs toxicity, bioavailability plays a crucial role in the toxicity induction of ENMs in nematodes [34, 35]. More importantly, intestinal barrier is very important for nematodes against ENMs toxicity and to block translocation of ENMs into secondary targeted organs [30, 36–38]. Nevertheless, the molecular basis for intestinal barrier against ENMs toxicity is still largely unclear in animals. We hypothesized that deficit in intestinal development at certain aspects may alter the function of intestinal barrier and affect the toxicity and the translocation of GO in nematodes.

In *C. elegans*, intestine is a powerful experimental system for different aspects of biological studies, including the stress response [39]. The intestine comprises approximately one third of the total somatic mass in nematodes. In *C. elegans*, intestine is structurally organized by several cellular domains: apical domain including brush border and terminal web, basolateral domain including basement membrane, and apical junctions joining enterocytes to their partners or to adjacent ints into the intestinal structure [39]. The molecular basis for different cellular domains of intestine was summarized in the Table 1. In the apical domain, ACT-5 is required for microvilli development [40], IFB-2 is required for terminal web development [41], ERM-1 is required for connection between actin cytoskeleton and plasma membrane [42], EPS-8 is required for microvilli length control and actin-capping function [43], PAR-3, PAR-6, and PKC-3 are required for apical-basal polarity [44, 45], GEM-4 is required for brush border development [46], and MTM-6 and EAT-3/dynamin are required for endocytosis [47, 48]. In the basolateral domain, LET-413 is required to confine the apical domain [49], NFM-1 acts as a cytoskeletal linker [50], INX-7 is required for cell adhesion [51], and UNC-64/syntaxin, a plasma membrane receptor for intracellular vesicles, regulates vesicle secretion [52]. In the apical junctions, DLG-1 is required for organization of epithelium to a coherent tube [53], AJM-1 is required for junctional integrity [54], EGL-8 is required for vesicle secretion [55], LIN-7 functions as an organizational center for large macromolecular complexes [56], and HMP-1, HMP-2, and HMR-1 are

Table 1 Information for genes required for the intestinal development in nematodes

Gene	Encoded protein	Function	Reference
act-5	Actin	Microvilli development	MacQueen et al., [73]
ifb-2	Intermediate filament protein	Terminal web development	Carberry et al., [41]
erm-1	Ezrin-radixin-moesin protein	Connection between actin cytoskeleton and plasma membrane	Gobel et al., [42]
eps-8	Cell signaling adaptor protein	Microvilli length control	Croce et al., [43]
par-3	PDZ-domain-containing protein	Apical-basal polarity	Nance and Priess, [44]
par-6	PDZ-domain-containing protein	Apical-basal polarity	Nance and Priess, [44]
pkc-3	Proetin kinase C	Apical-basal polarity	Wu et al., [45]
mtm-6	Myotubularin	Endocytosis	Xue et al., 2003
eat-3	Dynamin	Endocytosis	Labrousse et al., [48]
gem-4	Ca^{2+}-dependent phosphatidylserine binding protein	Bush border development	Church and Lambie, [46]
let-413	Scribble	Confine apical domain	Legouis et al., [49]
nfm-1	Neurofibrularin	Cytoskeletal linker	Culetto and Sattelle, [50]
unc-64	Syntaxin	Vesicle secretion	Saifee et al., [52]
inx-3	Gap junction channel	Cell adhesion	Altun et al., [51]
dlg-1	MAGUK protein	Organization of epithelium to a coherent tube	Segbert et al., [53]
ajm-1	Apical junction molecule	Junctional integrity	Koppen et al., [54]
egl-8	Phospholipase Cβ	Vesicle secretion	Lackner et al., [55]
lin-7	PDZ-domain-containing protein	Organization of large macromolecular complexes	Feng et al., [56]
hmp-2	β-catenin	Tissue integrity of intestinal tube	Segbert et al., [53]
hmp-1	α-catenin	Tissue integrity of intestinal tube	Segbert et al., [53]
hmr-1	Cadherin	Tissue integrity of intestinal tube	Segbert et al., [53]

required for tissue integrity of intestinal tube [53]. The aim of this study was to investigate the molecular basis for intestinal barrier against toxicity and translocation of GO using the *C. elegans* as a model animal. In this study, we first performed a genetic screen of genes required for the function of intestinal barrier against GO toxicity using the technique of intestine-specific RNA interference (RNAi). And then, we focused on the candidate gene of *pkc-3* to examine the underlying molecular mechanism for its role in regulating the function of intestinal barrier against GO toxicity. Our results will strengthen our understanding the molecular basis for developmental machinery of intestinal barrier against environmental ENMs in animals.

Results

Identification of intestinal-development related proteins required for the regulation of GO toxicity

VP303 strain is a tool for intestine-specific RNAi of certain genes [57]. Using the VP303 as an intestine-specific RNAi knockdown tool, we tried to identify the possible intestinal-development related genes required for the regulation of GO toxicity. Our previous study has indicated that acute exposure (from L4-larvae for 24 h) to GO at concentrations more than 10 mg/L could result in significant induction of intestinal reactive oxygen species (ROS) production and decrease in locomotion behavior in nematodes [28]. We here first selected the 10 mg/L as the working concentrations for GO exposure. L2-larvae were used to perform the RNAi treatment until the nematodes became L4-larvae. And then, the L4 larvae with RNAi knockdown of certain gene were exposed to GO for 24 h. We used the endpoint of intestinal ROS production to assess the potential toxic effect of GO exposure on the intestinal function. The data and the related information on the efficiency of RNAi of examined genes were shown in Additional file 1: Figure S1 and Table S1. Treatment with paraquat, a ROS generator, was used as a positive control of assay on intestinal ROS production (Additional file 1: Figure S2). Under normal conditions, intestine-specific RNAi knockdown of any examined gene required for the control of development of intestinal apical domain did not induce the significant intestinal ROS production (Fig. 1a). After acute exposure to GO, among the examined genes required for the control of development of intestinal apical domain, intestine-specific RNAi knockdown of *ifb-2*, *eps-8*, *par-3*, *par-6*, *mtm-6*, *eat-3*, or *gem-4* did not significantly affect the induction of intestinal ROS production (Fig. 1a). However, after acute exposure to GO, intestine-specific RNAi knockdown of *erm-1* or *pkc-3* enhanced the induction of intestinal ROS production, and intestine-specific RNAi knockdown of *act-5*

suppressed the induction of intestinal ROS production (Fig. 1a). After acute exposure to GO, RNAi knockdown of *ifb-2*, *eps-8*, *par-3*, *par-6*, *mtm-6*, *eat-3*, *erm-1*, *pkc-3*, or *gem-4* did not affect the survival of nematodes.

Similarly, under normal conditions, intestine-specific RNAi knockdown of any examined gene required for the control of development of intestinal basolateral domain did not induce the obvious intestinal ROS production (Fig. 1b). After acute exposure to GO, intestine-specific RNAi knockdown of *let-413*, *nfm-1*, *unc-64*, or *inx-3* could not significantly influence the induction of intestinal ROS production (Fig. 1b). After acute exposure to GO, RNAi knockdown of *let-413*, *nfm-1*, *unc-64*, or *inx-3* did not affect the survival of nematodes.

Under normal conditions, intestine-specific RNAi knockdown of any examined gene required for the control of development of intestinal apical junctions can not result in the induction of significant intestinal ROS production (Fig. 1c). After acute exposure to GO, among the examined genes required for the control of development of intestinal apical junctions, intestine-specific RNAi knockdown of *dlg-1*, *ajm-1*, *egl-8*, *lin-7*, *hmp-1*, or *hmr-1* did not significantly influence the induction of intestinal ROS production (Fig. 1c). In contrast, after acute exposure to GO, intestine-specific RNAi knockdown of *hmp-2* could cause the enhanced induction of intestinal ROS production (Fig. 1c). After acute exposure to GO, RNAi knockdown of *dlg-1*, *ajm-1*, *egl-8*, *lin-7*, *hmp-1*, *hmp-2*, or *hmr-1* did not affect the survival of nematodes.

Effects of intestine-specific RNAi knockdown of *act-5*, *erm-1*, *pkc-3*, or *hmp-2* on distribution and translocation of GO

We next examined the effects of intestine-specific RNAi knockdown of *act-5*, *erm-1*, *pkc-3*, or *hmp-2* on distribution and translocation of GO. After GO/Rho B exposure, GO/Rho B could be severely accumulated in the body of nematodes, including the pharynx, intestine, spermatheca, and tail in VP303 nematodes (Fig. 2). Compared with the accumulation and translocation of GO/Rho B in VP303 nematodes, intestine-specific RNAi knockdown of *erm-1*, *pkc-3*, or *hmp-2* significantly enhanced the accumulation of GO/Rho B in the body of nematodes; however, intestine-specific RNAi knockdown of *act-5* significantly inhibited the GO/Rho B in the body of nematodes (Fig. 2). The UV/Vis spectral data on GO/Rho B, GO, and Rho B demonstrated the binding of Rho B to GO in the obtained GO/Rho B, since we could observe both the UV/Vis peak of GO and the UV/Vis peak of Rho B in the obtained GO/Rho B (Additional file 1: Figure S3).

We next focused on the PKC-3 to investigate the underlying cellular and molecular mechanisms for its function in the regulation of toxicity and translocation

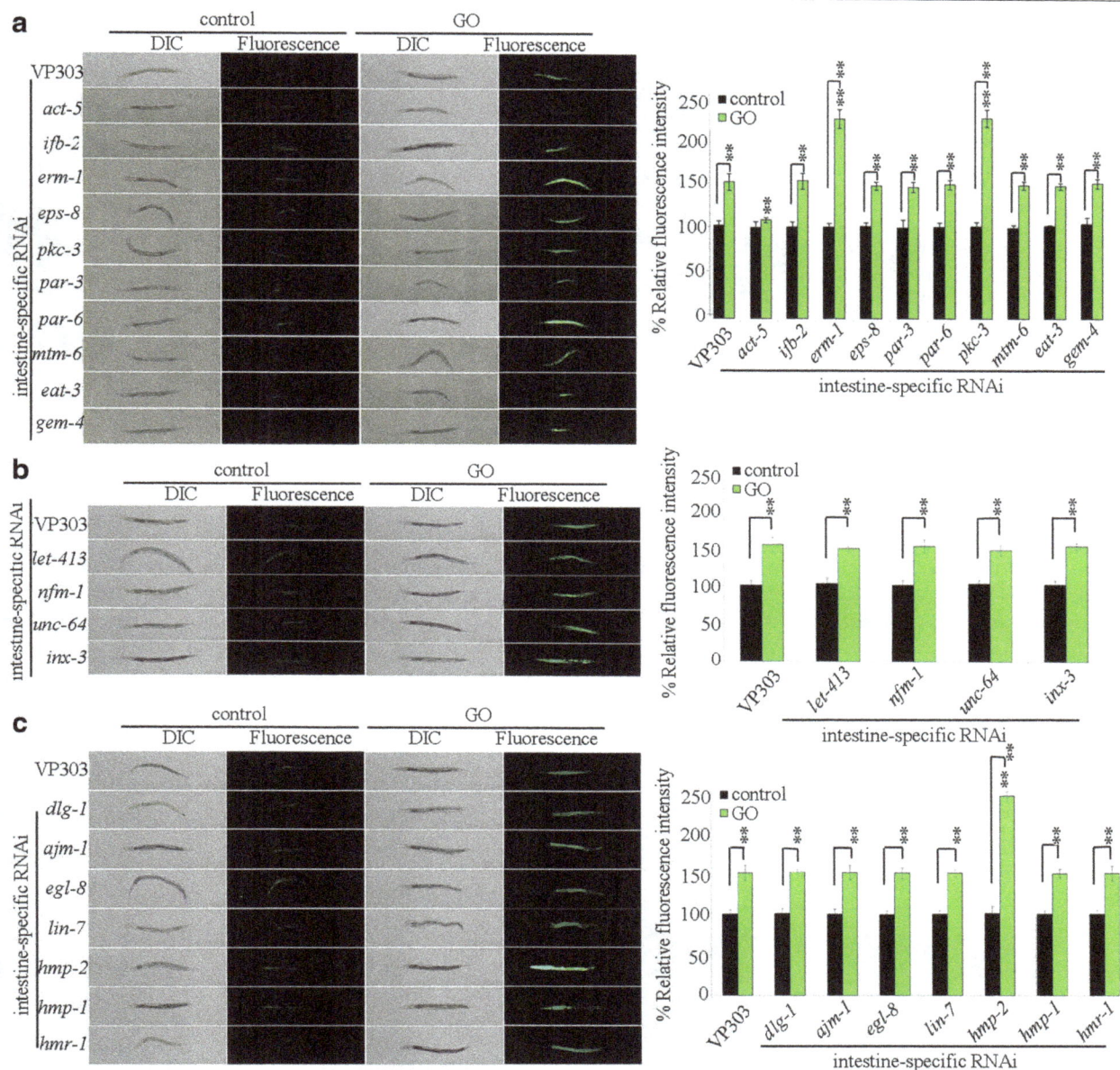

Fig. 1 Effects of intestine-specific RNAi knockdown of intestine-developmental related genes on GO toxicity. **a** Effects of intestine-specific RNAi knockdown of genes required for the control of development of intestinal apical domain on GO toxicity in inducing intestinal ROS production. **b** Effects of intestine-specific RNAi knockdown of genes required for the control of development of intestinal basolateral domain on GO toxicity in inducing intestinal ROS production. **c** Effects of intestine-specific RNAi knockdown of genes required for the control of development of intestinal apical junctions on GO toxicity in inducing intestinal ROS production. Acute exposure was performed from L4-larvae for 24 h. GO exposure concentration was 10 mg/L. Bars represent means ± SD. $^{**}P < 0.01$ vs VP303 (if not specially indicated)

of GO. We employed the molecular probe of Nile Red to analyze the possible effect of intestine-specific RNAi knockdown of *pkc-3* on intestinal permeability. Under normal conditions, the Nile Red signals were mainly located in the intestinal lumen in VP303 nematodes, whereas intestine-specific RNAi knockdown of *pkc-3* could cause the significant translocation of Nile Red into the intestinal cells in VP303 nematodes (Fig. 3a).

Moreover, after GO exposure, we observed the more severe translocation and accumulation of Nile Red signals into the intestinal cells and even the body cavity in nematodes with intestine-specific RNAi knockdown of *pkc-3* compared with that in VP303 (Fig. 3b). Meanwhile, under normal conditions, intestine-specific RNAi knockdown of *pkc-3* did not obviously affect the fat storage, because we observed the similar Sudan Black staining

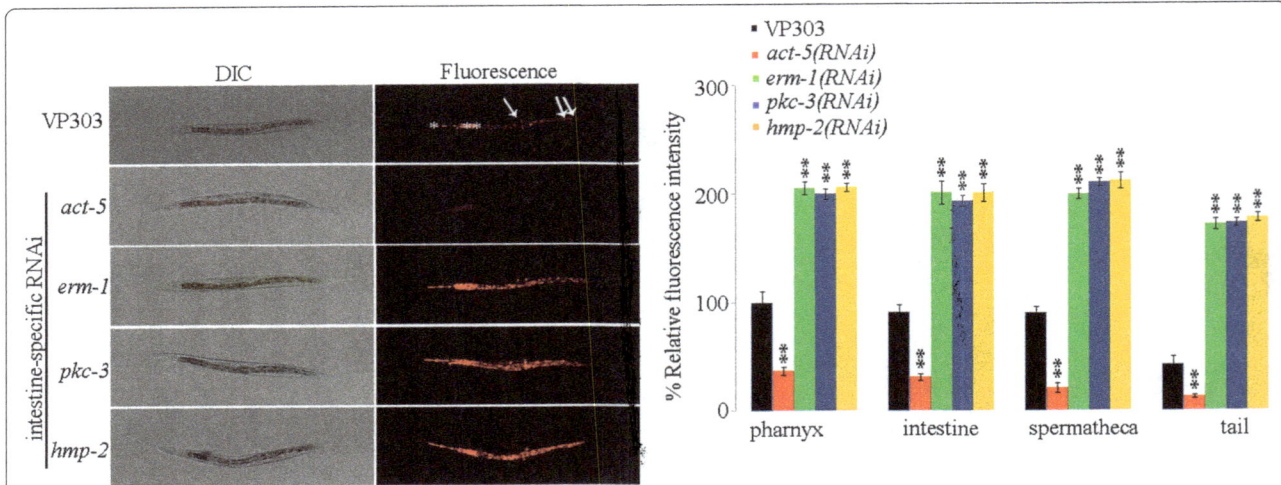

Fig. 2 Effects of intestine-specific RNAi knockdown of intestine-developmental related genes on distribution and translocation of GO. The pharynx (*) and the intestine (**) were indicated by asterisks. Single arrowhead indicates the spermatheca, and double arrowhead indicates the tail. Acute exposure was performed from L4-larvae for 24 h. GO exposure concentration was 10 mg/L. Bars represent means ± SD. **$P < 0.01$ vs VP303

results between nematodes with intestine-specific RNAi knockdown of *pkc-3* and VP303 nematodes (Fig. 3b). Additionally, after GO exposure, intestine-specific RNAi knockdown of *pkc-3* also did not obviously influence the fat storage (Fig. 3b). It has been reported that GO exposure could not alter the fat storage in wild-type nematodes [28]. Considering the fact that the Nile Red can also used to label the fat storage [58], our results suggest that PKC-3 is required for the regulation of intestinal permeability in nematodes.

Identification of downstream targets for intestinal PKC-3 in the regulation of toxicity and translocation of GO

In *C. elegans*, PAR-3, PAR-6, LGL-1, LIN-5, NLP-29, and SEC-8 may act as the potential targets for PKC-3 [59–64]. We further examined whether these proteins can act the downstream targets for intestinal PKC-3 in the regulation of GO toxicity. After GO exposure, intestine-specific RNAi knockdown of *pkc-3* did not significantly affect the transcriptional expressions of *par-1*, *par-6*, *lin-5*, and *nlp-29* (Fig. 4a). In contrast, after GO

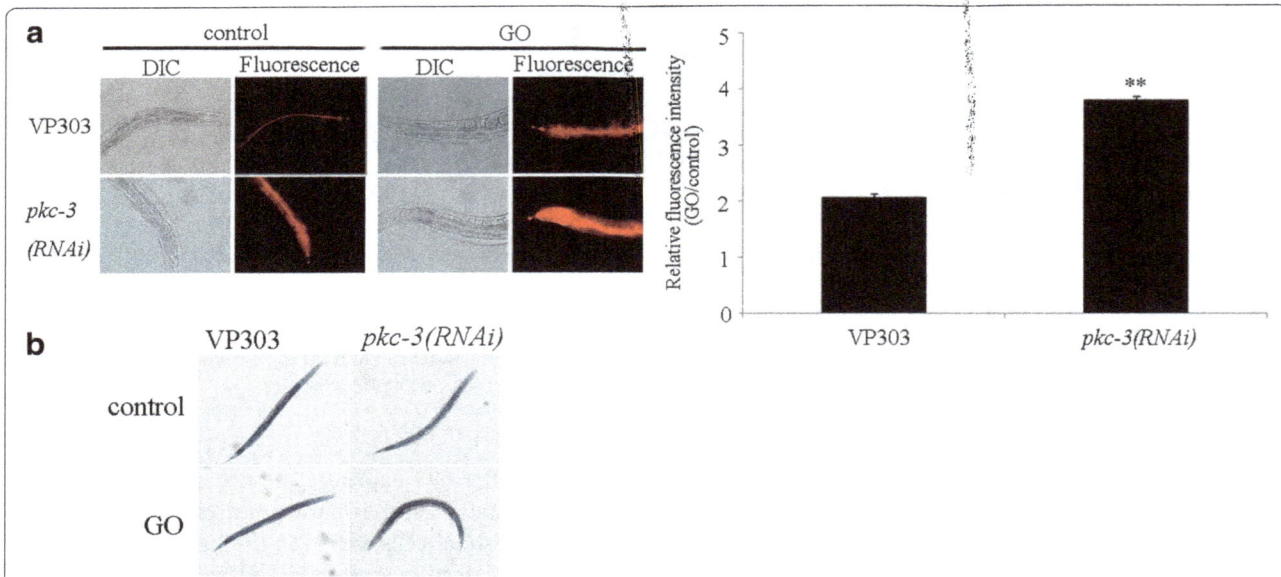

Fig. 3 Effect of intestine-specific RNAi knockdown of *pkc-3* on intestinal permeability in nematodes. **a** Effect of intestine-specific RNAi knockdown of *pkc-3* on intestinal permeability as indicated by the signals of Nile Red. The right shows the comparison of fluorescence intensity of Nile Red signals in intestinal cells. Bars represent means ± SD. **$P < 0.01$ vs VP303. **b** Effect of intestine-specific RNAi knockdown of *pkc-3* on fat storage labeled by Sudan Black. Acute exposure was performed from L4-larvae for 24 h. GO exposure concentration was 10 mg/L

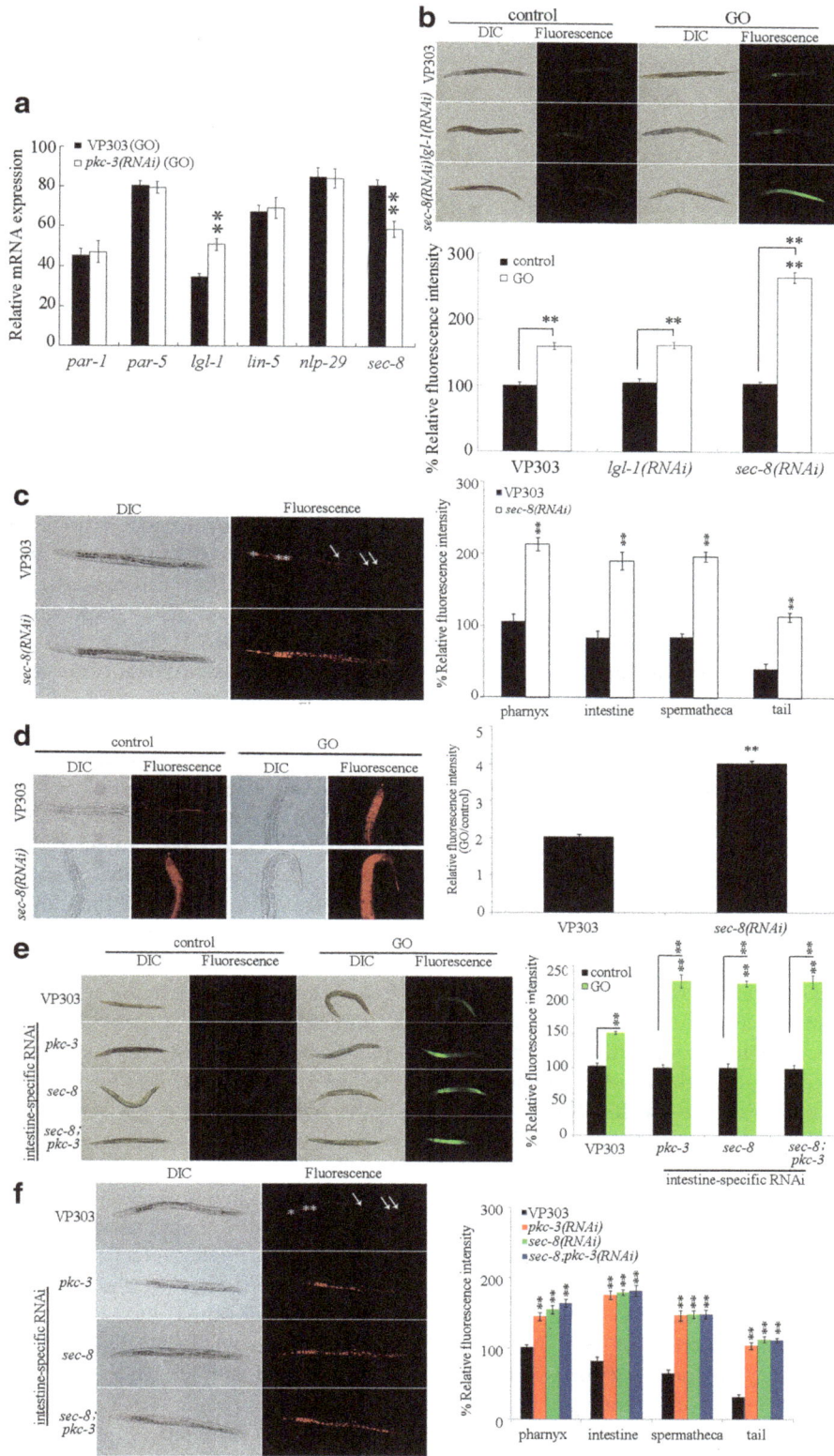

Fig. 4 (See legend on next page.)

(See figure on previous page.)
Fig. 4 Identification of downstream targets for intestinal PKC-3 in the regulation of GO toxicity and translocation. **a** Effects of intestine-specific RNAi knockdown of *pkc-3* on expressions of *par-1*, *par-5*, *lgl-1*, *lin-5*, *nlp-29*, and *sec-8* in GO exposed nematodes. **b** Effects of intestine-specific RNAi knockdown of *lgl-1* or *sec-8* on GO toxicity in inducing intestinal ROS production. **c** Effects of intestine-specific RNAi knockdown of *sec-8* on distribution and translocation of GO/Rho B. The pharynx (*) and the intestine (**) were indicated by asterisks. Single arrowhead indicates the spermatheca, and double arrowhead indicates the tail. **d** Effects of intestine-specific RNAi knockdown of *sec-8* on intestinal permeability as indicated by the signals of Nile Red. The right shows the comparison of fluorescence intensity of Nile Red signals in intestinal cells. **e** Genetic interaction between PKC-3 and SEC-8 in the regulation of toxicity and translocation of GO in inducing intestinal ROS production. **f** Genetic interaction between PKC-3 and SEC-8 in the regulation of toxicity and translocation of GO/Rho B. The pharynx (*) and the intestine (**) were indicated by asterisks. Single arrowhead indicates the spermatheca, and double arrowhead indicates the tail. Acute exposure was performed from L4-larvae for 24 h. GO or GO/Rho B exposure concentration was 10 mg/L. Bars represent means ± SD. **$P < 0.01$ vs VP303 (if not specially indicated)

exposure, intestine-specific RNAi knockdown of *pkc-3* significantly increased the transcriptional expression of *lgl-1*, and decreased the transcriptional expression of *sec-8* (Fig. 4a).

We next focused on the LGL-1 and SEC-8 to determine the effects of intestine-specific RNAi knockdown of *lgl-1* or *sec-8* on toxicity and translocation of GO. After GO exposure, intestine-specific RNAi knockdown of *sec-8* significantly enhanced the GO toxicity in inducing intestinal ROS production (Fig. 4b). However, intestine-specific RNAi knockdown of *lgl-1* did not significantly affect the GO toxicity in inducing intestinal ROS production (Fig. 4b). After acute exposure to GO, RNAi knockdown of *sec-8* did not affect the survival of nematodes. Moreover, we observed that intestine-specific RNAi knockdown of *sec-8* could noticeably strengthen the accumulation of GO/Rho B in the body of nematodes (Fig. 4c).

Furthermore, under normal conditions, we found that intestine-specific RNAi knockdown of *sec-8* caused the obvious translocation of Nile Red signals into the intestinal cells (Fig. 4d). Additionally, after GO exposure, intestine-specific RNAi knockdown of *sec-8* induced the more severe translocation and accumulation of Nile Red signals into the intestinal cells and even the body cavity (Fig. 4d). Meanwhile, intestine-specific RNAi knockdown of *sec-8* did not noticeably affect the fat storage under the normal conditions, and intestine-specific RNAi knockdown of *sec-8* also did not obviously influence the fat storage after GO exposure (Additional file 1: Figure S4). Therefore, like the PKC-3, SEC-8 may also function in the maintenance of normal intestinal permeability.

To further confirm the potential role of SEC-8 as the downstream target of PKC-3, we investigated the genetic interaction between PKC-3 and SEC-8 in the regulation of toxicity and translocation of GO. After GO exposure, the GO toxicity in inducing intestinal ROS production in nematodes with intestine-specific RNAi knockdown of both *pkc-3* and *sec-8* was similar to that observed in nematodes with intestine-specific RNAi knockdown of *pkc-3* or *sec-8* (Fig. 4e). Additionally, the accumulation and translocation of GO in nematodes with intestine-specific RNAi knockdown of both *pkc-3*

and *sec-8* was also similar to that observed in nematodes with intestine-specific RNAi knockdown of *pkc-3* or *sec-8* (Fig. 4f). Therefore, PKC-3 and SEC-8 may act in the same genetic pathway in the intestine to regulate the toxicity and the translocation of GO.

Identification of downstream targets for intestinal SEC-8 in the regulation of GO toxicity and translocation

In *C. elegans*, WTS-1 can act as a candidate target for SEC-8 [65]. After GO exposure, we found that intestine-specific RNAi knockdown of *sec-8* significantly decreased the transcriptional expression of *wts-1* (Fig. 5a). Intestine-specific RNAi knockdown of *wts-1* further significantly enhanced the GO toxicity in inducing intestinal ROS production (Fig. 5b), and strengthened the accumulation of GO/Rho B in the body of nematodes (Fig. 5c). After acute exposure to GO, RNAi knockdown of *wts-1* did not affect the survival of nematodes.

Under normal conditions, intestine-specific RNAi knockdown of *wts-1* induced the translocation of Nile Red signals into the intestinal cells (Fig. 5d). Moreover, after GO exposure, intestine-specific RNAi knockdown of *wts-1* caused the more severe translocation and accumulation of Nile Red signals into the intestinal cells and even the body cavity (Fig. 5d). Meanwhile, intestine-specific RNAi knockdown of *wts-1* did not noticeably affect the fat storage under the normal conditions or after GO exposure (Additional file 1: Figure S5). Therefore, WTS-1 may be also required for the maintenance of normal intestinal permeability. In *C. elegans*, *wts-1* encodes a serine/threonine protein kinase orthologous to members of the NDR/LATS family of protein kinases.

After GO exposure, we observed that the GO toxicity in inducing intestinal ROS production in nematodes with intestine-specific RNAi knockdown of both *sec-8* and *wts-1* was similar to that observed in nematodes with intestine-specific RNAi knockdown of *sec-8* or *wts-1* (Fig. 5e). Similarly, the accumulation and translocation of GO in nematodes with intestine-specific RNAi knockdown of both *sec-8* and *wts-1* was similar to that observed in nematodes with intestine-specific RNAi knockdown of *sec-8* or *wts-1* (Fig. 5f). These results

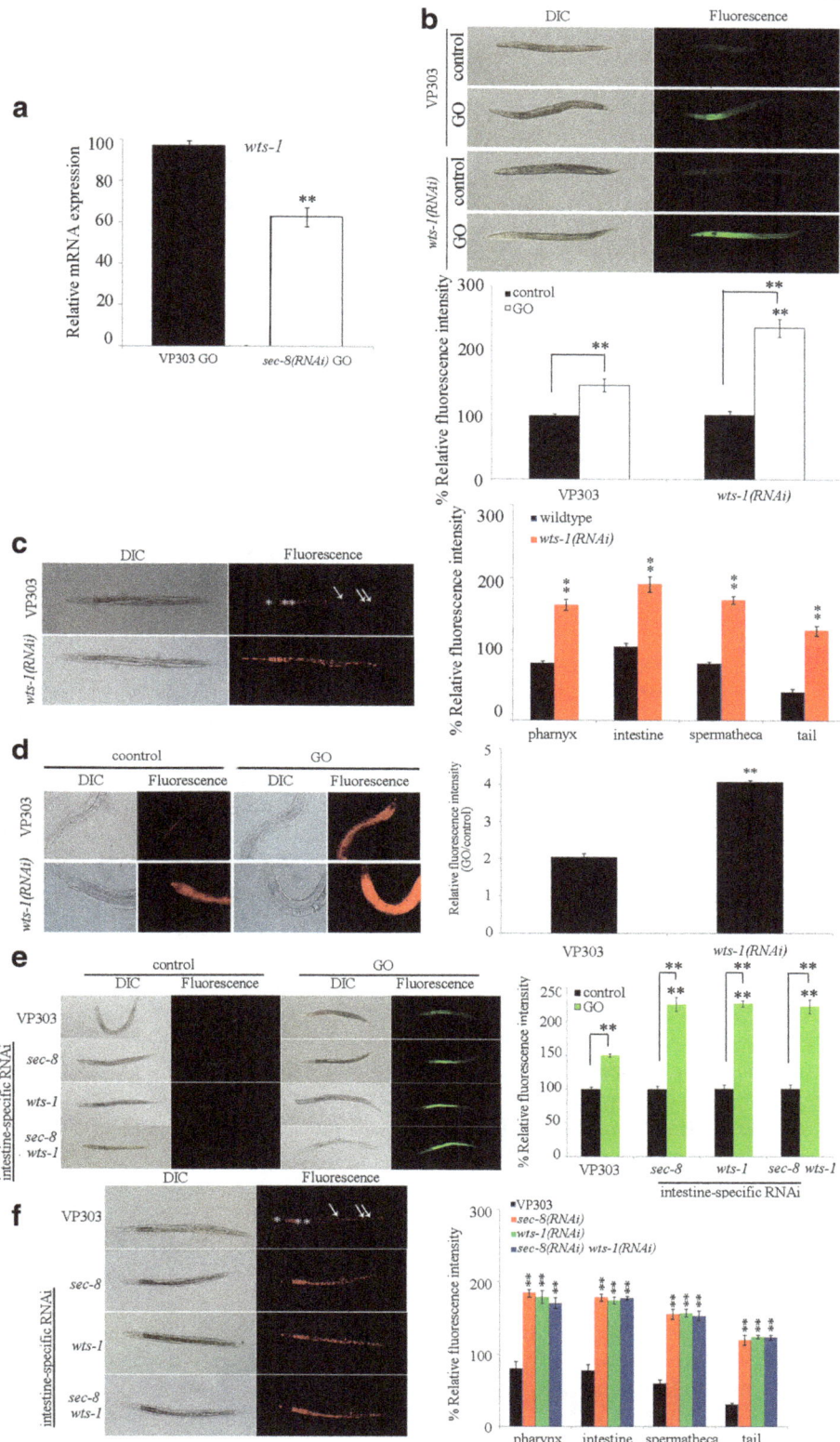

Fig. 5 (See legend on next page.)

(See figure on previous page.)
Fig. 5 Identification of downstream targets for intestinal SEC-8 in the regulation of GO toxicity and translocation. **a** Effects of intestine-specific RNAi knockdown of sec-8 on expressions of wts-1 in GO exposed nematodes. **b** Effects of intestine-specific RNAi knockdown of wts-1 on GO toxicity in inducing intestinal ROS production. **c** Effects of intestine-specific RNAi knockdown of wts-1 on distribution and translocation of GO/Rho B. The pharynx (*) and the intestine (**) were indicated by asterisks. Single arrowhead indicates the spermatheca, and double arrowhead indicates the tail. **d** Effects of intestine-specific RNAi knockdown of wts-1 on intestinal permeability as indicated by the signals of Nile Red. The right shows the comparison of fluorescence intensity of Nile Red signals in intestinal cells. **e** Genetic interaction between SEC-8 and WTS-1 in the regulation of toxicity and translocation of GO in inducing intestinal ROS production. **f** Genetic interaction between SEC-8 and WTS-1 in the regulation of toxicity and translocation of GO/Rho B. The pharynx (*) and the intestine (**) were indicated by asterisks. Single arrowhead indicates the spermatheca, and double arrowhead indicates the tail. Acute exposure was performed from L4-larvae for 24 h. GO or GO/Rho B exposure concentration was 10 mg/L. Bars represent means ± SD. **$P < 0.01$ vs VP303 (if not specially indicated)

suggest that SEC-8 and WTS-1 may further act in the same genetic pathway in the intestine to regulate the toxicity and the translocation of GO.

Effects of intestine-specific RNAi knockdown of *pkc-3* on molecular basis for oxidative stress

In *C. elegans*, *mev-1* encodes a subunit of mitochondrial complex II [66], *gas-1* encodes a subunit of mitochondrial complex I [67], *isp-1* encodes a subunit of the mitochondrial complex III [68], and *clk-1* encodes a ubiquinone biosynthesis protein COQ7 [69]. Under normal conditions, intestine-specific RNAi knockdown of *pkc-3* did not significantly affect the transcriptional expressions of *mev-1*, *gas-1*, *isp-1*, and *clk-1* (Fig. 6a). After GO exposure, although intestine-specific RNAi knockdown of *pkc-3* still did not significantly influence the transcriptional expressions of *mev-1*, *gas-1*, and *clk-1*, intestine-specific RNAi knockdown of *pkc-3* significantly increased the transcriptional expression of *isp-1* (Fig. 6a). In *C. elegans*, the *isp-1* mutant shows a decreased sensitivity to ROS [68].

In *C. elegans*, *sod* genes encode superoxide dismutases (SODs), which are required for the animals defending the oxidative stress [70, 71]. Under normal conditions, intestine-specific RNAi knockdown of *pkc-3* did not significantly affect the transcriptional expressions of all examined *sod* genes (Fig. 6b). After GO exposure, although intestine-specific RNAi knockdown of *pkc-3* still did not significantly influence the transcriptional expressions of *sod-1*, *sod-2*, *sod-4*, and *sod-5*, intestine-specific RNAi knockdown of *pkc-3* significantly increased the transcriptional expression of *sod-3* (Fig. 6b). In *C. elegans*, *sod-3* encodes a mitochondrial manganese SOD (Mn-SOD).

Moreover, we observed that intestine-specific RNAi knockdown of *isp-1* significantly suppressed the GO toxicity in inducing intestinal ROS production, whereas intestine-specific RNAi knockdown of *sod-3* enhanced the GO toxicity in inducing intestinal ROS production (Fig. 6c). After acute exposure to GO, RNAi knockdown of *sod-3* did not affect the survival of nematodes. These results imply that intestinal PKC-3 may further

regulate the GO toxicity by affecting the functions of ISP-1 and SOD-3.

Toxicity assessment of GO in nematodes with RNAi knockdown of *wts-1*, *sod-3*, or both after acute exposure

In nematodes, mutation of *isp-1* induced a resistance to GO toxicity [34, 72]; whereas mutation of *sod-3* induced a susceptibility to GO toxicity [72]. We next used intestinal ROS production as the toxicity assessment endpoint to investigate the effect of RNAi knockdown of *wts-1*, *sod-3*, or both on GO toxicity in nematodes acutely exposed to GO at different concentrations. After acute exposure to GO at the concentration of 10 mg/L, the more severe induction of intestinal ROS production was observed in nematodes with RNAi knockdown of *wts-1* or *sod-3* than that in VP 303 strain (Fig. 7a), and the more severe induction of intestinal ROS production was further detected in nematodes with RNAi knockdown of both *wts-1* and *sod-3* than that in nematodes with RNAi knockdown of *wts-1* or *sod-3* (Fig. 7a). After acute exposure to GO at the concentration of 1 mg/L, although we could not observe the significant induction of intestinal ROS production in VP303 strain, we detected the significant intestinal ROS production in nematodes RNAi knockdown of *wts-1* or *sod-3* than that in VP 303 strain (Fig. 7a). Additionally, we also observed the more severe induction of intestinal ROS production in nematodes with RNAi knockdown of both *wts-1* and *sod-3* than that in nematodes with RNAi knockdown of *wts-1* or *sod-3* after acute exposure to 1 mg/L of GO (Fig. 7a). After acute exposure to GO at the concentration of 0.1 mg/L, we could not observe the significant induction of intestinal ROS production in VP303 strain or nematodes RNAi knockdown of *wts-1* or *sod-3*; however, we could still detect the significant induction of intestinal ROS production in nematodes with RNAi knockdown of both *wts-1* and *sod-3* (Fig. 7a).

Genetic interaction between ACT-5 and PKC-3 in the regulation of the toxicity and the translocation of GO

To determine the underlying mechanism for the function of ACT-5 in regulating GO toxicity and translocation, we further investigated the genetic interaction between

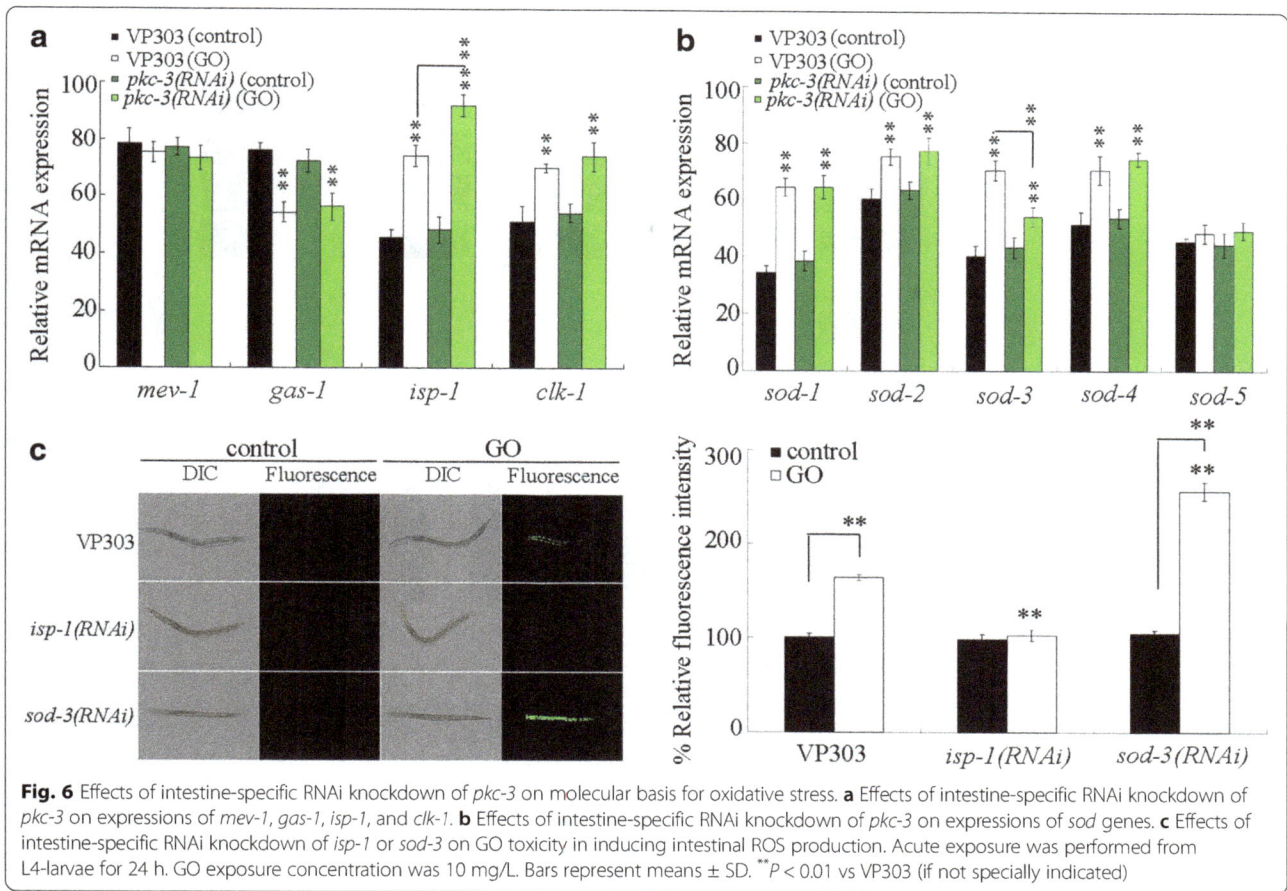

Fig. 6 Effects of intestine-specific RNAi knockdown of *pkc-3* on molecular basis for oxidative stress. **a** Effects of intestine-specific RNAi knockdown of *pkc-3* on expressions of *mev-1*, *gas-1*, *isp-1*, and *clk-1*. **b** Effects of intestine-specific RNAi knockdown of *pkc-3* on expressions of *sod* genes. **c** Effects of intestine-specific RNAi knockdown of *isp-1* or *sod-3* on GO toxicity in inducing intestinal ROS production. Acute exposure was performed from L4-larvae for 24 h. GO exposure concentration was 10 mg/L. Bars represent means ± SD. $^{**}P < 0.01$ vs VP303 (if not specially indicated)

ACT-5 and PKC-3 in the regulation of the toxicity and the translocation of GO. After acute exposure to GO at the concentration of 10 mg/L, intestine-specific RNAi knockdown of *pkc-3* significantly suppressed the resistance of nematodes with intestine-specific RNAi knockdown of *act-5* to GO toxicity in inducing ROS production (Fig. 8a). Moreover, intestine-specific RNAi knockdown of *pkc-3* could obviously disrupt the protection function for intestine-specific RNAi knockdown of *act-5* against translocation and accumulation of GO in targeted organs (Fig. 8b). These results suggest that, in intestinal cells, ACT-5 may act upstream of PKC-3 to regulate the toxicity and the translocation of GO in nematodes.

Discussion

In this study, with the aid of VP303 as an intestine-specific RNAi tool for certain genes, we identified the potential intestinal-development related genes required for the control of GO toxicity and translocation by performing a large screen. Based on the assays on the toxicity and translocation, we found that intestine-specific RNAi knockdown of *erm-1*, *pkc-3*, or *hmp-2* enhanced the GO toxicity and the accumulation of GO in the body of nematodes (Figs. 1 and 2). Our previous study has demonstrated that

prolonged exposure to GO from L1-larvae to young adults could significantly decrease the transcriptional expression of *pkc-3* [28]. In contrast, prolonged exposure to GO did not significantly alter the transcriptional expression of *erm-1* [28]. Although prolonged exposure to GO significantly decreased the transcriptional expression of *par-6* [28], intestine-specific RNAi knockdown of *par-6* did not obviously affect the GO toxicity in inducing intestinal ROS production (Fig. 1a). These results imply that the altered expression of some genes, such as *pkc-3*, may provide an important molecular basis for the involvement of developmental state of intestine in the regulation of GO toxicity and translocation.

Moreover, we found that intestine-specific RNAi knockdown of *act-5* could inhibit the GO toxicity and suppress the accumulation and translocation of GO in the body of nematodes (Figs. 1 and 2). This observation suggests that different deficits in intestinal development may have different or even opposite effects on toxicity and translocation of GO. ACT-5 is required for the microvilli development in the apical domain of intestine [73], implying that certain alterations in intestinal microvilli development caused by *act-5* mutation may be helpful for nematodes against the toxicity and the

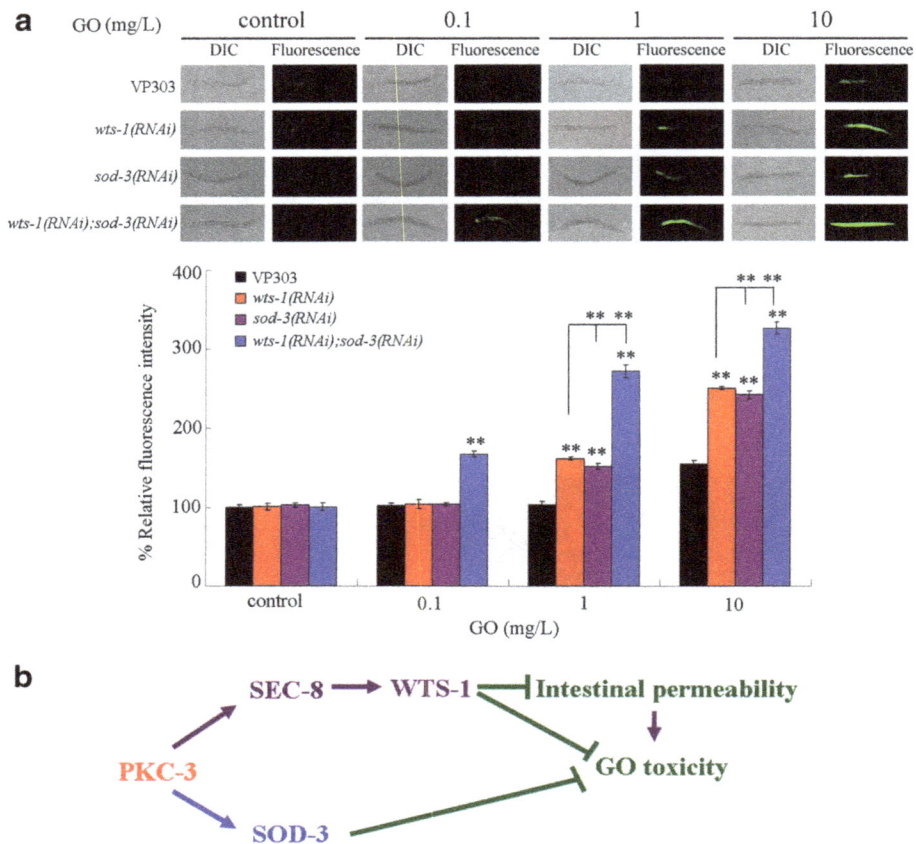

Fig. 7 Genetic interaction between WTS-1 and SOD-3 in the regulation of GO toxicity. **a** Toxicity assessment of GO at different concentrations in inducing intestinal ROS production in different strains. Acute exposure was performed from L4-larvae for 24 h. GO exposure concentration was 10 mg/L. Bars represent means ± SD. **$P < 0.01$ vs VP303 (if not specially indicated). **b** A diagram showing the molecular mechanism for PKC-3 in the regulation of GO toxicity

translocation of GO. In nematodes, it has been found that the ACT-5 can form coats around the membrane-bound vesicles containing environmental toxicants or pathogens to enhance their endocytosis into the targeted cells [74]. Therefore, the resistance of *act-5* mutant to GO toxicity may be formed by suppressing this coating around the membrane-bound vesicles containing environmental ENMs and the endocytosis process in nematodes. In the intestinal cells of nematodes, ACT-5 may further regulate the toxicity and the translocation of GO by suppressing the function of PKC-3 in nematodes (Fig. 8).

Among the identified four genes (*erm-1*, *pkc-3*, *hmp-2*, and *act-5*), *erm-1*, *pkc-3*, and *act-5* are required for the control of connection between actin cytoskeleton and plasma membrane, apical-basal polarity, or microvilli development in the apical domain of intestine [42, 44, 73], and *hmp-2* is required for the control of tissue integrity of intestinal tube in the apical junctions [53]. However, among the examined four genes (*let-413*, *nfm-1*, *unc-64*, and *inx-3*) required for the control of different aspects

of development of basolateral domain in the intestine, intestine-specific RNAi knockdown of any of these genes did not obviously affect the GO toxicity in inducing intestinal ROS production (Fig. 1b). Thus, at least the data obtained in this study do not support the potential involvement of developmental state of intestinal basolateral domain in the regulation of GO toxicity.

In *C. elegans*, *pkc-3* encodes an atypical protein kinase C, which is required for the normal progression of embryogenesis and viability [45]. In this study, we further observed that intestine-specific RNAi knockdown of *pkc-3* enhanced the intestinal permeability (Fig. 3). Moreover, after GO exposure, intestine-specific RNAi knockdown of *pkc-3* resulted in the more severe enhancement of intestinal permeability compared with VP303 nematodes (Fig. 3). In *C. elegans*, PKC-3 is localized to the outer, apical surfaces of intestinal epithelia [75]. These results imply that the integrity of intestinal epithelia in apical domain of intestine is necessary for the maintenance of normal intestinal permeability in nematodes. Once the nematodes lack the normal

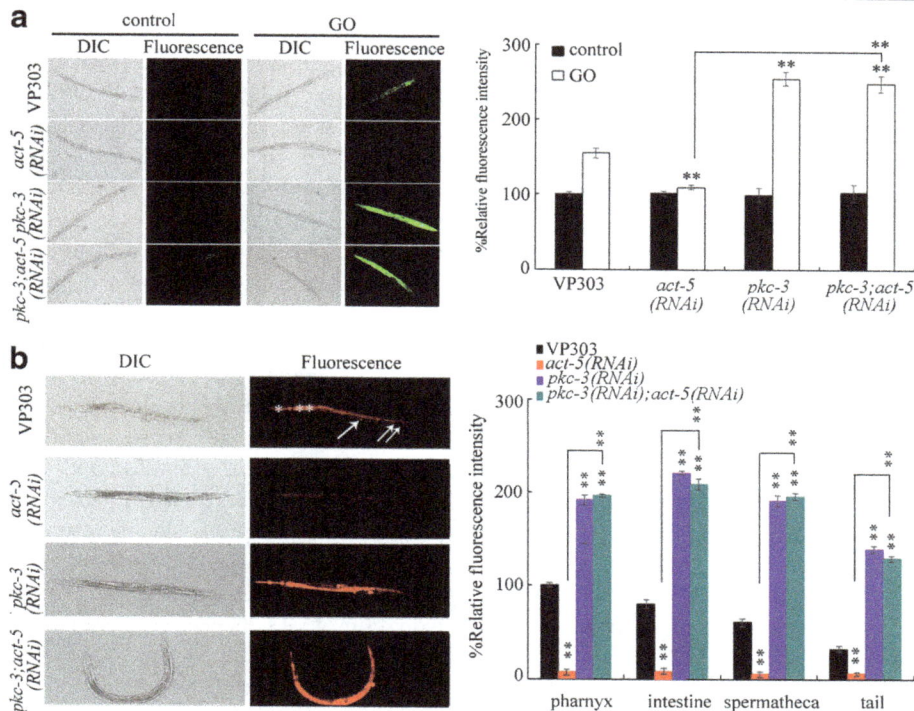

Fig. 8 Genetic interaction between ACT-5 and PKC-3 in the regulation of the toxicity in inducing ROS production (**a**) and the translocation (**b**) of GO in nematodes. Acute exposure was performed from L4-larvae for 24 h. GO or GO/Rho B exposure concentration was 10 mg/L. **P < 0.01 vs VP303 (if not specially indicated)

function of PKC-3, the development in the apical surfaces of intestinal epithelia may be disrupted, and the normal intestinal permeability may be difficult to be further maintained.

In this study, we provide several lines of evidence to prove the role of SEC-8 as the downstream target of PKC-3 in regulating toxicity and translocation of GO. Firstly, intestine-specific RNAi of pkc-3 altered the transcriptional expression of sec-8 (Fig. 4a). Secondly, intestine-specific RNAi of sec-8 resulted in the enhanced GO toxicity in inducing intestinal ROS production and GO accumulation in the body of nematodes (Fig. 4b and c). Thirdly, under the normal conditions, the nematodes with intestine-specific RNAi of sec-8 showed the increased intestinal permeability, which was similar to that observed in nematodes with intestine-specific RNAi of pkc-3 (Fig. 4d). Moreover, genetic interaction assay indicated that PKC-3 and SEC-8 acted in the same genetic pathway in the intestine to regulate the toxicity and the translocation of GO (Fig. 4e and f). In C. elegans, sec-8 encodes a subunit of exocyst complex, and may be involved in the endocytosis [76]. Therefore, our results imply that PKC-3 may regulate the intestinal permeability by affecting the function of SEC-8 in the regulation of the process of endocytosis, which in turn influences the response of nematodes to GO exposure.

Moreover, we provide several lines of evidence to further demonstrate the role of WTS-1 as the downstream of SEC-8 in the regulation of toxicity and translocation of GO. Intestine-specific RNAi of sec-8 decreased the transcriptional expression of wts-1 (Fig. 5a). Additionally, intestine-specific RNAi of wts-1 could also induce the enhanced GO toxicity in inducing intestinal ROS production and the more severe GO accumulation in the body of nematodes compared with those in VP303 nematodes (Fig. 5b and c). Moreover, nematodes with intestine-specific RNAi of wts-1 also exhibited the increased intestinal permeability, as observed in nematodes with intestine-specific RNAi of pkc-3 or sec-8 (Fig. 5d). Furthermore, SEC-8 and WTS-1 can act in the same genetic pathway in the intestine to regulate the toxicity and the translocation of GO (Fig. 5e and f). Therefore, in this study, we raise the intestinal signaling cascade of PKC-3-SEC-8-WTS-1 required for the maintenance of intestinal permeability and the regulation of toxicity and translocation of GO. In C. elegans, wts-1 is required for the integrity of the apical intestinal membrane by affecting localization of newly synthesized apical actins, and SEC-8-mediated exocyst complex is required for the mislocalization of apical actin in wts-1 mutant [65]. In this raised intestinal signaling cascade of PKC-3-SEC-8-WTS-1, PKC-3 may regulate the intestinal permeability and GO toxicity and translocation by affecting the function of SEC-8-mediated exocyst complex in controlling the role of WTS-1 in the maintenance of integrity of the apical intestinal membrane (Fig. 7b).

In this study, we further identified the ISP-1 and SOD-3 as the downstream targets for PKC-3 in the regulation of GO toxicity (Fig. 6). Moreover, we found that RNAi knockdown of both wts-1 and sod-3 led to a more severe GO toxicity in inducing intestinal ROS production than RNAi knockdown of wts-1 and sod-3 (Fig. 7a), suggesting a synergistic effect between WTS-1 and SOD-3 was formed in the regulation of GO toxicity (Fig. 7b). This observation further implies that, in nematodes with RNAi knockdown of pkc-3, the decrease in sod-3 could further enhance the susceptibility to GO toxicity caused by the expressional suppression of wts-1.

It is normally considered that the environmentally relevant concentrations of ENMs were in the range of ng/L or μg/L [77, 78]. In this study, we even found the significant induction of intestinal ROS production in nematodes with RNAi knockdown of both wts-1 and sod-3 after acute exposure to GO (100 μg/L) (Fig. 7a). Therefore, our results imply that acute exposure to GO in the range of μg/L may potentially cause the toxic effects on environmental organisms under certain genetic background(s).

Conclusions

In conclusion, we investigated the developmental basis for intestinal barrier against environmental GO toxicity using C. elegans as a model animal. Based on the genetic screen of genes required for intestinal development at different aspects, we identified four developmental genes (erm-1, pkc-3, hmp-2 and act-5) necessary for the function of intestinal barrier against GO toxicity. Erm-1, pkc-3, and act-5 are required for the connection between actin cytoskeleton and plasma membrane, apical-basal polarity, or microvilli development in apical domain of intestine, and hmp-2 is required for the tissue integrity of intestinal tube in the apical junctions. With the focus on the PKC-3, an atypical protein kinase C, we raised a signaling cascade of PKC-3-SEC-8-WTS-1 that is required for the regulation of both intestinal permeability and GO toxicity. ISP-1 and SOD-3, two proteins required for the control of oxidative stress, were further identified as downstream targets for PKC-3, and a synergistic effect between WTS-1 and SOD-3 was formed in the regulation of GO toxicity. Using the strain with RNAi knockdown of both wts-1 and sod-3 as a tool, we could detect the toxicity of GO in the range of μg/L after acute exposure. Our results will aid our understanding molecular mechanisms for the organization of intestinal barrier to defense the translocation and the toxicity of environmental ENMs in animals.

Methods
Preparation and characterization of GO

GO was prepared from natural graphite as described previously [79]. GO was finally obtained by ultrasonication of as-made graphite oxide in water for 1 h. GO was characterized by atomic force microscopy (AFM, SPM-9600, Shimadzu, Japan), Raman spectroscopy (Renishaw Invia Plus laser Raman spectrometer, Renishaw, UK), and X-ray photoelectron spectrum (XPS) (AXIS Ultra instrument, Kratos, UK) [34]. Based on the AFM assay, GO thickness was approximately 1.0 nm in topographic height, and sizes of most of the GO in K-medium after sonication (40 kHz, 100 W, 30 min) were mainly in the range of 40–60 nm [34]. Based on Raman spectroscopy measurement using a 632 nm wavelength excitation, a G band at 1573.7 cm^{-1} and a D band at 1350.2 cm^{-1} were detected in GO sheet [34]. Based on XPS assay, different oxygen functional groups exist in the GO structures (e.g. carbonyl, epoxy, hydroxyl groups), suggesting the considerable degree of oxidation of GO sheets [34].

C. elegans strains and culture

Nematode strains used in this study were wild-type N2 and transgenic strain of VP303/kbIs7[nhx-2p::rde-1], which were from Caenorhabditis Genetics Center. Nematodes were maintained on normal nematode growth medium (NGM) plates seeded with Escherichia coli OP50 as a food source at 20 °C [18]. Gravid hermaphrodite nematodes were collected and lysed with a bleaching mixture (0.45 M NaOH, 2% HOCl) in order to separate the eggs from the worms. The collected eggs were used to prepare the age synchronous L2-larvae populations.

Exposure and toxicity assessment

The stock solution of GO (1 mg/mL) was prepared in K medium by sonication for 30 min (40 kHz, 100 W). In this study, 0.1, 1, 10 mg/L were selected as the working concentrations for GO exposure. GO at the working concentrations were prepared by diluting the stock solution with K medium. Acute exposure (from L4-larvae for 24 h) to GO was performed in the liquid at 20 °C in the presence of food (OP50).

The endpoint of intestinal ROS production was used to reflect the functional state of the primary targeted organ of intestine [80]. ROS production was analyzed as described previously [81, 82]. After GO exposure, the examined nematodes were transferred to 1 μM 5′,6′-chloromethyl-2′,7′-dichlorodihydro-fluorescein diacetate (CM-H$_2$DCFDA; Molecular Probes) solution to incubate for 3 h in the dark. After labeling, the nematodes were mounted on a 2% agar pad and examined at 488 nm of excitation wavelength and at 510 nm of emission filter under a laser scanning confocal microscope

(Leica, TCS SP2, Bensheim, Germany). Relative fluorescence intensity of ROS signals in the intestine was semi-quantified, and expressed as the relative fluorescence units (RFU). Fifty nematodes were examined per treatment.

Distribution and translocation of GO in the body of nematodes

To investigate the translocation and distribution of GO in nematodes, Rho B was loaded on GO by mixing Rho B solution (1 mg/mL, 0.3 mL) with an aqueous suspension of GO (0.1 mg/mL, 5 mL) as previously described [72]. Unbound Rho B was removed by dialysis against distilled water over 72 h. The examined nematodes were incubated with GO/Rho B from L4-larvae for 24 h. After washing with M9 buffer for three times, the nematodes were observed under a laser scanning confocal microscope (Leica, TCS SP2, Bensheim, Germany). The UV/Vis spectral measurements were taken on a Perkin Elmer Lambda 25 spectrophotometer to examine the binding property of Rho B with GO.

Reverse-transcription and quantitative real-time polymerase chain reaction (qRT-PCR) assay

Total RNAs of nematodes were extracted using RNeasy Mini kit (Qiagen). The prepared total RNAs were reverse transcribed using PrimeScript ™ RT reagent kit (Takara, Otsu, Shiga, Japan). After cDNA synthesis, real-time PCR was performed using SYBR Premix Ex Taq™ (Takara) for the aim of amplification of PCR products. Real-time PCR was run at the optimized annealing temperature of 58 °C. Relative quantification of targeted genes in comparison to a reference *tba-1* gene encoding a tubulin protein was determined. The final results were expressed as relative expression ratio between targeted gene and reference gene. All reactions were performed in triplicate. The related primer information for qRT-PCR is shown in Additional file 1: Table S2.

RNAi assay

RNAi was performed by feeding nematodes with *E. coli* strain HT115 (DE3) expressing double-stranded RNA that is homologous to a target gene as described [83]. *E. coli* HT115 (DE3) grown in LB broth containing ampicillin (100 μg/mL) at 37 °C overnight was plated onto NGM containing ampicillin (100 μg/mL) and isopropyl 1-thio-β-D-galactopyranoside (IPTG, 5 mM). L2-larvae were placed on RNAi plates for 2 days at 20 °C until the nematodes became L4-larvae. The RNAi efficiency was confirmed by qRT-PCR (Additional file 1: Figure S1). The obtained L4-larvae with RNAi knockdown of certain gene were used for the further exposure to GO.

Nile red staining

Nile Red staining method was performed as described previously [35]. Nile Red (Molecular Probes, Eugene, OR) was dissolved in acetone to prepare a stock solution (0.5 mg/mL), and stored at 4 °C. The stock solution was freshly diluted in 1 x PBS buffer to obtain the working solution (1 mg/mL) for the Nile Red staining. Fifty nematodes were examined per treatment.

Sudan black staining

Sudan Black staining method was performed as described previously [58]. The examined nematodes were washed in M9 buffer and fixed with 1% paraformaldehyde. The nematodes were subjected to 3 freeze–thaw cycles and dehydrated through an ethanol series. The nematodes were then stained overnight in a 50% saturated solution of Sudan Black in 70% ethanol, rehydrated, and photographed. Fifty nematodes were examined per treatment.

Statistical analysis

Data in this article were expressed as means ± standard deviation (SD). Statistical analysis was performed using SPSS 12.0 software (SPSS Inc., Chicago, USA). Differences between groups were determined using analysis of variance (ANOVA), and probability level of 0.01 was considered statistically significant. Graphs were generated using Microsoft Excel software (Microsoft Corp., Redmond, WA).

Additional file

Additional file 1: Figure S1. Efficiency of RNAi of examined genes based on qRT-PCR assay. L4440, empty vector. Bars represent means ± SD. $^{**}P$ < 0.01 vs L4440. Figure S2. Comparison of intestinal ROS production in GO (10 mg/L) and paraquat (2 mM) exposed VP303 nematodes. Acute exposure was performed from L4-larvae for 24 h. Bars represent means ± SD. $^{**}P$ < 0.01 vs control. Figure S3. UV/Vis spectral analysis of GO/Rho B, GO, and Rho B. Figure S4. Effects of intestine-specific RNAi knockdown of *sec-8* on fat storage labeled by Sudan Black. Figure S5. Effects of intestine-specific RNAi knockdown of *wts-1* on fat storage labeled by Sudan Black. Table S1. Primers used for RNAi of certain genes. Table S2. Primer information for qRT-PCR. (DOC 1557 kb)

Funding

This work was supported by the grant from Bilateral Projects 2016 China-Bulgaria (no. 15-4).

Authors' contributions

DW conceived and designed the experiments. MR, LZ, XD, NK, and QR performed the experiments, and analyzed the data. DW wrote the paper. All authors read and approved the final manuscript.

Competing interests

The authors declare that they have no competing interests.

Author details

[1]Key Laboratory of Environmental Medicine Engineering in Ministry of Education, Medical School, Southeast University, Nanjing 210009, China. [2]College of Life Sciences, Nanjing Agricultural University, Nanjing 210095, China. [3]Institute of Biophysics and Biomedical Engineering, Bulgarian Academy of Science, 1113 Sofia, Bulgaria.

References

1. Geim AK. Graphene: status and prospects. Science. 2009;2009(324):1530–4.
2. Geim AK, Novoselov KS. The rise of graphene. Nat Mater. 2007;6:183–91.
3. Bitounis D, Ali-Boucetta H, Hong BH, Min D, Kostarelos K. Prospects and challenges of graphene in biomedical applications. Adv Mater. 2013;25: 2258–68.
4. Zhu X, Shan Y, Xiong S, Shen J, Wu X. Brianyoungite/graphene oxide coordination composites for high-performance Cu^{2+} adsorption and tunable deep-red photoluminescence. ACS Appl Mater Interfaces. 2016;8: 15848–54.
5. Cheng C, Wang D. Hydrogel-assisted transfer of graphene oxides into nonpolar organic media for oil decontamination. Angew Chem Int Ed. 2016; 55:6853–37.
6. Chang Y, Yang S, Liu J, Dong E, Wang Y, Cao A, Liu Y, Wang H. In vitro toxicity evaluation of graphene oxide on A549 cells. Toxicol Lett. 2011;200: 201–10.
7. Li Y-P, Wu Q-L, Zhao Y-L, Bai Y-F, Chen P-S, Xia T, Wang D-Y. Response of microRNAs to in vitro treatment with graphene oxide. ACS Nano. 2014;8: 2100–10.
8. Liao K, Lin Y, Macosko CW, Haynes CL. Cytotoxicity of graphene oxide and graphene in human erythrocytes and skin fibroblasts. ACS Appl Mater Interfaces. 2011;3:2607–15.
9. Liu Y, Wang X, Wang J, Nie Y, Du H, Dai H, Wang J, Wang M, Chen S, Hei TK, Deng Z, Wu L, Xu A. Graphene oxide attenuates the cytotoxicity and mutagenicity of PCB 52 via activation of genuine autophagy. Environ Sci Technol. 2016;50:3154–64.
10. Qu G, Zhang S, Wang L, Wang X, Sun B, Yin N, Gao X, Xia T, Chen J, Jiang G. Graphen oxide induces toll-like receptor 4 (TLR4)-dependent necrosis in macrophages. ACS Nano. 2013;7:5732–45.
11. Li B, Yang J, Huang Q, Zhang Y, Peng C, Zhang Y, He Y, Shi J, Li W, Hu J, Fan C. Biodistribution and pulmonary toxicity of intratracheally instilled graphene oxide in mice. NPG Asia Mater. 2013;5:e44.
12. Liang S, Xu S, Zhang D, He J, Chu M. Reproductive toxicity of nanosclae graphene oxide in male mice. Biomaterials. 2015;9:92–105.
13. Yang K, Li Y, Tan X, Peng R, Liu Z. Behavior and toxicity of graphene and its functionalized derivatives in biological systems. Small. 2013;9:1492–503.
14. Leung MC, Williams PL, Benedetto A, Au C, Helmcke KJ, Aschner M, Meyer JN. Caenorhabditis elegans: an emerging model in biomedical and environmental toxicology. Toxicol Sci. 2008;106:5–28.
15. Yu X-M, Guan X-M, Wu Q-L, Zhao Y-L, Wang D-Y. Vitamin E ameliorates the neurodegeneration related phenotypes caused by neurotoxicity of Al_2O_3-nanoparticles in C. elegans. Toxicol Res. 2015;4:1269–81.
16. Wu Q-L, Zhi L-T, Qu Y-Y, Wang D-Y. Quantum dots increased fat storage in intestine of Caenorhabditis elegans by influencing molecular basis for fatty acid metabolism. Nanomedicine. 2016;12:1175–84.
17. Zhao L, Wan H-X, Liu Q-Z, Wang D-Y. Multi-walled carbon nanotubes-induced alterations in microRNA let-7 and its targets activate a protection mechanism by conferring a developmental timing control. Part Fibre Toxicol. 2017;14:27.
18. Brenner S. The genetics of Caenorhabditis elegans. Genetics. 1974;77:71–94.
19. Zhao Y-L, Wu Q-L, Li Y-P, Wang D-Y. Translocation, transfer, and in vivo safety evaluation of engineered nanomaterials in the non-mammalian alternative toxicity assay model of nematode Caenorhabditis elegans. RSC Adv. 2013;3:5741–57.
20. Wang D-Y. Biological effects, translocation, and metabolism of quantum dots in nematode Caenorhabditis elegans. Toxicol Res. 2016;5:1003 11.
21. Mohan N, Chen C, Hsieh H, Wu Y, Chang H. In vivo imaging and toxicity assessments of fluorescent nanodiamonds in Caenorhabditis elegans. Nano Lett. 2010;10:3692–9.
22. Zhang W, Wang C, Li Z, Lu Z, Li Y, Yin J, Zhou Y, Gao X, Fang Y, Nie G, Zhao Y. Unraveling stress-induced toxicity properties of graphene oxide and the underlying mechanism. Adv Mater. 2012;24:5391–7.
23. Zanni Z, De Bellis G, Bracciale MP, Broggi A, Santarelli ML, Sarto MS, Palleschi C, Uccelletti D. Graphite nanoplatelets and Caenorhabditis elegans: insights from an in vivo model. Nano Lett. 2012;12:2740–4.
24. Chen P, Hsiao K, Chou C. Molecular characterization of toxicity mechanism of single-walled carbon nanotubes. Biomaterials. 2013;34:5661–9.
25. Yang J-N, Zhao Y-L, Wang Y-W, Wang H-F, Wang D-Y. Toxicity evaluation and translocation of carboxyl functionalized graphene in Caenorhabditis elegans. Toxicol Res. 2015;4:1498–510.
26. Shakoor S, Sun L-M, Wang D-Y. Multi-walled carbon nanotubes enhanced fungal colonization and suppressed innate immune response to fungal infection in nematodes. Toxicol Res. 2016;5:492–9.
27. Zhao Y-L, Yang J-N, Wang D-Y. A microRNA-mediated insulin signaling pathway regulates the toxicity of multi-walled carbon nanotubes in nematode Caenorhabditis elegans. Sci Rep. 2016;6:23234.
28. Wu Q-L, Yin L, Li X, Tang M, Zhang T, Wang D-Y. Contributions of altered permeability of intestinal barrier and defecation behavior to toxicity formation from graphene oxide in nematode Caenorhabditis elegans. Nanoscale. 2013;5:9934–43.
29. Qu M, Li Y-H, Wu Q-L, Xia Y-K, Wang D-Y. Neuronal ERK signaling in response to graphene oxide in nematode Caenorhabditis elegans. Nanotoxicology. 2017;11:520–33.
30. Xiao G-S, Zhi L-T, Ding X-C, Rui Q, Wang D-Y. Value of mir-247 in warning graphene oxide toxicity in nematode Caenorhabditis elegans. RSC Adv. 2017; 7:52694–701.
31. Zhao Y-L, Jia R-H, Qiao Y, Wang D-Y. Glycyrrhizic acid, active component from Glycyrrhizae radix, prevents toxicity of graphene oxide by influencing functions of microRNAs in nematode Caenorhabditis elegans. Nanomedicine. 2016;12:735–44.
32. Chatterjee N, Kim Y, Yang J, Roca CP, Joo SW, Choi J. A systems toxicology approach reveals the Wnt-MAPK crosstalk pathway mediated reproductive failure in Caenorhabditis elegans exposed to graphene oxide (GO) but not to reduced graphene oxide (rGO). Nanotoxicology. 2017;11:76–86.
33. Chen H, Li H-R, Wang D-Y. Graphene oxide dysregulates Neuroligin/NLG-1-mediated molecular signaling in interneurons in Caenorhabditis elegans. Sci Rep. 2017;7:41655.
34. Wu Q-L, Zhou X-F, Han X-X, Zhuo Y-Z, Zhu S-T, Zhao Y-L, Wang D-Y. Genome-wide identification and functional analysis of long noncoding RNAs involved in the response to graphene oxide. Biomaterials. 2016;102: 277–91.
35. Zhi L-T, Ren M-X, Qu M, Zhang H-Y, Wang D-Y. Wnt ligands differentially regulate toxicity and translocation of graphene oxide through different mechanisms in Caenorhabditis elegans. Sci Rep. 2016;6:39261.
36. Liu Z-F, Zhou X-F, Wu Q-L, Zhao Y-L, Wang D-Y. Crucial role of intestinal barrier in the formation of transgenerational toxicity in quantum dots exposed nematodes Caenorhabditis elegans. RSC Adv. 2015;5:94257–66.
37. Zhao Y-L, Yang R-L, Rui Q, Wang D-Y. Intestinal insulin signaling encodes two different molecular mechanisms for the shortened longevity induced by graphene oxide in Caenorhabditis elegans. Sci Rep. 2016;6:24024.
38. Zhi L-T, Fu W, Wang X, Wang D-Y. ACS-22, a protein homologous to mammalian fatty acid transport protein 4, is essential for the control of toxicity and translocation of multi-walled carbon nanotubes in Caenorhabditis elegans. RSC Adv. 2016;6:4151–9.
39. McGhee JD. The C. elegans intestine. WormBook. 2007; https://doi.org/10. 1895/wormbook.1.133.1.
40. Miyadera H, Amino H, Hiraishi A, Taka H, Murayama K, Miyoshi H, Sakamoto K, Ishii N, Hekimi S, Kita K. Altered quinone biosynthesis in the long-lived clk-1 mutants of Caenorhabditis elegans. J Biol Chem. 2001;276:7713–6.
41. Carberry K, Wiesenfahrt T, Geisler F, Stocker S, Gerhardus H, Uberbach D, Davis W, Jorgensen E, Leube RE, Bossinger O. The novel intestinal filament organizer IFO-1 contributes to epithelial integrity in concert with ERM-1 and DLG-1. Development. 2012;139:1851–62.
42. Gobel V, Barrett PL, Hall DH, Fleming JT. Lumen morphogenesis in C. elegans requires the membrane-cytoskeleton linker erm-1. Dev Cell. 2004;6: 865–73.

43. Croce A, Cassata G, Disanza A, Gagliani MC, Tacchetti C, Malabarba MG, Carlier MF, Scita G, Baumeister R, Di Fiore PP. A novel actin barbed-end-capping activity in EPS-8 regulates apical morphogenesis in intestinal cells of *Caenorhabditis elegans*. Nat Cell Biol. 2004;6:1173–9.

44. Nance J, Priess JR. Cell polarity and gastrulation in *C. elegans*. Development. 2002;129:387–97.

45. Wu SL, Staudinger J, Olson EN, Rubin CS. Structure, expression, and properties of an atypical protein kinase C (PKC3) from *Caenorhabditis elegans*. PKC3 is required for the normal progression of embryogenesis and viability of the organism. J Biol Chem. 1998;273:1130–43.

46. Church DL, Lambie EJ. The promotion of gonadal cell divisions by the *Caenorhabditis elegans* TRPM cation channel GON-2 is antagonized by GEM-4 copine. Genetics. 2003;165:563–74.

47. Xue Y, Fares H, Grant B, Li Z, Rose AM, Clark SG, Skolnik E. Genetic analysis of the myotubularin family of phosphatases in *Caenorhabditis elegans*. J Biol Chem. 2003;278:34380–6.

48. Labrousse AM, Shurland DL, van der Bliek AM. Contribution of the GTPase domain to the subcellular localization of dynamin in the nematode *Caenorhabditis elegans*. Mol Biol Cell. 1998;9:3227–39.

49. Legouis R, Gansmuller A, Sookhareea S, Bosher JM, Baillie DL, Labouesse M. LET-413 is a basolateral protein required for the assembly of adherens junctions in *Caenorhabditis elegans*. Nat Cell Biol. 2000;2:415–22.

50. Culetto E, Sattelle DB. A role for *Caenorhabditis elegans* in understanding the function and interactions of human disease genes. Hum Mol Genet. 2000;9:869–977.

51. Altun ZF, Chen B, Wang ZW, Hall DH. High resolution map of *Caenorhabditis elegans* gap junction proteins. Dev Dyn. 2009;238:1936–50.

52. Saifee O, Wei LP, Nonet ML. The *Caenorhabditis elegans* unc-64 locus encodes a syntaxin that interacts genetically with synaptobrevin. Mol Biol Cell. 1998;9:1235–52.

53. Segbert C, Johnson K, Theres C, van Furden D, Bossinger O. Molecular and functional analysis of apical junction formation in the gut epithelium of *Caenorhabditis elegans*. Dev Biol. 2004;266:17–26.

54. Koppen M, Simske JS, Sims PA, Firestein BL, Hall DH, Radice AD, Rongo C, Hardin JD. Cooperative regulation of AJM-1 controls junctional integrity in *Caenorhabditis elegans* epithelia. Nat Cell Biol. 2001;3:983–91.

55. Lackner MR, Nurrish SJ, Kaplan JM. Facilitation of synaptic transmission by EGL-30 Gqα and EGL-8 PLCβ: DAG binding to UNC-13 is required to stimulate acetylcholine release. Neuron. 1999;24:335–46.

56. Feng W, Long JF, Fan JS, Suetake T, Zhang M. The tetrameric L27 domain complex as an organization platform for supramolecular assemblies. Nat Struct Mol Biol. 2004;11:475–80.

57. Espelt MV, Estevez AY, Yin X, Strange K. Oscillatory Ca^{2+} signaling in the isolated *Caenorhabditis elegans* intestine: role of the inositol-1,4,5-trisphosphate receptor and phospholipases C β and γ. J Gen Physiol. 2005; 126:379–92.

58. Wu Q-L, Rui Q, He K-W, Shen L-L, Wang D-Y. UNC-64 and RIC-4, the plasma membrane associated SNAREs syntaxin and SNAP-25, regulate fat storage in nematode *Caenorhabditis elegans*. Neurosci Bull. 2010;26:104–16.

59. Tabuse Y, Izumi Y, Piano F, Kemphues KJ, Miwa J, Ohno S. Atypical protein kinase C cooperates with PAR-3 to establish embryonic polarity in *Caenorhabditis elegans*. Development. 1998;125:3607–14.

60. Lee I, Lehner B, Crombie C, Wong W, Fraser AG, Marcotte EM. A single gene network accurately predicts phenotypic effects of gene perturbation in *Caenorhabditis elegans*. Nat Genet. 2008;40:181–8.

61. Ziegler K, Kurz CL, Cypowyj S, Couillault C, Pophillat M, Pujol N, Ewbank JJ. Antifungal innate immunity in *C. elegans*: PKCdelta links G protein signaling and a conserved p38 MAPK cascade. Cell Host Microbe. 2009;5:341–52.

62. Beatty A, Morton D, Kemphues K. The *C. elegans* homolog of Drosophila lethal giant larvae functions redundantly with PAR-2 to maintain polarity in the early embryo. Development. 2010;137:3995–4004.

63. Galli M, Munoz J, Portegijs V, Boxem M, Grill SW, Heck AJ, van den Heuvel S. aPKC phosphorylates NuMA-related LIN-5 to position the mitotic spindle during asymmetric division. Nat Cell Biol. 2011;13:1132–8.

64. Armenti ST, Chan E, Nance J. Polarized exocyst-mediated vesicle fusion directs intracellular lumenogenesis within the *C. elegans* excretory cell. Dev Biol. 2014;394:110–21.

65. Kang J, Shin D, Yu JR, Lee J. Lats kinase is involved in the intestinal apical membrane integrity in the nematode *Caenorhabditis elegans*. Development. 2009;136:2705–015.

66. Ishii N, Fujii M, Hartman PS, Tsuda M, Yasuda K, Senoo-Matsuda N, Yanase S, Ayusawa D, Suzuki K. A mutation in succinate dehydrogenase cytochrome b causes oxidative stress and ageing in nematodes. Nature. 1998;394:694–7.

67. Kayser EB, Morgan PG, Hoppel CL, Sedensky MM. Mitochondrial expression and function of GAS-1 in *Caenorhabditis elegans*. J Biol Chem. 2001;276: 20551–8.

68. Feng J, Bussiere F, Hekimi S. Mitochondrial electron transport is a key determinant of life span in *Caenorhabditis elegans*. Dev Cell. 2001;1:633–44.

69. Miyadera H, Amino H, Hiraishi A, Taka H, Murayama K, Miyoshi H, Sakamoto K, Ishii N, Hekimi S, Kita K. Altered quinone biosynthesis in the long-lived *clk-1* mutant of *Caenorhabditis elegans*. J Biol Chem. 2001;276:7713–6.

70. Yanase S, Onodera A, Tedesco P, Johnson TE, Ishii N. SOD-1 deletions in *Caenorhabditis elegans* alter the localization of intracellular reactive oxygen species and show molecular compensation. J Gerontol A Biol Sci Med Sci. 2009;64:530–9.

71. Yanase S, Yasuda K, Ishii N. Adaptive responses to oxidative damage in three mutants of *Caenorhabditis elegans* (age-1, mev-1 and daf-16) that affect life span. Mech Ageing Dev. 2002;123:1579–87.

72. Zhao Y-L, Zhi L-T, Wu Q-L, Yu Y-L, Sun Q-Q, Wang D-Y. p38 MAPK-SKN-1/Nrf signaling cascade is required for intestinal barrier against graphene oxide toxicity in *Caenorhabditis elegans*. Nanotoxicology. 2016;10:1469–79.

73. MacQueen AJ, Baggett JJ, Perumov N, Bauer RA, Januszewski T, Schriefer L, Waddle JA. ACT-5 is an essential *Caenorhabditis elegans* actin required for intestinal microvilli formation. Mol Biol Cell. 2005;16:3247–59.

74. Szumowski SC, Estes KA, Popovich JJ, Botts MR, Sek G, Troemel ER. Small GTPases promote actin coat formation on microsporidian pathogens traversing the apical membrane of *Caenorhabditis elegans* intestinal cells. Cell Microbiol. 2016;18:30–45.

75. Izumi Y, Hirose T, Tamai Y, Hirai S, Nagashima Y, Fujimoto T, Tabuse Y, Kemphues KJ, Ohno S. An atypical PKC directly associates and colocalizes at the epithelial tight junction with ASIP, a mammalian homologue of *Caenorhabditis elegans* polarity protein PAR-3. J Cell Biol. 1998;143:95–106.

76. Fares H, Greenwald I. Genetic analysis of endocytosis in *Caenorhabditis elegans*: coelomocyte uptake defective mutants. Genetics. 2001;159:133–45.

77. Gottschalk F, Sonderer T, Scholz RW, Nowack B. Modeled environmental concentrations of engineered nanomaterials (TiO_2, ZnO, ag, CNT, fullerenes) for different regions. Environ Sci Technol. 2009;43:9216–22.

78. Mueller N, Nowack B. Exposure modeling of engineered nanoparticles in the environment. Environ Sci Technol. 2008;42:4447–53.

79. Kovtyukhova NI, Olivier PJ, Martin BR, Mallouk TE, Chizhik SA, Buzaneva EV, Gorchinskiy AD. Layer-by-layer assembly of ultrathin composite films from micron-sized graphite oxide sheets and polycations. Chem Mater. 1999;11:771–8.

80. Ren M-X, Zhao L, Lv X, Wang D-Y. Antimicrobial proteins in the response to graphene oxide in *Caenorhabditis elegans*. Nanotoxicology. 2017;11:578–90.

81. Ding X-C, Wang J, Rui Q, Wang D-Y. Long-term exposure to thiolated graphene oxide in the range of μg/L induces toxicity in nematode *Caenorhabditis elegans*. Sci Total Environ. 2018;616-617:29–37.

82. Zhi L-T, Qu M, Ren M-X, Zhao L, Li Y-H, Wang D-Y. Graphene oxide induces canonical Wnt/β-catenin signaling-dependent toxicity in *Caenorhabditis elegans*. Carbon. 2017;113:122–31.

83. Kamath RK, Martinez-Campos M, Zipperlen P, Fraser AG, Ahringer J. Effectiveness of specific RNA-mediated interference through ingested double stranded RNA in *C. elegans*. Genome Biol. 2001;2:1–10.

Group II innate lymphoid cells and microvascular dysfunction from pulmonary titanium dioxide nanoparticle exposure

Alaeddin Bashir Abukabda[1,2], Carroll Rolland McBride[1,2], Thomas Paul Batchelor[1,2], William Travis Goldsmith[1,2], Elizabeth Compton Bowdridge[1,2], Krista Lee Garner[1,2], Sherri Friend[3] and Timothy Robert Nurkiewicz[1,2,3*]

Abstract

Background: The cardiovascular effects of pulmonary exposure to engineered nanomaterials (ENM) are poorly understood, and the reproductive consequences are even less understood. Inflammation remains the most frequently explored mechanism of ENM toxicity. However, the key mediators and steps between lung exposure and uterine health remain to be fully defined. The purpose of this study was to determine the uterine inflammatory and vascular effects of pulmonary exposure to titanium dioxide nanoparticles (nano-TiO_2). We hypothesized that pulmonary nano-TiO_2 exposure initiates a Th2 inflammatory response mediated by Group II innate lymphoid cells (ILC2), which may be associated with an impairment in uterine microvascular reactivity.

Methods: Female, virgin, Sprague-Dawley rats (8–12 weeks) were exposed to 100 μg of nano-TiO_2 via intratracheal instillation 24 h prior to microvascular assessments. Serial blood samples were obtained at 0, 1, 2 and 4 h post-exposure for multiplex cytokine analysis. ILC2 numbers in the lungs were determined. ILC2s were isolated and phosphorylated nuclear factor kappa-light-chain-enhancer of activated B cells (NF-κB) levels were measured. Pressure myography was used to assess vascular reactivity of isolated radial arterioles.

Results: Pulmonary nano-TiO_2 exposure was associated with an increase in IL-1ß, 4, 5 and 13 and TNF- α 4 h post-exposure, indicative of an innate Th2 inflammatory response. ILC2 numbers were significantly increased in lungs from exposed animals (1.66 ± 0.19%) compared to controls (0.19 ± 0.22%). Phosphorylation of the transactivation domain (Ser-468) of NF-κB in isolated ILC2 and IL-33 in lung epithelial cells were significantly increased (126.8 ± 4.3% and 137 ± 11% of controls respectively) by nano-TiO_2 exposure. Lastly, radial endothelium-dependent arteriolar reactivity was significantly impaired (27 ± 12%), while endothelium-independent dilation (7 ± 14%) and α-adrenergic sensitivity (8 ± 2%) were not altered compared to control levels. Treatment with an anti- IL-33 antibody (1 mg/kg) 30 min prior to nano-TiO_2 exposure resulted in a significant improvement in endothelium-dependent dilation and a decreased level of IL-33 in both plasma and bronchoalveolar lavage fluid.

Conclusions: These results provide evidence that the uterine microvascular dysfunction that follows pulmonary ENM exposure may be initiated via activation of lung-resident ILC2 and subsequent systemic Th2-dependent inflammation.

Keywords: Engineered nanomaterials, Titanium dioxide nanoparticles, Microcirculation, Innate lymphoid cells, Inflammation

* Correspondence: tnurkiewicz@hsc.wvu.edu
[1]Department of Physiology and Pharmacology, West Virginia University School of Medicine, 64 Medical Center Drive, Robert C. Byrd Health Sciences Center - West Virginia University, Morgantown, WV 26505-9229, USA
[2]Toxicology Working Group, West Virginia University School of Medicine, Morgantown, WV, USA
Full list of author information is available at the end of the article

Introduction

Reproductive toxicity is increasingly becoming recognized as a critical aspect of ENM safety. However, the effects of ENM exposure on overall reproductive health have only recently been addressed and become a focus of intense study by numerous groups [1, 2]. As with other observations of systemic biologic effects after pulmonary ENM exposures, reproductive effects are equally susceptible but poorly understood. Our group has previously reported that nano-TiO_2 inhalation is associated with uterine microvascular dysfunction [3], potentially deleterious epigenomic alterations [4], and cognitive deficits in maternally exposed progeny [5]. While these studies highlight the importance of identifying the maternal effects of ENM exposure, the mechanisms linking such exposures to these negative reproductive and developmental outcomes have yet to be fully elucidated.

In the last decade, innate lymphoid cells (ILC) have emerged as a novel population of tissue-specific effector cells with the ability to initiate and regulate the innate and adaptive branches of the immune system [6, 7]. ILCs are now divided into 3 distinct groups according to the pattern of cytokine secretion; Group 1 ILC (ILC1) are predominantly tissue-resident cells capable of secreting interferon gamma (IFN- γ) in the liver, gut, spleen, skin, peritoneum, and salivary gland [8]. The role played by ILC1 in various immunological conditions remains unclear but is currently under investigation. Group 2 ILCs (ILC2, also known as nuocytes, natural helper cells) secrete IL-4, IL-5, IL-9, and IL-13 in response to damage-associated molecular patterns or "alarmins" and have been implicated in the immune response to parasitic infections and in allergic airway inflammation [9] to several environmental and anthropogenic agents [10, 11]. Lastly, group 3 ILCs (ILC3) produce IL-22 and or IL-17, are enriched at mucosal sites, contribute to the maintenance of the intestinal barriers, and may play a significant role in the promotion of the inflammatory response and etiology of inflammatory bowel diseases [12, 13]. One of the most important alarm signals secreted by cells is interleukin-33 (IL-33) [14]. IL-33 is a member of the IL-1 family of cytokines expressed by both non-immune cells such as epithelial, endothelial, smooth muscle cells, and fibroblasts [15], as well as immune effector cells including macrophages and dendritic cells. Its role in directing the inflammatory response following pulmonary exposure to carbon nanotubes [16–18], and ozone [19] have been previously reported. IL-33 has been demonstrated [20] to induce the release of Th2 cytokines by immune cells including ILC2s in asthmatic patients [21], and to induce airway hyperresponsiveness and increased pulmonary resistance [22, 23].

In view of the increasing number of studies indicating a crucial role for ILCs in the initiation of the acute inflammatory response to environmental agents, the goal of this work was to provide initial evidence of their potential involvement in the response to pulmonary ENM exposure. Therefore, the purpose of this study was threefold. First, we identified the inflammatory and uterine microvascular effects associated with acute pulmonary nano-TiO_2 exposure. Second, we determined the possible role played by ILC in the immune response mounted to acute pulmonary nano-TiO_2 exposure. Lastly, the microvascular and systemic effects of treatment with an IL-33 antibody (a key activator of ILC2) were determined. We hypothesized that pulmonary nano-TiO_2 exposure initiates a Th2 inflammatory response mediated involving IL-33 and potentially involving ILC2, which may be associated with a systemic impairment in uterine microvascular reactivity.

Results

SEM images and mass spectrometry of Nano-TiO_2

Figure 1 shows field-emission scanning electron microscope images (Hitachi S4800, Tokyo, Japan) of the nano-TiO_2 suspension used for this study. As seen in Fig. 1a, the suspended particles present significant agglomeration. Figure 1b shows the elemental composition of the nano-TiO_2 suspension (Bruker, Billerica, MA), indicating the prevalent presence of titanium.

Animal and vessel characteristics

No significant changes were observed in age, mean arterial pressure (MAP), heart rate and body weight between control and exposure groups (Table 1). Additionally, radial arteriolar inner and outer diameter, tone, passive diameter, wall thickness, wall to lumen ratio and calculated wall tension were not affected by nano-TiO_2 exposure and treatment with an anti-IL-33 antibody (Table 2). From these results we can infer that acute nano-TiO_2 exposure does not alter vascular tone or the balance of its contributing influences.

Acute plasma and BALF cytokine secretion patterns following pulmonary Nano-TiO_2 exposure

A time-course study was initially performed to identify the temporal effect of nano-TiO_2 on cytokine secretion. Plasma samples were obtained at 0,1,2, and 4 h following nano-TiO_2 exposure by tail vein puncture. Figure 2 shows the results of the multiplex analysis. No differences existed at time 0, 1 or 2 h post-exposure. However, significant differences were detected 4 h post-exposure in plasma levels of the pro-inflammatory cytokines IL-4, IL-5, IL-13, TNF-α, IL-1β, while no alterations in the cytokines IFN-γ, KC/GRO, TNF-α, IL-10, IL-6, MCP-1, TIMP-1, Lipocalin-2, and TSP-1 were noted (*Data not shown*).

In order to confirm the results observed in the plasma, the cytokine levels in the BALF were also measured 4 h post-exposure. Multiplex analysis of the BALF (Fig. 3)

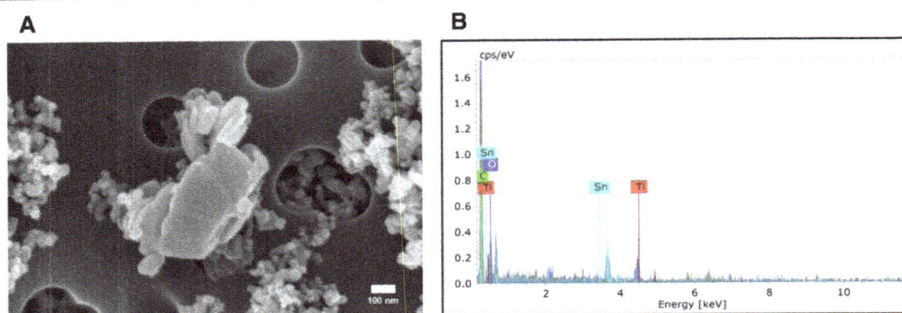

Fig. 1 Characterization of Nano-TiO₂. (**a**) SEM image and (**b**) Energy dispersive spectroscopy showing elemental composition of the nano-TiO₂ suspension used in this study

also showed an almost 5-fold increase in IL-5 and a 6-fold increase in IL-4, IL-13, TNF-α, and IL-1β, while no changes were seen in the other cytokines *(Data not shown)*. Based on the collective cytokine profile associated with this exposure paradigm, the results provide evidence that acute pulmonary nano-TiO₂ exposure may trigger a T-Helper cell type 2 (Th2) response beginning 4 h post-exposure.

IL-33 secretion by lung epithelial cells pre- and post- exposure and following treatment with an anti-IL-33 antibody

IL-33 plays a significant role in initiating and modulating lung inflammatory and immunological responses [24], by inducing the secretion of Th2 pro-inflammatory cytokines. It is constitutively present in mucosal epithelial cells and acts as a "danger" signal after tissue injury by activating immune cells. To determine the effect of nano-TiO₂ on pulmonary and plasma IL-33 levels, immunohistochemistry of tracheal sections was conducted 4 h post-exposure. In a separate cohort of control and exposed animals, multiplex analysis of plasma and BALF IL-33 was also performed 4 h post-exposure. Figure 4 shows representative images of lung sections from control and exposed rats stained for IL-33 4 h post-exposure and the quantitative measurements for both groups. Relative fluorescence intensity of IL-33 was significantly increased in exposed animals by $26.8 \pm 4.3\%$, while plasma and BALF levels indicated a $37.87 \pm 2.3\%$ and $171.26 \pm 13\%$ increase in IL-33 respectively (Fig. 5). Interestingly, treatment 1 h prior to exposure to nano-TiO₂ with pharmacological grade polyclonal anti-IL-33 antibody (EMD Millipore, Temecula, CA: intraperitoneal 1 mg/kg) resulted in a decrease in plasma and BALF IL-33 levels 4 h

post-exposure ($61.1 \pm 2.1\%$ in plasma and $149.7 \pm 7\%$ in BALF) when compared to nano-TiO₂ exposed and untreated animals. The results herein described provide evidence that reveals the critical role played by IL-33 in the initiation of the inflammatory response to ENM.

Flow cytometric analysis of ILC1 and ILC2

Polarization of T-cells requires several days [25], therefore, the early appearance of Th2 cytokines in the circulation after nano-TiO₂ suggests that other, more rapid immune effector cells may be involved. Previous work has indicated that both ILC1 and ILC2 [26, 27] reside in the lungs and may be involved in lung inflammatory responses and pathology. Therefore, we next wanted to determine the effect of nano-TiO₂ exposure on ILC1 and ILC2 levels in the lungs. For this reason, multi-parametric flow cytometric analysis was conducted on lung tissue from control and nano-TiO₂ exposed Sprague-Dawley rats for ILC1 *(Data not shown)* and ILC2 (Fig. 6) 4 h post-exposure. No significant differences were noted in ILC1 levels pre- and post- exposure while ILC2 levels increased from $0.19 \pm 0.22\%$ to $1.66 \pm 0.19\%$ (Fig. 7a and b).

NF-κB phosphorylation and Th2 cytokine secretion by isolated ILC2

Activation of the NF-κB pathway has been shown to play a role in inflammation through its ability to induce the transcription of proinflammatory genes [28, 29]. Specifically, phosphorylation of NF—κB at both serine residues 468 and 536 are associated with inflammatory response [29, 30]. Therefore, levels of phospho- NF—κB were measured in isolated ILC2 from control and nano-TiO₂

Table 1 Animal characteristics

	N	Age (weeks)	weight (grams)	Heart Rate (bpm)	Map (mm Hg)	Systolic Blood pressure (mm Hg)	Diastolic Blood Pressure (mm Hg)
Control	13	14 ± 1	232 ± 5	319 ± 13	85 ± 3	103 ± 4	73 ± 2
Exposed	14	15 ± 1	249 ± 12	330 ± 9	86 ± 4	110 ± 6	78 ± 4

Table showing characteristics of control ($N = 13$) and exposed groups ($N = 14$). Values shown are mean ± SEM. Statistics were analyzed with two-way ANOVA ($P \leq 0.05$), * Sham control group vs. nano-TiO₂ exposed groups

Table 2 Arteriolar characteristics

	n	Inner diameter (μm)	Outer diameter (μm)	Tone(%)	Passive diameter inner (μm)	Passive diameter outer (μm)	Wall Tension (Newton/meter)
Control	18	98 ± 5	152 ± 14	26 ± 7	152 ± 9	199 ± 15	0.33 ± 0.1
Exposed	16	102 ± 11	164 ± 13	21 ± 4	159 ± 15	207 ± 17	0.34 ± 0.1
Exposed + anti-L-33	12	97 ± 11	158 ± 19	21 ± 4	140 ± 14	187 ± 26	0.31 ± 0.6

Table showing characteristics of control and exposed radial arterioles ($n = 12$–18). All vascular assessments were performed 24 h post-exposure. Values shown are mean ± SEM. Statistics were analyzed with two-way ANOVA ($P \leq 0.05$), * Sham control group vs. nano-TiO$_2$ exposed groups

exposed animals (Fig. 8). No significant differences were noted in phosphorylation of the Serine-536 residue between the 2 groups, while phosphorylation of Serine-468 was increased after acute pulmonary nano-TiO$_2$ exposure ($128.6 \pm 7.24\%$ of control levels).

Lastly, isolated ILC2 were cultured overnight and IL-4, IL-5 and IL-13 levels in the cell-culture media were measured. Nano-TiO$_2$ resulted in a significant increase in IL-4, IL-5, and IL-13 ($122 \pm 7.2\%$, $141.4 \pm 9.1\%$, $158.8 \pm 7.6\%$ of control levels respectively) (Fig. 9).

Effect of acute pulmonary Nano-TiO$_2$ exposure and systemic immunotherapy on uterine radial arterioles
Endothelium-dependent dilation

In order to identify the acute reproductive effects associated with nano-TiO$_2$ exposure, radial arterioles were isolated from the uterus of control and exposed animals 24 h post-exposure and endothelium-dependent and

independent dilation along with adrenergic sensitivity were tested. Previous work by our group has shown that ENM exposure impacts vascular reactivity most severely within 24 h, a condition which has been shown to improve but not fully return to control levels after 168 h [30]. Based on these findings, all vascular assessments for this study were conducted 24 h post-exposure.

Endothelium-dependent dilation of radial arterioles was significantly impaired following intratracheal instillation of 100 μg of nano-TiO$_2$(Fig. 10), with a mean decrease in dilation of $49.23 \pm 6.5\%$ compared to controls and $24.35 \pm 10\%$ compared to anti-IL-33 antibody-treated rats. These results suggest that pulmonary nano-TiO$_2$ exposure disrupts normal physiological vascular endothelial function and that pre-treatment with an anti-IL-33 antibody partially attenuates the systemic acute inflammatory cascade triggered by lung-derived IL-33.

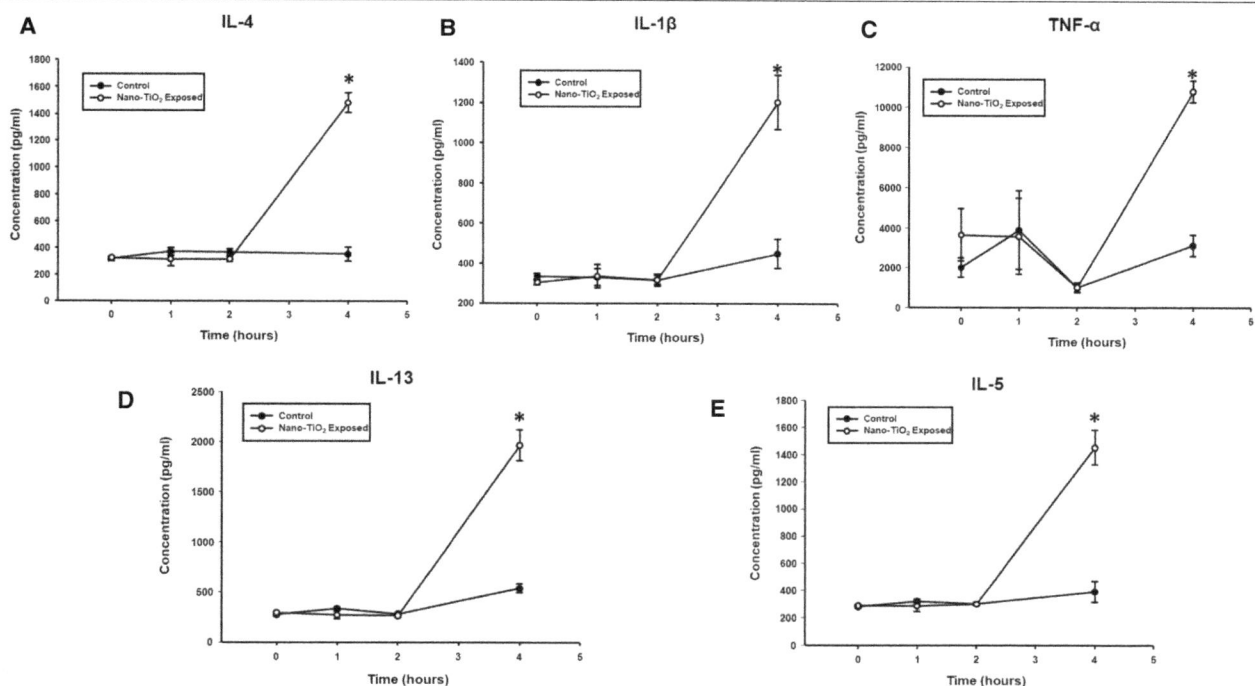

Fig. 2 Nano-TiO$_2$ exposure increases T-Helper type II cytokines 4 h post-exposure. Multiplex cytokine analysis showing concentrations of IL-4 (**a**), IL-1β (**b**), TNF-α (**c**), IL-13 (**d**) and IL-5 (**e**). Serum samples were obtained at 0, 1, 2 and 4 h post-exposure via tail-vein puncture ($N = 6$). Statistics were analyzed with two-way ANOVA ($P \leq 0.05$), * Sham control group vs. nano-TiO$_2$ exposed groups

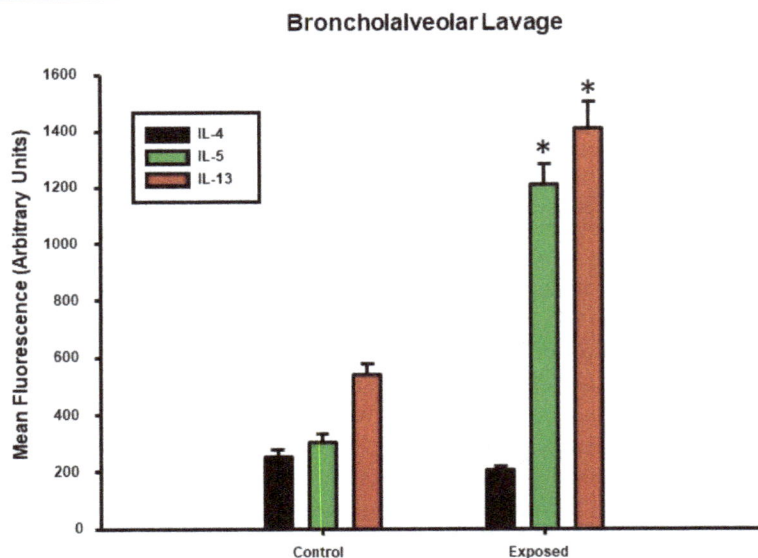

Fig. 3 Nano-TiO$_2$ exposure also increases T-Helper type II cytokines 4 h post-exposure in bronchoalveolar lavage fluid (BALF). Multiplex cytokine analysis showing concentrations of IL-4, IL-5, IL-13 in BALF from exposed and control animals 4 h post-exposure (N = 6). Statistics were analyzed with two-way ANOVA (P ≤ 0.05), * Sham control group vs. nano-TiO$_2$ exposed groups

In contrast to endothelium-dependent relaxation, no point to point differences were seen in α-adrenergic and endothelium-independent dilation between control, nano-TiO$_2$ exposed, and treated groups *(Data not shown)*.

Discussion

The inflammatory paradigm tested herein has been suggested by previous studies [16, 31, 32]. While these studies explored pulmonary responses to exogenously administered IL-33, carbon nanotubes and viral infection, our findings provide additional evidence of a similar link between acute pulmonary ENM exposure and subsequent inflammatory mechanisms with systemic microvascular consequences. Perhaps the most important finding of this study is the identification of IL-33 as a potential contributor to the systemic inflammatory phenotype and microvascular dysfunction resulting from acute pulmonary ENM exposure.

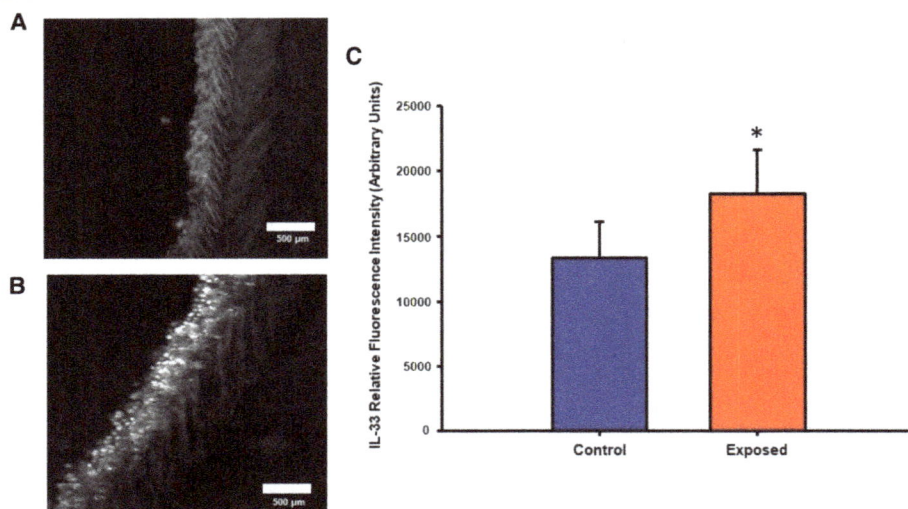

Fig. 4 Nano-TiO$_2$ exposure is associated with an increase in pulmonary interleukin-33 levels. Lung sections from control (**a**) and nano-TiO$_2$ exposed (**b**) animals obtained 4 h post-exposure were stained for interleukin-33. Fluorescence was achieved by staining tracheal sections with an anti-IL-33-FITC conjugated antibody. Relative fluorescence is shown in (**c**) tagged antibody (N = 6–7). Statistics were analyzed with two-way ANOVA (P ≤ 0.05), * Sham control group vs. nano-TiO$_2$ exposed groups

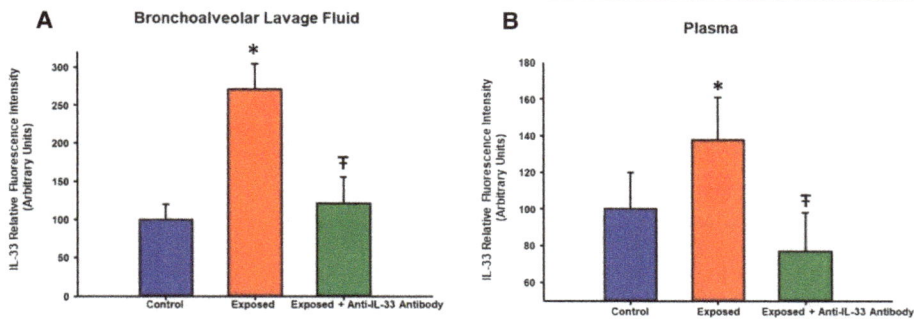

Fig. 5 Pre-treatment of nano-TiO$_2$ – exposed animals with an anti-IL-33 antibody lowers BALF and plasma IL-33. Interleukin-33 levels in (**a**) BALF and (**b**) plasma in control, nano-TiO$_2$ exposed groups and in rats pre-treated with an anti-IL-33 antibody. Rats were pre-treated with an anti-IL-33 antibody (1 mg/kg) 30 min prior to exposure. Plasma and BALF IL-33 levels were measured 4 h post-exposure. Statistics were analyzed with two-way ANOVA ($P \leq 0.05$). * Sham control group vs. nano-TiO$_2$ exposed groups, ⊤ $P < 0.05$ Exposed + Anti-IL-33 Antibody vs Exposed

We hypothesized that the innate response to pulmonary nano-TiO$_2$ exposure is triggered by the secretion of IL-33 by lung epithelial cells. IL-33, a member of the IL-1 family, plays a significant role in initiating and modulating lung inflammatory and immunological responses [33], by inducing the secretion of Th2 pro-inflammatory cytokines through the Suppression of Tumorigenicity 2 (ST2) receptor in a variety of immune cells [32, 34]. Previous studies have shown that exposure to multi-walled carbon nanotubes triggers the IL-33/ST2 axis leading to the activation of mast-cells and macrophages [20]. Interestingly, IL-33 is also required for the maturation, activation and egress of ILC2 lineage cells from the bone marrow to specific target

organs [35]. Several previous studies by our group and others have extensively investigated the cardiovascular effects of pulmonary ENM exposure [36, 37]. These studies consistently reveal that nano-TiO$_2$ exposure increases leukocyte activation [38], proinflammatory mediators [39], and oxidative stress [40]. Collectively, this results in endothelium-dependent dysfunction. ILCs are a recently identified subpopulation of immune effector cells [33, 41]. They are critical, non-cytolytic tissue-resident cells that can be activated and respond acutely to danger signals or "alarmins" such as IL-33 from mucosal tissue by producing a distinctive array of cytokines to maintain mucosal integrity. Group II ILCs specifically, secrete the cytokines

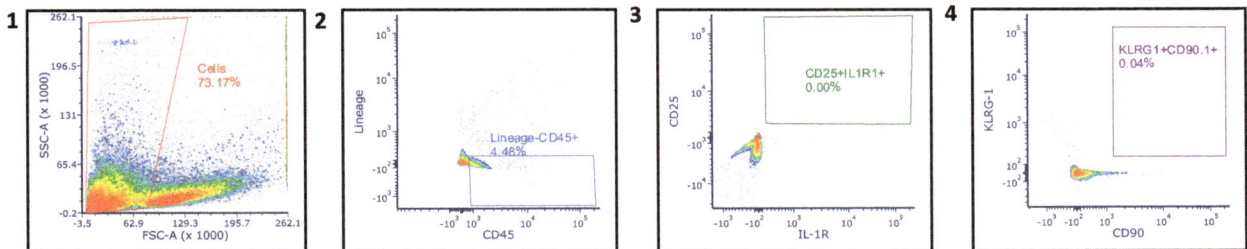

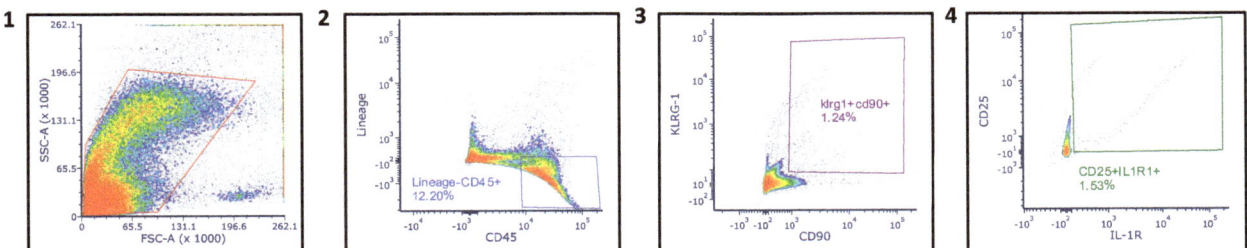

Fig. 6 Flow cytometric analysis of lung-resident Group II innate lymphoid cells. Flow cytometry of lung tissue 4 h post-exposure for Group II Innate Lymphoid Cells in (**a**) control and (**b**) nano-TiO$_2$ exposed animals ($N = 6$)

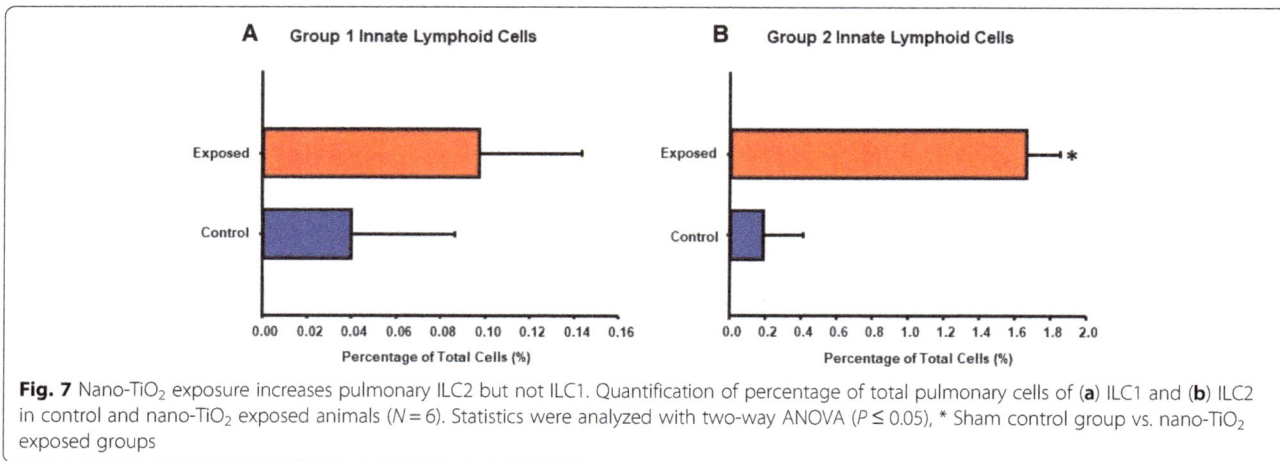

Fig. 7 Nano-TiO$_2$ exposure increases pulmonary ILC2 but not ILC1. Quantification of percentage of total pulmonary cells of (a) ILC1 and (b) ILC2 in control and nano-TiO$_2$ exposed animals (N = 6). Statistics were analyzed with two-way ANOVA (P ≤ 0.05), * Sham control group vs. nano-TiO$_2$ exposed groups

IL-5, IL-13, IL-9, amphiregulin, and low quantities of IL-4 [31] and have been linked to several lung-associated conditions including pathogen infections (viruses and helminths), asthma, and pulmonary fibrosis [42]. Lung ILC2 have an important role in regulating tissue remodeling and repair during acute epithelial injury and asthma [43]. Considered together, it is reasonable to speculate that the IL-33/ILC2 axis may impact systemic microvascular function after pulmonary ENM exposure.

Perhaps, the most significant finding of this study is the identification of a potential role for IL-33 in the initiation of an acute inflammatory response and the effects on systemic microvascular dysfunction (Fig. 10). This was achieved by interrupting the IL-33/ST2 signaling axis with an anti-IL-33 antibody treatment prior to ENM exposure. In these experiments, the control group (IT saline) did not receive the anti-IL-33 antibody. The scientific rationale for this decision was that the technique (isolated, perfused and pressurized arterioles) used to assess microvascular dysfunction is a plasma free system. As such, it was impossible to assess the role of the complete IL-33/ST2 axis on arteriolar tone and/or reactivity. Whereas,

this approach directly measured the impact that IL-33 inflammatory signaling has on microvascular function. It remains a distinct possibility that the IL-33/ST2 axis activated by pulmonary ENM exposure directly influences microvascular tone and/or reactivity. IL-33 expression has been identified in human vascular endothelial cells; whereas, is absent in murine vascular tissue [44]. This supports our postulate that IL-33 is impacting microvascular function via inflammation, rather than a direct activation of the ST2 receptor. Future in vivo studies must directly assess the impact of circulating IL-33 on microvascular tone, reactivity and blood flow.

While our study provides plausible mechanistic insights into both the inflammatory and microvascular effects associated with ENM exposure, additional considerations as well as the limitations must be kept in mind. ENM exposure has been shown to affect other innate immune effector cells such as neutrophils [45, 46], macrophages [47, 48], and dendritic cells [49]. Therefore, other mechanisms including local generation of reactive of oxygen species, secretion of chemokines and prostaglandins by macrophages and stimulation of the adaptive immune system by antigen-presenting cells

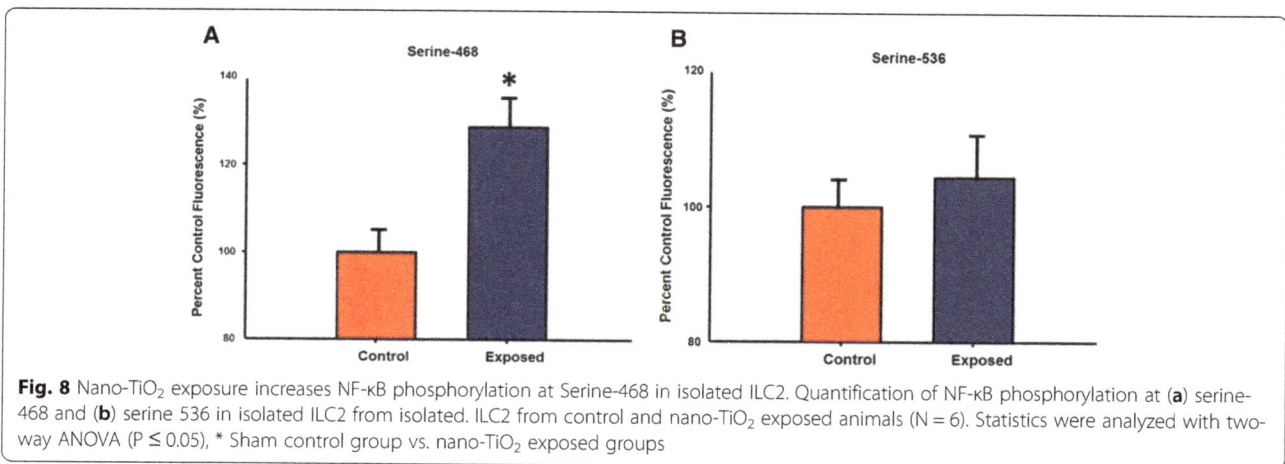

Fig. 8 Nano-TiO$_2$ exposure increases NF-κB phosphorylation at Serine-468 in isolated ILC2. Quantification of NF-κB phosphorylation at (a) serine-468 and (b) serine 536 in isolated ILC2 from isolated. ILC2 from control and nano-TiO$_2$ exposed animals (N = 6). Statistics were analyzed with two-way ANOVA (P ≤ 0.05), * Sham control group vs. nano-TiO$_2$ exposed groups

Cell Supernatant

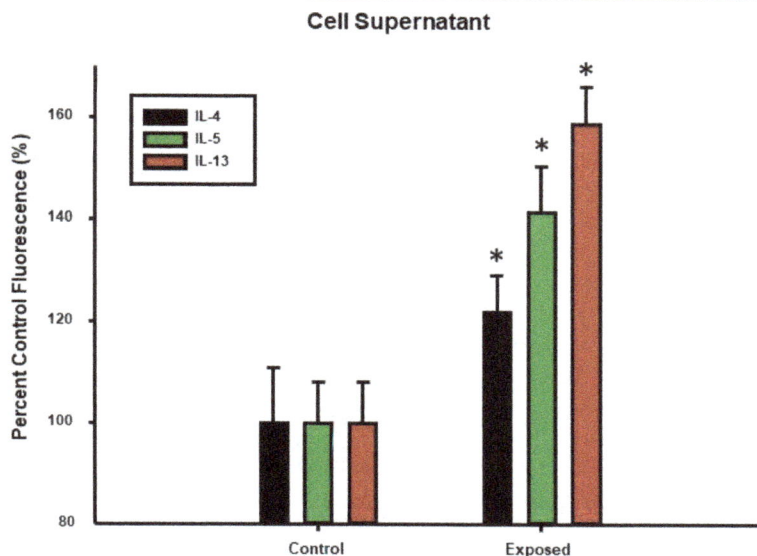

Fig. 9 Th2 cytokine secretion in isolated ILC2 is increased by nano-TiO$_2$ exposure. Multiplex cytokine analysis showing concentrations of IL-4, IL-5, IL-13 supernatant from isolated ILC2 cultured overnight from control and nano-TiO$_2$ exposed animals (N = 6). Statistics were analyzed with two-way ANOVA ($P \leq 0.05$), * Sham control group vs. nano-TiO$_2$ exposed groups

may play a role in the systemic inflammatory response and vascular effects seen in this study. It is also worth noting that in this study an immune response associated with pulmonary ENM exposure was observed as early as 4 h post-exposure, as evidenced not only by an increase in the proportion of lung-resident ILC2s (Fig. 7), but also by augmented levels of the Th2 cytokines IL-4, IL-5, and IL-13 (Figs. 2 and 3). This response timeframe is in agreement with previous studies, that have reported IL33, ILC2 numbers as well as lung and serum Th2 cytokines increase within 6–12 h of lung injury [50, 51]. Furthermore, isolated ILC2s have been shown to respond dose-dependently to transient or continuous stimulation with IL-2 and/or IL-33 within 3 h [52]. Similarly, nano-TiO$_2$ instillation at lung burdens of 40–160 μg/rat has also been shown to increase BALF inflammatory mediators within 4 h of exposure [53].

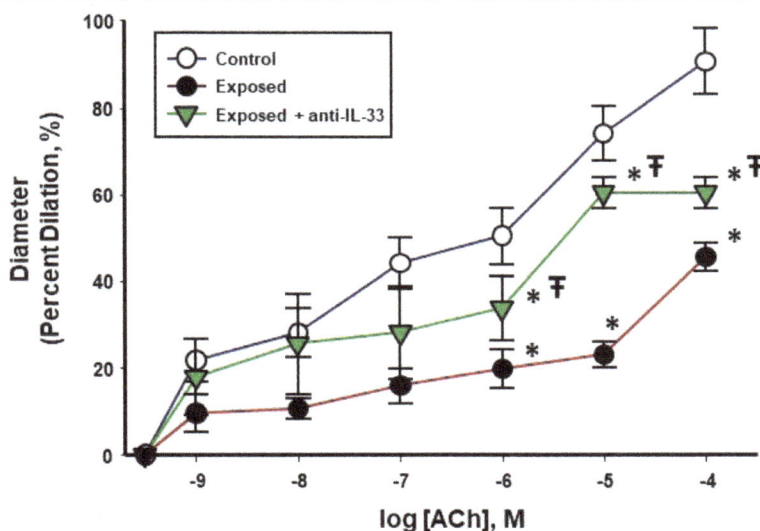

Fig. 10 Endothelium-dependent dilation of radial arterioles is blunted by nano-TiO$_2$ exposure and improved by pre-treatment with an anti-IL-33 antibody. Endothelium-dependent dilation of uterine radial arterioles from control, exposed and anti-IL-33 antibody treated animals was determined using pressure myography (n = 12–18). All vascular assessments were performed 24 h post-exposure. Statistics were analyzed with two-way ANOVA ($P \leq 0.05$). * Sham control group vs. nano-TiO$_2$ exposed groups, Ŧ $P < 0.05$ Exposed + Anti-IL-33 Antibody vs Exposed

We report herein a similar phenomenon as the lung burden used in this study was comparable at 100 µg/rat.

Our findings contribute consistent evidence for a role of ILC2s in the acute pulmonary response to ENM exposure. Due to the inherent limitations associated with our experimental in vivo model, we were unable to directly establish causality. In order to directly confirm such an observation, ILC2 deletion would be necessary. Our research program has a long-standing interest in the systemic microvascular consequences of pulmonary particle exposure. Rat models are primarily used in our in vivo studies as they are the most appropriate and widely used animals for microvascular research. However, they are not commonly or easily adapted for transgenic studies. As such, an ILC2 rat deletion model does not exist. If such a model were created in the future, it would then be possible to directly confirm a causative relationship between ENM exposure and ILC2 activation, proliferation and recruitment.

Lastly, to allow periodic blood sampling for cytokine analysis, intratracheal instillation was chosen as the preferred exposure method. The above-mentioned dose of nano-TiO$_2$ was selected based on previous studies conducted by our group which have shown that it is associated with significant microvascular impairment, oxidative and nitrosative stress and alveolar macrophage recruitment [36, 54]. Additionally, to better understand the relevance of the exposure paradigm used in this study to humans, alveolar surface areas must be known [55]. The rat alveolar surface area is 0.4 m^2/lung. Therefore, the rat burden of 50 µg/lung would result in 125 µg/m^2. Given that the human alveolar surface area is 102 m^2, the equivalent human burden of this exposure paradigm would be 12.75 mg. The next logical question is: How long would it take to achieve this burden in humans? In this regard, lung burden may be calculated as:

$$nano\text{-}TiO_2 aerosol\ concentration \cdot\ minute\ ventilation \cdot\ exposure\ duration\ deposition\ fraction,$$

with the following values:

$$25.5\ mg = nano\text{-}TiO_2 aerosol\ concentration \\ \cdot\ 7600\ ml/\ min\ (8\ hrh/day \cdot 60\ min/hr) \\ \cdot\ 14\%,$$

and therefore:

$$25.5\ mg = nano\text{-}TiO_2 aerosol\ concentration \\ \cdot\ 0.51\ m^3/day.$$

Considering both the National Institute for Occupational Safety and Health (NIOSH) and the Occupational Safety and Health Administration (OSHA) Permissible Exposure Limit (0.3 mg/m^3 and 5 mg/m^3 respectively) [4], it would require 0.34 working years or 122 working days for a human to achieve similar exposure levels to those used in this study.

Conclusion

In conclusion, the current study provides novel evidence that links acute pulmonary ENM exposure and systemic microvascular effects. Because this inflammatory link exists between the lung and the uterine microcirculation, it remains to be determined if such an axis extends to the placenta and or fetus.

Materials and methods
Nanomaterial characterization

Nano-TiO$_2$ P25 powder, obtained from Evonik (Aeroxide TiO$_2$, Parsippany, NJ), has previously been shown to be a mixture composed primarily of anatase (80%) and rutile (20%) TiO$_2$, with a primary particle size of 21 nm and a surface area of 48.08 m^2/g [54], and a Zeta-potential of − 56.6 mV [56]. Elemental composition analysis of the nano-TiO$_2$ suspension was conducted via energy dispersive spectroscopy.

Scanning electron microscopy was performed by diluting the nano-TiO$_2$ 1:100 with filtered distilled water. 0.5 ml of the diluted particle solution was filtered onto a 0.2 µm polycarbonate filter. A wedge-shaped portion of the polycarbonate filter was mounted onto carbon double stick tape which was affixed to a 13 mm aluminum stub. The sample was sputter coated with gold-palladium for two minutes. The sample was imaged using a Hitachi S4800 field-emission scanning electron microscope (Tokyo, Japan).

Experimental animals and exposure

Female (8–10 weeks) Sprague – Dawley rats were purchased from Hilltop Laboratories (Scottdale, PA) and housed in an AAALAC approved facility at West Virginia University (WVU) with 12:12 h light – dark cycle and regulated temperature. Rats were allowed ad libitum access to food and water. All procedures were approved by the Institutional Animal Care and Use Committee of WVU.

100 µg of nano-TiO$_2$ were suspended in 250 µL of vehicle (Normosol and 5% fetal bovine serum) for intratracheal instillation (IT) 24 h prior to experimentation. Nano-TiO$_2$ suspensions were sonicated for 1 min to ensure homogenous distribution of nanoparticles. Rats were anesthetized using 5% isoflurane and placed on a mounting stand. 250 µL of the nano-TiO$_2$ suspension was then instilled intratracheally. Sprague - Dawley rats instilled with 250 µL of vehicle were used as controls.

Mean arterial pressure (MAP) acquisition

Rats were anesthetized with isoflurane gas (5% induction, 2–3.5% maintenance). The animals were placed on a heating pad to maintain a 37 °C rectal temperature. The trachea was intubated to ensure an open airway and the right carotid artery was cannulated to acquire mean arterial pressure (MAP). The MAP was measured via a pressure transducer and recorded by PowerLab830 (AD Instruments, Colorado Springs, CO).

Multiplex cytokine panels of serum and Bronchoalveolar lavage fluid

Whole blood (1–2 ml) was collected via tail vein puncture from exposed and control animals at time 0, 1 h, 2 h, and 4 h after exposure into EDTA vacutainers and centrifuged (1000 x g) to collect plasma which was flash-frozen in liquid nitrogen and stored at − 80°C until analysis. Rats were euthanized and tissues harvested for further analysis. Multi-spot inflammatory assays were completed per manufacturer's directions (Meso Scale Diagnostics, Rockville, MD) for: lipocalin-2, TSP-1, TIMP-1, MCP-1, interferon (IFN-γ), interleukin (IL)-1β, IL-4, IL-5, IL-6, KC/GRO, IL-10, IL-13, and TNF-α.

Immunohistochemistry

Gelatin-coated cover slips of serial tissue sections were incubated with anti-rabbit (1:100) IL-33 (Cloud-Clone Corp., Katy, TX) overnight at 4°C, followed by 3 five-minute washes with cold PBS with 0.1% Triton-X. The sections were then incubated with a FITC conjugated goat anti-rabbit (1:100, Invitrogen, Carlsbad, CA) at 37°C for one hour, followed by 3 five-minute washes with cold PBS with 0.1% Triton-X. Cover slips were then mounted on slides for visualization on a Zeiss fluorescent microscope (Zeiss, Thornwood, NY).

Preparation of cell suspensions

Lungs were perfused with sterile PBS by injection into the right ventricle to remove remaining blood and then placed in PBS containing 20 mg/ml Collagenase A, 2.4 U/ml Dispase II solution, and 50 µl/ml DNAse (Roche, Indianapolis, IN) for 30 min.

The lung tissue was dissociated using the gentleMACS Octo Dissociator (Miltenyi Biotec, Auburn, CA) and then centrifuged (1100 x g for 10 min) to collect the sample material. The sample was resuspended with PBS and used for magnetic cell separation and flow cytometry.

Flow cytometry
Antibodies and reagents

ILC1 and ILC2 numbers 4 h after exposure to nano-TiO$_2$ from lung tissue were determined by flow cytometry as previously described [57–59]. Briefly, ILC1 were defined as Lin-CD45 + CD161 + CD335+, while ILC2 were defined as Lin-CD45 + CD90.1 + KLRG-1 + CD25 + IL1R1 + .

Monoclonal antibodies specific for CD90.1 (FITC), KLRG1 (APC EFLUOR 780), CD25 (APC), CD161 (PERCP EFLUOR 710), and CD335 (EFLUOR 450) were purchased from eBioscience (San Diego, CA). Lineage cocktail (Lin;

ALEXA FLUOR 700) was used to gate out (CD3, CD14, CD16, CD19, CD20, and CD56: Biorad, Hercules, CA) CD3 T lymphocytes, CD14 Monocytes, CD16 NK cells, granulocytes, CD19 B lymphocytes, CD20 B lymphocytes, and CD56 NK cells. Antibodies for CD45 (Cyanine 5) were from Invitrogen (Carlsbad, CA), while those for IL1R1 (PE) where from Sino Biologicals (North Wales, PA). Flow cytometry was performed on a FACSAria (BD Bioscience, Franklin Lakes, NJ). Data were analyzed with FCS Express 6 Software (De Novo Software, Glendale, CA).

Isolation of group II innate lymphoid cells

ILC2 were isolated as per manufacturer's instructions (Miltenyi Biotec, Auburn, CA). Briefly, lineage-positive cells were indirectly labeled with a cocktail of ALEXA FLUOR 700-conjugated antibodies, as primary labeling reagent, and antibodies conjugated to MicroBeads were used as secondary labeling reagents. In the second step, lineage-negative cells were labeled with CD45, CD90.1, KLRG-1, CD25, and IL1R1, labeled with MicroBeads and isolated by positive selection from the pre-enriched lineage negative cell-fraction by separation over a MACS Column (Miltenyi Biotec, Auburn, CA), which was placed in the magnetic field of a MACS Separator. After negative selection, the cells were subsequently eluted as the positively selected cell fraction containing ILC2.

Cytokine analysis of cell culture media and measurement of Phospho-NF-κB

Isolated ILC2s were incubated (37 °C, 90% humidity, 5% CO$_2$) overnight in supplemented (10% fetal bovine serum, 1% penicillin/streptomycin, 1% sodium pyruvate, 1% L-glutamine) Dulbecco's Modified Eagle Medium (Corning, Manassas, VA). The following day, the cell culture medium and cellular portion were separated via centrifugation (1100 x g for 10 min). IL-4, IL-5, and IL-13 levels were measured in the cell culture medium via multi-spot inflammatory assays per manufacturer's directions (Meso Scale Diagnostics, Rockville, MD). Lastly, isolated cells were lysed and phospho-NF-κB (Ser468 and Ser536) was measured (Meso Scale Diagnostics, Rockville, MD).

Systemic treatment with anti-Interleukin-33 antibody

Rats were treated 1 h prior to pulmonary nano-TiO$_2$ exposure with pharmacological grade polyclonal anti-IL-33 antibody (CAT#ABF108, EMD Millipore, Temecula, CA: intraperitoneal 1 mg/kg). The antibody and dosage were selected based on previous murine studies [60]. The antibody used was a polyclonal anti-IL-33 antibody developed in the rabbit with specific reactivity toward mouse IL-33 and expected cross reactivity due to the close homology to rat IL-33. We determined the interspecies homology of the anti-IL-33 target between rats and mice to be 87% (Additional file 1: Figure S1). Plasma, bronchoalveolar lavage fluid, and lung tissue were obtained 4 h post-exposure from treated animals for measurement of IL-33. Uterine microvascular assessments were conducted 24 h after treatment in a separate cohort of animals.

Pressure Myography microvessel preparation

After measuring MAP, the uterus was removed and placed in a dissecting dish with physiological salt solution (PSS) maintained at 4 °C. Radial arterioles were isolated, transferred to a vessel chamber, cannulated between two glass pipettes, and tied with silk sutures in the chamber (Living Systems Instrumentation, Burlington, VT). The chamber was superfused with fresh oxygenated (5% CO_2/21% O_2) PSS and warmed to 37 °C. Arterioles were pressurized to 60 mmHg using a servo control system and extended to their in situ length. Internal and external arteriolar diameters were measured using video calipers (Colorado Video, Boulder, CO).

Arteriolar reactivity

Previous work by our group has shown that ENM exposure impacts endothelium-dependent dilation most severely within 24 h, a condition which has been shown to improve but did not fully return to control levels after 168 h. Based on these findings, all vascular assessments for this study were conducted 24 h post-exposure [30].

Arterioles were allowed to develop spontaneous tone, defined as the degree of constriction experienced by a blood vessel relative to its maximally dilated state. Vascular tone ranges from 0% (maximally dilated) to 100% (maximal constriction). Vessels with a spontaneous tone ≥20% less than initial tone were included in this study. After equilibration, various parameters of arteriolar function were analyzed. Vessels that did not develop sufficient spontaneous tone were not included in the data analysis.

Endothelium-Dependent Dilation— arterioles were exposed to increasing concentrations of acetyl choline (ACh: 10^{-9} - 10^{-4} M) added to the vessel chamber.
Endothelium-Independent Dilation—increasing concentrations of sodium nitroprusside (SNP: 10^{-9} - 10^{-4} M) were used to assess arteriolar smooth muscle responsiveness.
Arteriolar Vasoconstriction—arterioles were exposed to increasing concentrations of phenylephrine (PE: 10^{-9} - 10^{-4} M). The steady state diameter of the vessel was recorded for at least 2 min after each dose. After each dose curve was completed, the vessel chamber was washed to remove excess chemicals by carefully removing the superfusate and replacing it with fresh warmed oxygenated PSS. After all experimental treatments were complete, the PSS was replaced with Ca^{2+}-free PSS until maximum passive diameter was established.

Pressure Myography calculations

Data are expressed as means ± standard error. Spontaneous tone was calculated by the following equation:

$$Spontaneous\ tone\ (\%) = \left\{ \frac{(Dm - Di)}{Di} \right\} x\ 100$$

, where Dm is the maximal diameter and Di is the initial steady state diameter recorded prior to the experiment. Active responses to pressure were normalized to the maximal diameter using the following formula:

$$Normalized\ diameter = Dss/Dm$$

, where Dss is the steady state diameter recorded during each pressure change. The experimental responses to ACh, PE, and SNP are expressed using the following equation:

$$\begin{aligned} Diameter\ &(percent\ maximal\ diameter) \\ &= \left\{ \frac{(Dss - Dcon)}{(Dm - Dcon)} \right\} x\ 100 \end{aligned}$$

, where DCon is the control diameter recorded prior to the dose curve, DSS is the steady state diameter at each dose of the curve. The experimental response to PE is expressed using the following equation:

$$\begin{aligned} Diameter\ &(percent\ maximal\ diameter) \\ &= \left\{ \frac{(Dcon - Dss)}{(Dcon)} \right\} x\ 100 \end{aligned}$$

Wall thickness (WT) was calculated from the measurement of both inner (ID) and outer (OD) steady state arteriolar diameters at the end of the Ca^{2+} free wash using the following equation:

$$WT = (OD - ID)/2$$

Wall-to-lumen ratio (WLR) was calculated using the following equation:

$$WLR = WT/ID$$

Statistics

Point-to-point differences in the dose response curves were evaluated using two-way repeated measures analysis of variance (ANOVA) with a Tukey's *post-hoc* analysis when significance was found. The slopes of the dose response curves were determined through a nonlinear regression. The animal characteristics, vessel characteristics and dose response curve slopes were analyzed using a one-way ANOVA with a Tukey *post-hoc* analysis when significance was found. All statistical analysis was completed with GraphPad Prism 5 (San Diego, CA) and SigmaPlot 11.0 (San Jose, CA). Significance was set at $p < 0.05$, n is the number of arterioles, and N is the number of animals.

Group II innate lymphoid cells and microvascular dysfunction from pulmonary titanium dioxide...

131

Abbreviations

ACh: Acetylcholine; ANOVA: Analysis of variance; APC: Allophycocyanin; BALF: Broncho alveolar lavage fluid; CD: Cluster of differentiation; Dcon: Control diameter; Di: Initial diameter; Dm: Maximal diameter; Dss: Steady state diameter; EDTA: Ethylenediaminetetraacetic acid; ENM: Engineered nanomaterials; FITC: Fluorescein isothiocyanate; ID: Inner diameter; IFN-γ: Interferon-gamma; IL: Interleukin; ILC: Innate lymphoid cells; KC/GRO: Keratinocyte chemoattractant/human growth-regulated oncogene; KLRG-1: Killer cell lectin-like receptor subfamily G member 1; Lin: Lineage; MCP-1: Monocyte chemoattractant protein 1; Nano-TiO$_2$: Titanium dioxide nanoparticles; NF-κB: Nuclear factor kappa-light-chain-enhancer of activated B cells; NIOSH: National Institute for Occupational Safety and Health; NK: Natural Killer; NO: Nitric oxide; OD: Outer diameter; OSHA: Occupational Safety and Health Administration; PBS: Phosphate buffered saline; PE: Phenylephrine; PE: Phycoerythrin; SEM: Scanning electron microscope; SEM: Standard error of the mean; Ser-468: Serine-468; SNP: Sodium nitroprusside; ST2: Suppressor of tumor tumorigenicity; Th2: T-helper type 2; TIMP-1: Tissue inhibitor of metalloproteinases 1; TNF- α: Tumor necrosis factor alpha; TSP-1: Thrombospondin 1; WLR: Wall-to-lumen ratio; WT: Wall thickness

Acknowledgments

We thank Kevin Engels from the West Virginia University (WVU) Department of Physiology and Pharmacology for his technical assistance in this study, and Dr. Kathleen Brundage from the Flow Cytometry & Single Cell Core Facility at WVU (FORTESSA S10 OD016165, FACSAria S10 RR020866). In addition, we would like to acknowledge our financial support: R01-ES015022 (TRN), and NSF-1003907 (TRN and ABA).

Disclaimer

The findings and conclusions in this report are those of the author(s) and do not necessarily represent the official position of the National Institute for Occupational Safety and Health, Centers for Disease Control and Prevention.

Authors' contributions

ABA conducted the vascular and immunological assessments, analyzed and interpreted the data, and was a major contributor in writing the manuscript. CRM assisted with the vascular assessments and was involved in drafting the manuscript and revising it critically for important intellectual content. TPB performed the tracheal immunohistochemistry and was involved in drafting the manuscript. WTG was involved in the animal exposures and was involved in the drafting of the manuscript. ECB and KLG were involved in the analysis and interpretation of the data and were major contributors in writing the manuscript. SF obtained the SEM images of the nano-TiO$_2$ and was involved in drafting of the manuscript. TRN made substantial contributions to the conception and design of the experiments, analysis and interpretation of the data and was a major contributor in writing of the manuscript. All the authors read and approved the final manuscript.

Competing interests

The authors declare that they have no competing interests.

Author details

[1]Department of Physiology and Pharmacology, West Virginia University School of Medicine, 64 Medical Center Drive, Robert C. Byrd Health Sciences Center - West Virginia University, Morgantown, WV 26505-9229, USA. [2]Toxicology Working Group, West Virginia University School of Medicine, Morgantown, WV, USA. [3]National Institute for Occupational Safety and Health, Morgantown, WV, USA.

References

1. Jackson P, et al. Prenatal exposure to carbon black (printex 90): effects on sexual development and neurofunction. Basic Clin Pharmacol Toxicol. 2011; 109(6):434–7.

2. Johansson HKL, et al. Airway exposure to multi-walled carbon nanotubes disrupts the female reproductive cycle without affecting pregnancy outcomes in mice. Part Fibre Toxicol. 2017;14(1):17.

3. Stapleton PA, et al. Maternal engineered nanomaterial exposure and fetal microvascular function: does the barker hypothesis apply? Am J Obstet Gynecol. 2013;209(3):227 e1–11.

4. Stapleton PA, et al. Maternal engineered nanomaterial inhalation during gestation alters the fetal transcriptome. Part Fibre Toxicol. 2018;15(1):3.

5. Engler-Chiurazzi EB, et al. Impacts of prenatal nanomaterial exposure on male adult Sprague-Dawley rat behavior and cognition. J Toxicol Environ Health A. 2016;79(11):447–52.

6. McKenzie AN. Type-2 innate lymphoid cells in asthma and allergy. Ann Am Thorac Soc. 2014;11(Suppl 5):S263–70.

7. Sonnenberg GF, et al. SnapShot: innate lymphoid cells. Immunity. 2013; 39(3):622–622 e1.

8. Artis D, Spits H. The biology of innate lymphoid cells. Nature. 2015; 517(7534):293–301.

9. Turner JE, et al. IL-9-mediated survival of type 2 innate lymphoid cells promotes damage control in helminth-induced lung inflammation. J Exp Med. 2013;210(13):2951–65.

10. Vercelli D, Gozdz J, von Mutius E. Innate lymphoid cells in asthma: when innate immunity comes in a Th2 flavor. Curr Opin Allergy Clin Immunol. 2014;14(1):29–34.

11. Spits H, et al. Innate lymphoid cells--a proposal for uniform nomenclature. Nat Rev Immunol. 2013;13(2):145–9.

12. Takatori H, et al. Lymphoid tissue inducer-like cells are an innate source of IL-17 and IL-22. J Exp Med. 2009;206(1):35–41.

13. Yasuda K, et al. Contribution of IL-33-activated type II innate lymphoid cells to pulmonary eosinophilia in intestinal nematode-infected mice. Proc Natl Acad Sci U S A. 2012;109(9):3451–6.

14. Shaw JL, et al. IL-33-responsive innate lymphoid cells are an important source of IL-13 in chronic rhinosinusitis with nasal polyps. Am J Respir Crit Care Med. 2013;188(4):432–9.

15. Marsland BJ, et al. Innate signals compensate for the absence of PKC-{theta} during in vivo CD8(+) T cell effector and memory responses. Proc Natl Acad Sci U S A. 2005;102(40):14374–9.

16. Katwa P, et al. A carbon nanotube toxicity paradigm driven by mast cells and the IL-(3)(3)/ST(2) axis. Small. 2012;8(18):2904–12.

17. Wang X, et al. Intravenously delivered graphene nanosheets and multiwalled carbon nanotubes induce site-specific Th2 inflammatory responses via the IL-33/ST2 axis. Int J Nanomedicine. 2013;8:1733–48.

18. Wang X, et al. Multi-walled carbon nanotube instillation impairs pulmonary function in C57BL/6 mice. Part Fibre Toxicol. 2011;8:24.

19. Michaudel C, et al. Inflammasome, IL-1 and inflammation in ozone-induced lung injury. Am J Clin Exp Immunol. 2016;5(1):33–40.

20. Beamer CA, et al. IL-33 mediates multi-walled carbon nanotube (MWCNT)-induced airway hyper-reactivity via the mobilization of innate helper cells in the lung. Nanotoxicology. 2013;7(6):1070–81.

21. Kabata H, et al. Group 2 innate lymphoid cells and asthma. Allergol Int. 2015;64(3):227–34.

22. Hams E, Fallon PG. Innate type 2 cells and asthma. Curr Opin Pharmacol. 2012;12(4):503–9.

23. Deckers J, Branco Madeira F, Hammad H. Innate immune cells in asthma. Trends Immunol. 2013;34(11):540–7.

24. Lai DM, Shu Q, Fan J. The origin and role of innate lymphoid cells in the lung. Mil Med Res. 2016;3:25.

25. Ley K. The second touch hypothesis: T cell activation, homing and polarization. F1000Res. 2014;3:37.

26. Halim TYF, McKenzie ANJ. New kids on the block: group 2 innate lymphoid cells and type 2 inflammation in the lung. Chest. 2013;144(5):1681–6.

27. Głobińska A, Kowalski ML. Innate lymphoid cells: The role in respiratory infections and lung tissue damage. Expert Rev Clin Immunol. 2017;13(10):991–9.

28. Pugazhenthi S, et al. Induction of an inflammatory loop by interleukin-1beta and tumor necrosis factor-alpha involves NF-kB and STAT-1 in differentiated human neuroprogenitor cells. PLoS One. 2013;8(7):e69585.

29. Pradere JP, et al. Negative regulation of NF-kappaB p65 activity by serine 536 phosphorylation. Sci Signal. 2016;9(442):ra85.

30. Stapleton PA, et al. Impairment of coronary arteriolar endothelium-dependent dilation after multi-walled carbon nanotube inhalation: a time-course study. Int J Mol Sci. 2012;13(11):13781–803.

31. Schmitz J, et al. IL-33, an interleukin-1-like cytokine that signals via the IL-1 receptor-related protein ST2 and induces T helper type 2-associated cytokines. Immunity. 2005;23(5):479–90.

32. Zeng S, et al. IL-33 receptor (ST2) Signalling is important for regulation of Th2-mediated airway inflammation in a murine model of acute respiratory syncytial virus infection. Scand J Immunol. 2015;81(6):494–501.

33. Mjosberg JM, et al. Human IL-25- and IL-33-responsive type 2 innate lymphoid cells are defined by expression of CRTH2 and CD161. Nat Immunol. 2011;12(11):1055–62.

34. Zoltowska AM, et al. The interleukin-33 receptor ST2 is important for the development of peripheral airway hyperresponsiveness and inflammation in a house dust mite mouse model of asthma. Clin Exp Allergy. 2016;46(3):479–90.

35. Stier MT, et al. IL-33 promotes the egress of group 2 innate lymphoid cells from the bone marrow. J Exp Med. 2018;215(1):263–81.

36. Nurkiewicz TR, et al. Nanoparticle inhalation augments particle-dependent systemic microvascular dysfunction. Part Fibre Toxicol. 2008;5:1.

37. Abukabda AB, et al. Heterogeneous vascular bed responses to pulmonary titanium dioxide nanoparticle exposure. Front Cardiovasc Med. 2017;4:33.

38. Stapleton PA, et al. Uterine microvascular sensitivity to nanomaterial inhalation: an in vivo assessment. Toxicol Appl Pharmacol. 2015;288(3):420–8.

39. Stapleton PA, et al. Estrous cycle-dependent modulation of in vivo microvascular dysfunction after nanomaterial inhalation. Reprod Toxicol. 2018;78:20–8.

40. LeBlanc AJ, et al. Nanoparticle inhalation impairs endothelium-dependent vasodilation in subepicardial arterioles. J Toxicol Environ Health A. 2009; 72(24):1576–84.

41. Spits H, Di Santo JP. The expanding family of innate lymphoid cells: regulators and effectors of immunity and tissue remodeling. Nat Immunol. 2011;12(1):21–7.

42. Hams E, et al. IL-25 and type 2 innate lymphoid cells induce pulmonary fibrosis. Proc Natl Acad Sci U S A. 2014;111(1):367–72.

43. Monticelli LA, et al. Innate lymphoid cells promote lung-tissue homeostasis after infection with influenza virus. Nat Immunol. 2011;12(11):1045–54.

44. Pichery M, et al. Endogenous IL-33 is highly expressed in mouse epithelial barrier tissues, lymphoid organs, brain, embryos, and inflamed tissues: in situ analysis using a novel Il-33-LacZ gene trap reporter strain. J Immunol. 2012;188(7):3488–95.

45. Sanfins E, et al. Nanoparticle effect on neutrophil produced myeloperoxidase. PLoS One. 2018;13(1):e0191445.

46. Thompson EA, et al. Innate immune responses to nanoparticle exposure in the lung. J Environ Immunol Toxicol. 2014;1(3):150–6.

47. Taylor AJ, et al. Atomic layer deposition coating of carbon nanotubes with aluminum oxide alters pro-fibrogenic cytokine expression by human mononuclear phagocytes in vitro and reduces lung fibrosis in mice in vivo. PLoS One. 2014;9(9):e106870.

48. Bonner JC, Hoffman M, Brody AR. Alpha-macroglobulin secreted by alveolar macrophages serves as a binding protein for a macrophage-derived homologue of platelet-derived growth factor. Am J Respir Cell Mol Biol. 1989;1(3):171–9.

49. Look M, et al. The nanomaterial-dependent modulation of dendritic cells and its potential influence on therapeutic immunosuppression in lupus. Biomaterials. 2014;35(3):1089–95.

50. Xu J, et al. IL33-mediated ILC2 activation and neutrophil IL5 production in the lung response after severe trauma: a reverse translation study from a human cohort to a mouse trauma model. PLoS Med. 2017;14(7):e1002365.

51. Yang Q, et al. Group 2 innate lymphoid cells mediate ozone-induced airway inflammation and hyperresponsiveness in mice. J Allergy Clin Immunol. 2016;137(2):571–8.

52. Yoda K, et al. Stochastic secretion response to transient stimulus of Goup-2 innate lymphoid cells (ILC2). Nagoya: IEEE; 2017. https://ieeexplore.ieee.org/document/8305219.

53. Baisch BL, et al. Equivalent titanium dioxide nanoparticle deposition by intratracheal instillation and whole body inhalation: the effect of dose rate on acute respiratory tract inflammation. Part Fibre Toxicol. 2014;11:5.

54. Nurkiewicz TR, et al. Pulmonary nanoparticle exposure disrupts systemic microvascular nitric oxide signaling. Toxicol Sci. 2009;110(1):191–203.

55. Stone KC, et al. Distribution of lung cell numbers and volumes between alveolar and nonalveolar tissue. Am Rev Respir Dis. 1992;146(2):454–6.

56. Nichols CE, et al. Reactive oxygen species damage drives cardiac and mitochondrial dysfunction following acute nano-titanium dioxide inhalation exposure. Nanotoxicology. 2018;12(1):32–48.

57. Drake LY, Kita H. Group 2 innate lymphoid cells in the lung. Adv Immunol. 2014;124:1–16.

58. Duerr CU, Fritz JH. Isolation of group 2 innate lymphoid cells from mouse lungs. Methods Mol Biol. 2017;1656:253–61.

59. Halim TY, Takei F. Isolation and characterization of mouse innate lymphoid cells. Curr Protoc Immunol. 2014;106:3 25 1–13.

60. Liu X, et al. Anti-IL-33 antibody treatment inhibits airway inflammation in a murine model of allergic asthma. Biochem Biophys Res Commun. 2009; 386(1):181–5.

Vasomotor function in rat arteries after ex vivo and intragastric exposure to food-grade titanium dioxide and vegetable carbon particles

Ditte Marie Jensen[1], Daniel Vest Christophersen[1], Majid Sheykhzade[2], Gry Freja Skovsted[3], Jens Lykkesfeldt[3], Rasmus Münter[4], Martin Roursgaard[1], Steffen Loft[1] and Peter Møller[1*]

Abstract

Background: Humans are continuously exposed to particles in the gastrointestinal tract. Exposure may occur directly through ingestion of particles via food or indirectly by removal of inhaled material from the airways by the mucociliary clearance system. We examined the effects of food-grade particle exposure on vasomotor function and systemic oxidative stress in an ex vivo study and intragastrically exposed rats.

Methods: In an ex vivo study, aorta rings from naïve Sprague-Dawley rats were exposed for 30 min to food-grade TiO_2 (E171), benchmark TiO_2 (Aeroxide P25), food-grade vegetable carbon (E153) or benchmark carbon black (Printex 90). Subsequently, the vasomotor function was assessed in wire myographs. In an in vivo study, lean Zucker rats were exposed intragastrically once a week for 10 weeks to vehicle, E171 or E153. Doses were comparable to human daily intake. Vasomotor function in the coronary arteries and aorta was assessed using wire myographs. Tetrahydrobiopterin, ascorbate, malondialdehyde and asymmetric dimethylarginine were measured in blood as markers of oxidative stress and vascular function.

Results: Direct exposure of E171 to aorta rings ex vivo increased the acetylcholine-induced vasorelaxation and 5-hydroxytryptamine-induced vasocontraction. E153 only increased acetylcholine-induced vasorelaxation, and Printex 90 increased the 5-hydroxytryptamine-induced vasocontraction, whereas Aeroxide P25 did not affect the vasomotor function. In vivo exposure showed similar results as ex vivo exposure; increased acetylcholine-induced vasorelaxation in coronary artery segments of E153 and E171 exposed rats, whereas E171 exposure altered 5-hydroxytryptamine-induced vasocontraction in distal coronary artery segments. Plasma levels of markers of oxidative stress and vascular function showed no differences between groups.

Conclusion: Gastrointestinal tract exposure to E171 and E153 was associated with modest albeit statistically significant alterations in the vasocontraction and vasorelaxation responses. Direct particle exposure to aorta rings elicited a similar type of response. The vasomotor responses were not related to biomarkers of systemic oxidative stress.

Keywords: Vasomotor function, E153, E171, Vegetable carbon, Titanium dioxide, Nanoparticles, Oxidative stress, Gastrointestinal exposure, Endothelial dysfunction

* Correspondence: pemo@sund.ku.dk
[1]Department of Public Health, Section of Environmental Health, Faculty of Health and Medical Sciences, University of Copenhagen, Øster Farimagsgade 5A, Building 5B, 2nd Floor, DK-1014 Copenhagen K, Denmark
Full list of author information is available at the end of the article

Background

Humans are continuously exposed to particles through the gastrointestinal (GI) tract. Particles are widely used in food products and drugs as pigments or as additives. Another important source of oral exposure is inhaled particles because particles in the upper respiratory tract are removed by the mucociliary clearance system and subsequently swallowed [1]. It has been estimated that 60% of the inhaled mass of particles is cleared to the stomach after 200 h [2]. Thus, inhalation of pigments such as TiO_2 inadvertently gives rise to GI exposure. Although there is an increase in the use of engineered nanoparticles as food additives, there is limited knowledge about the possible detrimental effects of oral exposure.

There is a relatively large body of literature showing that pulmonary exposure to particles is associated with vasomotor dysfunction and progression of atherosclerosis [3, 4], which are important intermediate steps in the development of cardiovascular disease. The underlying pathophysiological mechanisms are complex and poorly understood; however particle-generated oxidative stress seems to be a key component [5]. We have previously shown that oral exposure to nanosized carbon black in the form of Printex 90 was associated with endothelial dysfunction, which was observed as reduced acetylcholine (ACh)-induced vasorelaxation in the aorta, in both lean and obese Zucker rats [6]. Endothelial dysfunction, a hallmark in development of atherosclerosis, is characterized by endothelial nitric oxide synthase (eNOS) uncoupling and a concomitant shift from production of nitric oxide (NO) to superoxide anion radicals and peroxynitrite. This event results in decreased NO bioavailability, which is associated with vasomotor dysfunction. The increased production of superoxide anion radicals and peroxynitrite promotes a local milieu of oxidative stress in the endothelial cells. Uncoupling of eNOS can be caused by reduced bioavailability of tetrahydrobiopterin (BH_4), which is a cofactor for eNOS [7]. BH_4 reacts readily with reactive oxygen species and is thus susceptible to depletion during oxidative stress [7]. It has been shown that ascorbic acid improves the NO-dependent vasorelaxation in arteries via higher BH_4 bioavailability [8], further emphasizing the role of oxidative stress involved in vasomotor dysfunction. Systemic oxidative stress is also considered to be an important intermediate step in the development of vasomotor dysfunction. Decreased levels of antioxidants (e.g., ascorbic acid) or increased levels of lipid oxidation products such as malondialdehyde (MDA) are typically used as indicators of oxidative stress.

This study aimed to investigate the effect of repeated intragastric administration of food-grade particles on vasomotor function and systemic oxidative stress. Due to the analogy between air pollution particles and nanomaterials, we hypothesize that intragastric exposure to particles could result in similar effects as inhalation exposure. Carbon-based materials such as Printex 90 and other nanomaterials are not likely to be ingested on a regular basis by consumers. However, the European Food and Safety Authority (EFSA) has approved the use of carbon-based material from vegetable origin (E153) and TiO_2 (E171) as food coloring substances [9, 10] and there is no established upper threshold limit of intake. E153 is used as a black colorant in candy and as a pharmaceutical product for the treatment of acute poisoning and diarrhea. E171 is used as a white colorant in e.g., candy and dressings. It should be emphasized that these coloring agents are not nanomaterials per se, although there is a fraction of particles in the nanosize range in the samples. Nevertheless, they are highly relevant materials in particle toxicology because humans are exposed to these particles on a daily basis. First, we compared the effect of E171 and E153 to benchmark counterparts (Aeroxide P25 and Printex 90, respectively) on vasomotor function ex vivo in isolated aorta segments from naïve rats. Aeroxide P25 and Printex 90 have been used extensively in nanotoxicology and inhalation toxicology. We have used Aeroxide P25 and Printex 90 as benchmark particles, but there is not sufficient experimental evidence to regard them as positive controls for cardiovascular disease endpoints. Subsequently, we investigated in vivo effects, i.e., vasomotor function in the aorta and coronary arteries and systemic oxidative stress in lean Zucker rats after repeated oral administration of E171 and E153. The lean Zucker rat was chosen as an animal model, because of previous findings of endothelial dysfunction in the aorta in animals exposed to Printex 90 [6].

We have used one weekly exposure because repeated oral gavages may cause adverse effects in the rats. In addition, there is day-to-day variation in the exposure to E153 and E171, related to the intake of food (i.e. high exposure on certain days and little exposure on other days of the week). According to EFSA, the average daily intake of E171 is 1.8–10.4 mg/kg in children, whereas the 95% percentile is 4.9–32.4 mg/kg per day [10]. This corresponds to average weekly accumulated doses of 34 to 227 mg/kg for high-consumers. In comparison, the intake of E171 is lower in the elderly (mean: 0.4–4.5 mg/kg/day; 95% percentile: 1.2–10.7 mg/kg/day). The vegetable carbon doses were selected from an earlier study with Printex 90 [6]. It has been estimated that the mean dietary exposure to vegetable carbon is 3.0–29.7 and 3.7 mg/kg bw per day in children and adults respectively [9]. The high-level consumers have a daily intake of 15.3–79.1 and 28.1 mg/kg bw in children and adults, respectively [9]. Thus, the doses of E153 (i.e., 0.64 and 6.4 mg/kg) corresponds to the average daily dose in humans. The purpose of the ex vivo study was to compare the effect of the food-grade particles with their respective pigment-grade particles. Thus, the concentrations are rather high as compared to realistic concentrations after intake of E153 and E171. The concentrations of 10 and 100 µg/ml of E153 were identical to previous experiments on Printex 90 in aorta rings from mice [11]. The concentrations of TiO_2 in the ex vivo study was based on the average daily intake in children (i.e. 10.4 mg/kg/day), bodyweight (35 kg), blood volume (2500 ml) and either complete or 10% uptake of particles.

Results

Particle characterization

The particle size was assessed in dry form by transmission electron microscopy (TEM) (Fig. 1 and Table 1). Three size groups for E171 were observed from the TEM images; 135 ± 46 nm, 305 ± 61, 900 ± 247 nm and two size groups of E153; 50 ± 10 nm and 950 ± 200 nm.

The specific surface areas were 1935 and 7.9 m^2/g for E153 and E171, respectively (Table 1). Aeroxide P25 (identical to NM105 in the European Commission's Joint Research Centre) and Printex 90 have been thoroughly characterized in previous investigations [12, 13]. The specific surface areas are 295–338 and 46 m^2/g for Printex 90 and Aeroxide P25, respectively.

The zeta potentials of the E171 and E153 particles in PBS were measured using PALS (phase analysis light

Table 1 Primary particle size, charge and specific surface area of E171 and E153

	DLS Mean (nm)	Particle size (TEM) Mean (nm)	Surface area (BET) m^2/g	Zeta potential mV
E171	19 (1%)	135 ± 46 (27)	7.9	-37.2 ± 2.0
	880 ± 390 (94%)	305 ± 61 (12)		
	3200 (5%)	900 ± 247 (5)		
E153	283 ± 60	50 ± 10 (12)	1935	-24.7 ± 1.6
		950 ± 200 (20)		

Dry particle size was measured by TEM analysis. Three size groups were observed from E171 and two size groups from E153. Surface area was determined by BET analysis. Zeta potential was determined by PALS. The data on TEM, surface area, and zeta potential are expressed as the mean ± SD (number of particles is indicated in the brackets). The hydrodynamic size distribution was also measured by DLS. Three size distributions were observed for E171. Numbers in brackets indicate the intensity distribution

scattering) and M3-PALS. E171 had a zeta potential of -37.2 ± 2.0 mV and E153 of -24.7 ± 1.6 mV (Table 1). The results from single PALS measurements gave unusually high fluctuations; thus the hydrodynamic particle size was also measured with DLS on the same instrument. The DLS analysis showed a presence of microparticles (i.e. size of 6 µm and larger) and the suspension was not stable. The fluctuations in the zeta potential measurements might be caused by noise from aggregation of particles or sedimentation during the measurement.

The hydrodynamic particle size distribution was measured by the Nanoparticle Tracking Analysis (NTA)

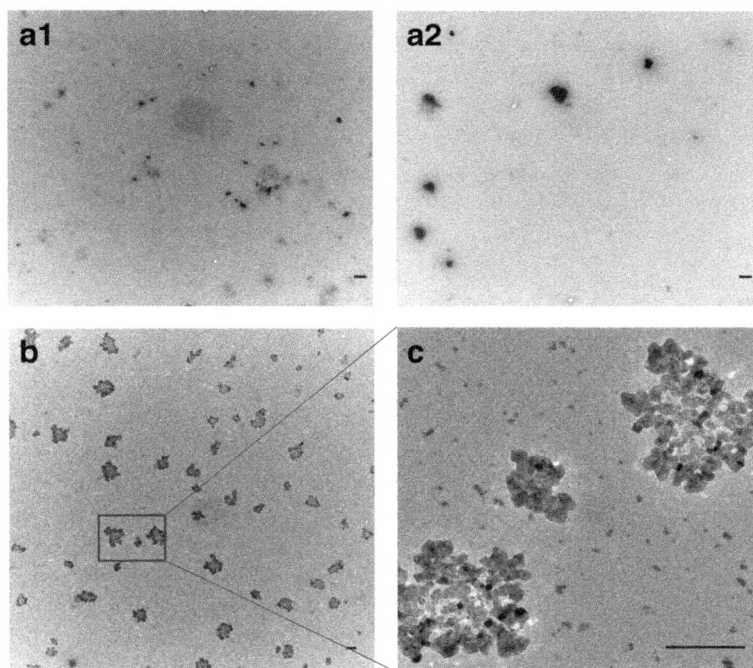

Fig. 1 TEM images of E153 and E171. Dry particle size and morphology of E153 and E171 was determined by TEM images. (**a1**) and (**a2**) are images of E171, magnification 5800×. Three size groups of E171 particles were observed in the pictures. (**b**) and (**c**) are images of E153, magnification 5800× (**b**) and 44,000× (**c**). Two size groups of particles were observed for E153. Scale bars are 500 nm

(Table 2). Particles were suspended in DMEM in the ex vivo study and filtered water + 2% fetal bovine serum (FBS) in the in vivo study. Graphs of the hydrodynamic particle size distribution analysis are shown in Fig. 2. E171 and E153, dispersed in DMEM or filtered water, had a similar hydrodynamic particle size (E171: 203 ± 75 nm in DMEM and 270 ± 25 nm in filtered water; E153, 204 ± 58 nm in DMEM and 230 ± 24 nm in filtered water) (Table 2). Only 10% of the food-grade particles in DMEM suspensions were below 100 nm, whereas 50% of the benchmark particles (Aeroxide P25 and Printex 90) were below 100 nm.

Ex vivo effect of food-grade and benchmark particles on the vasomotor function

Aorta rings from naïve rats were incubated for 30 min with E171 (14 µg/ml and 140 µg/ml), E153 (10 µg/ml and 140 µg/ml), Aeroxide P25 (14 µg/ml and 140 µg/ml) or Printex 90 (10 µg/ml and 100 µg/ml). We used a 30 min incubation period because it has been shown that ex vivo exposure to Printex 90 decreased ACh-induced vasorelaxation and increased the vasocontraction response to phenylephrine in aorta rings after exposure to 100 µg/ml for 30 min [11].

The vessel rings were exposed to cumulative increasing concentrations of vasoactive compounds to assess ACh-induced endothelium-dependent vasorelaxation (Fig. 3), nitroglycerine (NTG)-induced endothelium-independent vasorelaxation (Fig. 4) or 5-hydroxytryptamine (5-HT)-induced vasocontraction (Fig. 5). Log EC_{50} and E_{max} values of the vasomotor responses are shown in Table 3. The analysis demonstrated a slightly increased maximal effect value (E_{max}) of the ACh-dependent vasorelaxation in E171 and E153 exposed aorta rings (56.3%, 95% CI: 52.5–61.3%) and 57.5% (95% CI: 52.7–64.6%) respectively, compared to control group of 42.9% (95% CI: 38.7–48.6%) (Fig. 3). There were no differences in the NTG-mediated

endothelium-independent vasorelaxation response (Fig. 4). As expected, co-incubation with N^G-nitro-L-arginine methyl ester (L-NAME), an inhibitor of NOS, in the organ bath abolished the ACh-mediated vasorelaxation (Fig. 3). Thus, the results indicate an altered endothelium-dependent vasorelaxation response. The E171 and Printex 90 exposure also increased the E_{max} value of the 5-HT-mediated vasocontraction (Fig. 5). There was no effect on vasomotor when exposing rings with Aeroxide P25.

In vivo effect of food-grade particles on the vasomotor function in rats after intragastric administration of E171 and E153

The vasomotor function in coronary arteries and aorta were assessed in rats after intragastric administration of E171, E153 or vehicle, once a week for 10 weeks. The Log EC_{50} and E_{max} values are shown in Table 4. The maximal ACh-mediated endothelium-dependent vasorelaxation response was slightly increased in the proximal left anterior descending (LAD) artery of the low-dose E153 exposed rats (111.1%, 95% CI: 104.3–119.1%) compared to the control group of 98.2% (95% CI: 94.5–102.0%) (Fig. 6). There was also increased maximal ACh-mediated endothelium-dependent vasorelaxation response in the distal LAD in the high-dose E153 exposed rats (111.5%, 95% CI: 103.5–120.6%) compared to the control group of 93.3% (95% CI: 87.1–100.4%), and in the high-dose E171 exposed rats (112.0%, 95% CI: 101.9–124.7%), whereas there was no difference in the aorta (Fig. 6). The E_{max} value of the NTG-mediated endothelium-independent vasorelaxation response was unaffected (Fig. 7). The $LogEC_{50}$ of the E171 high-dose exposed rats was shifted to the left (– 7.8, 95% CI: -8.0 to – 7.7) compared to the control (– 7.5, 95% CI: -7.6 to – 7.4). This effect was not observed in any of the other exposures and segments. Overall, the findings on the NTG- and ACh- mediated responses suggest that the altered ACh-mediated vasorelaxation response is indeed an endothelium-dependent effect on the vasomotor function. The 5-HT-mediated vasocontraction response was increased in the distal (50 mg/kg) LAD (Fig. 8).

Biochemical parameters in plasma of rats after intragastric administration of E171 and E153

Plasma levels of vitamin C (calculated as ascorbate + dehydroascorbic acid (DHA; an oxidized form of ascorbate)), BH_4 and the oxidized form dihydrobiopterin (BH_2), asymmetric dimethylarginine (ADMA) and L-arginine (L-Arg) were measured to assess systemic oxidative stress and imbalances in the NO bioavailability. ADMA competes with arginine as a substrate for eNOS and functions as an endogenous eNOS inhibitor. Increased plasma levels of ADMA have been observed in

Table 2 Hydrodynamic particle size of E171 and E153 in suspension vehicle for the ex vivo and in vivo studies

	NTA				
	Mean (nm)	Mode (nm)	D10 (nm)	D50 (nm)	D90 (nm)
Ex vivo Study					
E171	203 ± 75	264 ± 135	77 ± 69	179 ± 84	363 ± 126
Aeroxide P25	101 ± 58	128 ± 120	27 ± 17	79 ± 56	204 ± 121
E153	204 ± 58	291 ± 130	79 ± 45	192 ± 70	340 ± 112
Printex 90	166 ± 27	224 ± 119	35 ± 20	13 ± 20	339 ± 72
In vivo Study					
E171	270 ± 25	298 ± 58	163 ± 19	266 ± 28	374 ± 26
E153	230 ± 24	227 ± 61	137 ± 17	211 ± 24	347 ± 33

Hydrodynamic size distribution of particles used in the ex vivo and the in vivo study was measured by the Nanoparticle Tracking Analysis (NTA). The data are expressed as the mean, mode, distribution fractions D10, D50 and D90, ± SD. Each experiment was repeated three times on different days

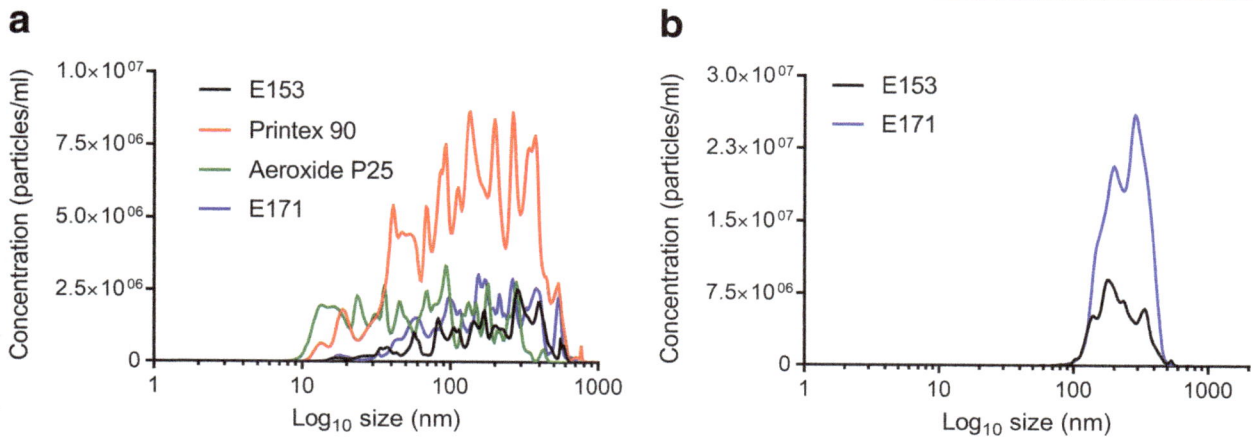

Fig. 2 Hydrodynamic particle size distribution. The hydrodynamic size of the particles was determined with NanoSight LM20 and the Nanoparticle Tracking Analysis software 3.0. Particles used in the ex vivo study was dispersed in DMEM (**a**). Particles used in the in vivo study was dispersed in 0.45 μm filtered sterile water added 2% FBS (**b**). The data are presented as the mean particle size (nm) from three independent experiments. On each experimental day the mean of five following measurements were used

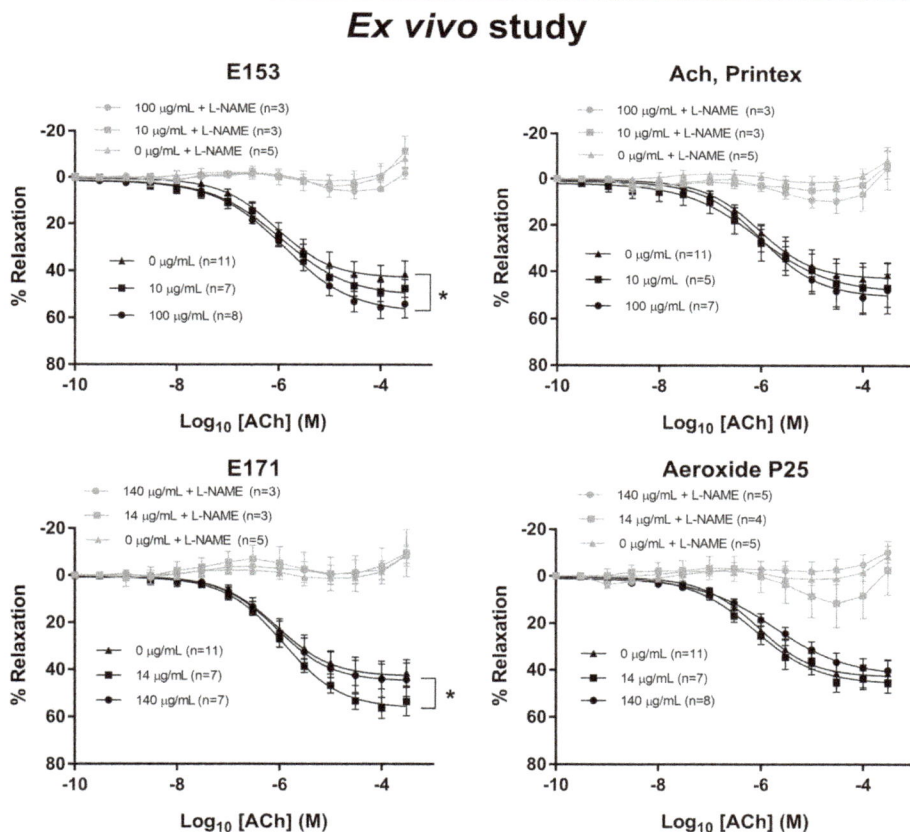

Fig. 3 Acetylcholine (ACh)-induced endothelium-dependent vasorelaxation of rat aorta segments exposed ex vivo to particles. The measurements were performed with and without the addition of the NOS inhibitor, L-NAME. The acetylcholine response is expressed as the % relaxation of the pre-contraction tension produced by PGF_{2a}. Each point on the curves represents the cumulative response at each concentration of acetylcholine. The data are presented as the mean ± SEM, n indicates the number of animals. An asterisk (*) denote a statistically significant effect on E_{max} compared to the control group ($P < 0.05$)

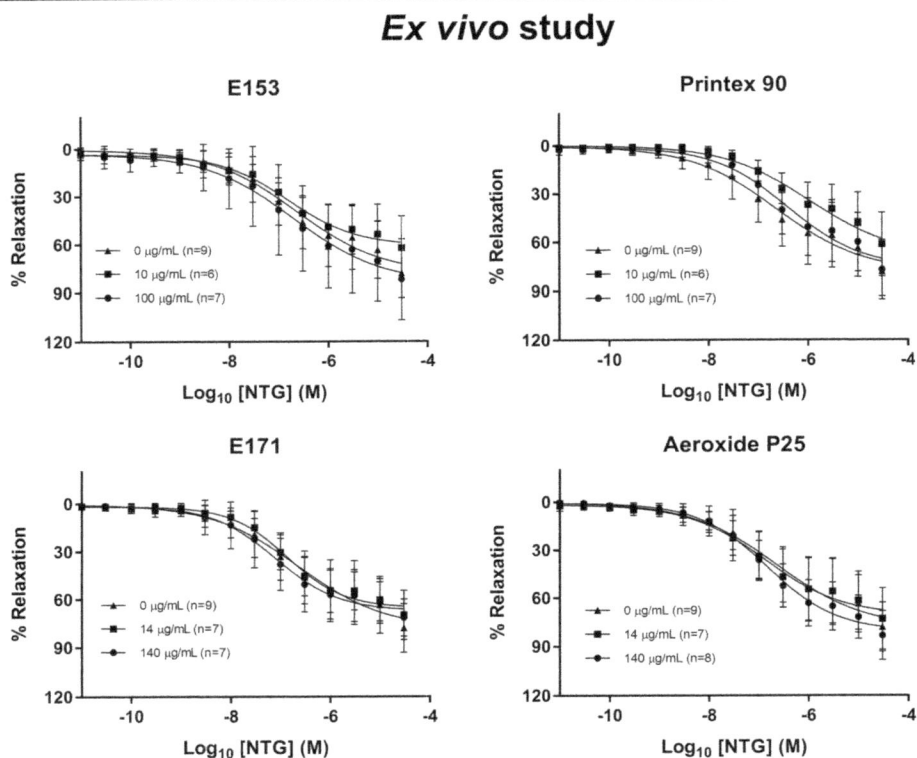

Fig. 4 Nitroglycerine (NTG)-induced endothelium-independent vasorelaxation of rat aorta segments exposed ex vivo to particles. The nitroglycerine response is expressed as the % relaxation of the pre-contraction tension produced by PGF_{2a}. Each point on the curves represents the cumulative response at each concentration of nitroglycerine. The data are presented as the mean ± SEM, n indicates the number of animals

rats after exposure to concentrated fine ambient air particles [14]. Malondialdehyde (MDA) is a lipid peroxidation product and was measured as a marker of oxidative stress.

In general, the plasma biomarkers were unaltered in particle-exposed rats as compared to controls (Table 5). Collectively, the results on plasma antioxidants (ascorbate and BH_4) and oxidants (i.e., MDA, and BH_2) demonstrated no change in systemic oxidative stress in response to the particle exposure in rats.

Discussion

The results of this study show that in vivo exposure to food-grade TiO_2 (E171) and vegetable carbon (E153) was associated with a slightly altered endothelium-dependent vasorelaxation and vasocontraction response in coronary arteries. The same effects were observed in aorta rings from naïve rats after direct exposure to E171 and E153. This consistency in ex vivo and in vivo responses should be noted, although it is equally important to note that the effects on vasomotor function did not occur in a dose-dependent manner. The study represents an exposure to "real-life" particles in the relevant route of exposure in humans after ingestion of either food or pharmaceuticals. In general, the exposure to

E153 and E171 is higher in children than adults and elderly [9, 10]. Nevertheless, the elderly, patients with pre-existing diseases and adults with cardiometabolic risk factors may be more suspectible to particle-induced cardiovascular disease than children and adolescents.

A systematic review has demonstrated that the majority of studies on particle exposure in animals and humans show reduced endothelium-dependent vasorelaxation and increased vasocontraction response in arteries [15]. The immediate consequence of this effect is an increased tone of the artery, which might be associated with elevated blood pressure. Thus, the increase in both the vasorelaxation and vasocontraction response, as found in the present study, is somewhat surprising, although other studies have demonstrated similar responses. It has been observed that amorphous nano silica particles induced vasorelaxation in thoracic aorta rings of rats ex vivo, which was mediated through NO by activation of PI3K/Akt/eNOS signaling [16]. Earlier studies on high-dose pulmonary exposure to ambient particulate matter also showed increased ACh-dependent vasorelaxation in aorta rings from spontaneously hypertensive rats [17]. The same type of exposure to ambient particulate matter provoked vasorelaxation in aorta rings after ex vivo exposure [18, 19]. In our

Ex vivo study

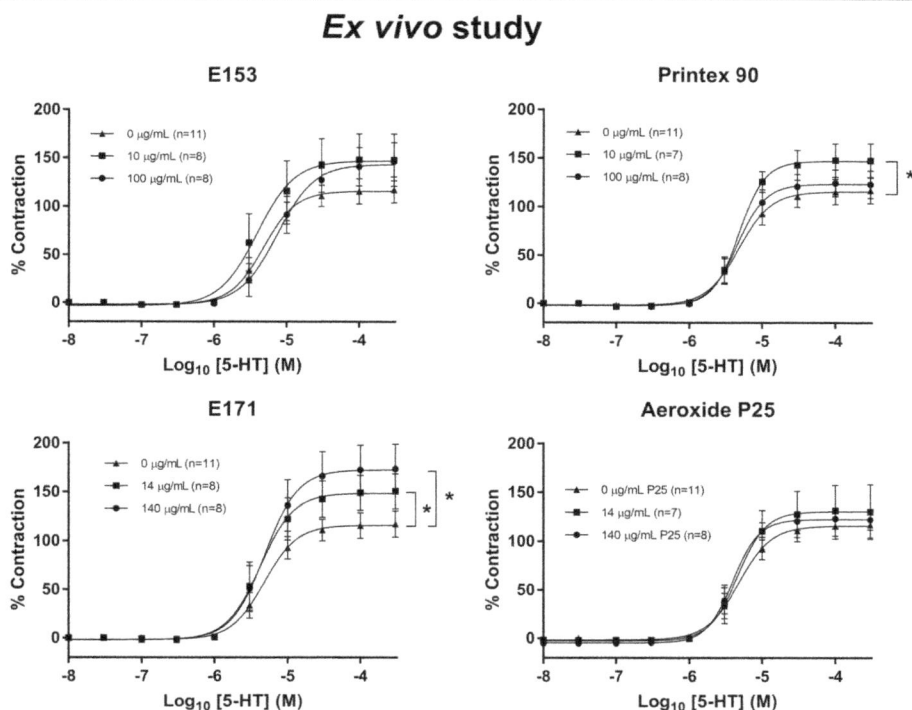

Fig. 5 5-hydroxytryptamine(5-HT)-induced receptor-dependent vasocontraction of rat aorta segments exposed ex vivo to particles. The 5-HT response is expressed as the % maximal contraction induced by stimulation with K^+ before the dose-response measurements. Each point on the curve represents the cumulative response at each concentration of 5-HT. The data are presented as the mean ± SEM, n indicates the number of animals. An asterisk (*) denote a statistically significant effect on E_{max} compared to the control group ($P < 0.05$)

study, the increased vasorelaxation after ACh exposure to vessels may originate from an eNOS-dependent pathway since L-NAME abolished the effect in the ex vivo study and the NTG-mediated vasorelaxation was unaltered. It is possible that the concurrent increase in both vasorelaxation and vasocontraction occur by different mechanisms, although they may also be the product of compensation in the vessel. The effect on vasomotor function was seen in resistance arteries, whereas the aorta (i.e., a conductance artery) was not affected. The endothelium-dependent vasorelaxation in conductance arteries is mainly driven by NO, whereas resistance arteries also use endothelium-derived hyperpolarization factor [20].

The effects on vasomotor function responses in the in vivo study were in the range of 20–40% difference in the distal LAD. To the best of our knowledge, there are no observations on vasomotor function in humans after oral exposure to particles. It has been shown that gastric exposure to nanosized CeO_2 produced a smaller impairment of microvascular function in Sprague-Dawley rats compared to the same dose administered by intratracheal instillation [21]. However, a larger induction of oxidatively damaged DNA has been observed in the liver after oral exposure to Printex 90 compared to the same dose administered by intratracheal instillation to Fisher

F344 rats [22]. Previously, we have obtained less than 10% difference in microvascular function in humans after controlled inhalation exposure to particulate matter and the effect has been strongest in risk groups of cardiovascular disease and elderly [23–29]. The magnitude of the effects on vasomotor function in the present study is modest, but they are also realistic, considering the magnitude of exposure.

The toxicity of nanosized particles is typically considered to be related to inflammation and oxidative stress. We chased this mechanism by analysis of plasma levels of the lipid peroxidation products (MDA) and antioxidants (ascorbate and BH_4). However, these results did not indicate a systemic oxidative stress reaction. It is important to emphasize that MDA was measured with a validated HPLC assay. Likewise, care was taken to secure plasma from spurious oxidation during sampling and processing for the ascorbate and BH_4 assays. It should be noted that some studies have shown associations between exposure to particles and altered vasomotor function without systemic inflammation and oxidative stress [3]. Still, oxidative stress and inflammation may occur in the vascular wall as shown in a study where inhalation of TiO_2 generated microvascular dysfunction, concurrently with increased production of reactive oxygen species and nitrosative stress [30]. Unfortunately, the lack of

Table 3 Log EC_{50} and E_{max} values of concentration-response curves in naïve aorta rings from wild-type rats

	Concentration (μg/ml)	Log EC_{50} (M)			E_{max} (%)		
		ACh	NTG	5-HT	ACh	NTG	5-HT
Control	0	−6.1 (−6.3 to −5.8)	−6.6 (−7.0 to −5.7)	−5.3 (−5.5 to −5.2)	42.9 (38.7–48.6)	78.3 (66.7–113.2)	115.8 (105.1–127.5)
E171	14	−5.9 (−6.1 to −5.7)	−6.9 (−7.1 to −6.6)	−5.4 (−5.6 to −5.2)	56.3* (52.5–61.3)	65.3 (59.9–73.5)	148.5* (131.3–168.2)
	140	−6.1 (−6.4 to −5.6)	−7.1 (−7.4 to −6.7)	−5.3 (−5.5 to −5.1)	44.9 (38.9–55.2)	67.2 (60.4–79.3)	172.7* (151.4–197.3)
Aeroxide P25	14	−6.1 (−6.4 to −5.8)	−6.9 (−7.3 to −6.1)	−5.3 (−5.6 to −5.1)	45.9 (41.8–51.8)	70.8 (61.0–98.8)	130.6 (111.3–152.5)
	140	−5.7 (−6.0 to −5.3)	−6.8 (−7.0 to −6.6)	−5.4 (−5.5 to −5.3)	42.4 (37.7–51.4)	80.5 (73.7–91.3)	122.5 (114.0–131.4)
E153	10	−6.0 (−6.2 to −5.7)	−6.8 (−7.1 to −6.2)	−5.4 (−5.7 to −5.1)	50.4 (45.9–57.5)	61.0 (53.3–79.6)	147.0 (122.7–179.5)
	100	−5.9 (−6.1 to −5.7)	−6.7 (−7.3 to 0.2)	−5.1 (−5.3 to −4.9)	57.5* (52.7–64.6)	84.1 (67.5–514.0)	143.4 (125.7–166.5)
Printex 90	10	−6.1 (−6.7 to −2.1)	−6.0 (−6.5 to −3.4)	−5.3 (ND to −5.2)	48.7 (39.3–161.2)	68.7 (53.0–188.8)	147.1* (134.8–160.0)
	100	−6.0 (−6.3 to −5.6)	−6.4 (−6.8 to −5.6)	−5.3 (−5.5 to −5.2)	50.8 (45.3–59.3)	75.6 (63.9–109.5)	123.6 (112.5–135.4)

The concentration-response curves were performed for acetylcholine (ACh), nitroglycerine (NTG) and 5-hydroxytryptamine (5-HT) on aorta from rats exposed ex vivo to E171, Aeroxide P25, E153 or Printex 90 for 30 min. The data are presented as the mean and 95% CI. The number of animals in each group varied; specified in Figs. 3, 4 and 5. Asterisk (*) denotes statistically significant effects on E_{max} when compared to the effect in the control group ($P < 0.05$), ND: the value could not be determined by non-linear regression analysis

Table 4 Log EC$_{50}$ and E$_{max}$ values of concentration-response curves in aorta and left anterior descending coronary artery (LAD)

	Dose (mg/kg bw/week)	Log EC$_{50}$ (M)			E$_{max}$ (%)		
		Aorta	LAD proximal	LAD distal	Aorta	LAD proximal	LAD distal
ACh							
Control	0	−5.8 (−6.1 to −5.4)	−7.3 (−7.4 to −7.2)	−7.5 (−7.7 to −7.3)	38.9 (34.6–46.0)	98.2 (94.5–102.0)	93.3 (87.1–100.4)
E171	50	−6.0 (−6.7 to −2.3)	−7.5 (−7.6 to −7.4)	−7.6 (−7.7 to −7.4)	43.1 (35.2–131.6)	101.1 (97.6–104.7)	98.0 (92.3–104.5)
	500	−6.1 (−6.6 to −5.1)	−7.2 (−7.4 to −7.1)	−7.6 (−7.9 to −7.3)	49.5 (42.4–75.0)	101.4 (96.1–107.4)	112.0* (101.9–124.7)
E153	0.64	−5.9 (−6.2 to −5.5)	−7.1 (−7.2 to −6.9)	−7.4 (−7.6 to −7.3)	34.6 (30.7–41.4)	111.1* (104.3–119.1)	101.4 (95.9–107.6)
	6.4	−5.9 (−6.4 to −4.3)	−7.5 (−8.0 to −7.2)	−7.4 (−7.6 to −7.2)	40.2 (33.2–74.1)	98.9 (88.5–116.1)	111.5* (103.5–120.6)
NTG							
Control	0	−7.5 (−7.6 to −7.4)	−5.4 (−6.1 to −3.0)	−6.7 (−7.1 to −6.1)	91.0 (87.2–95.6)	153.1 (115.7–365.2)	111.1 (96.8–144.3)
E171	50	−7.5 (−7.7 to −7.2)	−5.2 (−6.0 to −0.1)	−5.9 (−6.4 to −4.7)	89.0 (82.2–99.3)	166.2 (118.7–902.1)	143.0 (117.2–226.7)
	500	−7.8* (−8.0 to −7.7)	−6.6 (−7.3 to 2.6)	−6.2 (−6.7 to −4.9)	94.1 (90.5–98.2)	125.8 (98.9–1086.0)	115.3 (94.8–188.8)
E153	0.64	−7.8 (−8.0 to −7.6)	−5.0 (−5.9 to 0.8)	−6.3 (−6.9 to −6.1)	90.2 (85.1–96.8)	176.0 (122.9–1208.0)	126.4 (98.3–480.6)
	6.4	−7.7 (−7.9 to −7.5)	−6.2 (−6.6 to −5.5)	−6.2 (−7.0 to 17.1)	89.2 (83.8–96.3)	129.5 (111.4–171.2)	142.5 (107.8–26,498.0)
5-HT							
Control	0	−5.2 (−5.3 to −5.0)	−6.2 (−6.4 to −6.0)	−6.0 (−6.2 to −5.9)	125.8 (117.7–135.4)	158.9 (147.5–171.5)	112.2 (104.4–120.9)
E171	50	−5.1 (−5.2 to −5.0)	−6.3 (−6.4 to −6.1)	−6.2 (−6.4 to −6.0)	128.4 (120.7–137.8)	152.2 (144.1–160.7)	155.4* (141.5–171.3)
	500	−5.2 (−5.4 to −5.0)	−6.2 (−6.6 to −5.8)	−6.1 (−6.3 to −5.8)	113.9 (100.4–132.5)	126.9 (111.5–149.5)	113.7 (102.6–126.7)
E153	0.64	−5.0 (−5.1 to −4.9)	−6.3 (−6.6 to −5.9)	−6.2 (−6.4 to −5.9)	130.8 (122.2–141.1)	172.4 (152.6–201.3)	115.1 (102.6–128.7)
	6.4	−5.1 (−5.3 to −6.0)	−6.3 (−6.6 to −6.0)	6.1 (−6.3 to −5.9)	123.5 (115.2–133.6)	132.8 (119.4–148.9)	112.2 (103.9–121.9)

The concentration-response curves were performed for acetylcholine (ACh), nitroglycerine (NTG) and 5-hydroxytryptamine (5-HT) on the aorta and coronary arteries from rats exposed intragastrically to E171 or E153 once a week for 10 weeks. The data are presented as mean and 95% CI. The number of animals in each group varied; specified in the concentration-response curves (Figs. 6, 7 and 8). An asterisk (*) denotes statistically significant effects when compared to the effect in the control group ($P < 0.05$)

In vivo study

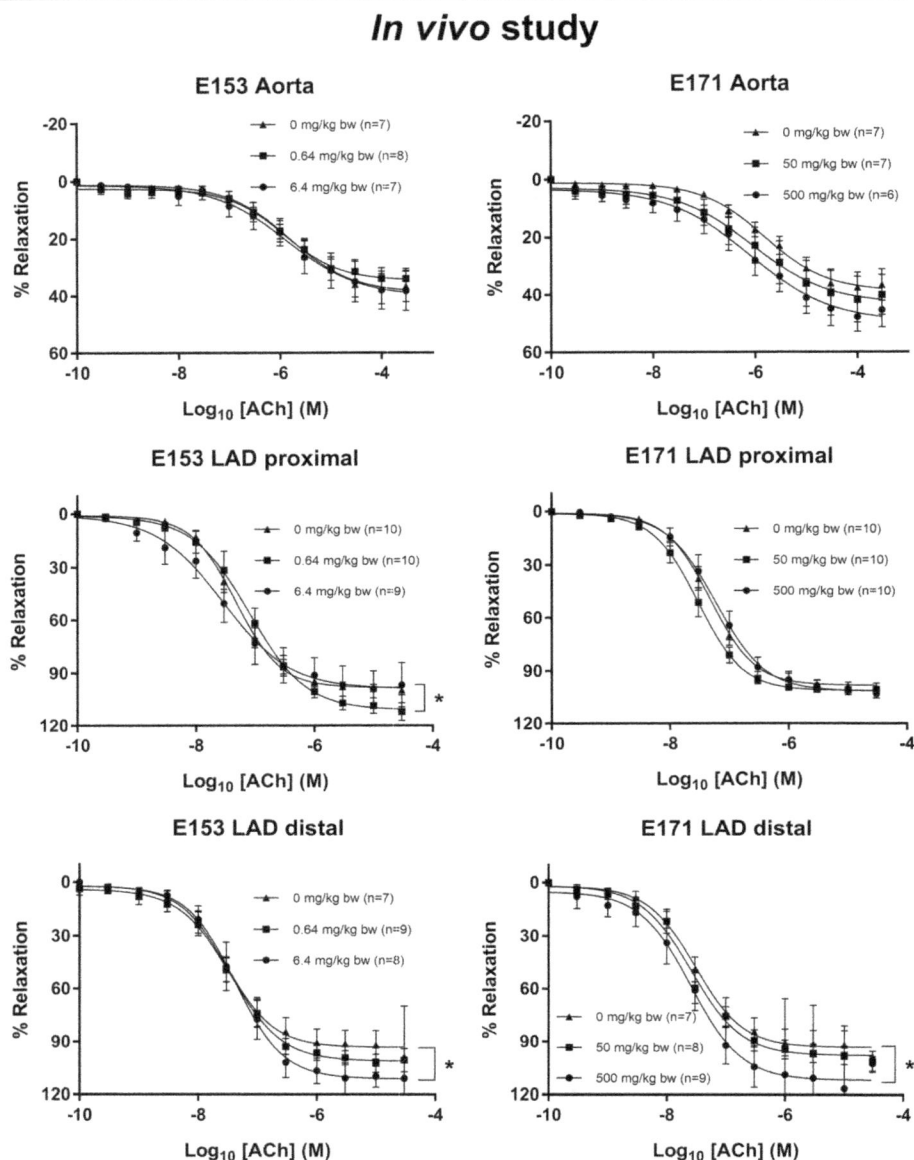

Fig. 6 Acetylcholine (ACh)-induced endothelium-dependent vasorelaxation of artery segments from rats exposed intragastrically to particles. The acetylcholine response is expressed as the % relaxation of the pre-contraction tension produced by PGF_{2a}. Each point on the curves represents the cumulative response at each concentration of acetylcholine. The data are presented as the mean ± SEM, n indicates the number of animals. An asterisk (*) denote a statistically significant effect on E_{max} compared to the control group ($P < 0.05$)

oxidative stress indicators in plasma leaves the study without a link in the causal pathway from external exposure to the observed vasomotor function response in the in vivo study. Nevertheless, we speculate that the altered vasomotor response may be due to bioactive components in plasma that interact with the cellular signaling (e.g., NO production or delivery from endothelial cells to smooth muscle cells) or increases the response to vasoactive drugs. Previously, we have shown that plasma from Printex 90 exposed mice caused vasocontraction in aorta rings from naïve mice [31]. This type of

bioactivity has been described in various studies on pulmonary exposure to particulate matter [32]. Unfortunately, we did not have sufficient plasma to measure plasma bioactivity.

The ex vivo experiments indicated that E171 and E153 could generate the same effects as observed in vivo after oral exposure. In a previous study, we observed that fine, nanosized and photocatalytic TiO_2 increased the surface expression of cell adhesion molecules in human umbilical vein endothelial cells without concurrent generation of reactive oxygen species [33]. We used Printex 90 as a

In vivo study

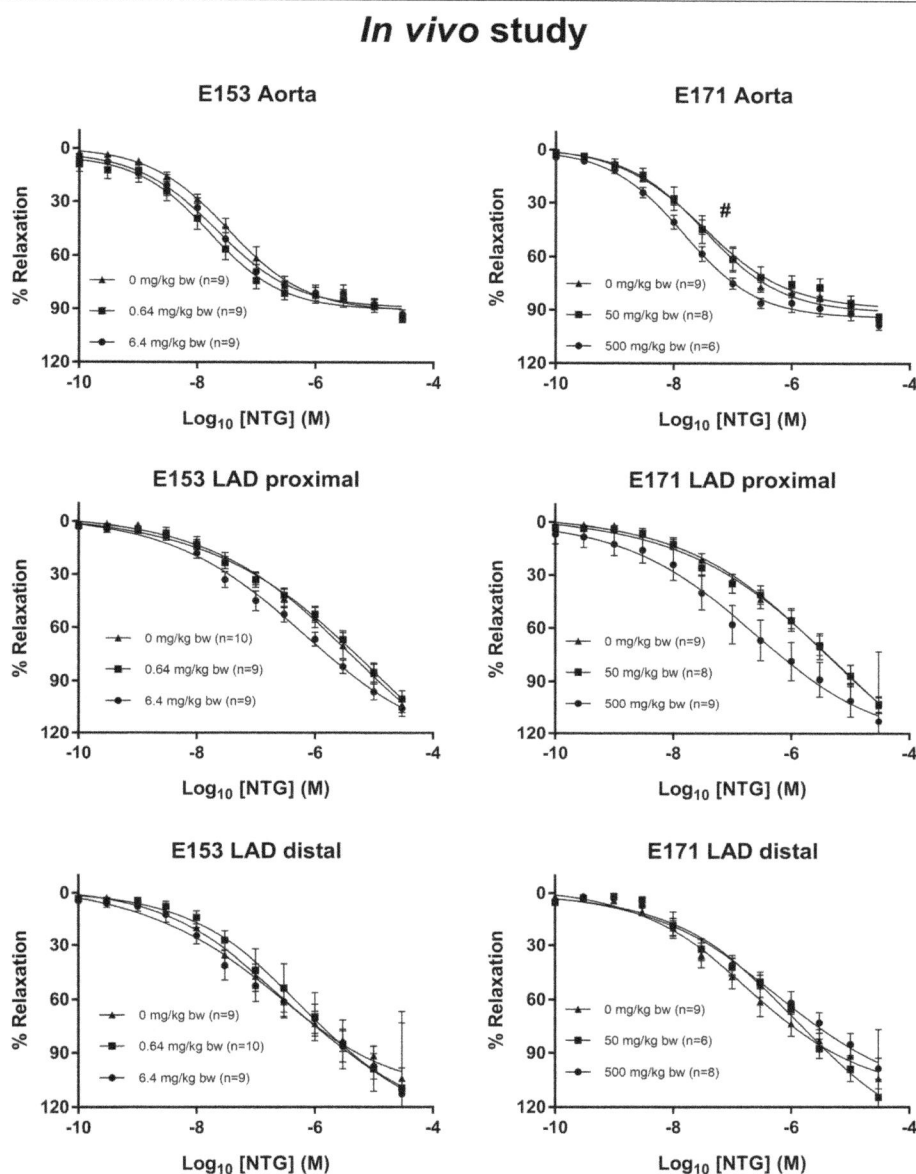

Fig. 7 Nitroglycerine-induced endothelium-independent vasorelaxation of artery segments from rats exposed intragastrically to particles. The nitroglycerine response is expressed as the % relaxation of the pre-contraction tension produced by PGF_{2a}. Each point on the curves represents the cumulative response at each concentration of nitroglycerine. The data are presented as the mean ± SEM, *n* indicates the number of animals. # denotes a statistically significant effect on log EC_{50} compared to the control group ($P < 0.05$)

benchmark particle, which previously demonstrated increased phenylephrine-mediated vasocontraction in mice aorta rings following exposure to 100 μg/ml [11]. The ACh-vasorelaxation response was mixed in the sense that it was associated with a decreased response at 10 μg/ml and increased response at 100 μg/ml [11]. However, it should be noted that the exposure conditions were different as the aorta rings were exposed directly in the organ bath in the mouse study while in the present study, rat aorta rings were exposed to particles before they were mounted in the organ bath. Also, there

is a clear difference in species. In our previous study, we also exposed rat mesenteric arteries to Printex 90 in a pressure myograph, which demonstrated a decrease in the vessel diameter, indicating an overall vasocontraction response to Printex 90.

We did not measure cytotoxicity in the ex vivo study because the exposure only lasted 30 min, which is too short to detect a reliable response by conventional techniques such as the lactate dehydrogenase activity and WST-1 assays. In a previous study we did not observe statistically significant increases in cytotoxicity in human

In vivo study

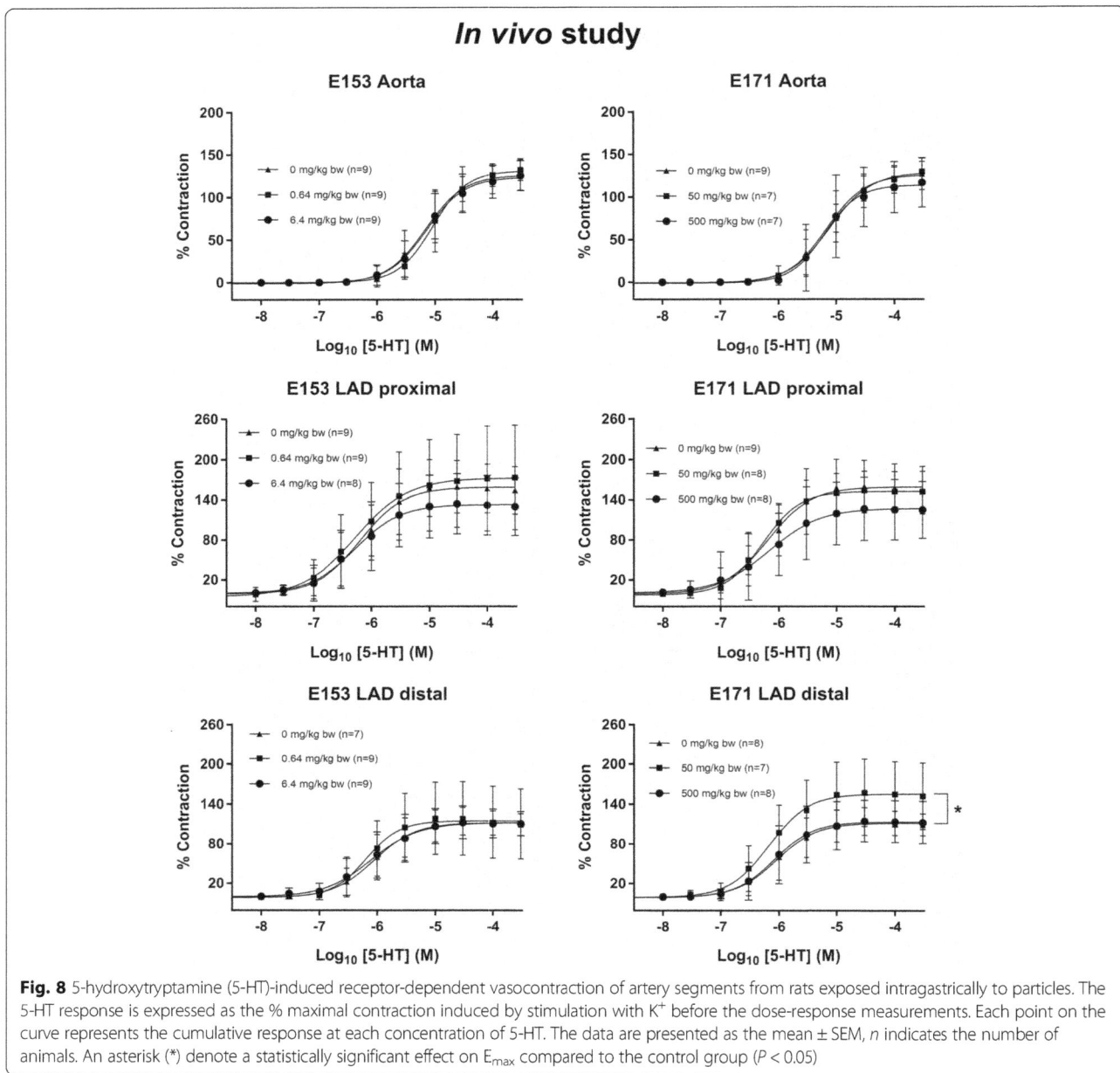

Fig. 8 5-hydroxytryptamine (5-HT)-induced receptor-dependent vasocontraction of artery segments from rats exposed intragastrically to particles. The 5-HT response is expressed as the % maximal contraction induced by stimulation with K^+ before the dose-response measurements. Each point on the curve represents the cumulative response at each concentration of 5-HT. The data are presented as the mean ± SEM, n indicates the number of animals. An asterisk (*) denote a statistically significant effect on E_{max} compared to the control group ($P < 0.05$)

Table 5 Biochemical parameters in lean Zucker rats after repeated exposure to E171 and E153 by oral gavage

In vivo Study	Control (n = 9)	E171 (n = 9)	E171 (n = 10)	E153 (n = 10)	E153 (n = 8)
Dose (mg/kg bw/week)	0	50	500	0.64	6.4
Vitamin C (μM) (ascorbate + DHA)	19.6 ± 2.9	20.3 ± 2.6	21.0 ± 4.6	20.5 ± 3.9	18.9 ± 2.9
MDA (μM)	0.20 ± 0.05	0.19 ± 0.08	0.22 ± 0.07	0.20 ± 0.07	0.19 ± 0.05
BH_4 (nM)	150.1 ± 20.4	149.2 ± 18.9	154.8 ± 43.7	151.5 ± 20.5	134.5 ± 27.4
BH_4/BH_2 ratio (nM)	0.20 ± 0.04	0.18 ± 0.04	0.19 ± 0.04	0.17 ± 0.05	0.21 ± 0.05
ADMA (μM)	178.1 ± 31.8	192.3 ± 41.0	179.1 ± 47.0	219.8 ± 118.1	215.1 ± 89.4
L-arginine (μM)	51.0 ± 8.8	61.8 ± 15.8	58.3 ± 16.9	75.5 ± 54.1	75.1 ± 35.5

All biochemical parameters were measured in plasma samples taken at the time of sacrifice. bw: body weight, *DHA* dehydroascorbic acid, *MDA* malondialdehyde, *BH4* tetrahydrobiopterin, *BH2* dihydrobiopterin, *ADMA* asymmetric dimethylarginine. Data are represented as mean ± SD

umbilical vein endothelial cells (HUVECs) after 3 or 24 h exposure to Printex 90 [34]. Equivocal results on Printex 90 in HUVECs were observed after 24-h exposure periods as there was 20% increase in lactate dehydrogenase (LDH) activity assay, whereas the WST-1 assay was unaltered after exposure to 100 µg/ml) [11]. On the other hand, a fine size carbon black (Flammrus 101) did not generate cytotoxicity in the LDH assay [33]. TiO_2 has low toxicity as compared to other nanomaterials [35]. We have obtained mixed results with TiO_2 in HUVECs; one study showed no effect of fine and photocatalytic TiO_2 particles, whereas a nanosized sample generated approximately 20% cytotoxicity (LDH assay) [33]. Another study actually showed a rather large effect in the WST-1 assay after exposure to 7 nm anatase TiO_2 and some rutile forms [36]. It should be noted that HUVECs are adherent cells and the exposure may increase during the incubation period because of sedimentation of particles, whereas the aorta rings were exposed in suspension in the present study. In addition, there is no consensus about the role of cytotoxicity in ex vivo studies on vasomotor function. In genotoxicology, it is recommended that the level of cytotoxicity should not increase more than 30% in assays for DNA damage such as the comet assay [37].

There is no consistency in the available literature concerning the uptake of TiO_2 to the circulation [38]. Earlier studies on micro size (500 nm) TiO_2 in rats demonstrated a relatively high fraction of absorption (approximately 6.5% of the administered dose) after exposure by oral gavage to 12.5 mg/kg per day for 10 days [39]. However, a recent study demonstrated only 0.6% absorption after a single small dose of radioactively labeled 70 nm TiO_2 nanoparticles in rats [40]. E171 mainly consists of micro-sized TiO_2 particles, with less than 3.2% of the mass in the nanoscale range [10]. Taking the dose level and particle size into consideration, the exposure in our study may be more similar to the observations of translocation of micro-sized particles in rats.

Nevertheless, it appears safe to assume that the translocation is low. Uptake of TiO_2 to the systemic circulation has been described in humans [41]. It is even more unclear whether carbon-based particles translocate to the systemic circulation because it is more difficult to measure carbon material than metals in tissues.

Conclusion

This study shows that 10 weeks of intragastric exposure to vegetable carbon (E151) or food-grade TiO_2 (E171) was associated with modest albeit statistically significant alterations in the vasomotor response in coronary arteries, without evidence of systemic oxidative stress.

Methods
Particles

E153 (Norit N.V., Amersfoort, The Netherlands, distributed by Medic Team A/S, Allerød, Denmark) was purchased as an over-the-counter drug in a local pharmacy. Each package contained 30 gelatine capsules with 200 mg vegetable carbon powder. Norit is marketed as a drug for treatment of acute poisoning and diarrhea; it is commonly described as "activated charcoal" or "activated carbon". The gelatine capsule was discharged, and the internal powder content was stored in a sterile container. Food-grade TiO_2 was bought as a white coloring agent (E171) at a Danish webshop (www.bolsjehuset.dk). Aeroxide P25 was obtained from Sigma-Aldrich (product number 718467, declared primary particle size of 21 nm). Printex 90 was kindly supplied from Degussa-Hüls, Frankfurt, Germany (declared primary particle size of 14 nm).

We characterized E171 and E153 with both transmission electron microscopy and specific surface areas. The latter used nitrogen adsorption according to the Brunauer, Emmet and Teller method [42]. The analysis was performed at Quantachrome Instruments (LabQMC, Boynton Beach, FL, USA). Particles were suspended in water with 2% FBS in a concentration of 100 µg/ml for the visualization in TEM. A few drops of the suspension were applied on TEM grids and dried [43]. Afterwards the TEM grids were inspected in a Phillips CM20 transmission microscope at 5800 and 44,000 magnification. We measured the size of individual particles using ImageJ software (https://imagej.nih.gov) on digital images from two different grids, which were prepared on the same day of analysis.

Zeta potential was measured on a Brookhaven ZetaPALS (Brookhaven Instruments, Holtsville NY, USA) and a Zetasizer Nano ZS (Malvern Instruments, Malvern, UK). E171 and E153 were sonicated for 30 min at 60 Hz using a VWR UltraSonic Cleaner (VWR, Radnor PA, USA) and diluted to 0.2 mg/mL in PBS (P4417, Sigma). Measurements were on both instruments performed using a dip cell. On the ZetaPALS instrument, ten runs on three different particle suspensions were done, on the Zetasizer, three runs were done on the same samples. Reported values in Table 1 are from the Zetasizer, the encountered fluctuations in signal were observed on the ZetaPALS.

The hydrodynamic particle size in suspension was determined by the Nanoparticle Tracking Analysis (NTA). The particles were sonicated as described below and diluted to a final concentration of approximately 10 µg/ml. The samples were analyzed on a NanoSight LM20 (Nanosight Ltd., Malvern Instruments, Malvern, UK) with a blue (450 nm) laser. All measurements were repeated on three different days. On each experimental day, five consecutive measurements on the same particle suspension were assessed, and the mean was used for data analysis.

For the ex vivo and in vivo study particle stock suspensions were prepared by dispersing particles in either 0.45 μm filtered sterile water added 2% FBS (ref. 10,500–064, Gibco®) (in vivo study) or DMEM cell culture medium (Dulbecco's modified eagle medium, D5796, Sigma) (ex vivo study), using a Branson Sonifier mounted with a disruptor horn (Model S-450D, Branson Ultrasonics Corp., Danbury, CT, USA) in the in vivo study or using a Vibra Cell Vc50t, Ultrasonic Processor 20 kHz (R125136, Sonics & Materials, Newtown, Connecticut, USA) in the ex vivo study. Stock suspensions were sonicated for 16 min without pause and continuously cooled on ice, according to the recommendations in the protocol that was developed for the EU Framework 7 project "Risk assessment of engineered nanoparticles" (ENPRA; http://www.enpra.eu). Stock suspension concentrations were in the ex vivo study 1.4 mg/ml for E171 and Aeroxide P25 and 1.0 mg/ml for E153 and Printex 90. Stock suspensions for the in vivo study were 120 mg/ml for E171 and 1.6 mg/ml for E153. The stock solutions were prepared the same day of use and used immediately after sonication (vortexed before use) after dilution with dispersion media to final concentrations.

Animal model and study design

Ex vivo study

Eleven female Sprague-Dawley rats were purchased from Taconic (Ejby, Denmark). The rats were aged between 14 and 17 weeks when sacrificed and weighed 297 ± 21 g. The rats were acclimatized for minimum 1 week before entering the study. The rats were housed in pairs, in an enriched environment, with free access to tap water and standard chow. The cages were housed in an animal facility with a 12 h day-night cycle in a temperature (20–24 °C) and moisture (55%) controlled room. At the day of the experiment, one rat was sacrificed. The rat was anesthetized with a subcutaneous injection (in the lower back) of a combination of hypnorm (fentanyl 0.315 mg/ml and fluanisone 10 mg/ml) and dormicum (midazolam, 5 mg/ml) (0.3 ml/100 g bw), and decapitated following deep anesthesia and concomitant disappearance of voluntary reflexes. The heart with the aorta was isolated and put in a glass vial containing ice-cold PSS buffer, until dissection in the laboratory facilities immediately thereafter. PSS had the following composition: 119.0 mM NaCl, 4.7 mM KCl, 1.5 mM $CaCl_2$, 1.2 mM $MgSO_4$, 1.2 KH_2PO_4 mM, 0.027 EDTA mM, 6.05 mM glucose, 25.0 mM $NaHCO_3$. pH was 7.4 when the solution was gassed with 95% O_2 and 5% CO_2 mixture. The aorta was dissected free of fat- and connective tissue in a petri dish containing ice cold PSS and cut into segments of approximately 2 mm in length and incubated for 30 min in particle suspension (DMEM) (in a 12-well plate/2 ml per well) at 37 °C with 5% CO_2. Particles and concentrations were either E171 (14 or 140 μg/ml), Aeroxide P25 (14 or 140 μg/ml), E153 (10 or 100 μg/ml) or Printex 90 (10 or 100 μg/ml). After the exposure to particles, the aorta rings were carefully washed in a physiological saline solution (PSS) and mounted in a wire myograph. Each segment was normalized to a standard pressure of 13.3 kPa, and an internal circumference (IC) set to 90% (IC_{90}) of the IC_{100} (pressure at 100 mmHg). After a 30 min equilibration period, the rings were stimulated with a high potassium concentration to test their viability and then preconstricted with prostaglandin $F_{2\alpha}$ ($PGF_{2\alpha}$) before vasorelaxation studies. There was no difference between the precontraction ability of aorta rings that had been exposed to particles or vehicle (results not shown). The rings were challenged with vasoactive compounds as described below.

In vivo study

Lean Zucker rats were used because of previous findings of endothelial dysfunction in aorta rings in this strain after exposure to Printex 90 [6]. The study showed similar vasomotor dysfunction response in both lean and obese Zucker rats, and therefore the less expensive lean Zucker rat was chosen as a model animal in this study. The obese Zucker rat is an animal model for metabolic syndrome, and it develops vasomotor dysfunction [6, 44].

Fifty, female lean Zucker rats (Crl:ZUC-Lepr^{fa}, strain code 138), were purchased from Charles River (distributed in Denmark by Scanbur, Karlslunde, Denmark). The rats were between 8 and 13 weeks of age and acclimatized for at least 1 week before entering the study. All rats were randomly assigned to one of five exposure groups; vehicle, low-dose E153 (0.64 mg/kg bw/week), high-dose E153 (6.4 mg/kg bw/week), low-dose E171 (50 mg/kg bw/week) or high-dose E171 (500 mg/kg bw/week). Each exposure group included ten rats. The group size was based on a power calculation of previous results on vasomotor function in the aorta of Printex 90 exposed lean Zucker rats [6] (calculations not shown). The rats were housed in pairs in cages with standard bedding and nesting materials. Rats, living in the same cage, were assigned to the same exposure, to avoid the possibility of cross-contamination of particles via, e.g., ingestion of stool pellets. The rats had unlimited access to standard rodent chow (Altromin no. 1319) and tap water. None of the rats were euthanized before the end of the exposure period due to discomfort, assessed as excessive loss of body weight (exceeding 20% over a week). The bodyweights before (188 ± 20 g) and after (239 g ± 15 g) the exposure period were not different between groups (mean and standard deviation). Particles were administered to the rat by oral gavage of 1 ml particle suspension or vehicle, with the use of a plastic feeding tube (15ga × 100 mm, Instech Laboratories, Winsum, the Netherlands). The rats were weighed the day before exposure, and the particle stock suspension was adjusted to individual weight. Control rats received a bolus of 1 ml dispersion media, sonicated as described above, but without particles. Animals were exposed once a week, for 10 weeks. Oral gavage was executed on the same weekday and time a day for each animal. The procedure was performed by an experienced animal technician to minimize stress and discomfort in the rats. At the day of the experiment, two rats, from different exposure groups, was sacrificed. The rat was anesthetized 24 h after the last exposure, with a subcutaneous injection (in the lower back) of a combination of hypnorm (fentanyl 0.315 mg/ml and fluanisone 10 mg/ml) and dormicum (midazolam, 5 mg/ml) (0.3 ml/100 g bw), following death by exsanguination due to blood collection.

Biochemical parameters in plasma

Blood was collected by abdominal aortic puncture using a 21 gauge needle equipped with a syringe (without anticoagulant). Approximately 4 ml blood was immediately transferred to an ethylenediamine-tetraacetic acid (EDTA) K3 tube (2.1 mg/ml EDTA K3, Venosafe®) and plasma was collected after centrifugation (2000 g, 4 °C for 5 min). The remaining blood was set to coagulate in an Eppendorf tube, and serum was collected by centrifugation (2000 g, 4° for 5 min). Plasma from EDTA treated blood was used to measure concentrations of MDA and ADMA. For measurement of BH_4, EDTA treated blood was added 4% dithioerythritol and plasma were collected by centrifugation (1500 g, 4 °C for 1 min). For measurement of vitamin C, 10% metaphosphoric acid was added to plasma from EDTA tubes and stored at − 80 °C until analyzed. Plasma concentrations of BH_4, vitamin C, MDA, and AMDA were measured by HPLC with fluorescent detection [45–48].

Vasomotor function assessed by the wire myograph method

The procedure for assessing vasomotor function was similar in the ex vivo- and the in vivo study. In the ex vivo study, segments of the aorta was incubated with particles for 30 min and then assessed for vasomotor responses. In both the ex vivo- and in vivo study segments of the aorta was used. In the in vivo study, we also chose to include segments of both the proximal and distal segments of the LAD. This was due to possible differences in vasomotor responses in LAD segments compared to the aorta. LAD mainly resembles resistance arteries whereas the aorta is a conductance artery, in addition, coronary arteries are a common site for

atheroma formation. The vasomotor function was analyzed immediately after the rats were sacrificed and blood was collected. The heart with aorta was excised from the rats and kept in ice-cold PSS before dissection. Before dissection, the heart and aorta were secured gently with entomology pins in a petri dish with a thick layer of clear silicone gel in the base. The tissue was covered with Ca^{2+}free PSS buffer. This buffer had the same composition as PSS, only $CaCl_2$ was omitted, and 1 μM ethylene glycol tetraacetic acid was added. The dissection was done in Ca^{2+}free PSS buffer to avoid unnecessary vessel contraction. The aortic root and arch were gently trimmed free of connective- and fat tissue under a dissecting microscope. One segment of the ascending aorta cut immediately before the three large side branches of the aortic arch, was cut into a ring-shaped segment of approximately 2 mm in length. The vessel was carefully cannulated with two stainless steel wires (40 μm in diameter) and mounted in the organ bath of a Multi-Wire Myograph 620 M (Danish Myo Technology, Aarhus, Denmark) interfaced to a PowerLab4/35 recorder (ADInstruments). The organ bath was filled with cold, oxygenated Ca^{2+}free PSS buffer (5 ml) and continuously perfused with a 95% O_2 and 5% CO_2 gas mixture. Perfusion with the gas mixture was continuously done throughout the entire experimental procedure. In the in vivo study, we also included two segments of the LAD artery. The LAD artery was dissected free from the heart by carefully removing a part of the myocardial tissue. One segment of the LAD proximal to the aortic root, and one segment distal to the aortic root (nearer the apex) were cut into ring-shaped segments of approximately 2 mm in length. The LAD segments were mounted in organ baths as described for the aorta but cannulated with a stainless steel wire of 25 μm in diameter. When finished mounting, Ca^{2+}free PSS buffer was removed from the organ bath, and replaced by cold PSS. The heat was turned on to 37 °C, and the segments were allowed to equilibrate for 30 min. All baths were maintained at 37 °C throughout the experiment. The DMT LabChart normalization procedure was used, to set vessels to standard initial conditions. Normalization was done to ensure that the physiological responses of the vessels were assessed reliably. With normalization, the internal circumference a vessel would have if relaxed and under a transmural pressure of 100 mmHg (IC_{100}), is determined. The maximal active tension was set to 90% (IC1) of IC_{100}, which is optimal at this point. After normalization, the vessel viability was confirmed by the use of a "wake-up" protocol. The protocol consisted of stimulation with 37 °C potassium physiological salt solution (KPSS). KPSS had the same constituents as PSS but without NaCl and the concentration of KCl was 125 mM. KPSS induces non-receptor mediated vasocontraction, due to depolarization of the cell by enhancing extracellular influx of calcium. The contraction was allowed to stabilize and reach a plateau before adding PSS. The stimulation was repeated three times, and only responsive vessels were used in the further experiments. ACh (acetylcholine chloride, Sigma Aldrich) was used to assess the endothelium-dependent vasorelaxation in $PGF_{2\alpha}$ (3–10 µM) (dinoprost trometamol 5 mg/mL, Glostrup apotek, Denmark) precontracted vessels. The particle exposure did not alter the precontraction ability with $PGF_{2\alpha}$ (results not shown). ACh was cumulatively added to the organ bath (0.1 nM - 0.3 mM in aorta, 0.1 nm - 0.03 mM in LAD), each concentration was allowed to reach a plateau before adding the next concentration. To assess if the ACh-induced relaxation were dependent on eNOS, some of the arteries in the ex vivo study ($n = 3–5$) were incubated with the NOS inhibitor L-NAME (N5751, Sigma-Aldrich) for 15 min (10^{-5} M), before an additional concentration-response curve with acetylcholine were assessed.

To assess the endothelium-independent vasorelaxation, the NO donor nitroglycerin (NTG) (glyceryl nitrate 5 mg/mL, Region H's Apotek, Herlev, Denmark) was added to the organ bath in a cumulative manner (ex vivo: 0.01 nm - 0.03 mM; in vivo: 0.1 nm 0.03 mM) after inducing a stable contraction in the vessels with $PGF_{2\alpha}$. The arteries responses to receptor-dependent vasocontraction were assessed with 5-hydroxytryptamine (5-HT, serotonin hydrochloride, H9523, Sigma Aldrich) (ex vivo: 10 nm - 0.3 mM; in vivo: 3.0 nm 0.3 mM).

Between the cumulative concentration-response curves with ACh, NTG, and 5-HT, the vessels were washed with PSS and contracted once with KPSS. The precontraction response with $PGF_{2\alpha}$ was expressed as the percentage of the maximal contraction when stimulating the vessels with K⁺ (125 mM). Vessels precontracted to 10–150% of the maximal K⁺ induced contraction was included in the study. There was no difference between groups in the precontraction response. The vasorelaxation caused by ACh and NTG were expressed as the percentage relaxation of the precontraction tension produced by $PGF_{2\alpha}$. The contraction caused by 5-HT were expressed as the percentage of the maximal contraction obtained when stimulating the vessel segments with K⁺ (125 mM) before the 5-HT concentration-response curve. Data on vasomotor response were excluded from the study if segments did not respond to K⁺ stimulation, there were missing values in the cumulative concentration-response curves, data could not be fitted to a sigmoid curve with nonlinear regression analysis or if the segment could not be mounted in the organ bath due to technical difficulties. Animals from different exposure groups were analyzed on the same experimental day.

Statistical analysis

All concentration-response curves were analyzed by nonlinear regression analysis using GraphPad Prism version 7 (San Diego, CA, USA). The data were fitted to sigmoid curves with varying slopes according to the following equation: $Y = \text{Bottom} + (\text{Top} - \text{Bottom})/ (1 + 10^{((\text{Log } EC50 - X) * \text{Hill Slope}))}$, where X is the logarithm of concentration and Y is the response. Y starts at Bottom and goes to Top with a sigmoid shape. The data points on each curve are expressed as mean ± SEM and n denotes the number of rats. Non-overlapping confidence intervals were considered to be statistically different. Values of E_{max} (top value) and Log EC_{50} values were compared.

Data on biomarkers measured in plasma was analyzed by one-way ANOVA with Dunnett's post-tests. All statistical analyses were considered significant when $P < 0.05$.

Abbreviations
5-HT: 5-hydroxytryptamine; ACh: Acetylcholine; ADMA: Asymmetric dimethylarginine; BH_2: Dihydrobiopterin; BH_4: Tetrahydrobiopterin; BW: Body weight; DHA: Dehydroascorbic acid; DLS: Dynamic light scattering; EDTA: Ethylenediamine tetraacetic acid; E_{max}: Maximal effect value; eNOS: Endothelial nitric oxide synthase; FBS: Foetal bovine serum; HUVEC: Human umbilical vein endothelial cell; KPSS: Potassium physiological salt solution; LAD: Left anterior descending; L-arg: L-arginine; L-NAME: N^G-nitro-L-arginine methyl ester, Log EC_{50}; MDA: Malondialdehyde; NO: Nitric oxide; NTA: Nanoparticle tracking analysis; NTG: Nitroglycerin; $PGF_{2\alpha}$: Prostaglandin $F_{2\alpha}$; PSS: Physiological saline solution

Acknowledgements
The authors would like to thank Julie Hansen, Lisbeth Bille Carlsen, Camilla Skånstrøm Dall, Joan Frandsen and Annie Bjergby Kristensen for their technical assistance.

Funding
The project was funded by an internal PhD-fellowship grant at the Faculty of Medical Sciences, University of Copenhagen. The funding body has not been involved in the design of the study and collection, analysis, and interpretation of data, and in writing the manuscript.

Authors' contributions
DMJ, MS, JL, GFS, SL, and PM contributed to the idea and design of the study. DMJ was responsible for the particle characterization, supervised by MR. RM performed the Zeta potential and DLS measurements. DMJ carried out the animal experiments. DVC assisted DMJ in the animal facility at the day of sacrifice and organ removal in the in vivo study. DMJ carried out the experiments on vasomotor function assisted and supervised by MS in the in vivo study and assisted and supervised by GFS in the ex vivo study. DMJ wrote the draft manuscript, which was revised by PM. All authors critically read and approved the final manuscript.

Competing interests
The authors declare that they have no competing interests.

Author details

[1]Department of Public Health, Section of Environmental Health, Faculty of Health and Medical Sciences, University of Copenhagen, Øster Farimagsgade 5A, Building 5B, 2nd Floor, DK-1014 Copenhagen K, Denmark. [2]Department of Drug Design and Pharmacology, Section of Molecular and Cellular Pharmacology, Faculty of Health and Medical Sciences, University of Copenhagen, Universitetsparken 2, 22, 2100 Copenhagen, Denmark. [3]Experimental Animal Models, Department of Veterinary and Animal Sciences, Faculty of Health and Medical Sciences, University of Copenhagen, Ridebanevej 9, DK-1870 Frederiksberg C, Denmark. [4]Colloids and Biological Interfaces, Department of Micro- and Nanotechnology, Technical University of Denmark, 2800 Kongens Lyngby, Denmark.

References

1. Oberdörster G, Oberdörster E, Oberdörster J. Nanotoxicology: an emerging discipline evolving from studies of ultrafine particles. Environ Health Perspect. 2005;113:823–39.
2. Sturm R. A computer model for the clearance of insoluble particles from the tracheobronchial tree of the human lung. Comput Biol Med. 2007;37:680–90.
3. Møller P, Christophersen DV, Jacobsen NR, Skovmand A, Gouveia ACD, Andersen MHG, et al. Atherosclerosis and vasomotor dysfunction in arteries of animals after exposure to combustion-derived particulate matter or nanomaterials. Crit Rev Toxicol. 2016;46:437–76.
4. Donaldson K, Duffin R, Langrish JP, Miller MR, Mills NL, Poland CA, et al. Nanoparticles and the cardiovascular system: a critical review. Nanomedicine. 2013;8:403–23.
5. Miller MR. The role of oxidative stress in the cardiovascular actions of particulate air pollution. Biochem Soc Trans. 2014;42:1006–11.
6. Folkmann JK, Vesterdal LK, Sheykhzade M, Loft S, Møller P. Endothelial dysfunction in normal and prediabetic rats with metabolic syndrome exposed by oral gavage to carbon black nanoparticles. Toxicol Sci. 2012;129:98–107.
7. Laursen JB, Somers M, Kurz S, Mccann L, Warnholtz A, Freeman BA, et al. Implications for interactions between Peroxynitrite. Circulation. 2001;103:1282–9.
8. Mortensen A, Lykkesfeldt J. Does vitamin C enhance nitric oxide bioavailability in a tetrahydrobiopterin-dependent manner? In vitro, in vivo and clinical studies. Nitric Oxide. 2014;36:51–7.
9. EFSA Journal. EFSA panel on food additives and nutrient sources added to food (ANS); scientific opinion on the re-evaluation of vegetable carbon (E 153) as a food additive. 2012.
10. EFSA Journal. EFSA panel on food additives and nutrient sources added to food (ANS); scientific opinion on the re-evaluation of titanium dioxide (E 171) as a food additive. 2016.
11. Vesterdal LK, Mikkelsen L, Folkmann JK, Sheykhzade M, Cao Y, Roursgaard M, et al. Carbon black nanoparticles and vascular dysfunction in cultured endothelial cells and artery segments. Toxicol Lett. 2012;214:19–26.
12. Saber AT, Jensen KA, Jacobsen NR, Birkedal R, Mikkelsen L, Møller P, et al. Inflammatory and genotoxic effects of nanoparticles designed for inclusion in paints and lacquers. Nanotoxicology. 2012;6:453–71.
13. Rasmussen K, Mast J, De Temmerman P-J, Verleysen E, Waegeneers N, Van SF, et al. Titanium dioxide, NM-100, NM-101, NM-102, NM-103, NM-104, NM-105: characterisation and Physico- chemical properties. JRC. 2014;86291:1–218.
14. Dvonch JT, Brook RD, Keeler GJ, Rajagopalan S, D'Alecy LG, Marsik FJ, et al. Effects of concentrated fine ambient particles on rat plasma levels of asymmetric dimethylarginine. Inhal Toxicol. 2004;16:473–80.
15. Møller P, Mikkelsen L, Vesterdal LK, Folkmann JK, Forchhammer L, Roursgaard M, et al. Hazard identification of particulate matter on vasomotor dysfunction and progression of atherosclerosis. Crit Rev Toxicol. 2011;41:339–68.
16. Onodera A, Yayama K, Tanaka A, Morosawa H, Furuta T, Takeda N, et al. Amorphous nanosilica particles evoke vascular relaxation through PI3K/Akt/eNOS signaling. Fundam Clin Pharmacol. 2016;30:419–28.
17. Bagate K, Meiring JJ, Gerlofs-Nijland ME, Vincent R, Cassee FR, Borm PJA. Vascular effects of ambient particulate matter instillation in spontaneous hypertensive rats. Toxicol Appl Pharmacol. 2004;197:29–39.
18. Bagaté K, Meiring JJ, Cassee FR, Borm PJA. The effect of particulate matter on resistance and conductance vessels in the rat. Inhal Toxicol. 2004;16:431 6.
19. Knaapen AM, den Hartog GJ, Bast A, Borm PJ. Ambient particulate matter induces relaxation of rat aortic rings in vitro. Hum Exp Toxicol. 2001;20:259–65.
20. Félétou M, Köhler R, Vanhoutte PM. Nitric oxide: orchestrator of endothelium-dependent responses. Ann Med. 2012;44:694–716.
21. Minarchick VC, Stapleton PA, Fix NR, Leonard SS, Sabolsky EM, Nurkiewicz TR. Intravenous and gastric cerium dioxide nanoparticle exposure disrupts microvascular smooth muscle signaling. Toxicol Sci. 2015;144:77–89.
22. Danielsen PH, Loft S, Jacobsen NR, Jensen KA, Autrup H, Ravanat JL, et al. Oxidative stress, inflammation, and DNA damage in rats after intratracheal instillation or oral exposure to ambient air and wood smoke particulate matter. Toxicol Sci. 2010;118:574–85.
23. Bräuner EV, Forchhammer L, Møller P, Barregard L, Gunnarsen L, Afshari A, et al. Indoor particles affect vascular function in the aged: an air filtration-based intervention study. Am J Respir Crit Care Med. 2008;177:419–25.
24. Bräuner EV, Møller P, Barregard L, Dragsted LO, Glasius M, Wåhlin P, et al. Exposure to ambient concentrations of particulate air pollution does not influence vascular function or inflammatory pathways in young healthy individuals. Part Fibre Toxicol. 2008;5:1–9.
25. Forchhammer L, Moller P, Riddervold IS, Bonlokke J, Massling A, Sigsgaard T, et al. Controlled human wood smoke exposure: oxidative stress, inflammation and microvascular function. Part Fibre Toxicol. 2012;9:7.
26. Karottki DG, Spilak M, Frederiksen M, Gunnarsen L, Brauner EV, Kolarik B, et al. An indoor air filtration study in homes of elderly: cardiovascular and respiratory effects of exposure to particulate matter. Environ Health. 2013;12:116.
27. Karottki DG, Bekö G, Clausen G, Madsen AM, Andersen ZJ, Massling A, et al. Cardiovascular and lung function in relation to outdoor and indoor exposure to fine and ultrafine particulate matter in middle-aged subjects. Environ Int. 2014;73:372–81.
28. Olsen Y, Karottki DG, Jensen DM, Bekö G, Kjeldsen BU, Clausen G, et al. Vascular and lung function related to ultrafine and fine particles exposure assessed by personal and indoor monitoring: a cross-sectional study. Environ Health. 2014;13:1–10.
29. Hemmingsen JG, Rissler J, Lykkesfeldt J, Sallsten G, Kristiansen J, Møller PP, et al. Controlled exposure to particulate matter from urban street air is associated with decreased vasodilation and heart rate variability in overweight and older adults. Part Fibre Toxicol. 2015;12:1–15.
30. Nurkiewicz TR, Porter DW, Hubbs AF, Stone S, Chen BT, Frazer DG, et al. Pulmonary nanoparticle exposure disrupts systemic microvascular nitric oxide signaling. Toxicol Sci. 2009;110:191–203.
31. Christophersen DV, Jacobsen NR, Jensen DM, Kermanizadeh A, Sheykhzade M, Loft S, et al. Inflammation and vascular effects after repeated intratracheal instillations of carbon black and lipopolysaccharide. PLoS One. 2016;11:1–24.
32. Aragon M, Chrobak I, Brower J, Roldan L, Fredenburgh LE, Mcdonald JD, et al. Inflammatory and vasoactive effects of serum following inhalation of varied complex mixtures. Cardiovasc Toxicol. 2016;16:163–71.
33. Mikkelsen L, Jensen KA, Koponen IK, Saber AT, Wallin H, Loft S, et al. Cytotoxicity, oxidative stress and expression of adhesion molecules in human umbilical vein endothelial cells exposed to dust from paints with or without nanoparticles. Nanotoxicology. 2013;7:117–34.
34. Frikke-Schmidt H, Roursgaard M, Lykkesfeldt J, Loft S, Nøjgaard JK, Møller P. Effect of vitamin C and iron chelation on diesel exhaust particle and carbon black induced oxidative damage and cell adhesion molecule expression in human endothelial cells. Toxicol Lett. 2011;203:181–9.
35. Kermanizadeh A, Gosens I, MacCalman L, Johnston H, Danielsen PH, Jacobsen NR, et al. A multilaboratory toxicological assessment of a panel of 10 engineered nanomaterials to human health - ENPRA project - the highlights, limitations, and current and future challenges. J Toxicol Environ Heal - Part B Crit Rev. 2016;19:1–28.
36. Danielsen PH, Cao Y, Roursgaard M, Møller P, Loft S. Endothelial cell activation, oxidative stress and inflammation induced by a panel of metal-based nanomaterials. Nanotoxicology. 2015;9:813–24.
37. Møller P, Jacobsen NR. Weight of evidence analysis for assessing the genotoxic potential of carbon nanotubes. Crit Rev Toxicol. 2017;47:867–884.
38. Warheit DB, Donner EM. Risk assessment strategies for nanoscale and fine-sized titanium dioxide particles: recognizing hazard and exposure issues. Food Chem Toxicol. 2015;85:138–47.
39. Jani PU, McCarthy DE, Florence AT. Titanium dioxide (rutile) particle uptake from the rat GI tract and translocation to systemic organs after oral administration. Int J Pharm. 1994;105:157–68.
40. Kreyling WG, Holzwarth U, Schleh C, Kozempel J, Wenk A, Haberl N, et al. Quantitative biokinetics of titanium dioxide nanoparticles after oral application in rats: part 2. Nanotoxicology. 2017;11:443–53.

41. Pele LC, Thoree V, Bruggraber SFA, Koller D, Thompson RPH, Lomer MC, et al. Pharmaceutical/food grade titanium dioxide particles are absorbed into the bloodstream of human volunteers. Part Fibre Toxicol. 2015;12:1–6.

42. Brunauer S, Emmett PH, Teller E. Adsorption of gases in multimolecular layers. J Am Chem Soc. 1938;60:309–19.

43. Skovmand A, Damiao Gouveia AC, Koponen IK, Møller P, Loft S, Roursgaard M. Lung inflammation and genotoxicity in mice lungs after pulmonary exposure to candle light combustion particles. Toxicol Lett. 2017;276:31–8.

44. Løhr M, Folkmann JK, Sheykhzade M, Jensen LJ, Kermanizadeh A, Loft S, et al. Hepatic oxidative stress, genotoxicity and vascular dysfunction in lean or obese Zucker rats. PLoS One. 2015;10:e0118773.

45. Mortensen A, Hasselholt S, Tveden-Nyborg P, Lykkesfeldt J. Guinea pig ascorbate status predicts tetrahydrobiopterin plasma concentration and oxidation ratio in vivo. Nutr Res. 2013;33:859–67.

46. Lykkesfeldt J. Determination of ascorbic acid and dehydroascorbic acid in biological samples by high-performance liquid chromatography using subtraction methods: reliable reduction with Tris[2-carboxyethyl]phosphine hydrochloride. Anal Biochem. 2000;282:89–93.

47. Lykkesfeldt J. Determination of malondialdehyde as dithiobarbituric acid adduct in biological samples by HPLC with fluorescence detection: comparison with ultraviolet-visible spectrophotometry. Clin Chem. 2001;47:1725–7.

48. Ekeloef S, Larsen MHH, Schou-Pedersen AMV, Lykkesfeldt J, Rosenberg J, Gögenür I. Endothelial dysfunction in the early postoperative period after major colon cancer surgery. Br J Anaesth. 2017;118:200–6.

The unrecognized occupational relevance of the interaction between engineered nanomaterials and the gastro-intestinal tract

Antonio Pietroiusti[1]*[†] (ID), Enrico Bergamaschi[2], Marcello Campagna[3], Luisa Campagnolo[1], Giuseppe De Palma[4], Sergio Iavicoli[5], Veruscka Leso[6], Andrea Magrini[1], Michele Miragoli[7], Paola Pedata[8], Leonardo Palombi[1] and Ivo Iavicoli[6†]

Abstract

Background: There is a fundamental gap of knowledge on the health effects caused by the interaction of engineered nanomaterials (ENM) with the gastro-intestinal tract (GIT). This is partly due to the incomplete knowledge of the complex physical and chemical transformations that ENM undergo in the GIT, and partly to the widespread belief that GIT health effects of ENM are much less relevant than pulmonary effects. However, recent experimental findings, considering the role of new players in gut physiology (e.g. the microbiota), shed light on several outcomes of the interaction ENM/GIT. Along with this new information, there is growing direct and indirect evidence that not only ingested ENM, but also inhaled ENM may impact on the GIT. This fact, which may have relevant implications in occupational setting, has never been taken into consideration.
This review paper summarizes the opinions and findings of a multidisciplinary team of experts, focusing on two main aspects of the issue: 1) ENM interactions within the GIT and their possible consequences, and 2) relevance of gastro-intestinal effects of inhaled ENMs. Under point 1, we analyzed how luminal gut-constituents, including mucus, may influence the adherence of ENM to cell surfaces in a size-dependent manner, and how intestinal permeability may be affected by different physico-chemical characteristics of ENM. Cytotoxic, oxidative, genotoxic and inflammatory effects on different GIT cells, as well as effects on microbiota, are also discussed.
Concerning point 2, recent studies highlight the relevance of gastro-intestinal handling of inhaled ENM, showing significant excretion with feces of inhaled ENM and supporting the hypothesis that GIT should be considered an important target of extrapulmonary effects of inhaled ENM.

Conclusions: In spite of recent insights on the relevance of the GIT as a target for toxic effects of nanoparticles, there is still a major gap in knowledge regarding the impact of the direct versus indirect oral exposure. This fact probably applies also to larger particles and dictates careful consideration in workers, who carry the highest risk of exposure to particulate matter.

Keywords: Ingested nanoparticles, Inhaled nanoparticles, Direct toxicity, Indirect toxicity, Workers' exposure, Gastrointestinal tract, Microbiota

* Correspondence: pietroiu@uniroma2.it
[†]Equal contributors
[1]Department of Biomedicine and Prevention, University of Rome Tor Vergata, Via Montpellier 1, 00133 Rome, Italy
Full list of author information is available at the end of the article

Background

Despite the large and growing number of ENM used in agri-food products [1–5], oral ingestion has received significantly less attention than the pulmonary route and therefore there is relatively lower information on the possible toxic effects of ENM on the gastro-intestinal tract (GIT). This may be due to the fact that the study of the impact of ENM on the GIT (and vice versa) is a rather complicated issue: both food and the processes that break down and transform food ingredients (e.g., physical forces, osmotic concentration and pH gradients, digestive enzyme, redox conditions and salinity levels) may in fact transform, aggregate and dissolve ENMs in ways that alter their naive and inherent properties, therefore potentially affecting their biological reactivity as well as their toxicological profiles.

This picture is however changing: It is becoming clear that the gut micro-organisms (the microbiota) play a pivotal role in maintaining both local (intestinal) and systemic homeostasis and that they may influence ENM and be influenced by them [6, 7]. Very recent in vitro and in vivo data, discussed in the first section of the present review, have shown that ingested ENM may induce substantial adverse effects unrecognized in past studies; last but not least, there is indirect growing evidence that inhaled ENM, representing the most common pathway of exposure in workers, may have a substantial impact on the GIT, as shown in the second section of the review.

In September 2016, the Italian Society of Occupational Medicine and Industrial Hygiene (SIMLII) hosted a research workshop in order to exchange and merge knowledge and expert point of view on the above-mentioned topics. In the following sections, we outline how these topics have been developed and summarize the state of the evidence about their possible impact on future research in the field of nanotoxicology.

Interaction of ingested ENM with the GIT
Aggregation, agglomeration and dissolution

The fate and bioavailability of ENM in the gastrointestinal system may be affected, at least partly, by their primary characteristics, such as size, surface chemistry and charge, or, in turn, by properties acquired through the transit via the GIT. Several factors, such as pH gradients, gastrointestinal transit time, nutritional status, meal quality, level of mucosal and enzymatic secretions, as well as the intestinal microflora, may all influence ENM physical and chemical reactivity [8]. There is limited information on the physical changes of some metallic ENM (Ag, TiO2, SiO2 and ZnO) once in contact with the gastro-intestinal fluids. It seems that ion release may occur in the gastric environment, along with size-dependent aggregation and agglomeration. For example, it has been shown that in gastric juice ZnO and Ag

undergo dissolution [9–14]. Agglomeration has been shown for TiO2 and also for Ag ENM, dependently from size [9–13, 15, 16]. Conflicting data have been obtained as far as aggregation/agglomeration in the intestinal environment is concerned: agglomeration has been reported for SiO_2 [17] and de-agglomeration for Ag [9]. Probably the chemical composition of ENM, their surface charge and the fasting/fed state may be important components of the final outcome. Clearly, more data are needed in order to understand how different variables such as previous transit in different environments, fasting and fed state may each contribute to the final physical status of ENM travelling along the GIT. In addition, a higher number of ENM and of gastro-intestinal physiological states should be investigated.

ENM uptake and absorption

Although limited information is available on the toxicokinetics of orally administered ENM [18], available data suggest that uptake and absorption of ENM in the GI tract may have relevant implications for their local and systemic effects [19, 20].

A detailed description of the GIT cellular and extracellular structures involved in the uptake and absorption of ENMs, and of the mechanisms of uptake are beyond the scope of this review, however a brief presentation of the main players is needed in order to understand the fate of ENM in the intestine.

In this regard, the key cell types are a) the enterocytes, which are by far the most represented cell type along the intestine and are connected each other by tight junctions, which prevent the unselected intercellular access to the luminal content; b) the antigen sampling M cells, overlying organized lymphoid structures such as the Peyer's patches and other gut-associated lymphoid tissue (GALT). Although representing only 1% of the intestinal cells, M cell are covered by a much thinner mucus layer than enterocytes, and are very relevant for the uptake of foreign substances, which are subsequently delivered to the underlying lymphoid cells; c) the mucus producing goblet cells (about 10% of the total intestinal cells), secreting the mucus lining the whole surface of the small and large intestine.

The first barrier encountered by ingested ENM is indeed represented by mucus, which has been reported to be efficient in trapping larger ENM [21], this factor being a possible explanation for the less pronounced toxic effects of 200 nm Ag ENM in comparison to 20 nm Ag ENM observed in in vitro experiments on a co-culture of CaCo 2 cells and mucus producing cells [22]. Ingested ENM may on the other hand influence mucus secretion, in both quantitative and qualitative terms. For example, sub-chronic (28-days) oral exposure to 60 nm Ag ENM in rats [23] promoted the secretion of mucus in the ileum and rectum, and changes in mucin composition (amounts of neutral and acidic mucins and proportions of sulfated and sialylated mucins). This may be interpreted as a non-specific inflammatory response.

Once crossed the mucus barrier, ENM come in contact with the intestinal cells: the main mechanism through which they may cross the intestinal barrier is represented by transcellular transport. Available in vitro studies suggest that smaller particles may traverse enterocyte cell membranes, mediating changes in membrane fluidity, resulting in altered signaling or increased permeability and cytotoxicity; conversely, as particle size increases or as agglomeration occurs, uptake is predominantly performed by M cells, which are already specialized for this function [20]. Of note, the immunologic responses by lymphoid tissue beneath M cells is typically oriented to hypo-responsiveness (oral tolerance). It is not known, however, whether environmental ENM can have similar mucosal immunologic effects. Evidence for this possibility arises from the observation that agglomerates of endogenous calcium-phosphate nanoparticles (of similar size to ENM in biological media) and dietary TiO_2 can bind gut microbial-derived molecules (e.g. peptidoglycan, lipopolysaccharide) and traffic these to GALT, with influence on tolerance or immunogenicity [24–27].

In vivo studies in rodents suggest that a low percentage of ENM present in the gut lumen is actually absorbed. For example, in a long term study (24 or 84 days) of orally administered amorphous silica (7 nm or 10–25 nm), absorption was 0.25% [28]. A higher uptake was reported in another 10 day administration study, in which 500 nm TiO_2 particles, given by gavage, were taken up in percentages ranging from 0.11%, in the stomach, to 4% in the large intestine, and the vast majority of the ENM accumulated in the Peyer's patches [29]. Although the size of TiO_2 particles in the above-mentioned study was beyond the conventional size limit of ENM (100 nm), the findings of another report, showing the presence of 12 nm TiO_2 particles in Peyer's patches soon after a single administration by gavage, suggest that early absorption of ENM occurs [15]. Of relevance, available information from in vitro experiments suggests that uptake of ENM may be decreased by food components, as shown for silica and polystyrene [17]. Some data regarding TiO_2 upake and absorption, after a single administration, are available also for humans, and they range from no evidence of absorption (TiO_2 size: 10–1800 nm; dose range 315–620 mg) [30] to detectable elemental Ti in blood after the administration of 100 mg of 260 nm particles [31].

Data regarding chronic low dose exposure are of course needed in order to clarify the presence and extent of intestinal absorption in humans under real life exposure settings.

Toxic effects

In the following paragraphs the most relevant available in vitro and in vivo studies on ENM toxicity on the GIT are summarized.

In vitro studies

Cell damage In Caco-2 cells, TiO_2 ENM exposure caused loss and morphological changes in microvilli and disorganization of the brush border [32], while rutile-cored aluminum hydroxide and polydimethylsiloxane-surface treated TiO_2 ENM did not cause any damage [33]. Epithelial alterations, consisting of plasma membrane disruption and tight junction loosening, have been demonstrated also by Mahler et al. [34] in a tri-culture gut model including enterocytes, goblet cells and M cells, treated with 50 and 200 nm polystyrene beads.

Changes in permeability Changes in permeability of the epithelial barrier may be interpreted as the result of functional damage to the integrity of the intestinal barrier, sometimes preceding the development of evident cellular damage. Ag ENM treatment of T84 human colonic epithelial cells, characterized by polarized monolayers naturally producing mucus, induces size- and dose-dependent changes in the expression of genes involved in anchoring tight junctions, which results in increased intestinal permeability [35]. A significant increase in epithelial permeability of Caco-2 tight monolayers was reported also for TiO_2 ENM [36] and a reversible effect was also observed for differently functionalized fullerenes and single walled carbon nanotubes (SWCNTs) [37].

However, other studies performed on Caco-2 monolayers as well as on Caco-2/HT29-MTX co-culture models failed to detect such alterations both for TiO_2 [15], SiO_2 [17] and Ag ENM [38].

These conflicting findings may be explained by the different doses, in vitro models, methods of detection and physico-chemical characteristics of the tested ENM. As in other experimental settings regarding the study of toxicity of ENM, grouping of ENM and standardized experimental conditions may help to clarify the role of different ENM in inducing alterations of intestinal permeability.

Cell viability and proliferation Different culture methods have been used in order to study the effects of ENM on viability of cells of the GIT. Since different models may show different sensitivity, we are presenting separately data regarding undifferentiated and differentiated monocultures and those regarding co-culture models.

Studies in undifferentiated mono-cultures These studies generally show alterations in cell viability induced by metal based ENM, with high cytotoxicity induced by

ZnO [39–43], SiO$_2$ [17, 44, 45], and Ag ENM [46]. Milder cytotoxic effects have been reported for Au [47–49], TiO$_2$ ENM [15, 32, 33, 40, 48, 50–56], and carbon nanotubes [37, 51, 57, 58] in short-term studies.

Studies in fully differentiated Caco-2 cells cultures
Relatively few studies are available in fully differentiated Caco-2 cells, which, however, better reflect the native GIT and are generally less sensitive to cytotoxic injuries [45, 59]. Nevertheless, some ENM such as Ag and ZnO ENM [45] are equally toxic to both undifferentiated and differentiated cultures. It remains to be defined whether the effect is attributable to ENM themselves, or to ion release or to both [60].

Studies in co-culture models Toxicity of nanomaterials (TiO$_2$ NM101, Ag NM300, Au) has been evaluated in non-inflamed and inflamed co-cultures, and also compared to non-inflamed Caco-2 monocultures. The inflamed co-cultures released higher amounts of IL-8 compared to Caco-2 monocultures, but the cytotoxicity of Ag NP was higher in Caco-2 monocultures than in 3D co-cultures [48]. However, other investigations failed to detect such differential vulnerability of Caco-2 monocultures to Ag ENM [22, 39, 61–64]. Nevertheless Ag ENM were found to be more toxic than TiO2 or Au ENM [48], while negligible toxic effects have been reported for Carbon nanotubes [65, 66]. More complex in vitro intestinal models have been proposed, such as organoid cultures; these seem very promising for studies on diseased gut, however such models are not completely characterized yet [20].

When investigating in vitro the potential toxicity of ENM on the GIT, several in vivo occurring phenomena should be considered and reproduced to more faithfully mimic the in vivo conditions. As already discussed, there is an ongoing debate on the contribution of the time-dependent dissolution and ion release from metal based ENM to cytotoxic effects [60].

Moreover, the modifications induced to ENM after the interactions with different GIT compartments should be carefully addressed. For instance, acid treatment simulating quantum dots (QD) exposure to gastric juice increased the toxicity of PEG-coated QDs on Caco-2 cells, as a consequence of coating removal, which enabled dissolution into Cd^{2+} ions [67]. Conversely, simulation of Ag ENM digestion, with or without organic and food components, did not significantly affect cytotoxicity and only caused minor agglomeration of particles [13, 38]. Therefore, considering that pH in vivo varies across different gut compartments and with composition of ingesta, future research should aim to clarify whether and to what extent these conditions may affect ENM toxicity. The effect of food

should also be considered. A paradigmatic example is that of micronutrients; whereas phenolic compounds (namely, quercetin and kaempferol), present in fruits and vegetables, can protect Caco-2 cells from Ag ENM induced toxicity and thus maintained the integrity of the epithelial barrier, resveratrol do not exert such effects [68, 69]. This protective action may be attributed to the potent anti-oxidant properties of flavonoids. Another study failed to detect differences in cytotoxicity between digested or undigested Ag ENM on Caco-2 cells when the digestion process was implemented with the presence of the main food components, i.e. carbohydrates, proteins and fatty acids [38, 59]. Native TiO$_2$ ENM and TiO$_2$ ENM pretreated with digestion simulation fluid or bovine serum albumin did not show significant different toxicity in Caco-2 cells [59]. The administration of ZnO NPs in combination with fatty acids, on the other hand, increased their cytotoxic effects [70]. Overall, these data strongly support the relevance, when investigating the potential toxicity of orally ingested ENM, of developing in vitro models which take into account the possible ENM transformation after contact with food or food components, with acidic pH, and GIT constituents in order to mimic in vivo realistic scenarios.

Studies regarding effects of ENM on cell viability are detailed in Table 1, where doses, and physico-chemical characteristics of tested ENM are also reported. For a more complete overview of the available literature, the table includes also studies that have not been discussed in the text.

Overall, in vitro data are seemingly discordant, however, as discussed above, different experimental conditions (doses, exposure duration, cell types, functionalization) may at least in part explain the different results. An important potential causal factor is represented by the effective dose cells are challenged with, which may be quite different in experiments using the same nominal dose: ENM administration under static conditions to cells cultured at the bottom of a culture plate may lead to different interaction rate of the materials with the medium and therefore with cells in different experiments, leading to different cellular concentrations. For example, a fraction of ENM may aggregate in liquid suspension and come in contact with cells at relatively fast rate, whereas those suspended may remain in suspension for the whole duration of the experiment and never get in contact with the cellular surface. Even small changes in the proportion between aggregated and suspended ENM may lead to quite different dose-response curves. The ultimate fate of ENM in a fluid is then dictated by its mass density, i.e. nanomaterials will settle if their mass density is greater than that of the fluid [71]. Suggestions to overcome these limitations have recently been discussed [72].

Table 1 Studies addressing the effects of different NPs on viability of gastro-intestinal cellular models

Nanoparticles	Physico-chemical NP properties	Cell line	Experimental design	Cytotoxic effects	Reference
SW-CNTs	Surface functionalization: SW-CNTs modified with COOH-functional groups.	SW480	Up to 24 h exposure to CNTs (0.5–2 µg per well)	After 4 and 24 h of exposure, CNTs did not have any cytotoxic effect, however there was a reduction in viability at 48 h and for the highest dose employed.	Kulamarva et al. 2008 [58]
CdSe-QDs; CdSe-ZnS-PEG coated QDs	Surface characterization: ZnS shell and poly-ethylene glycol hydrophilic coating.	Caco-2	Twenty four h exposure to native QDs or QDs incubated acidic medium (0–105 nmol/ml)	A dose dependent cytotoxicity for CdSe-QDs was detected. Toxic effects increased with increasing the Cd/Se ratio during synthesis. PEG-coated QDs had less effects. The relative viability of Caco-2 cells dropped from 90% when incubating with 4.2 nmol/ml CdSe-ZnS-PEG-QDs to 53% when incubating with acid medium treated QDs. This result was not confirmed for CdSe- QDs incubated into acid medium.	Wang et al. 2008 [67]
Au-nanorods	CTAB capped and PAA and PAH-coated Au-nanorods.	HT-29	Four days exposure to Au-nanorods (0.4 nM)	CTAB-capped Au-nanorods displayed a significant cytotoxicity (65–75% loss of viability), independent of the aspect ratio. PAA- and PAH-coated gold nanorod solutions were found relatively nontoxic	Alkilany et al. 2009 [49]
SW- CNTs	Size: average diameter of individual SW-CNT is 1.4 ± 0.1 nm, bundle dimensions are 4–5 nm × 0.5–1.5 µm Surface functionalization: carboxylic acid.	Caco-2	Twenty-four h exposure to CNTs (5 and 1000 µg/ml)	A significant decrease in cell viability was detected at the higher concentrations: 500 and 1000 µg/ml.	Jos et al. 2009 [57]
MW-CNTs	Impurities: traces of cobalt, nickel, zinc and lead	Caco-2	Seventy-two h exposure to MW-CNTs (0–100 µg/ml)	No significant difference in CFE dose-effect relationship in comparison to controls.	Ponti et al. 2010 [65]
ZnO-NPs	Size: 50–70 nm; Average diameter: 196 nm; Surface area: 3 m²/g.	Lovo	Up to 72 h exposure to ZnO, (0–23 µg/ml)	ZnO-NPs induced a time- and dose-dependent decrease of cell number. Ten, 20 and 40 µg/cm² induced <5% cell survival after 24 h. Dose-dependent apoptotic cell death was evident.	De Berardis et al. 2010 [42]
TiO₂-NPs	Size: <40 nm; Crystal form: a mixture of rutile and anatase; Surface area: 20–40 m²/g; Hydrodynamic diameter (water): 220 ± 20 nm.	Caco-2	Twenty-four h, or 10 days chronic exposure to TiO₂-NPs (0–1000 µg/ml)	Little indication of any cell fatality compared to the controls was reported at both time points for all concentrations employed.	Koeneman et al. 2010 [32]
Ag-NPs	–	Caco-2	Twenty-four h exposure to Ag-NPs (0–10 µg/ml)	At 1 µg/ml cells did not show a significant viability decrease (LD₅₀: ~5 µg Ag/ml).	Lamb et al. 2010 [62]

Table 1 Studies addressing the effects of different NPs on viability of gastro-intestinal cellular models (*Continued*)

Nanoparticles	Physico-chemical NP properties	Cell line	Experimental design	Cytotoxic effects	Reference
Ag-NPs	Size (mean ± SD): 20 ± 2–113 ± 8 nm; Hydrodinamic diameter (mean ± SD): - MQ water (24 h followed by sonication): 94 ± 4–177 ± 8 nm; - DMEM (24 h followed by sonication): 118 ± 8–189 ± 9; Impurities in NP suspensions: none. Elementary Ag + in supernatant: 17.4; 15.8; 5.8; and 7.6% for 20, 34, 61, 113 nm NPs, respectively.	Caco-2 and Raji B cells in co-culture	Twenty-four h exposure to Ag-NPs (0–50 μg/ml)	No significant viability alterations were observed.	Bouwmeester et al. 2011 [61]
Fe₂O₃, TiO₂, SiO₂, and ZnO nano-powders	Size: 3, 5, 10 and 8–10 for Fe₂O₃, TiO₂, SiO₂, and ZnO- NPs, respectively. Agglomerate mode (DMEM culture media): 1300, 1000, 600, 650 nm, respectively. Surface area: 222, 240, 124, 24 m²/g, respectively.	Caco-2 and RKO	Twenty-four h exposure to SiO₂, TiO₂, ZnO and Fe₂O₃ nano-powders (0–100 μg/cm²) in the presence or absence of TNF-α.	TiO₂, SiO₂, and Fe₂O₃ had minimal toxicity below 100 μg/cm². ZnO displayed the most relevant toxicity (LC₅₀ 27 ± 3.6 and 28 ± 4.6 μg/cm² for RKO and Caco-2, respectively). TNF-α pretreatment did not induce differences in cell viability.	Moos et al. 2011 [41]
Fullerenes; SW-CNTs	Surface functionalization: polyhydroxy small-gap fullerenes (OH-fullerenes), COOH-SW-CNTs; PEG-SW-CNTs. Size: 0.7 (fullerenes); 1.4 ± 0.1 nm in diameter, 4–5 nm × 0.5–1.5 μm bundle dimension (COOH-SW-CNTs); 1.4 ± 0.1 nm in diameter, 4–5 nm × 0.5–0.6 μm in bundle dimension (PEG-SW-CNTs). Purity: >90% (COOH-SW-CNTs); >80% (PEG-SW-CNTs).	Caco-2 cells	Twenty-four h exposure to carbon nanomaterials (0–1000 μg/ml)	All three carbon nanomaterials had minimum cytotoxicity on Caco-2 cells (range of 15.6–1000 μg/mL), and no significant difference was observed compared to the vehicle control.	Coyuco et al. 2011 [37]
Ag-NPs	Size: 20, 40 nm; Surface coating: peptide L-cysteine L-lysine L-lysine	Caco-2	Up to 48 h exposure to Ag-NPs (0–100 μg/ml).	Time-, concentration- and particle size-dependent decrease in cell viability. More toxic effects for 20 nm compared to 40 nm sized Ag-NPs.	Böhmert et al. 2012 [141]
SiO₂-NPs; ZnO-NPs	Size: 14 and <10 nm for SiO₂- and ZnO-NPs, respectively; Surface area: 200 and ≥70 m²/g for SiO₂- and ZnO-NPs, respectively; Shape: near-spherical and needle-like ZnO-NPs; Spherical SiO₂-NPs	Caco-2	Up to 24 h exposure to 0–80 μg/cm² native or digestion simulated (DS) SiO₂, and ZnO-NPs.	SiO₂-NPs and DS- SiO₂-NPs reduced cell viability only in undifferentiated Caco-2 cells (even at 5 μg/cm²). ZnO-NPs and DS-ZnO-NPs were cyto-toxic to both undifferentiated and dif-ferentiated cells (24 h)	Gerloff et al. 2013 [45]
TiO₂-surface treated NPs	T-light SF NPs, a rutile core surrounded by an Al hydroxide layer, vs degradation residues generated after exposure to UV light (T light-DL) or acidic medium (T light-DA). Rutile core size: 7 ± 2 nm × 50 ± 10 nm) Hydrodynamic diameter: T light (347 ± 69); T light-DA (688 ± 209 nm); T light-DL (237 ± 26 nm).	Caco-2	Up to 72 h exposure to TiO2-surface treated NPs (0–100 μg/ml)	No cytotoxic effects were reported using Tripan blue, ATP, XTT and assays	Fisichella et al. 2012 [33]

Table 1 Studies addressing the effects of different NPs on viability of gastro-intestinal cellular models (*Continued*)

Nanoparticles	Physico-chemical NP properties	Cell line	Experimental design	Cytotoxic effects	Reference
ZnO- NPs; TiO$_2$-NPs	Size: 50–70 nm for ZnO-NPs and <25 nm for anatase TiO$_2$-NPs. Purity: 99.7% for TiO$_2$-NPs. Mean hydrodynamic diameter in ethanol and serum-free culture medium, respectively: 340.2 ± 12.04, 941.6 ± 118.3 nm for ZnO-NPs; 771.9 ± 110 and 1080 ± 190.5 nm for TiO$_2$-NPs. Shape: spherules to rod-like or irregularly shaped particles. Impurities: 0.47% of Cu and traces of Ni, and Pb in ZnO-NPs; 4.0% of Sc, 0.6% of Sb and 0.5% of B in TiO$_2$-NPs.	Caco-2	Six and 24 h exposure to ZnO, and TiO$_2$-NPs (0–140 µg/ml) with or without inactivated foetal calf serum.	A dose-dependent decrease of cell viability after ZnO-NP exposure. The presence of the foetal calf serum strongly reduced ZnO NP toxic effects. No effect on cell viability was reported after treatment with TiO$_2$-NPs either in presence or in absence of foetal calf serum.	De Angelis et al. 2013 [40]
Ag-NPs; TiO$_2$-NPs; ZnO-NPs	Size: 20–30, 21, 20 for Ag, TiO$_2$, and ZnO-NPs, respectively; Purity: >99.5% for all NPs; Specific surface area: ~20, 50 ± 15, 50 m^2/g for Ag, TiO$_2$, and ZnO-NPs, respectively. Size in Caco-2 media: 202–227, 311–305, and 212–260 nm for Ag, TiO$_2$, and ZnO-NPs, respectively. Size in SW480 media: 207–221, 306–300, and 288–303 nm, respectively.	Caco-2 and SW480	Up to 48 h exposure to Ag, TiO$_2$, and ZnO-NPs (0–100 µg/ml).	ZnO-NPs (10 and 100 µg/ml) were cytotoxic to both cell lines at 24 and 48 h exposure. No alterations were induced by Ag- and TiO$_2$-NPs.	Abbot and Schwab, 2013 [39]
TiO$_2$- nanobelts; MW-CNTs	TiO$_2$ anatase nanobelts size: length (7 µm), width (0.2 µm), thickness (0.01 µm); Hydrodynamic size (water): 2897 ± 117 nm; Surface area: 17.94 m^2/g. MW-CNTs size: length (5–10 nm), diameter (20–30 nm). Hydrodynamic size (water): 858 ± 58 nm. Surface area: 513 m^2/g; Impurities: 1.8% Ni and 0.1% Fe.	Caco-2/HT29-MTX co-culture	One and 24 h exposure to TiO$_2$-nanobelts; MW-CNTs (10 and 100 µg/ml)	TiO$_2$-nanobelts: only low levels of toxicity were observed. MW-CNTs: no toxicity at 1 h post exposure, and a low level of toxicity (<20% compared to controls) at 24 h post exposure (only for 100 µg/ml).	Tilton et al. 2014 [51]
TiO$_2$-NPs	Size: 21 nm (P25 Degussa); 10–25 nm (anatase); 30 nm (rutile); Hydrodynamic diameter (Milliq water): 7.1 ± 4.1, 42.3 ± 14.4 and 88.3 ± 34.1 nm for P25, anatase and rutile, respectively.	Caco-2	Twenty-four h exposure to TiO$_2$-NPs (1 µg/ml).	No alterations in cell viability were detected by low LDH leak, and normal cell morphology.	Gitrowski et al. 2014 [53]
TiO$_2$-NPs	Size: 12 ± 3 nm anatase NPs (95%); Hydrodynamic diameter (water): 132 ± 0.8 nm.	Caco-2 mono-culture, Caco-2 and HT-29 and Caco-2 and Raji co-cultures.	Forty-eight h exposure to TiO$_2$-NPs (0–200 µg/ml).	Exposure to TiO$_2$-NPs did not cause overt cytotoxicity. No apoptosis was observed.	Brun et al. 2014 [15]

Table 1 Studies addressing the effects of different NPs on viability of gastro-intestinal cellular models (*Continued*)

Nanoparticles	Physico-chemical NP properties	Cell line	Experimental design	Cytotoxic effects	Reference
Ag-NPs, ZnO-NPs	Size: ~90 nm for both NPs.	Caco-2	Twenty-four h exposure to Ag- and ZnO-NPs (0–200 µg/ml).	Ag- and ZnO-NPs significantly inhibited cell proliferation, with greater effects induced by ZnO-NPs (LD_{50} for ZnO-NPs: 0.431 µg/ml).	Song et al. 2014 [43]
Ag-NPs; Au-NPs	Size: < 100 nm	Caco-2	Twenty-four h exposure to Ag- and Au-NPs (0–1000 µg/ml).	A dose-dependent toxic effect of Ag-NPs, with IC_{50} values of 16.7 and14.9 µg/ml derived from the MTT and trypan blue exclusion assays, respectively. Au-NPs did not cause any significant decrease in the cell viability.	Aueviriyavit et al. 2014 [47]
Ag-NPs	Mean primary size: 7.02 ± 0.68 nm; Hydrodynamic diameter in acqueous suspension: 14.7 ± 0.2 nm.	Caco-2	Up to 48 h exposure to primary or digested Ag-NPs (0–100 µg/ml).	Digested and undigested Ag-NPs decreased the cell viability of Caco-2 cells in a concentration-dependent manner. No differences emerged between NPs.	Böhmert et al. 2014 [13]
Ag-NPs	Size: 10–100 nm; Size distribution: less than 10% deviation from the primary size; Shape and surface chemistry: spherical NPs stabilized with citrate; Impurities in NP suspensions: none; Agglomeration status: none in culture medium.	LoVo	Up to 48 h exposure to Ag-NPs (0–10 µg/ml).	Cell viability (24 h): At 10 µg/ml, the mitochondrial activity significantly decreased to 53% and to 85% compared to controls for cells exposed to 10 and 20 nm Ag-NPs, respectively. Cell viability (48 h): At 10 µg/ml, 10 nm Ag-NPs mitochondrial activity was reduced to 8% compared to controls. On average, 20–100 nm Ag-NPs resulted in a decrease to 40%.	Miethling-Graff et al. 2014 [105]
Ag-NPs	Size: 20 nm; Hydrodynamic size of Ag-NPs by (A) intensity-weighted distribution (27.3 nm) and (B) by volume-weighted distribution (21.4 nm); Average size by TEM: 20.4 nm.	Caco-2	Three h exposure to Ag-NPs (0–20 µg/ml).	A significant concentration (10–20 µg/ml) -dependent decrease in cell viability compared with controls.	Sahu et al. 2014 [142]
Ag-NPs	Size: < 20 nm	Caco-2 and Raji B cells in co-culture	Twenty-four h exposure to Ag-NPs (0–90 µg/ml) with or without phenolic compounds.	Ag-NPs decreased significantly cellular viability starting from 30 µg/ml with an EC_{50} of ca. 40 µg/ml. Kaempferol (10 or 50 mM) had a protective effect at lower concentrations of Ag-NPs (up to 14%). Resveratrol had no effect.	Martirosyan et al. 2014 [69]
SiO₂-NPs	Size: 50, 100, 200 nm;	Caco-2	Six h exposure to SiO_2-NPs incubated in fasting or fed state simulated gastric fluids (0–10 mg/ml).	Up to 6 h time point, no cytotoxicity was observed for all sized NPs. During additional incubation time with fresh medium (24 and 48 h), only 50 nm NPs dispersed in PBS or in fasting simulated fluids, induced a significant cytotoxicity.	Sakai-Kato et al. 2014 [17]

Table 1 Studies addressing the effects of different NPs on viability of gastro-intestinal cellular models (*Continued*)

Nanoparticles	Physico-chemical NP properties	Cell line	Experimental design	Cytotoxic effects	Reference
SiO$_2$-NPs	Size: 15 and 55 nm; Size distribution range by TEM: 10.8–29.8 and 41–121 for 15 and 55 nm NPs; Shape: spherical.	Caco-2	Twenty-four h exposure to SiO$_2$-NPs (0–256 μg/ml).	SiO$_2$-NPs (55 nm): a decrease in cell viability (30%) was only observed at the highest tested dose (256 μg/ml). SiO$_2$-NPs (15 nm): viability was 80% of controls at 32 μg/ml and 20% at 256 μg/ml. IC50: 43 μg/ml.	Tarantini et al. 2015a [44]
TiO$_2$-NPs	Size: 12 ± 3 nm (anatase), 22 ± 4 nm (rutile); Surface area: 82 ± 3 and 73 ± 5 g/m^2 for anatase and rutile, respectively Hydrodynamic diameter (water): 132 ± 1 nm (anatase); >1000 nm (rutile)	Caco-2	Twenty-four h exposure to TiO$_2$-NPs (0–200 μg/ml).	Neither anatase, nor rutile NPs induced overt cell toxicity.	Dorier et al. 2015 [55]
TiO$_2$-NPs; SiO$_2$-NPs	Size: 22–26 nm ± 10 nm (hydrophilic and hydrophobic TiO$_2$-NPs); 14 ± 7, and 13 ± 6 nm for SiO$_2$-NPs. Surface areas: 51, 56 (TiO$_2$-NPs); 189.2 and 203.9 (SiO$_2$-NPs) m^2/g.	Caco-2	Three and 10 day exposure to TiO$_2$-NPs and SiO$_2$-NPs (100 μg/ml)	Three day exposure: TiO$_2$-NPs did not induce significant changes in the CFE of cells compared to controls. Cytotoxic effects were registered only for 13 ± 6 nm for SiO$_2$-NPs (99% SiO$_2$), with values of cytotoxicity (CFE = 66% ± 4) Ten day exposure: significant cytotoxic effects were detected after hydrophilic TiO$_2$-NPs (CFE = 72% ± 5) and 13 ± 6 nm SiO$_2$-NP exposure (CFE = 43% ± 4).	Farcal et al. 2015 [56]
TiO$_2$-NPs; ZnO-NPs	Size: 50–70 for ZnO-NPs, and <25 nm for TiO$_2$-NPs; Size by TEM: 45–170 (ZnO-NPs) 20–60 nm (TiO$_2$-NPs) Hydrodynamic diameter in in cell culture medium without foetal calf serum: 942 ± 118 (ZnO-NPs); 1080 ± 190 nm (TiO$_2$-NPs). Purity: 99.7% for anatase TiO$_2$-NPs.	Caco-2	Six and 24 h exposure to ZnO, and TiO$_2$-NPs (0–128 μg/ml)	Only ZnO-NPs exert a strong cytotoxic effect on cells as determined by replication indexes.	Zijno et al. 2015 [60]
ZnO-NPs	TEM size: 20 to 250/50 to 350 nm; Size in medium: 306 nm; Surface area: 14 m2/g.	Caco-2	Exposure to ZnO-NPs and ZnO-NPs in co-exposure to palmitic acid or free fatty acids	Dose dependent cytotoxic effects were detected for ZnO-NPs (EC50: 25 μg/ml MTT assay). Co-exposure of ZnO-NPs and palmitic acid to cells showed the largest cytotoxic effects as indicated by the lowest EC$_{50}$ value (19 μg/ml), whereas free fatty acids had a higher EC$_{50}$ value (24 μg/ml).	Cao et al. 2015 [70]

Table 1 Studies addressing the effects of different NPs on viability of gastro-intestinal cellular models (*Continued*)

Nanoparticles	Physico-chemical NP properties	Cell line	Experimental design	Cytotoxic effects	Reference
TiO$_2$-NPs	Size: 99 ± 30 and 26 ± 12 nm anatase NPs; Hydrodynamic diameter in water: 233 ± 12 and 497 ± 137 nm for the larger and smaller NPs, respectively. Hydrodynamic diameter in culture medium: 719 ± 56 and 727 ± 9 nm for the larger and smaller NPs, respectively. Purity: over 99%.	Caco-2	Twenty-four h exposure to Native NPs and pretreated with digestive fluids (50 and 200 μg/ml)	After 24 h exposure, native NPs do not induce any clear loss of viability on cells. Pretreated NPs are non-toxic to differentiated Caco-2 cells, while can induce a decrease in viability of the undifferentiated Caco-2 cells after 24 h exposure, although the viability remains higher than 86%.	Song et al. 2015 [59]
SW-CNTs; MW-CNTs; MWCNT-OH, and MWCNT-COOH.	Size: SW-CNTs ranged between 1.04–1.71 nm; the layer of MW-CNTs is about 8.4 (± 0.9) graphite layers.	Caco-2	Up to 72 h exposure to CNTs (0–100 μg/ml).	No significant decrease of cell viability was observed at 0.1, 1 and 10 μg/mL doses of four types of CNTs from 4 to 8 h, but the long-lasting treatment (>24 h) increased the cytotoxicity	Chen et al. 2015 [66]
Ag-NPs	Size (untreated NPs): mean radius: 3.2 ± 0.1 nm; width: 1.1 ± 0.3 nm; Size in culture medium (untreated NPs): mean radius: 3.6 ± 0.1 nm; width: 1.2 ± 0.6 nm; Size (digested NPs): 16.0 ± 0.1 nm and 6.6 ± 1.3 nm (with) and 16.6 ± 0.2 and 7.3 ± 1.7 nm (without cell culture medium).	Caco-2	Twenty-four h exposure to untreated or digested Ag-NPs (0–100 μg/ml).	In up to 40 μg/ml Ag no reduction of viability was observed for both NPs. At concentrations higher than 40 μg/ml digested and undigested particles were almost equally cytotoxic.	Lichtenstein et al. 2015 [38]
Ag-NPs	Size: 50 nm; The average size of Ag-NPs by TEM and DLS was 44.7and 54.9 nm, respectively; TEM images demonstrated no noticeable aggregation, agglomeration.	Caco- 2	Four h and 24 h exposure to Ag-NPs (0–50 μg/ml).	A significant concentration (10–50 μg/ml) -dependent decrease in cell viability compared with controls.	Sahu et al. 2016 [143]
Ag-NPs	Size: < 20 nm.	Caco-2 and Raji B cells in co-culture	Three h exposure to Ag-NPs (0–90 μg/ml) with or without a phenolic compound.	Ag-NPs induced a dose-dependent decrease in cell viability. Co-administration with Quercetin protected the cells from the toxic effects of Ag-NPs.	Martirosyan et al. 2016 [68]
Ag-NPs	Size: 10–110 nm.	T84	Fourty-eight h exposure to Ag-NPs (20 and 100 μg/ml).	Little to no change in cell viability compared to controls (acridine orange/ ethidium bromide staining). Significant decrease in cell viability only after 100 μg/ml Ag-NPs doses (ATP-based luminescence assay)	Williams et al. 2016 [35]
Ag-NPs	Size: 20 and 200 nm. Hydrodynamic diameter: 129 and 308 for 20 and 200 nm sized Ag-NPs.	Caco-2/TC7/HT29-MTX co-culture	Twenty-four h exposure to Ag-NPs (0–100 μg/ml).	Ag-NPs did not induce cytotoxicity at any of the tested concentrations in single cell lines or in co-culture.	Georgantzopoulou et al. 2016 [22]

Table 1 Studies addressing the effects of different NPs on viability of gastro-intestinal cellular models *(Continued)*

Nanoparticles	Physico-chemical NP properties	Cell line	Experimental design	Cytotoxic effects	Reference
PVP capped Ag-NPs; TiO₂-NPs; Phosphine capped Au-NPs.	Ag, TiO₂, and Au-NP size: < 20; 7–10 and 15, 80 nm, respectively. Mean hydrodynamic diameter in DMEM culture medium: 120 ± 4, 896 ± 133 and 51 ± 6, 116 ± 5 nm, respectively.	Caco-2 mono-, and co-culture with THP-1, MUTZ-3 cells in a 3D model of intestinal mucosa	Twenty-four h exposure to NPs (0–625 μg/cm²) in both inflamed and not-inflamed conditions	Au-NPs and TiO₂-NPs did not affect cell viability. Ag-NPs: the highest concentration induced a significant cytotoxicity in Caco-2 mono-culture > than in co-culture, with no influence due to the in-flammatory status.	Susewind et al. 2016 [48]
TiO₂-NPs	TiO₂-NP size: 50 and 100 nm (anatase); 50 nm (rutile); 21 nm (P25Degussa); Hydrodynamic diameter (DMEM): 227.78 ± 3.62 (anatase 50); 253.40 ± 4.11 (anatase 100); 194.20 ± 2.14 (rutile 50); 193.85 ± 1.86 nm (P25 Degussa).	Caco-2 cells	Twenty-four, and 72 h exposure to NPs (0–50 μg/ml)	No change in Caco-2 cell viability was evident at 24 h-exposure. 72 h exposure: 50 nm anatase (10, 25, 50 μg/ml), 100 nm anatase (50 μg/ml), 50 nm rutile (50 μg/ml), and P25 Degussa TiO₂-NPs (25, 50 μg/ml) reduced cell viability.	Tada-Oikawa et al. 2016 [52]
TiO₂-NPs	Size: < 25 nm anatase NPs (99%); Surface area: 45–55 m²/g; Hydrodynamic diameter (water): 604 ± 24 nm.	HT-29	Up to 48 h exposure to TiO₂-NPs (0–36 μg/ml).	No significant cytotoxic effect of TiO₂-NPs was observed in LDH and MTT assays at all concentrations after 6, 24, and 48 h exposure.	Ammendolia et al. 2017 [50]

Caco-2 cells human colorectal adenocarcinoma cells, *CFE* colony forming efficiency, *COOH- SW-CNTs* carboxylic acid functionalized single walled carbon nanotubes, *CTAB* cetyltrimethylammonium bromide, *DLS* dynamic light scattering, *DS* digestion simulated, *EC₅₀* half maximal effective concentration, *HT-29* human colon carcinoma cells, *HT29-MTX* human adenocarcinoma mucus secreting cells, *IC* inhibition concentration, *LD50* Lethal dose, *LoVo* human colon carcinoma cell line, *MUTZ-3* human dendritic cells, *MW-CNTs* multi-walled carbon nanotubes, *PAA* polyacrylic acid, *PAH* polyelectrolyte poly(allylamine) hydrochloride, *PEG* poly-ethylene glycol, *PEG-SW-CNTs* poly(ethylene glycol) functionalized single walled carbon nanotubes, *Raji B line* human Burkitt's lymphoma cells, *RKO* human colon adenocarcinoma cells, *SW- CNTs* single walled- carbon nanotubes, *SW480* human colon adenocarcinoma cells, *T84* human colonic epithelial cells, *TEM* transmission electron microscopy, *THP-1* Human macrophages

In vivo studies

Only a few studies have investigated toxicity of ENM in vivo. Studies focusing on *Ag ENM* provided evidence for liver inflammatory infiltration after acute and chronic administration [73–76], although studies demonstrating no toxic effects have also been reported [77–79]. However, the difference is mainly related to the dose used. Indeed, in one of the studies demonstrating ENM adverse effects on the GIT [74], a NOAEL (no observable adverse effect level) of 30 mg/kg and LOAEL (lowest observable adverse effect level) of 125 mg/kg were calculated. In studies showing no toxicity, doses lower than the calculated LOAEL were used.

Interestingly, in positive studies, the liver damage was elicited at comparatively lower doses in mice than in rats.

TiO₂ ENM were found to induce inflammatory changes in the small bowel [80] and also to enter the systemic circulation to accumulate and cause inflammation and oxidative damage in the liver, kidney and spleen [81–86]. However, other studies did not detect any adverse effect after oral administration of titanium dioxide, even at very high doses [87–89].

In order to reconcile the contradictory data regarding TiO_2 ENM, Warheit and Donner [88] noted that negative studies had been performed according to OECD test guidelines, whereas those showing adverse effects were "experimental-type" studies, and highlighted the predominant use of mice in studies indicating adverse effects and of rats in those showing no effects, suggesting that differences in susceptibility of exposed animals may contribute to the final result. In addition, commercial test materials were used in studies showing no effects, whereas "home-made" particles were more often used in studies in which adverse effects were observed. However, the presence of substantial adverse effects at doses as low as 1 mg/kg/bw reported by Tassinari et al. [86], and their absence at doses three order of magnitude higher reported by Warheit et al. [88] remains hard to be explained.

Local intestinal damage was reported after oral ingestion of *Carbon nanotubes* (*CNTs*). Indeed, multiple necrotic foci in the small intestine were observed after a 30-days treatment with multi-walled carbon nanotubes (MWCNTs) in mice, maybe related to the direct CNT-mediated mechanical damage to the enterocytes [90]; whereas a 6 month chronic exposure to MWCNTs in rats induced a dose-dependent decrease in the number of villi in the small intestine characterized by apical necrosis [91]. Ingested *ZnO ENM* were reported to undergo size-dependent intestinal absorption with accumulation in multiple organs and damage to liver and pancreas [92–95]. Finally, ingested *SiO₂ ENM* caused low-level hepatotoxicity in rats following a 10-week exposure [96]. As highlighted above, no observed adverse effect levels (NOAEL), which might be extrapolated to exposed workers, were calculated for some of the studies following OECD guidelines [73, 87–89, 92]: for silver ENM a NOAEL of 30 mg/kg per day was extrapolated [73], whereas for ZnO the calculated NOAEL was 268 mg/kg. NOAEL ranging from 1000 mg/kg to 24,000 mg/kg have been proposed for titanium dioxide [88].

Mechanisms of toxicity

Mechanisms of ENM induced toxicity have been recently reviewed [20, 97] and will not be reported in detail here. We will, however, discuss two developing new fields represented by the interaction of ENM with the gut microbiota and by the contribution that the "omics" technique may give to detect effects which are not observed by using traditional approaches. In the second section of this review, we will also discuss the possible different toxicity mechanisms occurring after direct ingestion of ENM or indirect ingestion, following ENM inhalation.

Effects on intestinal microbiota

Most of the functions of the gastrointestinal tract are facilitated, influenced or modulated by the vast resident collection of microbes, known collectively as the intestinal microbiota [98]. The intestinal microbiome has been a major topic of research in the fields of microbiology and medicine [46, 99, 100] and only recently it has been considered in the context of potential toxicological effects of ingested metals, including their nanoforms [64, 78]. Given that a disruption of the normal intestinal microbiota, also known as dysbiosis, has been linked to severe medical conditions like colitis, inflammatory bowel disease, diabetes and metabolic syndrome, determining whether ENM have an impact on commensal gut microbiota is an essential step in evaluating their overall safety [101].

Few data are available from human. For instance, Das et al. [102] found that the human microbiota (evaluated in stool samples) could be significantly impacted in metabolic activity, as demonstrated by the reduced total gas produced by the stool microbial ecosystem as well as in phylogenetic assemblages, since the anaerobe, Gram negative abundance was significantly reduced by a subacute 48 h exposure to 25–200 μg/ml Ag ENM.

Studies in rodents evaluated the effects of ingested Ag ENM on the gut microbiota, although with non-univocal results [78, 100]. Williams et al. [64] reported a significant decrease in colony-forming units of indigenous ileal microbial populations of rats sub-chronically gavaged with 10–110 nm PVP-coated Ag ENM at doses of 9, 18 and 36 mg/kg bw/day for 13 weeks. The most pronounced effects on cultivable bacteria were observed at lower doses and with smaller diameter particles. Importantly, when real-time PCR was utilized to amplify DNA extracts, i.e. 16 s universal bacterial gene, to measure the relative expression of bacteria, no significant differences could be detected in any of the treatment groups. This may be due to the fact that 16 s–based real-time PCR technique, although proposed as the most suitable method for the quantification of specific microbial communities compared to the traditional culture strategy or the next generation sequencing, is not able to distinguish live bacteria from uncultivable dead or non-proliferating microbes. Therefore, caution should be paid in the interpretation of such kind of data. They also compared the ratio of Bacteroidetes to Firmicutes, the two major phyla of the intestinal microbiome, showing that 110 nm Ag ENM at the highest dose induced a significant increased ratio due to a decrease in Firmicutes. However, no clear description was available concerning the physiologic effect, either detrimental or beneficial, of these alterations in animals.

Another in vivo study [103] performed in mice, showed that Ag ENM could affect the gut microbiota at doses relevant for human dietary exposure (0.046–4.6 mg/kg). In fact, a 28 day oral exposure to Ag ENM mixed in food increased the ratio between Firmicutes and Bacteroidetes phyla inducing a dose-dependent decrease in Bacteroides and an increase in Firmicutes as assessed by the next generation sequencing technique [103]. The trend in Firmicutes alterations reported in this study [103] was different compared to that emerged in Williams et al. [64], maybe in relation to the different techniques employed to analyse the microbiota. Interestingly, when 4 or 8 month aged Ag ENM were used to treat animals, microbiome alterations could not be confirmed. These ENM, in fact, induced a less evident, if any, inversion of the Firmicutes to Bacteroidetes ratio. Ag ENM sulfidation, as a major transformation process for ENM in contact with organic materials, was demonstrated to be responsible for the reduction of aged Ag NP ENM solubilization and Ag + ion release, that may all prevent the gut microbiota alterations observed with freshly prepared Ag ENM.

A polydisperse mixture of 60–100 nm Ag ENM (0–100 µg Ag/kg for 4 h) incubated with ileal contents sampled from weaned piglets, induced a dose-dependent reduction in intestinal coliforms [104]. However, in the same study, when pigs were treated with 20–40 mg Ag/Kg for 2 weeks, only a non-significant trend toward coliform reduction could be detected.

These results were in contrast with those obtained by Hadrup et al. [78] in Wistar rats and Wilding et al. [100] who found in C57BL/6NCrl mice that 28 days gavage administration of 14–110 nm Ag ENM (2.25–10 mg/kg bw/day) irrespective of their coatings, i.e. PVP or silver

acetate, did not affect the balance and number of the two major bacterial phyla in the gut [78].

Interspecies differences in intestinal pH, gut microbiota, diet as well as pathological conditions, which may affect microbial composition generating significant inter-individual variation, even in genetically identical animals with identical starting microbial populations, may explain such different outcomes. Certainly the ENM physico-chemical diversity, in terms of size, coating, or other physicochemical properties may have a different antimicrobial activity [7]. Additionally, the chemical transformations undergone by ENM in aging consumer products as well as during digestion processes may all affect the potential risk for microbial alterations in real human conditions of exposure, particularly in relation to the ENM solubilization ability. In this perspective, to assess the degree, rate and duration of ion release over time, also in in vitro models, should be verified as an interesting instrument to predict the fresh or aged ENM potential to affect microbial communities. Finally, the experimental methodologies utilized in microbiota investigations should be considered as a possible confounding issue for the direct comparison of the data [103].

Sample type, collection site, the employment of a culture strategy or not, lab techniques for the microbiota analysis based on totally different approaches may all affect the final outcomes of the studies and should be carefully considered for an adequate interpretation of the results.

Effects detected by "omic" techniques

To gain insights into potential mechanisms of action of ENM exposure on intestinal cells, biochemical changes have been investigated by using "omics-" aproaches. By using this technique, transcriptional effects involving an enrichment of gene ontology categories related to unfolded proteins, chaperons and stress responses were detected after $5 \, \mu g/cm^2$ ZnO ENM exposure for 4 h of Caco2 cells [41]. As far as epithelium permeability is concerned, Brun et al. [15] demonstrated a significant up-regulation in the expression of genes encoding proteins involved in the maintenance of cell junctions in Caco-2 and Caco-2-HT29-MTX models exposed to 50 µg/mL of TiO2 ENM for 6 h or 48 h; similar findings, showing up-regulation of several genes involved into tight junction and desmosome formation were reported after exposure of T84 cells to Ag ENM (100 µg/mL for 48 h) [35]; by contrast a significant down-regulation of genes encoding junctional proteins was observed by Brun et al. [15] in the ileum of mice exposed to a single gavage of 12.5 mg/kg TiO_2 ENM, and sacrificed 6 h after the gavage. These seemingly conflicting results may at least in part be related to the different times of exposure, which may allow, in the case of relatively protracted exposure, the induction of compensatory mechanisms of repair.

In terms of nanosafety implications, genes whose expression levels change significantly in a manner that correlates with the effects of the ENM-exposure might be useful as early nanotoxicity biomarkers.

As far as the mechanisms involved in the oxidative stress are concerned, it has been reported the concomitant down regulation of mammalian mitochondrial proteins, and the up-regulation of those involved into the cellular redox systems after exposure of LoVo cells to 10 µg/ml for 24 h Ag ENM [105]. On the other hand, up-regulation of cytosolic proteins associated with anti-oxidant activities has been found, this finding being probably related to the development of compensatory mechanisms [106].

Promising results have been obtained when using the omics technique in order to discriminate between the effects related to metallic ENM and those due to the release of ions: as an example, a higher number of deregulated proteins was detected after exposure to Ag NPs compared to the ionic form [107].

Whether or not distinct pathways may be activated in response to specific ENM has been investigated by Tilton et al. [51], who performed global transcriptome and proteome analyses of intestinal (Caco-2/HT29-MTX) co-cultured cells, exposed to 10 and 100 µg/ml TiO_2 nanobelts (TiO2-NBs) and multi-walled carbon nanotubes (MWCNT). Interestingly, the early 1 h post-exposure transcriptional response was primarily independent of ENM type, showing similar expression patterns in response to both TiO_2-NB and MWCNTs, while the 24 h response was unique to each nanomaterial type. TiO_2-NB treatment affected several pathways, such as those associated with inflammation, apoptosis, cell cycle arrest, DNA replication stress and genomic instability, while MWCNTs regulated pathways involved in cell proliferation, DNA repair and anti-apoptosis.

Finally, the "omics" technique has also been exploited in order to identify the mechanisms underlying the different responses sometimes elicited by ENM of different size. It has been recently reported that 20 nm sized Ag ENM (1 µg/ml for 24 h) regulated different sets of proteins, principally involved in pathogen-like response and in the maintenance of the intestinal barrier function and integrity, with a distinct pattern of cellular responses compared to 200 nm Ag particles at the same experimental conditions in a co-culture of Caco-2/HT29-MTX cells [22].

Impact of the inhaled enm on the git and occupational implications

GIT is a relevant target for extrapulmonary effects of inhaled ENM

Inhalation is the main route through which people, in particular workers, may come in contact with ENM, and the lung is therefore the most obvious target of their possible toxic effects. However, in recent years, a lot of

extrapulmonary effects of inhaled ENM, regarding almost all organs and organ systems, have been reported [108]. As summarized in Fig. 1, these effects may be related to direct mechanisms (i.e. due to nanoparticles crossing the alveolo-capillary barrier) or to indirect mechanisms (i.e. due to the release of toxic mediators following nanoparticles/lung interaction). It is important to note that translocation to the systemic circulation is very low, below 0.5% of the exposure concentration [109], however, in the case of chronic exposure, accumulation of nanoparticles in target organs might reach a critical threshold causing injury.

GIT: An important overlooked target of extrapulmonary effects of inhaled ENM

Among extrapulmonary effects, those on the gastrointestinal tract have not explored yet. This is surprising, because inhaled nanoparticles may reach the gastrointestinal tract at a much larger amount than other organs. In fact, like other organs and organ systems, the GI tract can be exposed to nanoparticles crossing the alveolar barrier and reaching the systemic circulation, as suggested by the substantial fecal excretion of intravenously-injected ENM [93]. The amount of ENM reaching the gut through the systemic circulation is probably greater than that reaching other sites, as shown by Lee et al. who found that silver ENM were transferred from systemic circulation into the gut at a much higher rate than into the kidney or other biological sites [110]. In addition to ENM crossing the aveolar-capillary barrier (the only mechanism of direct effect for other organs), the GIT may be also exposed a) to inhaled ENM cleared from the lung through the mucociliary escalator (which is a major clearance pathway for ENM from the lung as compared with translocation through the alveolo-capillary barrier [111] and b) to nanoparticles directly ingested while breathing air (the so called "aerophagia"). People affected by this common disorder ingest air (and its content) at a much higher rate than normal persons [112].

The relevance of gastro-intestinal exposure following ENM inhalation is strongly supported by the recent finding that after pulmonary exposure of rats to CeO2 ENM, the highest amount of ENM was recovered from feces (71–90%), ENM recovered from the lungs being 7–18%, whereas urine and other extra-pulmonary organs both contributed between 4 and 6% of the total recovered mass [113]. Of note, the presence of ENM in feces is by itself the proof of a significant interaction with the GIT, since it implies a contact with the intestinal microbiome/microbiota, a major player in GI physiology and pathology [114, 115].

As reported for other organs and organ systems, there is evidence that the gut may be sensitive to mediators released by the inflamed lung, the so-called lung-gut axis.

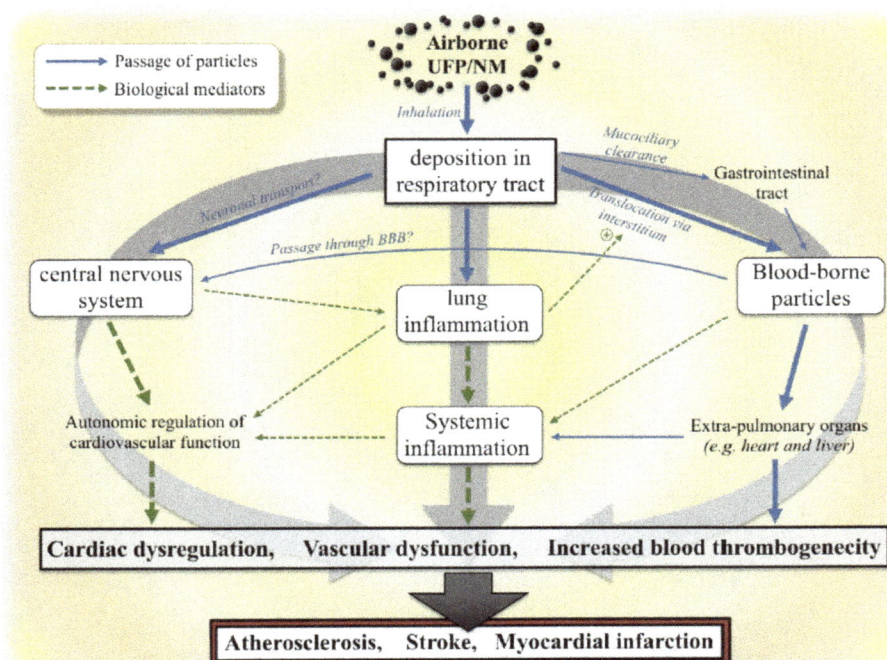

Fig. 1 Mechanisms of extrapulmonary effects of inhaled ENM. Legend: UFP = Ultrafine particles; NM = Nanomaterials. Reproduced from Environmental Health Perspective [140] (https://ehp.niehs.nih.gov/EHP424/)

This may be the case for interleukin-6 (IL-6), which is systemically elevated in patients with emphysema [116] and is implicated in the pathogenesis of inflammatory bowel disease [117, 118]. In patients with asthma, histopathological and functional alterations of the gastro-intestinal tract have been described [119], probably related to the circulation of activated lymphocytes between the mucosal tissues of the lungs and of the gastrointestinal tract [120].

As shown in Fig. 1, systemic inflammation has been reported after pulmonary exposure to ENM [121], and it is considered a major pathophysiological mechanism in order to explain the extrapulmonary effects of ENM. On the basis of the above reported evidence, these effects are to be expected also for the GI tract after inhalation of nanoparticles.

In summary, on the basis of the currently available evidence, not only the direct and the indirect mechanisms evoked for the effects on other extrapulmonary sites are plausible for the gastro-intestinal tract, but their impact might be even greater for this biological site in comparison to others.

Peculiar effects on GIT of inhaled ENM in comparison to ingested ENM

The reasons why the possible effects of inhaled ENM on the GI tract have been neglected until now are probably two: from one side the lack of substantial epidemiological evidence of relevant gastrointestinal effects in workers inhaling particles of larger size; from the other one, the fact that the very large amounts of nanoparticles ingested with food and drinks seem not to cause substantial damage.

As far as the first argument is concerned, only sparse data linking exposure to particulate and functional [122] or organic [123] GI diseases are available. Indeed, a systematic investigation of this possible association has not been performed. In any case, it should be considered that ENM may have enhanced or novel toxic properties in comparison to the same material in the bulk form, therefore the lack of robust epidemiological data for the inhaled bulk form cannot be translated to inhaled nanoparticles.

The assumption that ingested ENM are not harmful (second point), is questioned by recent experiments showing that ingested ENM may cause important consequences on the homeostasis of the GI tract, in particular on the gut microbiome, starting a chain of events leading to significant physiological and anatomical alterations [7].

In addition, it should be considered that the biocorona of inhaled nanoparticles is quite different in comparison to that of ingested nanoparticles: the first are primarily covered by biomolecules of the fluid lining the respiratory tract, whereas the biocorona of the second ones is mainly determined by the proteins, lipids and carbohydrates present in the food, which they are usually ingested with. The different biological identity between

Table 2 Different bio-corona and biological effects of nanoparticles reaching the gastro-intestinal tract through different modalities

Modality	Primary bio-corona (before coming in contact with the GI tract)	Available information on changes of biocorona during GI Transit	Effects on biokinetics/activity	Relative amount of nanoparticles
Ingested with food	Derived from interaction with food	Biocorona formed with the milk protein beta-lactoglobulin may be replaced by biliary salts in small intestine	The complex nano-particle/biliary salts may be efficiently absorbed in the small intestine.	High
Ingested with air (aerophagia)	No primary biocorona	A pepsin biocorona is formed in the stomach.	May affect the agglomeration status of nanoparticles	Low
Ingested after muco-ciliary clearance	Formed with surfactant phospholipids and proteins in the lung.	Unknown	Unknown	Substantial
Reaching the GI tract through systemic circulation (after lung crossing)	Formed with surfactant phospholipids and proteins in the lung. It may be partly modified by the contact with blood proteins (128) and by the contact with bile before being excreted in the gut	Unknown	Unknown	Low

inhaled and ingested nanoparticles may be associated with quite different biological effects, given the increasing awareness of the role of biocorona in governing the activity of nanoparticles in living organisms [124].

As an example, in experiments exploring the biological fate of nanoparticles ingested with food, it was found that gold nanoparticles ingested with milk are decorated with beta lactoglobulin, a protein of bovine milk, and that the protein is totally displaced by bile salts in the small intestine (whose excretion from the gallbladder into the intestine is in turn stimulated by food ingestion) so that a complex formed by a core of gold nanoparticles and a surface of bile salts is formed [125]. This complex resembles the complex lipid droplet/bile salts, which allows the absorption of lipids through the intestinal epithelium, otherwise not permeable to them. It can therefore be speculated that a similar phenomenon may occur for inorganic nanoparticles ingested with milk, allowing their transport through the intestinal epithelial cells.

On the other hand, the bio-corona of inhaled nanoparticles is characterized by a relatively fixed pattern of phospholipids derived from the contact with the pulmonary surfactant, whereas the protein composition changes according to the surface properties of the inhaled particles [126]. Nothing is known about the interaction of this nanoparticle/biocorona complex with the biological fluids of the gastrointestinal tract, (which are in any case of different composition than those encountered by nanoparticles ingested with food, due to the lack of food-related stimulation of biliary and pancreatic secretions) and we suggest that this topic should be explored (see recommendations).

As highlighted above, pristine nanoparticles (i.e. nanoparticles without a pre-formed biocorona) can also be ingested with aerophagia. These nanoparticles are covered in the stomach with a protein corona mainly composed by pepsin, a proteolytic protein secreted by the gastric chief cells. This protein seems to influence the aggregation status of silver nanoparticles, which may have implications on their toxicity [127]. Furthermore, the presence of a pepsin corona might explain the reported lack of antimicrobial effect of silver nanoparticles in the distal murine intestine [100].

A third type of biocorona may characterize ENM reaching the GIT through the blood after pulmonary pulmonary exposure: in this case ENM are covered with a biocorona primarily formed in the lung and subsequently modified in the blood [128]. Table 2 summarizes the different biocorona composition of nanoparticles reaching the gastro-intestinal tract through different modalities, and highlights possible biological effects.

Another important point to be taken into consideration is that nanoparticles reaching the gut following inhalation may have a synthetic identity different from that of ingested nanoparticles. As an example, some nanoparticles at high risk of being inhaled (e.g. carbon nanotubes) have a low chance to reach the gastrointestinal tract through ingestion. Therefore, not only the same nanoparticle may have different effects on the GI tract, depending on the modality of exposure, but also some nanoparticles reaching the gut following inhalation may have a low chance to do so by ingestion with food and may therefore cause biological responses which cannot be observed with ingested nanoparticles.

Discussion

The increasing interest in nanomaterials for advanced technologies, consumer products, and biomedical applications has led to great excitement about potential benefits, but also concerns over the potential for adverse human health effects. The gastrointestinal tract represents a likely route of entry for many nanomaterials. In occupational settings, gastrointestinal exposure may result from the mucociliary clearance of inhaled nanomaterials, or from a direct exposure in case of accidental events or when proper standards of personal and industrial hygiene are not met [129].

The gastrointestinal epithelium and supporting elements primarily act as a physical and biochemical barrier between the luminal compartment and the interior of the human body [130]. A key factor important to understand the gastrointestinal toxicological profile of ENM is the complex "interplay" between the great variability in ENM physico-chemical properties and the absolutely changeable conditions found along the gastrointestinal system. ENM chemical composition, structure/cristallinity, size and size distribution, shape, concentration, surface area, functionality and charge may all vary according to the methods of ENM production, preparation processes, and storage, but may also be modified when ENM are introduced into biological compartments. A number of gastrointestinal luminal parameters, such as physical forces, osmotic concentration, pH, digestive enzymes, (i.e. buccal amylase, gastric pepsin, and intestinal pancrease and lipase), together with different gastrointestinal transit time, dietary status, other biochemicals and commensal microbes may potentially impact ENM properties therefore affecting their toxicological profile. In this scenario, future researches should provide a systematic and deeper characterization of both the primary physico-chemical features of ENM and those secondarily acquired through the interactions occurring along the gastrointestinal tract, e.g. the degree of aggregation or agglomeration and the percentage of available ions for those ENM undergoing dissolution, known influencing factors of NP toxicity. Moreover, investigations focused on the possible toxic impact of ENM on the gastrointestinal system should elucidate which parameters are the strongest inducers of any changes in ENM features, and, on the other side, whether the full range of nanomaterials may be modified in the gastrointestinal milieu, or if only certain categories of ENM are subjected to such modifications [97]. Due to their intrinsically increased surface/mass ratio, ENM may adsorb biomolecules on their surface upon contact with food and/or biological fluids in gastrointestinal compartments, resulting in the formation of a biomolecular "corona" which may affect the uptake, bioaccumulation and biotransformation of NPs possibly leading to unanticipated, reduced or augmented, toxicities [131, 132]. All these aspects should be carefully considered to better correlate ENM primary and acquired properties and biological effects, in order to support the production of "ENM safe by design" that, while maintaining most of the innovative and revolutionary ENM features may, at the same time, be characterized by lower toxicity [133].

Additionally, M cell- targeting of ENMs should be carefully considered as another possible pathway of interaction between ENMs and the intestinal milieu which may have possible systemic implications. M cells are specialized epithelial cells of the gut-associated lymphoid tissues (GALT) that can play an immunosensing and surveillance role by delivering luminal antigens through the follicle-associated epithelium to the underlying immune cells. Recent evidence has supported the critical function of endogenous and synthetic nanomineral chaperones in the efficient transport of molecules across the epithelial barrier of the lymphoid follicles in the small intestine [27, 31]. In this perspective, further investigation should be focused to assess whether ENMs may be involved in protecting molecules from the GI degradation, favoring an effective M-cell delivery, and a greater transfection efficacy, therefore promoting tolerogenic or stimulatory immunological responses. Overall, this may be important to define the role of ENMs in vaccine delivery systems for priming more effective humoral and mucosal immune responses in the hosts [134].

A challenging issue relates also on the difficulties to extrapolate experimental data to realistic human/occupational exposure contexts. In vitro studies demonstrated the ability of several types of ENM to induce cytotoxic, inflammatory, oxidative stress as well as genotoxic responses in exposed cells. However, in vitro models may not accurately resemble the complexity of the in vivo response [135]. Therefore, in the attempt to improve physiological relevance of in vitro models and better mimic in vivo gastrointestinal situations, including conditions of inflamed mucosa, multi-cellular cultures have been proposed. These may incorporate mucus secreting goblet cells [34], microfold-cells [61], and even immunecompetent macrophages and dendritic cells [136] and have shown a diverse, as well as more predictive of in vivo response, susceptibility to the ENM injuries compared to

the cellular monolayers [48]. Moreover, for the assessment of the toxicity of orally ingested ENM, additional refinements, for instance, pre-treatment or co-administration of particles with gastrointestinal reconstituted bio-fluids or food matrix components, may be employed in order to achieve more meaningful in vitro tests, with the aim to deeply understand how protein corona changes may affect ENM uptake, metabolism and toxicological behavior.

In vivo studies, on the other hand, can provide information concerning ENM toxico-kinetics in gastrointestinal and extra-intestinal tissues and ENM toxico-dynamic behaviors in relation to their physicochemical properties. In this regard, future in vivo studies should overcome the difficulty to extrapolate findings from the generally, higherdoses, short-term investigations on animal models, to real low-dose, long-term conditions of exposure experienced in general living and occupational settings, through the adoption of more realistic experimental designs. Moreover, in vivo studies should provide useful data to identify possible biomarkers of exposure and early effect as well as indicators of susceptibility to greater ENM induced adverse health outcomes. Macrophage-mediated mucociliary escalation followed by fecal excretion is a pathway for clearing the inhaled NPs from the body [129, 137]. Although it is rather difficult to routinely employ feces as a suitable biological matrix for occupational biomonitoring, on the account of the aforementioned clearance mechanism, in the case of metal- or metal oxide-NP exposure, the measurement of the elemental metal content in feces should be viewed as a means to evaluate the recent/current exposure to this kind of NPs [129]. Moreover, future investigations should explore possible biomarkers of early effect, particularly as concerns mucosal inflammatory alterations, which may be detected in fecal matrix. Clinical experience, carried out with inflammatory bowel diseases, Chron's disease or ulcerative colitis, in this sense, may provide useful suggestions for potential biomarkers to be investigated and validated in the nano-toxicological gastrointestinal field [138]. Additionally, taking advantage of more innovative "omics techniques", a comprehensive analysis of differential gene and protein expression should be performed to derive molecular profiles indicative of NP exposure or early effect which may also explain possible early modes of cellular response to NPs. This may be helpful to understand also biological processes affected by ENM or possibly involved in their toxico-dynamic behavior to identify potential parameters of individual susceptibility to ENM adverse effects [139]. Importantly, in the attempt to define conditions of greater susceptibility to ENM adverse outcomes, intra- and inter-individual differences in normal physiology as well as in specific diseases should be deeply analyzed. These conditions, in fact, may alter the gastrointestinal environments affecting ENM stability and movement as well as epithelial permeability.

Age, gender-specific differences, pregnancy status, malnutrition, sleep cycle and stress, as well as inflammatory bowel diseases can all result in increased lining permeability and can augment the susceptibility to the absorption of some types of ENM and to the induction of possible toxic effects.

An emerging aspect that deserves deep attention regards the potential interactions of ingested ENM with the gut microbiota [7].

Few studies are still available concerning such interesting issue, and some of them showed conflicting results. In this field, some knowledge gaps should be overcome by future investigations, particularly concerning which pathological consequences may derive from microbiota alterations induced by ENM. In an opposite perspective, alterations in ENM toxico-kinetic and dynamic profile caused by the same microbiota as well as by pre-existing altered microbial states, such as gram negative bacterial overgrowth, should be clarified. To deeply assess such issues, fecal samples as representative models of the microbiota of the colon, together with samples of the human small intestine microbiota obtained from ileostomies of people undergoing colon surgery, may be used. Moreover, the employment of «humanized» models by the inoculation of human gut microbiota to gnotobiotic animals should be carefully considered as an ideal model to study in vivo effects of ENM in order to transfer animal data to humans. The study of the interactions between ENM and the gastrointestinal tract may provide the identification of innovative biomarkers based on the possible specific modifications induced by ENM on the gut microbiota. However, confounding effects related to individual characteristics, pathological statuses, diet, drugs and co-exposure to other xenobiotics should be taken into careful consideration to adequately interpret these results.

Overall, this information would provide deep insight into possible ENM toxicological aspects that have not been sufficiently explored up to date, with the aim to reach a suitable assessment of risks in general living and occupational ENM exposure settings.

In this perspective, another crucial aspect which needs to be adequately explored in the future is represented by the possible gastro-intestinal effects and gastrointestinal-mediated systemic effects of inhaled ENM. There is evidence that GIT may be a relevant target for extra-pulmonary effects of inhaled ENM, and that these effects may be different (and possibly more relevant) than those induced by ingested ENM. In this respect, experimental studies focused to this specific topic are needed. We recommend in particular:

1. Assessing the impact of GI fluids and (gut) microbiome on the biocorona of particles that are deposited in the respiratory tract and after

mucociliary clearance being swallowed versus nanoparticles ingested with food and how this affects the biodistribution

2. Assessing the toxic effects of inhaled nanoparticles (i.e. incubated with pulmonary surfactant) on gastric cells, cells of the small intestine and cells of the colon (including the interaction with the microbiome), as compared with toxic effects of nanoparticles ingested with food using in vitro methods

3. Perform a systematic comparison of effects of inhaled nanoparticles on the gastrointestinal tract and on intestinal microbiome compared with ingested nanoparticles.

The results of these studies might be the basis for refining the focus on possible effects of ENM on human at high risk of lung exposure (i.e. workers directly or indirectly involved in nanotechnology).

Conclusions

The gastro-intestinal tract (GIT) is considered to be a potential target of ENM ingested with food and water. It is believed that the possible biological effects on the gastrointestinal tract (GIT) deriving from ENM ingestion involve mainly the consumers, whereas workers may be only marginally affected, the inhalation being the main way through which they may come in contact with ENM. The biological effects of ENM on this organ are poorly known both because of inherent difficulties in their assessment due to the complex GIT environment and because most available experimental studies suggest the lack of overt toxicity.

In this review we discussed the most relevant gaps in the knowledge of the biological effects of ENM on the GIT and demonstrate that, by logically connecting the available sparse information on this topic, it is possible to identify sequential key processes, spanning from the alterations of intestinal permeability to functional and organic cellular damage, which may shed light on the pathophysiological mechanisms of the gut/ENM interaction.

We also re-interpreted the results of some experiments, such as, for example, the presence in the stools of almost the total amount of ingested ENM, a finding generally considered to be an indicator of the lack of substantial local and systemic effects of the ingested ENM; however, the recent evidence that ENM may have a relevant impact on the gut microbiota, even in the absence of substantial contact with GIT cells, indicates that local and systemic biological effects mediated by changes in gut microbiota are possible even in this situation.

Last but not least, we challenged the common belief that the possible biological effects of ENM on the GIT are confined to consumers, showing that inhaled ENM, which represent the main route of ENM exposure for workers, may induce peculiar and substantial effects on the GIT: these effects may be different (and potentially more important) than those related to ingested ENM.

Taken together, our findings suggest that the GIT should have a primary role in the future research on the biological effects of ENM. In this light, we identified and suggested proper experimental protocols aimed to verify this hypothesis.

Acknowledgements
Not applicable.

Funding
Not applicable.

Authors' contributions
II and AP conceived the study, reviewed the literature, wrote and edited the manuscript, provided overall guidance to the development of the manuscript; EB critically reviewed and edited the manuscript; VL reviewed the literature and wrote the manuscript; MC, LC, GDP, SI, AM, MM, PP critically reviewed the manuscript and contributed to various sections; LP critically reviewed and edited the manuscript. All authors read and approved the final manuscript.

Competing interests
The authors declare that they have no competing interests.

Author details
[1]Department of Biomedicine and Prevention, University of Rome Tor Vergata, Via Montpellier 1, 00133 Rome, Italy. [2]Department of Sciences and Public Health and Pediatrics, University of Turin, Turin, Italy. [3]Department of Medical Sciences and Public Health, University of Cagliari, Cagliari, Italy. [4]Department of Medical and Surgical Specialties, Radiological Sciences, and Public Health, Section of Public Health and Human Sciences, University of Brescia, Brescia, Italy. [5]Department of Occupational and Environmental Medicine, Epidemiology and Hygiene, Italian Workers' Compensation Authority (INAIL), Rome, Italy. [6]Department of Public Health, University of Naples Federico II, Naples, Italy. [7]Department of Medicine and Surgery, University of Parma, Parma, Italy. [8]Department of Experimental Medicine- Section of Hygiene, Occupational Medicine and Forensic Medicine, University of Campania Luigi Vanvitelli, Naples, Italy.

References
1. Martirosyan A, Schneider YJ. Engineered nanomaterials in food: implications for food safety and consumer health. Int J Environ Res Public Health. 2014; 11:5720–50.
2. Chen H, Seiber JN, Hotze M. ACS select on nanotechnology in food and agriculture: a perspective on implications and applications. J Agric Food Chem. 2014;62:1209–12.
3. Athinarayanan J, Alshatwi AA, Periasamy VS, Al-Warthan AA. Identification of nanoscale ingredients in commercial food products and their induction of mitochondrially mediated cytotoxic effects on human mesenchymal stem cells. J Food Sci. 2015;80:N459–64.
4. Lim JH, Sisco P, Mudalige TK, Sánchez-Pomales G, Howard PC, Linder SW. Detection and characterization of SiO2 and TiO2 nanostructures in dietary supplements. J Agric Food Chem. 2015;63:3144–52.
5. Shahabi-Ghahfarrokhi I, Khodaiyan F, Mousavi M, Yousefi H. Preparation of UV-protective kefiran/nano-ZnO nanocomposites: physical and mechanical properties. Int J Biol Macromol. 2015;72:41–6.
6. Hollister EB, Gao C, Versalovic J. Compositional and functional features of the gastrointestinal microbiome and their effects on human health. Gastroenterology. 2014;146:1449–58.
7. Pietroiusti A, Magrini A, Campagnolo L. New frontiers in nanotoxicology: gut microbiota/microbiome-mediated effects of engineered nanomaterials. Toxicol Appl Pharmacol. 2016;299:90–5.
8. Fröhlich E, Roblegg E. Models for oral uptake of nanoparticles in consumer products. Toxicology. 2012;291:10–7.
9. Walczak AP, Fokkink R, Peters R, Tromp P, Herrera Rivera ZE, Rietjens IM, et al. Behaviour of silver nanoparticles and silver ions in an in vitro human gastrointestinal digestion model. Nanotoxicology. 2013;7:1198–210.
10. Axson JL, Stark DI, Bondy AL, Capracotta SS, Maynard AD, Philbert MA, et al. Rapid kinetics of size and pH-dependent dissolution and aggregation of silver nanoparticles in simulated gastric fluid. J Phys Chem C Nanomater Interfaces. 2015;119:20632–41.
11. Rogers KR, Bradham K, Tolaymat T, Thomas DJ, Hartmann T, Ma L, et al. Alterations in physical state of silver nanoparticles exposed to synthetic human stomach fluid. Sci Total Environ. 2012;420:334–9.
12. Mwilu SK, El Badawy AM, Bradham K, Nelson C, Thomas D, Scheckel KG, et al. Changes in silver nanoparticles exposed to human synthetic stomach fluid: effects of particle size and surface chemistry. Sci Total Environ. 2013;447:90–8.
13. Böhmert L, Girod M, Hansen U, Maul R, Knappe P, Niemann B, et al. Analytically monitored digestion of silver nanoparticles and their toxicity on human intestinal cells. Nanotoxicology. 2014;8:631–42.
14. Cho WS, Kang BC, Lee JK, Jeong J, Che JH, Seok SH. Comparative absorption, distribution, and excretion of titanium dioxide and zinc oxide nanoparticles after repeated oral administration. Part Fibre Toxicol. 2013;10:9.
15. Brun E, Barreau F, Veronesi G, Fayard B, Sorieul S, Chanéac C, et al. Titanium dioxide nanoparticle impact and translocation through ex vivo, in vivo and in vitro gut epithelia. Part Fibre Toxicol. 2014;11:13.
16. Wang Y, Chen Z, Ba T, Pu J, Chen T, Song Y, et al. Susceptibility of young and adult rats to the oral toxicity of titanium dioxide nanoparticles. Small. 2013;9:1742–52.
17. Sakai-Kato K, Hidaka M, Un K, Kawanishi T, Okuda H. Physicochemical properties and in vitro intestinal permeability properties and intestinal cell toxicity of silica particles, performed in simulated gastrointestinal fluids. Biochim Biophys Acta. 2014;1840:1171–80.
18. Antunović B, Barlow S, Chesson A, Flynn A, Hardy A, Jany K-D, et al. Guidance on the risk assessment of the application of nanoscience and nanotechnologies in the food and feed chain. EFSA J. 2011;9:2140.
19. Bellmann S, Carlander D, Fasano A, Momcilovic D, Scimeca JA, Waldman WJ, et al. Mammalian gastrointestinal tract parameters modulating the integrity, surface properties, and absorption of food-relevant nanomaterials. Wiley interdisciplinary reviews-nanomedicine and. NanoBiotechnology. 2015;7:609–22.
20. Bouwmeester H, van der Zande M, Jepson MA. Effects of food-borne nanomaterials on gastrointestinal tissues and microbiota. Epub ahed of print: Wiley Interdiscip Rev Nanomed Nanobiotechnol; 2017 May 26.
21. Behrens I, Pena AI, Alonso MJ, Kissel T. Comparative uptake studies of bioadhesive and non-bioadhesive nanoparticles in human intestinal cell lines and rats: the effect of mucus on particle adsorption and transport. Pharm Res. 2002;19:1185–93.
22. Georgantzopoulou A, Serchi T, Cambier S, Leclercq CC, Renaut J, Shao J, et al. Effects of silver nanoparticles and ions on a co-culture model for the gastrointestinal epithelium. Part Fibre Toxicol. 2016;13:9.
23. Jeong GN, Jo UB, Ryu HY, Kim YS, Song KS, Yu YJ. Histochemical study of intestinal mucins after administration of silver nanoparticles in Sprague-Dawley rats. Arch Toxicol. 2010;84:63–9.
24. Ashwood P, Thompson RP, Powell JJ. Fine particles that adsorb lipopolysaccharide via bridging calcium cations may mimic bacterial pathogenicity towards cells. Exp Biol Med (Maywood). 2007; 232:107–17.
25. Evans SM, Ashwood P, Warley A, Berisha F, Thompson RP, Powell JJ. The role of dietary microparticles and calcium in apoptosis and interleukin-1beta release of intestinal macrophages. Gastroenterology. 2002;123:1543–53.
26. Powell JJ, Faria N, Thomas-McKay E, Pele LC. Origin and fate of dietary nanoparticles and microparticles in the gastrointestinal tract. J Autoimmun. 2010;34:J226–33.
27. Powell JJ, Thomas-McKay E T, Thoree V, Robertson J, Hewitt LE, Skepper JN, et al. An endogenous nanomineral chaperones luminal antigen and peptoglycan to intestinal immune cells. Nat Nanotechnol. 2015;10:361–9.

28. McMellen ME, Wakeman D, Longshore SW, McDuffie LA, Warner BW. Growth factors: possible roles for clinical management of the short bowel syndrome. Semin Pediatr Surg. 2010;19:35–43.

29. Jani PU, McCarthy DE, Florence AT. Titanium dioxide (rutile) particle uptake from the rat GI tract and translocation to systemic organs after oral administration. Int J Pharm. 1994;105:157–68.

30. Jones K, Morton J, Smith I, Jurkschat K, Harding AH, Evans G. Human in vivo and in vitro studies on gastrointestinal absorption of titanium dioxide nanoparticles. Toxicol Lett. 2015;233:95–101.

31. Pele LC, Thoree V, Bruggraber SF, Koller D, Thompson RP, Lomer MC, et al. Pharmaceutical/food grade titanium dioxide particles are absorbed into the bloodstream of human volunteers. Part Fibre Toxicol. 2015;12:26.

32. Koeneman BA, Zhang Y, Westerhoff P, Chen Y, Crittenden JC, Capco DG. Toxicity and cellular responses of intestinal cells exposed to titanium dioxide. Cell Biol Toxicol. 2010;26:225–38.

33. Fisichella M, Berenguer F, Steinmetz G, Auffan M, Rose J, Prat O. Intestinal toxicity evaluation of TiO2 degraded surface-treated nanoparticles: a combined physico-chemical and toxicogenomics approach in caco-2 cells. Part Fibre Toxicol. 2012;9:18.

34. Mahler GJ, Esch MB, Tako E, Southard TL, Archer SD, Glahn RP, et al. Oral exposure to polystyrene nanoparticles affects iron absorption. Nat Nanotechnol. 2012;7:264–71.

35. Williams KM, Gokulan K, Cerniglia CE, Khare S. Size and dose dependent effects of silver nanoparticle exposure on intestinal permeability in an in vitro model of the human gut epithelium. J Nanobiotechnology. 2016;14:62.

36. Ruiz PA, Morón B, Becker HM, Lang S, Atrott K, Spalinger MR, et al. Titanium dioxide nanoparticles exacerbate DSS-induced colitis: role of the NLRP3 inflammasome. Gut. 2017;66:1216–24.

37. Coyuco JC, Liu Y, Tan BJ, Chiu GN. Functionalized carbon nanomaterials: exploring the interactions with Caco-2 cells for potential oral drug delivery. Int J Nanomedicine. 2011;6:2253–63.

38. Lichtenstein D, Ebmeyer J, Knappe P, Juling S, Böhmert L, Selve S, et al. Impact of food components during in vitro digestion of silver nanoparticles on cellular uptake and cytotoxicity in intestinal cells. Biol Chem. 2015;396:1255–64.

39. Abbott CTE, Schwab KJ. Toxicity of commercially available engineered nanoparticles to Caco-2 and SW480 human intestinal epithelial cells. Cell Biol Toxicol. 2013;29:101–16.

40. De Angelis I, Barone F, Zijno A, Bizzarri L, Russo MT, Pozzi R, et al. Comparative study of ZnO and TiO2 nanoparticles: physicochemical characterization and toxicological effects on human colon carcinoma cells. Nanotoxicology. 2013;7:1361–72.

41. Moos PJ, Olszewski K, Honeggar M, Cassidy P, Leachman S, Woessner D, et al. Responses of human cells to ZnO nanoparticles: a gene transcription study. Metallomics. 2011;3:1199–211.

42. De Berardis B, Civitelli G, Condello M, Lista P, Pozzi R, Arancia G, et al. Exposure to ZnO nanoparticles induces oxidative stress and cytotoxicity in human colon carcinoma cells. Toxicol Appl Pharmacol. 2010;246:116–27.

43. Song Y, Guan R, Lyu F, Kang T, Wu Y, Chen X. In Vitro cytotoxicity of silver nanoparticles and zinc oxide nanoparticles to human epithelial colorectal adenocarcinoma (Caco-2) cells. Mutat Res. 2014;769:113–8.

44. Tarantini A, Huet S, Jarry G, Lanceleur R, Poul M, Tavares A, et al. Genotoxicity of synthetic amorphous silica nanoparticles in rats following short-term exposure. Part 1: oral route. Environ Mol Mutagen. 2015;56:218–27.

45. Gerloff K, Pereira DI, Faria N, Boots AW, Kolling J, Förster I, et al. Influence of simulated gastrointestinal conditions on particle-induced cytotoxicity and interleukin-8 regulation in differentiated and undifferentiated Caco-2 cells. Nanotoxicology. 2013;7:353–66.

46. Wilding LA, Bassis CM, Walacavage K, Hashway S, Leroueil PR, Morishita M, et al. Repeated dose (28-day) administration of silver nanoparticles of varied size and coating does not significantly alter the indigenous murine gut microbiome. Nanotoxicology. 2016;10:513–20.

47. Aueviriyavit S, Phummiratch D, Maniratanachote R. Mechanistic study on the biological effects of silver and gold nanoparticles in Caco-2 cells–induction of the Nrf2/HO-1 pathway by high concentrations of silver nanoparticles. Toxicol Lett. 2014;224:73–83.

48. Susewind J, De Souza Carvalho-Wodarz C, Repnik U, Collnot EM, Schneider-Daum N, Griffiths GW, et al. A 3D co-culture of three human cell lines to model the inflamed intestinal mucosa for safety testing of nanomaterials. Nanotoxicology. 2016;10:53–62.

49. Alkilany AM, Nagaria PK, Hexel CR, Shaw TJ, Murphy CJ, Wyatt MD. Cellular uptake and cytotoxicity of gold nanorods: molecular origin of cytotoxicity and surface effects. Small. 2009;5:701–8.

50. Ammendolia MG, Iosi F, Maranghi F, Tassinari R, Cubadda F, Aureli F, et al. Short-term oral exposure to low doses of nano-sized TiO2 and potential modulatory effects on intestinal cells. Food Chem Toxicol. 2017;102:63–75.

51. Tilton SC, Karin NJ, Tolic A, Xie Y, Lai X, Hamilton RF Jr, et al. Three human cell types respond to multi-walled carbon nanotubes and titanium dioxide nanobelts with cell-specific transcriptomic and proteomic expression patterns. Nanotoxicology. 2014;8:533–48.

52. Tada-Oikawa S, Ichihara G, Fukatsu H, Shimanuki Y, Tanaka N, Watanabe E, et al. Titanium dioxide particle type and concentration influence the inflammatory response in Caco-2 cells. Int J Mol Sci. 2016;17:576.

53. Gitrowski C, Al-Jubory AR, Handy RD. Uptake of different crystal structures of TiO2 nanoparticles by Caco-2 intestinal cells. Toxicol Lett. 2014;226:264–76.

54. Onishchenko GE, Erokhina MV, Abramchuk SS, Shaitan KV, Raspopov RV, Smirnova VV, et al. Effects of titanium dioxide nanoparticles on small intestinal mucosa in rats. Bull Exp Biol Med. 2012;154:265–70.

55. Dorier M, Brun E, Veronesi G, Barreau F, Pernet-Gallay K, Desvergne C, et al. Impact of anatase and rutile titanium dioxide nanoparticles on uptake carriers and efflux pumps in Caco-2 gut epithelial cells. Nano. 2015;7:7352–60.

56. Farcal L, Torres Andón F, Di Cristo L, Rotoli BM, Bussolati O, Bergamaschi E, et al. Comprehensive in vitro toxicity testing of a panel of representative oxide nanomaterials: first steps towards an intelligent testing strategy. PLoS One. 2015;10:e0127174.

57. Jos A, Pichardo S, Puerto M, Sánchez E, Grilo A, Cameán AM. Cytotoxicity of carboxylic acid functionalized single wall carbon nanotubes on the human intestinal cell line Caco-2. Toxicol in Vitro. 2009;23:1491–6.

58. Kulamarva A, Bhathena J, Malhotra M, Sebak S, Nalamasu O, Ajayan P, et al. In Vitro cytotoxicity of functionalized single walled carbon nanotubes for targeted gene delivery applications. Nanotoxicology. 2008;2:184–8.

59. Song ZM, Chen N, Liu JH, Tang H, Deng X, Xi WS, et al. Biological effect of food additive titanium dioxide nanoparticles on intestine: an in vitro study. J Appl Toxicol. 2015;35:1169–78.

60. Zijno A, De Angelis I, De Berardis B, Andreoli C, Russo MT, Pietraforte D, et al. Different mechanisms are involved in oxidative DNA damage and genotoxicity induction by ZnO and TiO2 nanoparticles in human colon carcinoma cells. Toxicol in Vitro. 2015;29:1503–12.

61. Bouwmeester H, Poortman J, Peters RJ, Wijma E, Kramer E, Makama S, et al. Characterization of translocation of silver nanoparticles and effects on whole-genome gene expression using an in vitro intestinal epithelium coculture model. ACS Nano. 2011;5:4091–103.

62. Lamb JG, Hathaway LB, Munger MA, Raucy JL, Franklin MR. Nanosilver particle effects on drug metabolism in vitro. Drug Metab Dispos. 2010;38:2246–51.

63. Gaiser BK, Fernandes TF, Jepson MA, Lead JR, Tyler CR, Baalousha M, et al. Interspecies comparisons on the uptake and toxicity of silver and cerium dioxide nanoparticles. Environ Toxicol Chem. 2012;31:144–54.

64. Williams K, Milner J, Boudreau MD, Gokulan K, Cerniglia CE, Khare S. Effects of subchronic exposure of silver nanoparticles on intestinal microbiota and gut-associated immune responses in the ileum of Sprague-Dawley rats. Nanotoxicology. 2015;9:279–89.

65. Ponti J, Colognato R, Rauscher H, Gioria S, Broggi F, Franchini F, et al. Colony forming efficiency and microscopy analysis of multi-wall carbon nanotubes cell interaction. Toxicol Lett. 2010;197:29–37.

66. Chen H, Wang B, Zhao R, Gao D, Guan M, Zheng L, et al. Coculture with low-dose SWCNT attenuates bacterial invasion and inflammation in human enterocyte-like Caco-2 cells. Small. 2015;11:4366–78.

67. Wang L, Nagesha DK, Selvarasah S, Dokmeci MR, Carrier RL. Toxicity of CdSe nanoparticles in Caco-2 cell cultures. J Nanobiotechnology. 2008;6:11.

68. Martirosyan A, Grintzalis K, Polet M, Laloux L, Schneider YJ. Tuning the inflammatory response to silver nanoparticles via quercetin in Caco-2 (co-)cultures as model of the human intestinal mucosa. Toxicol Lett. 2016;253:36–45.

69. Martirosyan A, Bazes A, Schneider YJ. In Vitro toxicity assessment of silver nanoparticles in the presence of phenolic compounds–preventive agents against the harmful effect? Nanotoxicology. 2014;8:573–82.

70. Cao Y, Roursgaard M, Kermanizadeh A, Loft S. Møller P. Synergistic effects of zinc oxide nanoparticles and fatty acids on toxicity to caco-2 cells. Int J Toxicol 2015;34:67–76.

71. Balog S, Rodriguez-Lorenzo L, Monnier CA, Obiols-Rabasa M, Rothen-Rutishauser B, Schurtenberger P, et al. Characterizing nanoparticles in complex biological media and physiological fluids with depolarized dynamic light scattering. Nano. 2015;7:5991–7.

72. Cohen JM, Teeguarden JG, Demokritou P. An integrated approach for the in vitro dosimetry of engineered nanomaterials. Part Fibre Toxicol. 2014;11:20.

73. Cha K, Hong H-W, Choi Y-G, Lee MJ, Park JH, Chae H-K, et al. Comparison of acute responses of mice livers to short-term exposure to Nano-sized or micro-sized silver particles. Biotechnol Lett. 2008;30:1893–9.

74. Kim YS, Song MY, Park JD, Song KS, Ryu HR, Chung YH, Chang HK, Lee JH, KH O, Kelman BJ, Hwang IK, Yu IJ. Subchronic oral toxicity of silver nanoparticles. Part Fibre Toxicol. 2010;7:20.

75. Park E-J, Bae E, Yi J, Kim Y, Choi K, Lee SH, et al. Repeated-Dosetoxicity and inflammatory responses in mice by oral administration of silver nanoparticles. Environ Toxicol Pharmacol. 2010;30:162–8.

76. Kim YS, Kim JS, Cho HS, Rha DS,Kim JM et al. Twenty-eight-day oral toxicity, genotoxicity, and gender-related tissue distribution of silver nanoparticles in Sprague-Dawley rats. Inhal Toxicol. 2008;20:575–83.

77. van der Zande M, Vandebriel RJ, Van Doren E, Kramer E, Herrera Rivera Z, Serrano-Rojero CS, Gremmer ER, Mast J, Peters RJ, Hollman PC, Hendriksen PJ, Marvin HJ, Peijnenburg AA, Bouwmeester H. Distribution, elimination, and toxicity of silver nanoparticles and silver ions in rats after 28-day oral exposure ACS Nano. 2012;6:7427–42.

78. Hadrup N, Loeschner K, Bergström A, Wilcks A, Gao X, Vogel U, et al. Subacute oral toxicity investigation of nanoparticulate and ionic silver in rats. Arch Toxicol. 2012;86:543–51.

79. Bergin IL, Wilding LA, Morishita M, Walacavage K, Ault AP, Axson JL, et al. Effects of particle size and coating on toxicologic parameters, fecal elimination kinetics and tissue distribution of acutely ingested silver nanoparticles in a mouse model. Nanotoxicology. 2016;10:352–60.

80. Nogueira CM. Titanium dioxide induced inflammation in the small intestine. World J Gastroenterol. 2012;18:4729.

81. Cui Y, Liu H, Zhou M, Duan Y, Li N, Gong X, et al. Signaling pathway of inflammatory responses in the mouse liver caused by TiO2 nanoparticles. J Biomed Mater Res A. 2011;96:221–9.

82. Duan Y, Liu J, Ma L, Li N, Liu H, Wang J, et al. Toxicological characteristics of nanoparticulate anatase titanium dioxide in mice. Biomaterials. 2010;31:894–9.

83. Sycheva LP, Zhurkov VS, Iurchenko VV, Daugel-Dauge NO, Kovalenko MA, Krivtsova EK, et al. Investigation of genotoxic and cytotoxic effects of micro- and nanosized titanium dioxide in six organs of mice in vivo. Mutat Res. 2011;726:8–14.

84. Gui S, Zhang Z, Zheng L, Cui Y, Liu X, Li N, et al. Molecular mechanism of kidney injury of mice caused by exposure to titanium dioxide nanoparticles. J Hazard Mater. 2011;195:365–70.

85. Bu Q, Yan G, Deng P, Peng F, Lin H, Xu Y, et al. NMR-based metabonomic study of the sub-acute toxicity of titanium dioxide nanoparticles in rats after oral administration. Nanotechnology. 2010;21:125105.

86. Tassinari R, Cubadda F, Moracci G, Aureli F, D'Amato M, Valeri M, et al. Oral, short-term exposure to titanium dioxide nanoparticles in Sprague-Dawley rat: focus on reproductive and endocrine systems and spleen. Nanotoxicology. 2014;8:654–62.

87. OECD Guideline for the Testing of Chemicals e Repeated Dose 90-Oral Toxicity Study in Rodents e OECD 408, 1998. Adopted 21st September 1998.

88. Warheit DB, Donner EM. How meaningful are risk determinations in the absence of a complete dataset? Making the case for publishing standardized test guideline and "no-effect" studies for evaluating the safety of nanoparticulates versus spurious "high effect" results from single investigative studies. Sci Technol Adv Mater. 2015;16:034603.

89. Warheit DB, Hoke RA, Finlay C, Donner EM, Reed KL, Sayes CM. Development of a base set of toxicity tests using ultrafine TiO2 particles as a component of nanoparticle risk management. Toxicol Lett. 2007;171:99–110.

90. Masyutin AG, Erokhina MV, Sychevskaya KA, Gusev AA, Vasyukova IA, Tkachev AG, et al. Multiwalled carbon nanotubules induce pathological changes in the digestive organs of mice. Bull Exp Biol Med. 2016;161:125–30.

91. Belyaeva NN, Sycheva LP, Savostikova ON. Structural and functional analysis of the small intestine in rats after six-month-long exposure to multiwalled carbon nanotubes. Bull Exp Biol Med. 2016;161:826–8.

92. Seok SH, Cho WS, Park JS, Na Y, Jang A, Kim H, et al. Rat pancreatitis produced by 13-week administration of zinc oxide nanoparticles: biopersistence of nanoparticles and possible solutions. J Appl Toxicol. 2013; 33:1089–96.

93. Choi J, Kim H, Kim P, Jo E, Kim HM, Lee MY, et al. Toxicity of zinc oxide nanoparticles in rats treated by two different routes: single intravenous injection and single oral administration. J Toxicol Environ Health A. 2015;78:226–43.

94. Li CH, Shen CC, Cheng YW, Huang SH, Wu CC, Kao CC, et al. Organ biodistribution, clearance, and genotoxicity of orally administered zinc oxide nanoparticles in mice. Nanotoxicology. 2012;6:746–56.

95. Esmaeillou M, Moharamnejad M, Hsankhani R, Tehrani AA, Maadi H. Toxicity of ZnO nanoparticles in healthy adult mice. Environ Toxicol Pharmacol. 2013;35:67–71.

96. So SJ, Jang IS, Han CS. Effect of micro/nano silica particle feeding for mice. J Nanosci Nanotechnol. 2008;8:5367–71.

97. Bergin IL, Witzmann FA. Nanoparticle toxicity by the gastrointestinal route: evidence and knowledge gaps. Int J Biomed Nanosci Nanotechnol. 2013;3(1–2)

98. Robles Alonso V, Guarner F. Linking the gut microbiota to human health. Br J Nutr. 2013;109(Suppl 2):S21–6.

99. Wikoff WR, Anfora AT, Liu J, Schultz PG, Lesley SA, Peters EC, et al. Metabolomics analysis reveals large effects of gut microflora on mammalian blood metabolites. Proc Natl Acad Sci U S A. 2009;106:3698–703.

100. Lynch SV, Pedersen O. The human intestinal microbiome in health and disease. N Engl J Med. 2016;375:2369–79.

101. Winter SE, Lopez CA, Bäumler AJ. The dynamics of gut-associated microbial communities during inflammation. EMBO Rep. 2013;14:319–27.

102. Das P, McDonald JAK, Petrof EO, Allen-Vercoe E, Walker VK. Nanosilver-mediated change in human intestinal microbiota. J Nanosci Nanotechnol. 2014;5:5.

103. van den Brule S, Ambroise J, Lecloux H, Levard C, Soulas R, De Temmerman PJ, et al. Dietary silver nanoparticles can disturb the gut microbiota in mice. Part Fibre Toxicol. 2016;13:38.

104. Fondevila M, Herrer R, Casalbas MC, Abecia L, Ducia JJ. Silver nanoparticles as a potential antimicrobial additive for weaned pigs. Anim Feed Sci Technol. 2009;150:259–69.

105. Miethling-Graff R, Rumpker R, Richter M, Verano-Braga T, Kjeldsen F, Brewer J, et al. Exposure to silver nanoparticles induces size- and dose-dependent oxidative stress and cytotoxicity in human colon carcinoma cells. Toxicol in Vitro. 2014;28:1280–9.

106. Verano-Braga T, Miethling-Graff R, Wojdyla K, Rogowska-Wrzesinska A, Brewer JR, Erdmann H, et al. Insights into the cellular response triggered by silver nanoparticles using quantitative proteomics. ACS Nano. 2014;8:2161–75.

107. Oberemm A, Hansen U, Böhmert L, Meckert C, Braeuning A, Thünemann AF, et al. Proteomic responses of human intestinal Caco-2 cells exposed to silver nanoparticles and ionic silver. J Appl Toxicol. 2016;36:404–13.

108. Bakand S, Hayes A, Dechsakulthorn F. Nanoparticles: a review of particle toxicology following inhalation exposure. Inhal Toxicol. 2012;24:125–35.

109. Braakhuis HM, Park MVDZ, De Jong W, Cassee F. Physicochemical characteristics of nanomaterials that affect pulmonary inflammation. Part Fibre Toxicol. 2014;11:18.

110. Lee Y, Kim P, Yoon J, Lee B, Choi K, Kil KH, et al. Serum kinetics, distribution and excretion of silver in rabbits following 28 days after a single intravenous injection of silver nanoparticles. 2013;7:1120–30.

111. Geiser M, Kreyling WG. Deposition and biokinetics of inhaled nanoparticles. Part Fibre Toxicol. 2010;7:2.

112. Hemmink GJ, Weusten BL, Bredenoord AJ, Timmer R, Smout AJ. Aerophagia: excessive air swallowing demonstrated by esophageal impedance monitoring. Clin Gastroenterol Hepatol. 2009;7:1127–9.

113. Li D, Morishita M, Wagner JG, Fatouraie M, Wooldridge M, Eagle WE, et al. In Vivo biodistribution and physiologically based pharmacokinetic modeling of inhaled fresh and aged cerium oxide nanoparticles in rats. Part Fibre Toxicol. 2016;13:45.

114. Bennett BJ, Hall KD, FB H, McCartney AL, Roberto C. Nutrition and the science of disease prevention: a systems approach to support metabolic health. Ann N Y Acad Sci. 2015;1352:1–12.

115. Marchesi JR, Adams DH, Fava F, Hermes GD, Hirschfield GM, Hold G, et al. The gut microbiota and host health: a new clinical frontier. Gut. 2016;65: 330–9.

116. Xiong Z, Leme AS, Ray P, Shapiro SD, Lee JS. CX3CR1+ lung mononuclear phagocytes spatially confined to the interstitium produce TNF-alpha and IL-6 and promote cigarette smoke-induced emphysema. J Immunol. 2011;186:3206–14.

117. Atreya R, Neurath MF. Involvement of IL-6 in the pathogenesis of inflammatory bowel disease and colon cancer. Clin Rev Allergy Immunol. 2005;28:187–96.

118. Eastaff-Leung N, Mabarrack N, Barbour A, Cummins A, Barry S. Foxp3+ regulatory T cells, Th17 effector cells, and cytokine environment in inflammatory bowel disease. J Clin Immunol. 2010;30:80–9.

119. Vieira WA, Pretorius E. The impact of asthma on the gastrointestinal tract. Journal of Asthma and Allergy. 2010;3:123–30.

120. Wallaert B, Desreumaux P, Copin MC, Tillie I, Benard A, Colombel JF, et al. Immunoreactivity for interleukin 3 and 5 and granulocyte/macrophage colony-stimulating factor of intestinal mucosa in bronchial asthma. J Exp Med. 1995;182:1897–904.

121. Donaldson K, Brown D, Clouter A, Duffin R, MacNee W, Renwick L, et al. The pulmonary toxicology of ultrafine particles. J Aerosol Med. 2002;15(2):213–20.

122. Coppeta L, Pietroiusti A, Magrini A, Somma G, Bergamaschi A. Prevalence and characteristics of functional dyspepsia among workers exposed to cement dust. Scand J Work Environ Health. 2008;34:396–402.

123. Sjödahl K, Jansson C, Bergdahl IA, Adami J, Boffetta P, Lagergren J. Airborne exposures and risk of gastric cancer: a prospective cohort study. Int J Cancer. 2007;120:2013–8.

124. Gunawan C, Lim M, Marquis CP, Amal R. Nanoparticle-protein corona complexes govern the biological fates and functions of nanoparticles. J Mat Chem B. 2014;2:2060–83.

125. Winuprasith T, Suphantharika M, McClements DJ, He L. Spectroscopic studies of conformational changes of β-lactoglobulin adsorbed on gold nanoparticle surfaces. J Colloid Interface Sci. 2014;416:184–9.

126. Raesch SS, Tenzer S, Storck W, Rurainski A, Selzer D, Ruge A, Perez-Gil J, Schaefer UF, Lehr C-M. Proteomic and lipidomic analysis of nanoparticle corona upon contact with lung surfactant reveals differences in protein, but not lipid composition. ACS Nano. 2015;9:11872–85.

127. Ault AP, Stark DI, Axson JL, Keeney JN, Maynard AD, Bergin IL, et al. Protein corona-induced modification of silver nanoparticle aggregation in simulated gastric fluid. Environ Sci Nano. 2016;3:1510–20.

128. Monopoli MP, Aberg C, Salvati A, Dawson KA. Biomolecular coronas provide the biological identity of nanosized materials. Nat Nanotech. 2012;7:779–86.

129. Iavicoli I, Leso V, Manno M, Schulte PA. Biomarkers of nanomaterial exposure and effect: current status. J Nanopart Res. 2014;16:2302.

130. Pietroiusti A, Campagnolo L, Fadeel B. Interaction of engineered nanoparticles with organs protected by internal biological barriers. Small. 2013;9:1557–72.

131. Lundqvist M, Stigler J, Elia G, Lynch I, Cedervall T, Dawson KA. Nanoparticle size and surface properties determine the protein corona with possible implications for biological impacts. Proc Natl Acad Sci U S A. 2008;105:14265–70.

132. Lynch I, Cedervall T, Lundqvist M, Cabaleiro-Lago C, Linse S, Dawson KA. The nanoparticle-protein complex as a biological entity; a complex fluids and surface science challenge for the 21st century. Adv Colloid Interf Sci. 2007;134-135:167–74.

133. Leso V, Fontana L, Mauriello MC, Iavicoli I. Occupational risk assessment of engineered nanomaterials: limits, challenges and opportunities. Curr Nanosci. 2017;13:55–78.

134. Farris E, Brown DM, Ramer-Tait AE, Pannier AK. Micro- and nanoparticulates for DNA vaccine delivery. Exp Biol Med (Maywood). 2016;241:919–29.

135. Eisenbrand G, Pool-Zobel B, Baker V, Balls M, Blaauboer BJ, Boobis A, et al. Methods of in vitro toxicology. Food Chem Toxicol. 2002;40:193–236.

136. Leonard F, Collnot EM, Lehr CMA. Three-dimensional coculture of enterocytes, monocytes and dendritic cells to model inflamed intestinal mucosa in vitro. Mol Pharm. 2010;7:2103–19.

137. Oberdörster G, Oberdörster E, Oberdörster J. Nanotoxicology: an emerging discipline evolving from studies of ultrafine particles. Environ Health Perspect. 2005;113:823–39.

138. Ltopez RN, Leach ST, Lemberg DA, Duvoisin G, Gearry RB, Day AS. Fecal biomarkers in inflammatory bowel disease. J Gastroenterol Hepatol. 2017;32:577–82.

139. Iavicoli I, Leso V, Schulte PA. Biomarkers of susceptibility: state of the art and implications for occupational exposure to engineered nanomaterials. Toxicol Appl Pharmacol. 2016;299:112–24.

140. Stone V, Miller MR, Clift MJ, Elder A, Mills NL, Møller P, et al. Nanomaterials vs ambient ultrafine particles: an opportunity to exchange toxicology knowledge. Environ Health Perspect. 2016 Nov 4;

141. Böhmert L, Niemann B, Thünemann AF, Lampen A. Cytotoxicity of peptide-coated silver nanoparticles on the human intestinal cell line Caco-2. Arch Toxicol. 2012;86:1107–15.

142. Sahu SC, Roy S, Zheng J, Yourick JJ, Sprando RL. Comparative genotoxicity of nanosilver in human liver HepG2 and colon Caco2 cells evaluated by fluorescent microscopy of cytochalasin B-blocked micronucleus formation. J Appl Toxicol. 2014;34:1200–8.

143. Sahu SC, Roy S, Zheng J, Ihrie J. Contribution of ionic silver to genotoxic potential of nanosilver in human liver HepG2 and colon Caco2 cells evaluated by the cytokinesis-block micronucleus assay. J Appl Toxicol. 2016; 36:532–42.

Effects of urban coarse particles inhalation on oxidative and inflammatory parameters in the mouse lung and colon

Cécile Vignal[1], Muriel Pichavant[2], Laurent Y. Alleman[3], Madjid Djouina[1], Florian Dingreville[1], Esperanza Perdrix[3], Christophe Waxin[1], Adil Ouali Alami[2], Corinne Gower-Rousseau[1], Pierre Desreumaux[1] and Mathilde Body-Malapel[1]* (iD)

Abstract

Background: Air pollution is a recognized aggravating factor for pulmonary diseases and has notably deleterious effects on asthma, bronchitis and pneumonia. Recent studies suggest that air pollution may also cause adverse effects in the gastrointestinal tract. Accumulating experimental evidence shows that immune responses in the pulmonary and intestinal mucosae are closely interrelated, and that gut-lung crosstalk controls pathophysiological processes such as responses to cigarette smoke and influenza virus infection. Our first aim was to collect urban coarse particulate matter (PM) and to characterize them for elemental content, gastric bioaccessibility, and oxidative potential; our second aim was to determine the short-term effects of urban coarse PM inhalation on pulmonary and colonic mucosae in mice, and to test the hypothesis that the well-known antioxidant N-acetyl-L-cysteine (NAC) reverses the effects of PM inhalation.

Results: The collected PM had classical features of urban particles and possessed oxidative potential partly attributable to their metal fraction. Bioaccessibility study confirmed the high solubility of some metals at the gastric level. Male mice were exposed to urban coarse PM in a ventilated inhalation chamber for 15 days at a concentration relevant to episodic elevation peak of air pollution. Coarse PM inhalation induced systemic oxidative stress, recruited immune cells to the lung, and increased cytokine levels in the lung and colon. Concomitant oral administration of NAC reversed all the observed effects relative to the inhalation of coarse PM.

Conclusions: Coarse PM-induced low-grade inflammation in the lung and colon is mediated by oxidative stress and deserves more investigation as potentiating factor for inflammatory diseases.

Keywords: Particulate matter, Coarse PM, Oxidative stress, Inflammation, Gut-lung axis, N-acetyl-L-cysteine

Background

Episodic increases in ambient air contaminant levels have been demonstrated to modulate the pathogenesis of an increasing number of chronic diseases, from asthma to cancer and stroke [1]. Exposure to ambient air pollution, especially to particulate matter (PM), is a major risk factor for pulmonary diseases such as asthma, chronic bronchitis, and pneumonia [2]. Numerous epidemiological studies indicate that long- and short-term exposure to coarse PM is associated with adverse health effects on the human respiratory system [3].

Although research on airborne pollutants has focused mostly on cardiovascular and respiratory effects, emerging epidemiological and experimental evidence suggests that air pollutants can also cause adverse effects on the gastrointestinal tract. Recent epidemiological studies have reported that exposure to air pollution may be associated with various gastrointestinal diseases including inflammatory bowel diseases [4, 5], appendicitis [6], irritable bowel syndrome [7], and enteric infections in children [8]. Notably, a correlation has been reported between ambient air

* Correspondence: mathilde.body@univ-lille2.fr
[1]Inserm, CHU Lille, U995-LIRIC-Lille Inflammation Research International Center, Univ. Lille, F-59000 Lille, France
Full list of author information is available at the end of the article

pollution and hospitalizations for inflammatory bowel diseases in Wisconsin [9].

To date, only one study has assessed the effects of PM inhalation on the gastrointestinal tract in an animal model [10]. Li et al. reported that in Ldlr$^{-/-}$ mice, inhalation of ultrafine PM led to shortened villus length, which was accompanied by prominent macrophage and neutrophil infiltration into the ileum. Ultrafine PM exposure also increased the concentrations of intestinal free oxidative fatty acids and lysophosphatidic acids. This study was the first to report that inhaled particles can trigger a deleterious effect at the intestinal level, which justifies the value of exploring this topic further.

Investigations of the mechanisms responsible for air pollution exposure-induced toxicity are challenging because of the complexity of air pollutants. Reactive gases such as ozone, nitrogen oxides, carbon monoxide, sulfur dioxide, volatile organic compounds and PM of varying size are part of the air pollutant mixture. The physicochemical characteristics of this complex matrix of gases and PM are also highly variable depending on the generation mode and sources (e.g., point industrial sources, automotive combustion, natural processes such as wildfires and volcanic eruptions, and atmospheric conditions) [11]. Air particles are known sinks for various organics molecules and a number of inorganic chemicals including physiologically active transition metals.

Our study focused on coarse PM, which has an aerodynamic diameter between 2.5 and 10 μm. It therefore includes an extra-thoracic particulate fraction (particles from 5 to 10 μm in size) and a thoracic particulate fraction (particles from 2.5 to 5 μm in size) [12]. The particulate fraction deposited into the extra-thoracic region becomes trapped in the nasal cavity, mouth, and pharynx. The vast majority of particules deposited in the extrathoracic region are removed via a combination of nose-blowing, sneezing, and mucociliary transport to the gastrointestinal tract [13]. Ingestion is therefore the dominant exposure pathway to particles deposited in the extra-thoracic region. Meanwhile, the thoracic particulate fraction deposits in the tracheobronchial region. This region consists of trachea, bronchi and terminal bronchioles. These particles, trapped in the mucus produced by the bronchial epithelial cells are typically cleared by mucociliary transport into the throat, and then expectored or swallowed [14, 15]. Moreover, for both fractions, soluble particles can be absorbed directly via the airway epithelium and cleared into the blood or lymphatic system [13, 16]. Therefore, coarse PM appears to be a relevant PM fraction to study, because it comes into direct contact with the digestive tract and has several input pathways allowing it to affect both the pulmonary and intestinal mucosae.

The first objective of this study was to characterize metal content of urban coarse PM collected in the French city of Douai, hereafter called coarse PM^D (cPM^D) and to assess its gastric metal bioaccessibility. Because oxidative stress is a major mechanism of PM toxicity, the oxidative potential of cPM^D was quantified. The second aim was to assess the effects of inhalation of cPM^D at a concentration relevant to episodic elevation peak of air pollution in mice. The third aim was to evaluate the effect of the administration of a well-known antioxidant, the N-acetyl-L-cysteine (NAC), on the effects of cPM^D inhalation in mice.

Methods
Sample collection
Aerosol samples were collected with a High-Vol (35 m^3/h) six- stages (10.2, 4.2, 2.1, 1.4, 0.73, 0.41 μm) cascade impactor (Tisch Environmental Inc.). Particles were collected during the warm season from July 13 to October 9, 2013, in Douai, a small city in a densely urbanized region in the north of France, located about 100 km from the English Channel coast (Additional file 1: Figure S1). Daily meteorological data during the sampling period were retrieved from the nearest weather station of the French meteorological service *Météo-France*, located 20 km north of the sampling site at the airport of Lille-Lesquin. PM was collected onto each impactor plate covered with adhesive Teflon stripes, which allowed the particles to be easily swiped with a Teflon tip, and then transferred directly into acid-cleaned sterile tubes, weighed, homogenized, and kept at 4 °C until later sampling for chemical and biological assays. The particle fraction size of the cPM^D used in this study was between 2.1 and 10.2 μm.

Total metal concentration
Particulate trace element mineralization and analysis were performed in triplicate, following a previously published method [17]. About 3 mg of cPM^D was acid digested in a microwave oven (Milestone ETHOS) at 220 °C. Digests were diluted to 50 mL with ultrapure water and analyzed by inductively coupled plasma mass spectrometry (ICP-MS) (NeXion 300XX, PerkinElmer) for trace elements (As, Ba, Bi, Cd, Ce, Co, Cr, Cs, Cu, Hg, La, Li, Mn, Mo, Ni, Pb, Rb, Sb, Sc, Se, Sn, Sr, Th, Ti, Tl, U, V, Zn) and major elements (Al, Ca, Fe, K, Mg, Na). An internal mixed standard (69Ga, 103Rh) was added (1 μg/L) to all analyzed solutions to correct the drift of the ICP-MS signal. Reagent blanks, quality controls and standard reference materials (NIST 1648a and ERM CZ-120) were also analyzed repeatedly to validate the entire analytical procedure, as previously described [18]. The total metal concentration is expressed in micrograms of metal per gram of cPM^D.

Metals bioaccessibility

Gastric bioaccessible fractions of cPM^D were characterized after in vitro extraction using a synthetic gastric juice (SGJ), according to the previously described procedures [19]. The gastric extractions were performed using three aliquots of 1–5 mg of cPM^D by agitating the PM suspensions for 2 h at 37 °C in accordance with the estimated physiological residence time. The separation of the particles from the synthetic fluid was performed by centrifugation for 10 min at 14,600 rpm at 6 °C. The supernatant was analyzed after a HNO$_3$ digestion on a hot plate, evaporation to dryness, and dilution to 10 mL (1% HNO$_3$). The results are expressed in micrograms of solubilized metal in the supernatant per gram of cPM^D. To check the consistency of the measured concentrations, the residual fraction was acid digested in a microwave oven at 220 °C according to the method of Alleman et al. [17]. Elemental analyses were performed in triplicate. Trace and major elements were validated through repeated analysis of reagent blanks, quality controls and standard reference materials (NIST 1648a and 2584). The bioaccessible fractions are presented as the ratio (expressed as a percentage) of metal concentration measured in the gastric leaching solutions to the total metal concentration.

Oxidative potential of cPM^D measured in ascorbic acid (AA) depletion assays

Oxidative potential is defined as a measure of the capacity of PM to oxidize target molecules, here AA, by generating reactive oxygen species in an acellular assay [20]. The AA depletion assay was performed under physiological conditions: at 37 °C and pH 7.4 in potassium Phosphate-buffered saline (PBS) at 10^{-2} mol/L, containing 30% KH$_2$PO$_4$ and 70% K$_2$HPO$_4$ on a molar basis, that had been pretreated with Chelex resin to remove all potential metallic contaminants. Ten milligrams of cPM^D was solubilized in 300 mL of PBS 10^{-2} mol/L in an ultrasonic bath for 30 min and then agitated at 37 °C for 24 h. The cPM^D suspension was prefiltered through a 0.45 µm syringe filter and divided into three cPM^D extracts of 100 mL each. Next, 0.5 mL of AA at 4.10^{-2} mol/L in PBS was added to each cPM^D extract and the sample was mixed. The absorbance was measured at 265 nm for different times up to 1 h for both the cPM^D extract solution test and the blank samples without cPM^D. The molar concentration of AA was then calculated from the absorbance at 265 nm using a preestablished calibration curve. A faster AA depletion rate in the presence of cPM^D extract compared with the blank indicates that cPM^D promotes the oxidation of AA. A similar assay using 10 mg of cPM^D in 300 mL of PBS 10^{-2} mol/L was performed in the presence of 87.5 mg of EDTA, a transition metal chelating agent, before introducing the AA reactant to examine the effect of metal redox activity on AA depletion (Zielinski et al., 1999). All experiments were performed in triplicate. Oxidative potential is expressed as the maximum AA depletion rate in micromoles per liter per minute (i.e., the depletion rate calculated during the first hour) calculated after subtracting the blank for a solid-to-liquid ratio of 10 mg-to-300 mL.

Animals

The animal treatment protocol was approved by the regional bioethics committee (committee no.75; authorization no.CEEA2016072517274040) and all of the animals received human care in accordance with the Guide for the Care and the Use of Laboratory Animals (National Research Council (US) Committee 2011).

Male C57BL/6 mice (aged 7 weeks) were purchased from Janvier Labs and housed under standard conventional conditions. The room relative humidity was 55% and the temperature was 21 °C. Mice were randomly divided into the different exposure groups ($n = 10$/group), as described in Scheme 1 and Fig. 4a.

Inhalation exposures

For inhalation experiments, mice were placed 4 h/day, 5 days/week for 2 weeks and for one additional day in a ventilated whole-body inhalation chamber that allowed free movement (InExpose, Scireq®) [21]. Nebulization was achieved using an Aeroneb Lab™ ultrasonic nebulizer directly connected to a 5 l–chamber and controlled through the flexiWare software v.6 according to the following parameters: bias flow of 2 l/min, nebulization rate of 0.083 ml/min, which were measured and controlled throughout the experiment. The Aeroneb Lab™ ultrasonic nebulizer produced droplets with a volume median diameter of 11 µm characterized by laser diffraction using the Spraytec system from Malvern Instruments. Mice were exposed to a solution of 40 µg cPM^D/ml or to the soluble or insoluble fractions of cPM^D. The dose concentration of the aerosol achieved with these conditions was 1.66 µg/L. Control mice were exposed to sterile water under the same conditions. cPM^D suspension was fractionated into soluble and insoluble fractions by centrifugation for 5 min at 13000 g as previously described [22, 23]. Soluble and insoluble fractions were diluted in the same volume of sterile water as the total fraction.

N-acetyl-L-cysteine (NAC) administration

Mice were administrated NAC (Sigma-Aldrich) in drinking water (15 µg/kg/day), from the beginning of the PM exposure until the day of sacrifice as described in Scheme 1.

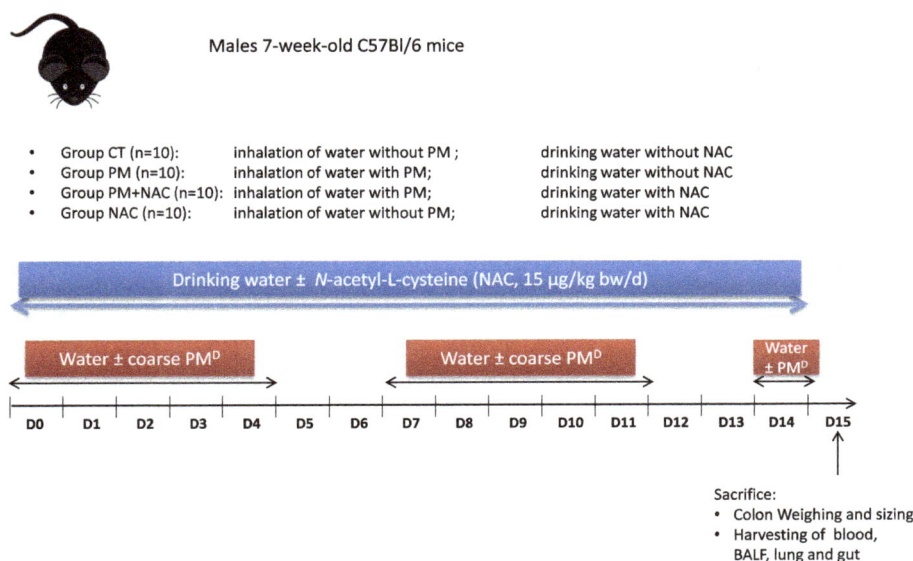

Scheme 1 Experimental design of the mouse model

Biological samples

Mice were euthanized the morning following the final exposure day. The colon was dissected and measured. Then, the colon was emptied by pushing the stool outwards using a dissecting forceps, and weighed. Bronchoalveolar lavage fluid (BALF) and samples of the lungs, colon, and blood were collected and kept on ice for FACS analysis or immediately frozen at −80 °C.

Flow cytometry

Cells harvested from BALF or extracted from lung tissue were washed in PBS and incubated with antibodies (BD, Franklin Lakes, NJ, USA) for 30 min in PBS and then washed twice and suspended in PBS with 2% fetal calf serum. The antibodies used were: fluorescein isothiocyanate (FITC)-conjugated anti-I-A[b]; phycoerythrin (PE)-conjugated anti-F4/80; peridinin chlorophyll protein complex (PerCP)/Cy5-conjugated anti-CD103; PE/Cy7-conjugated anti-CD11c; allophycocyanin (APC)-conjugated anti-CCR2; Alexa 700-conjugated anti-CD86; APC-H7-conjugated anti-Ly6G; V450-conjugated anti-CD11b; V500-conjugated anti-CD45; BV605-conjugated anti-Ly6C; FITC-conjugated anti-CD5; PE-conjugated anti-CD1d tetramer; PerCP/Cy5-conjugated anti-NK1.1; APC-conjugated anti-CD25; Alexa 700-conjugated anti-CD69; APC-H7-conjugated anti-CD4; V450-conjugated anti-T-cell receptor-β; V500-conjugated anti-CD8, and BV605-conjugated CD45. Cells were analyzed on an LSR Fortessa cell analyzer (BD). The generated data were analyzed using FlowJo 8.7 (TreeStar, Stanford, CA, USA).

Gene expression in tissues

Total mRNA from lung and colon tissues was extracted using a Nucleospin RNA II kit (Macherey Nagel). Reverse transcription was performed using a High Capacity cDNA Archive Kit and quantitative polymerase chain reaction (PCR) with SYBR Green (Life Technologies). The primer sequences were designed using Primer Express 3 (Life Technologies) and are available upon request. Melting curve analyses were performed for each sample and gene to confirm the specificity of the amplification. Because the exposure to PM did not cause any significant alterations in *Polr2a* mRNA expression, the relative expression of each gene of interest was normalized to the relative expression of this gene. The quantification of the target gene expression was based on the comparative cycle threshold (Ct) value. The fold changes in the target genes were analyzed by the $2^{-\Delta\Delta Ct}$ method [24].

Serum malondialdehyde (MDA) analysis

Serum samples (50 μL) were incubated with acetic acid and SDS at 95 °C for 1 h, followed by centrifugation at 800 g for 10 min. Supernatants were transferred to a 96-well plate and the absorbance was measured at $\lambda_{ex} = 532$ and $\lambda_{em} = 553$ nm. 1,1,3,3-Tetramethoxypropane (Sigma-Aldrich) was used as a standard. Protein concentration in samples was determined using a DC™ protein assay (Bio-Rad Laboratories). Serum MDA concentration was corrected by the sample protein concentration and is expressed as nanomoles per milliliter of serum.

Myeloperoxidase activity assay

Neutrophil influx into colon was analyzed by measuring the enzymatic activity of myeloperoxidase (MPO). Mice colons were homogenized in 0.5% hexadecyltrimethylammonium bromide (Sigma-Aldrich) in 50 mM PBS, freeze-thawed three times, and centrifuged. MPO was analyzed in the clear supernatant by adding 1 mg/mL of dianisidine dihydrochloride (Sigma-Aldrich) and 5.10^{-4}% hydrogen peroxide (H_2O_2), and the change in optical density was measured at 450 nm. Human neutrophil MPO (Sigma-Aldrich) was used as a standard. One unit of MPO activity was defined as the amount that degraded 1 μmol of peroxide per min at 25 °C. Readings from tissue samples were normalized to total protein content as detected in the DC™ protein assay (Bio-Rad).

Statistical analysis

Results are expressed as mean ± SEM. The statistical significance of differences between experimental groups was calculated using the Mann–Whitney U test (GraphPad, San Diego, CA).

Results

Characteristics of cPM^D

The meteorological conditions during the sampling period were typical for summertime under the oceanic climate of the northwestern European coast. The daily averages were a temperature of 17.7 °C (Additional file 1: Figure S2A), 71% relative humidity (Additional file 1: Figure S2B), 1017 hPa atmospheric pressure and cumulated rain of 172 mm over the whole period (Additional file 1: Figure S2C). These relatively high pressures and sparse rainfall conditions were observed throughout the period, and a continuing decrease in temperature and increase in relative humidity were recorded from summer to mid-autumn. The average wind speed was 3.3 m/s (Additional file 1: Figure S2D) and winds came mostly (39%) from the west sector (marine air masses from the English Channel and Atlantic Ocean) and secondarily (28%) from the north sector (more continental air masses toward the regional *Scarpe-Escaut* natural park and the south of Belgium (Additional file 1: Figure S2E).

The concentrations of elements in cPM^D varied from 1 to 57,312 μg/g in the following order: U < Tl < Cs < Th < Sc < Hg < Bi < Se < La < Li < Cd < Co < As < Ce < Mo < Rb < V < Ni < Sb < Sn < Cr < Sr < Pb < Ba < Cu < Mn < Ti < Zn for trace elements and Mg < K < Al < Fe < Na < Ca for major elements (Fig. 1a). Enrichment factors relative to the upper continental crust with Th as the reference element [25] were applied to assess the anthropogenic influence on cPM^D content (Fig. 1b). Enrichment factors >10 were observed for As, Mo, Sn, Pb, Cu, Bi, Zn, Cd, and Sb. All of these elements are commonly associated with traffic nonexhaust emissions (i.e., brakes and tire wear), particularly Cu,

which is predominant in coarse PM in Europe [26], and Sb, which showed the highest enrichment factor, and confirmed the urban typology of the sampling site. Cd, Zn, Bi, and Pb are known tracers of nonferrous smelting [27–29] and their enrichment may indicate the influence of a nearby Zn smelter located 3 km north of our sampling site. To characterize cPM^D better, we sought to assess their features in relation to other urban coarse PM. For this purpose, the elemental concentrations in cPM^D were compared with those measured in other European cities: an urban site in Helsinki, Finland [30] and a traffic site in Budapest, Hungary [31] (Additional file 1: Figure S3). Globally, the elemental concentrations were very similar, except for the highest levels of Cd, Zn and Bi in Douai, in accordance with a significant influence of the nearby Zn smelter.

Gastric bioaccessibility of cPM^D

Simulation of solubilization pathways was performed using the SGF to approximate gastric conditions (Fig. 1c). Metals showing the higher gastric bioaccessibility were Pb > Sb > Cd > Co > Sr, with values ranging from 90% for Pb to 70% for Sr. The lowest gastric bioaccessibility were observed for Cr (9%) and Fe (11%).

Oxidative potential of cPM^D

The oxidative potential of cPM^D was assessed using an AA depletion assay (Fig. 1d); AA is an antioxidant naturally present in the human body. The rates of AA depletion measured showed the effective oxidative potential of cPM^D. To examine the effects of metal redox activity on AA depletion, the same experiment was performed in the presence of EDTA, a transition metal chelating agent. In the presence of EDTA, AA depletion was significantly lower (– 42%) although not totally depleted, which indicates a role of metals in the oxidative potential of cPM^D.

Effects of cPM^D inhalation on oxidative stress and inflammation in mice

We then exposed mice to this cPM^D by inhalation in a whole body inhalation chamber. By this physiological way of exposure, as in real-life, coarse PM is expected to deposit primarily in the upper respiratory tract, and then to be transported from the conducting airways to the gastrointestinal tract by mucociliary clearance [12, 32]. We first aimed to assess the effects of an environmentally relevant episodic increase in ambient PM exposure on pulmonary and intestinal mucosal tissues. Following 14 days of exposure to inhaled cPM^D, serum MDA concentration was significantly higher in the PM mice compared with CT mice that inhaled only water. This finding reflects the appearance of systemic oxidative stress (Fig. 2a). More cells were obtained in BALF from PM mice

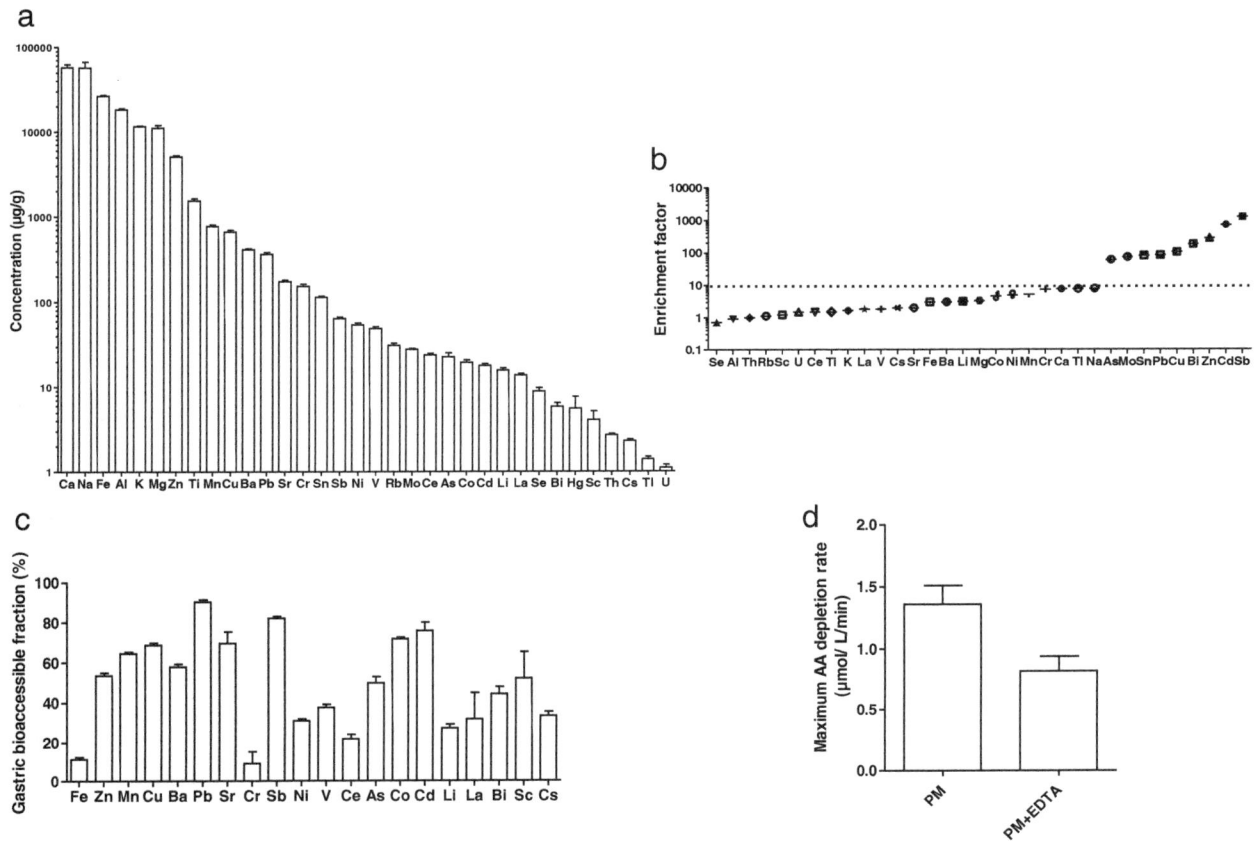

Fig. 1 Coarse PM^D characterization. **a** Mean concentrations of trace and major elements (μg/g). **b** Enrichment factors relative to Thorium. **c** Gastric bioaccessibility in SGJ (%). **d** Measurement of oxidative potential of cPM^D in the AA depletion assay with or without EDTA, and for a solid-to-liquid ratio of 10 mg/300 mL, expressed as the maximum rate of AA depletion (μmol/L/min)

compared with CT mice (Fig. 2b). The numbers of neutrophils and alveolar macrophages in the lung did not differ significantly between PM and CT mice (Fig. 2c). By contrast, more conventional T cells and invariant natural killer (iNKT) cells were observed in the lung of PM mice, and these increased cell numbers were associated with higher *Tnfα*, *Il5*, *Il22*, and *Il10* mRNA levels (Fig. 2d). At the intestinal level, the colon weight size ratio did not differ between PM and CT mice (Fig. 2e). A trend toward an increase in MPO activity was observed in the colons of PM mice (Fig. 2f). The gene expression levels of markers of neutrophils (*Csf3r*), macrophages (*Cd68*), conventional T cells (*Cd247*), and iNKT cells (*Vα14*) did not differ between PM and CT mice (Fig. 2g). By contrast, significantly greater expression of *Tnfα*, *Ifnγ*, *Il10* and *Cxcl10*, and lower expression of *Il5* were found in the colons of PM mice compared with CT mice (Fig. 2h). Together, these results suggest that cPM^D inhalation led to low-grade inflammation in both the lungs and gut.

Effects of NAC administration on cPM^D-induced deleterious effects

Oral administration of NAC has been shown to protect against oxidative stress in the lung [33, 34]. We evaluated the consequences of NAC administration on the previously observed PM-induced effects. NAC was added to drinking water of mice that inhaled PM (PM + NAC mice). A group of mice that inhaled PM and did not receive NAC in drinking water was also included (PM mice). Serum MDA concentration was lower in PM + NAC mice than in PM mice (Fig. 3a). Fewer cells were found in BALF from PM + NAC mice than in that from PM mice (Fig. 3b). In the lungs, less iNKT recruitment (Fig. 3c) and lower *Ifnγ*, *Il5* and *Cxcl10* expression levels were observed (Fig. 3d). The mRNA levels of several oxidative stress markers such as *Nos2*, *COX2*, *Sod2*, *Cat*, and *Hmox1* were markedly lower in the lungs of PM + NAC mice compared with those from PM mice (Fig. 3e). The colons of PM + NAC mice showed lower MPO activity (Fig. 3f) and reduced *Tnfα*, *Ifnγ* and *Cxcl10* mRNA expression compared

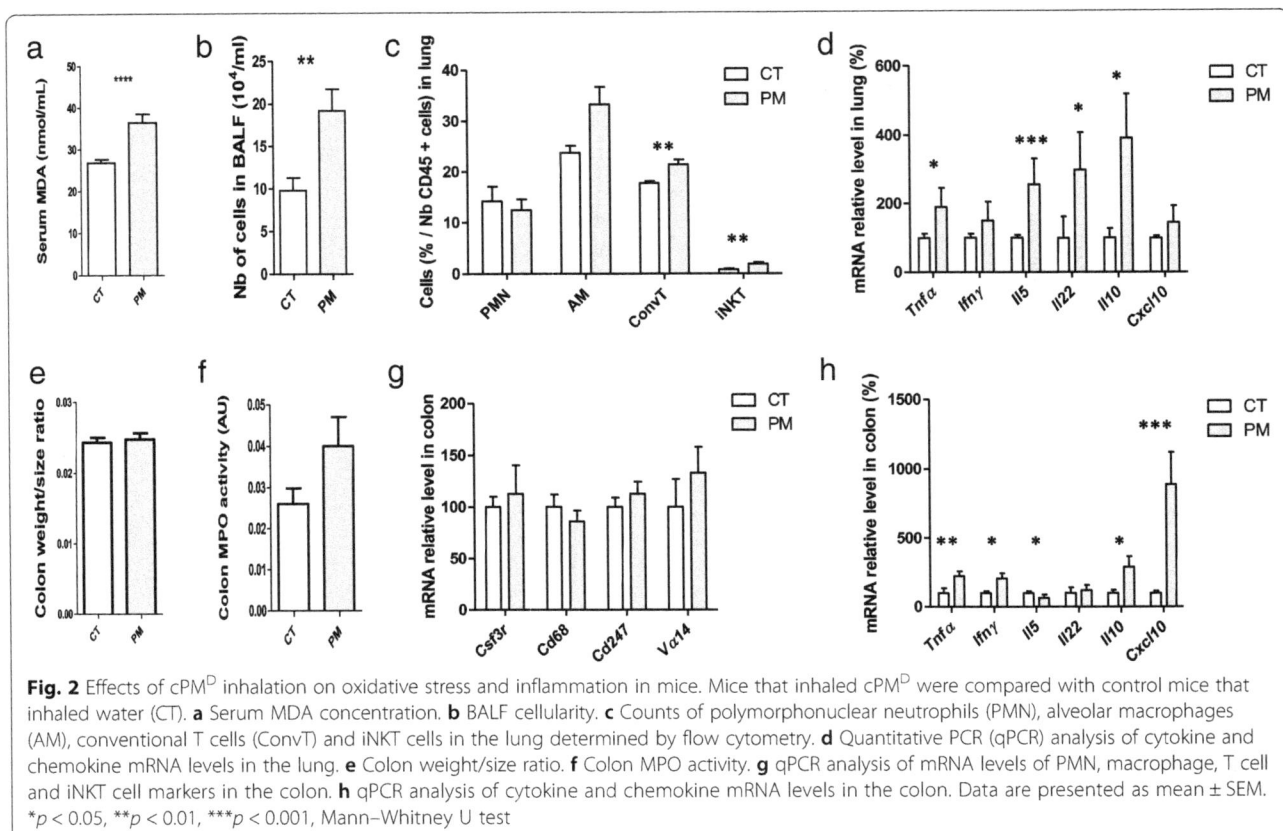

Fig. 2 Effects of cPM^D inhalation on oxidative stress and inflammation in mice. Mice that inhaled cPM^D were compared with control mice that inhaled water (CT). **a** Serum MDA concentration. **b** BALF cellularity. **c** Counts of polymorphonuclear neutrophils (PMN), alveolar macrophages (AM), conventional T cells (ConvT) and iNKT cells in the lung determined by flow cytometry. **d** Quantitative PCR (qPCR) analysis of cytokine and chemokine mRNA levels in the lung. **e** Colon weight/size ratio. **f** Colon MPO activity. **g** qPCR analysis of mRNA levels of PMN, macrophage, T cell and iNKT cell markers in the colon. **h** qPCR analysis of cytokine and chemokine mRNA levels in the colon. Data are presented as mean ± SEM. *$p < 0.05$, **$p < 0.01$, ***$p < 0.001$, Mann–Whitney U test

with those from PM mice (Fig. 3g). Taken together, these data show that NAC administration reversed the deleterious effects induced by PM inhalation. NAC did not alter the basal condition because NAC treatment did not modify inflammatory and oxidative stress parameters in serum, lung, or colon of CT mice that inhaled water (Additional file 1: Figure S4).

Involvement of water-soluble and insoluble fractions on cPM^D-induced low-grade inflammation

To assess if the solubilization of PM in water during nebulization is involved in the observed low-grade inflammation, an experiment was performed including in addition to the 2 previously described groups [mice exposed to water (CT group), and mice exposed to cPM^D (total fraction, FT group)], a group exposed to the soluble fraction of cPM^D (Soluble Fraction, SF group) and a group exposed to the insoluble fraction of cPM^D (Insoluble Fraction, IF group) (Fig. 4a). The increased number of cells in BALF in TF-exposed mice compared to CT mice was found also in IF-exposed mice, and not in SF-exposed mice (Fig. 4b). Similarly, the enhancement of iNKT cells in lungs of TF-exposed mice compared to CT mice was also found in IF-exposed mice, and not in SF-exposed mice (Fig. 4c). In the colon, an unexpected decrease of *Tnfa* levels was quantified in IF-exposed

mice compared to CT mice (Fig. 4d). Most interestingly, no increase of *Tnfa* and *Cxcl2* mRNA levels was detected in the colons of SF-exposed mice, while the transcription of both genes was increased in TF-exposed mice. Taken together, these results show that the water-soluble fraction of cPM^D is not sufficient to induce the low-grade inflammation associated to cPM^D inhalation.

Discussion

The cPM^D used in this study comprised urban particles collected over 4 months of the warm season in northern France, and ranged in size from 2.1 to 10,2 μm. Fe, Cu, and Zn were among the most concentrated metals quantified in cPM^D, and their high concentrations are of concern because of their pro-oxidative potential [35]. The most enriched element was Sb, which is consistent with the main traffic-related origin of cPM^D. Another metal of concern is Pb, which is highly toxic and is enriched by 86 times in cPM^D [36, 37]. Both Sb and Pb concentrations were similar to those reported for other urban areas [30, 38, 39]. The strong enrichment for Cd and As in cPM^D compared with the upper crust is likely to contribute to their negative health impact. Cd exposure is known to induce pulmonary damage such as emphysema and lung cancer [40, 41] and to cause intestinal inflammation in mice [42]. Similarly, As exposure has

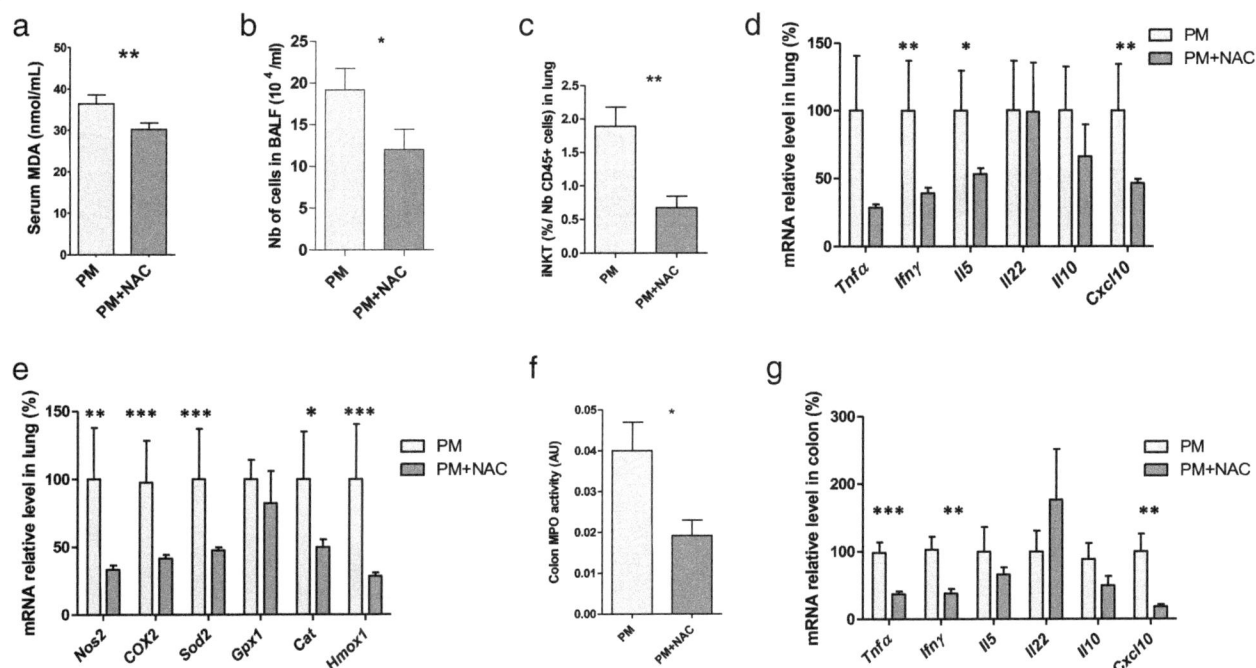

Fig. 3 Effects of NAC administration on cPM^D-induced damage. All mice inhaled PM. Mice that received NAC (15 µg/kg/day for 14 days) in drinking water were compared with CT mice that did not receive NAC in drinking water. **a** Serum MDA concentration. **b** BALF cellularity. **c** iNKT cell count in the lung measured by flow cytometry. **d** qPCR analysis of cytokine and chemokine mRNA levels in the lung. **e** qPCR analysis of mRNA levels of oxidative stress markers in the lung. **f** Colon MPO activity. **g** qPCR analysis of cytokine and chemokine mRNA levels in the colon. Data are presented as mean ± SEM. *$p < 0.05$, **$p < 0.01$, ***$p < 0.001$, Mann–Whitney U test

been repeatedly associated with lung carcinogenesis [43] and has been shown to perturb the gut microbiome in mice [44].

Furthermore, Pb, Sr, Sb, Co and Cd presented both high concentration in cPM^D and high gastric bioaccessibility. A substantial proportion of these elements is therefore likely to be found in the bloodstream during air pollution peak in urban areas. The diffusion of these metals in the bloodstream could lead to both directly cytotoxic effects on circulatory monocytes [45], but also to indirectly aggravating effects on inflammation in peripheral tissues: notably, lead and cadmium levels in PM have been found negatively associated with miR-146a expression in blood leukocytes RNA from foundry workers [46]. Mir-146a is involved in limiting inflammatory responses triggered through the innate immune system [47]. Moreover, miR-146a-mediated NOD2-SHH signaling regulates gut inflammation in murine model of inflammatory bowel diseases [48].

The main objective of the current study was to assess the effects of cPM^D inhalation at both the pulmonary and colonic levels. Our in vivo study was conducted in conditions as close as possible to real life, and aimed to determine the effects of a realistic inhalation of coarse PM. Exposure in an inhalation chamber was preferred to oral or intratracheal administration. For their

aerosolization, the cPM^D were solubilized in sterile water; the impact of solubilization on the observed effects seems negligible, since the mice that inhaled the water-soluble fraction of the cPM^D did not exhibit pulmonary and colon low-grade inflammation. The dosage of PM nebulized in the inhalation chamber is close to that breathed during pollution peaks by inhabitants of megacities strongly affected by particulate pollution. In urban areas, the mean daily concentration of PM of ≤10 µm in diameter (PM$_{10}$) ranges from <10 µg/m^3 to >200 µg/m^3 [49]. In 2002, the US Environmental Protection Agency reported a range of maximal city PM concentrations of 26–534 µg/m^3 [50]. Extreme hourly concentrations of PM$_{10}$ reaching 800 µg/m^3 have been measured at a traffic site in London [51]. PM$_{10}$ pollution peaks at >250 µg/m^3 were measured in megacities in India, Pakistan and China in 2010 [52, 53]. Therefore, the dose used here is fairly representative of high pollution episodes in the most affected megacities worldwide.

The studies performed until now that assess the effects of coarse PM at the pulmonary level were performed using intratracheal instillation or oropharyngeal aspiration [54–57]; these two modes of coarse PM administration partially or totally excluded the physiological exposure of the mouth, nose, larynx and pharynx. They revealed in most of the cases pulmonary inflammation, which the

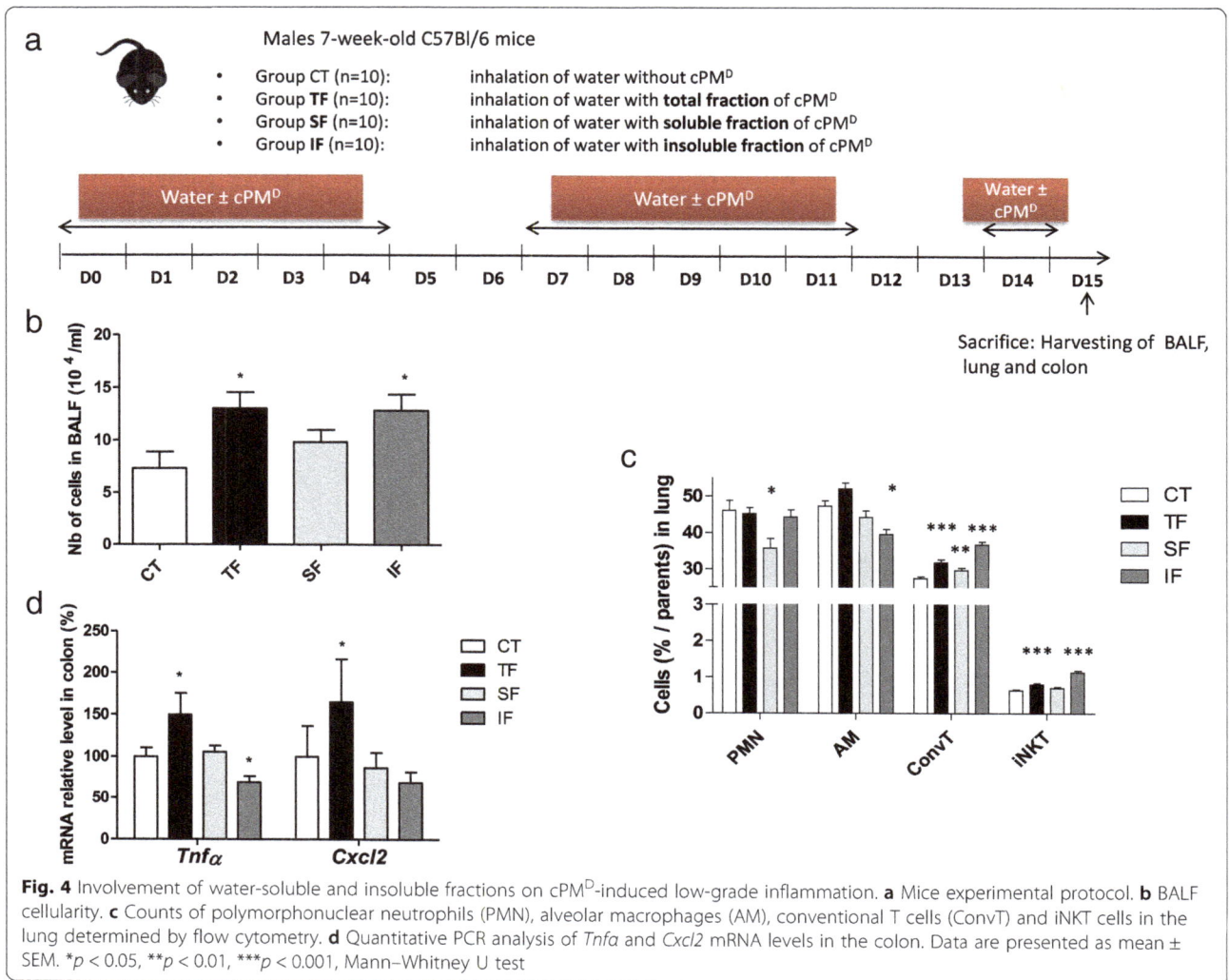

Fig. 4 Involvement of water-soluble and insoluble fractions on cPM^D-induced low-grade inflammation. **a** Mice experimental protocol. **b** BALF cellularity. **c** Counts of polymorphonuclear neutrophils (PMN), alveolar macrophages (AM), conventional T cells (ConvT) and iNKT cells in the lung determined by flow cytometry. **d** Quantitative PCR analysis of *Tnfα* and *Cxcl2* mRNA levels in the colon. Data are presented as mean ± SEM. *$p < 0.05$, **$p < 0.01$, ***$p < 0.001$, Mann–Whitney U test

players were variable regarding the type of PM, the timing and the dose of exposure. Some consistencies can however be found with our study assessing the effects of coarse PM following inhalation. Tumor necrosis factor (TNFα) produced by activated alveolar macrophages and by epithelial cells is a master cytokine of the inflammation induced by PM in the lung [58, 59]. As for TNFα, increased levels of interleukin 5 (IL-5), IL-10, and IL-22 are in agreement with previous studies. Overexpression of both IL-5 and IL-10 in the lung has been shown following early life exposure to combustion-derived PM [58]. IL-22 upregulation may be linked to activation of the aryl hydrocarbon receptor (AHR), as reported by previous work showing the ability of urban dust PM to induce Th17 polarization and IL-22 production in an AHR-dependent manner [60]. The most pronounced effects on the recruitment of immune cells involved in pulmonary inflammation induced by cPM^D seemed to involve iNKT cells. Our report is the first to show that this immune population is associated with PM exposure, although its key role has been demonstrated in the pulmonary response to ozone [61] and cigarette smoke [62].

Few studies have assessed the effects of PM inhalation at the intestinal level. As expected because of the low dose of cPM^D used, we did not find evidence of colitis clinical manifestation in the PM-exposed mice, as reflected by the lack of effect on the colon weight size ratio. Accordingly, some major intestinal immune populations, namely neutrophils, macrophages, lymphocytes and iNKT cells, do not seem to be significantly affected by PM inhalation. However, the increase in colon MPO activity, which almost reached significance, as well as the strong increase in the colonic expression of *Tnfα*, *Ifnγ* and *Cxcl10* argue in favor of a low-grade inflammation generated in colon following PM inhalation. The large production of *Il10* may be indicative of a regulatory response, although the decrease in *Il5* level remains unexplained.

It is the first time that the effects of coarse PM administration on mice are studied by natural ventilation in an inhalation chamber. Nevertheless, when a high dose of coarse PM was administered to mice by gavage during 14 days, an increase of pro-inflammatory cytokines (*Il12a, Il17,* and *Il2*) has been described [63]. Moreover, increases in colon TNFα and IFNγ protein levels have also been reported following 10 and 14 weeks of oral coarse PM intoxication in mice starting from the neonatal period [64]. Taken as a whole, the experimental protocols used to explore the effects of coarse PM on the gastrointestinal tract consistently describe low-grade intestinal inflammation, but are too diverse to reveal the common immune cells or molecular pathways implicated in the colonic effects of PM. Notably, it remains to be determined whether the observed effects on the gastrointestinal tract are mediated through a topical effect of PM, which comes into direct contact with intestinal epithelium, or through a systemic mechanism.

The triggering of low-grade intestinal inflammation could contribute in part to many health issues. Low-grade intestinal inflammation is a feature of irritable bowel syndrome [65]. It could also exacerbate Inflammatory Bowel Diseases [66], and promote colon carcinogenesis [67]. Moreover, a huge body of evidence indicates that low-grade intestinal inflammation participates in whole-body metabolism, and therefore to the metabolic syndrome that embraces cardiovascular diseases, type 2 diabetes, and non-alcoholic liver disease [68, 69]. It has also been speculated that intestinal low-grade inflammation associated with dysbiosis may play a pathophysiological role in human brain diseases, including autism spectrum disorder, anxiety, depression, and chronic pain [66, 70]. Intestinal low-grade inflammation has also been associated with chronic obstructive pulmonary disease [71]. Because of its critical role in health, any disturbance of intestinal immune homeostasis should be considered as a serious health threat.

A prominent finding of our study is that oxidative stress was a key mechanism for PM-induced deleterious effects. The AA depletion assay showed the oxidative potential of cPM[D] and the involvement of metal content in this property. Consistently, PM metal chelation prevents the systemic inflammatory response induced in mice by repeated PM intratracheal instillations [72]. Quinones [73] and polycyclic aromatic hydrocarbons [74] present in PM are likely to also contribute to the oxidative potential of cPM[D]. The increase in serum MDA concentrations that we observed in cPM[D]-exposed mice reflects systemic oxidative stress, which is a well-known effect of PM in rats [75] and in humans [76]. NAC has been used for several years as an antioxidant agent [77–79]. In our study, NAC administration led to a normalization of pulmonary and systemic phenotypes. Our results lead us to hypothesize a

similar mechanism to that demonstrated in chronic obstructive pulmonary disease induced in mice by cigarette smoke exposure [34]: that the protective effects of NAC are mediated through reduced accumulation and activation of iNKT cells. Most noticeably, NAC administration led to obvious protective effects in the colon, such as downregulation of MPO activity and complete reversal of the phenotype observed in PM-exposed mice compared with control mice, i.e., extinction of *Tnfα, Ifnγ,* and *Il10* upregulation. Because the concentration of NAC shown to induce significant improvement in colitis following oral administration (150 mg/kg body weight (bw)/day [80] or 160 mg/kg bw/day [81]) is much higher than that used in our study (15 μg/kg bw/day), these effects are not likely to be attributed to a topical effect of NAC.

NAC has been also described as a metal-chelating agent, able to increase urine gold excretion in rheumatoid arthritis patients treated with gold sodium thiomalate [82]. Moreover, intraperitoneal administration of NAC was very effective in increasing the urinary excretion of chromium and borate, but not lead, in rats intoxicated with potassium dichromate, boric acid and lead tetracetate respectively [83]. On the other hand, when NAC is administrated orally, its anti-oxidative properties are not systematically associated with chelating effects. By instance, in lead-exposed mice, oral administration of NAC (5.5 mmol/kg) reduced several indices of oxidative stress in both brain and liver samples, but not tissue lead levels [84]. Similarly, NAC treatment of arsenic-exposed rats (1 mmoml/kg) did not reduce significantly blood and liver arsenic levels, but reversed the elevation of brain MDA levels observed in untreated animals exposed to arsenic [85]. Especially, if the effects observed are mediated by the bioaccessible metal fraction of PM, it can be hypothesized that the attenuating effects of NAC are partly due to its metal chelating properties, but it is unlikely that this is the major mode of action of NAC.

Taken together, our results suggest that PM inhalation induces a succession of oxidative and inflammatory reactions that involve immune populations in the blood and in the pulmonary and gastrointestinal mucosae. Our work did not allow us to determine how these populations communicate but highlight an involvement of the gut-lung axis. This concept is strengthened by several lines of evidence showing the pathophysiological relevance of the immune crosstalk between the gut and lung. For example, house dust mite aeroallergens induce inflammation in the respiratory mucosa and reduce the gut epithelial barrier integrity [86]. In allergic airway disease, gut microbiota metabolism of dietary fibers influences the severity of allergic inflammation [87]. The importance of the gut microbiota has also been reported during respiratory influenza virus infection [88] and pneumococcal pneumonia [89]. The effects of cigarette smoke on the small intestine and colon, as evidenced by epithelial barrier defects, inflammatory cell recruitment, and microbial shifts, have been well described [62, 90, 91]. Therefore, our data demonstrating the deleterious effects of inhaled PM on both the pulmonary and colonic mucosae constitute additional evidence for the gut-lung axis, which deserves further investigation.

Conclusions

In healthy mice, inhalation of urban coarse PM which presented with significant oxidative potential induced a low-grade inflammation that affected both the pulmonary and colonic mucosae. The development of this low-grade inflammation was at least partly driven by an oxidative stress mechanism, as evidenced by its reversal by concomitant administration of the antioxidative compound NAC. Our results provide further demonstration of a gut-lung axis, and highlight the importance of understanding the mechanisms of crosstalk between the pulmonary and colonic mucosae. Together with previous experimental and epidemiological observations, our study strongly suggests that coarse PM inhalation may trigger or accelerate the development of both pulmonary and gastrointestinal inflammatory diseases, particularly in genetically susceptible individuals.

Additional file

Additional file 1: Figure S1. Location of the sampling site. **Figure S2.** Meteorological conditions during the sampling period. **A** Temperature. **B** Relative humidity. **C** Rain. **D** Wind speed. **E** Wind direction and frequency. **Figure S3.** Comparison of trace element concentrations in cPM^D collected at Douai and coarse PM collected in Helsinki, Finland [30] and Budapest, Hungary [31]. **Figure S4.** Effects of NAC in the basal condition. All mice inhaled sterile water. Mice that received NAC (15 μg/kg/day for 14 days) in drinking water were compared with CT mice that did not receive NAC in drinking water. **A** Serum MDA levels. **B** iNKT cell count measured by flow cytometry. **C** Quantitative PCR (qPCR) analysis of cytokine and chemokine mRNA levels in the lung. **D** qPCR analysis of mRNA levels of oxidative stress markers in the lung. **E** MPO activity in the colon. **F** qPCR analysis of cytokine and chemokine mRNA levels in the colon. Data are presented as mean ± SEM. *$p < 0.05$, Mann-Whitney U test. (DOCX 1064 kb)

Abbreviations

AA: Ascorbic acid; AHR: Aryl hydrocarbon receptor; AM: Alveolar macrophage; APC: Allophycocyanin; BALF: Bronchoalveolar lavage fluid; Cat: Catalase; Cd: Cluster of differentiation; ConvT: Conventional T cell; COX2: Cytochrome c oxidase subunit II; cPM^D: Coarse particulate matter from Douai; Csf3r: Colony stimulating factor 3 receptor; CT: Control; Cxcl10: C-X-C motif chemokine 10; Cxcl2: C-X-C motif chemokine 2; FITC: Fluorescein isothiocyanate; Gpx1: Glutathione peroxidase 1; Hmox1: heme oxygenase 1; ICP-MS: Inductively coupled plasma mass spectrometry; Ifnγ: Interferon gamma; Il: Interleukin; iNKT: Invariant Natural Killer T cell; MDA: Malondialdehyde; MPO: Myeloperoxidase; NAC: N-acetyl-L-cysteine; Nos2: Nitric Oxide Synthase 2; PE: Phycoerythrin; PerCP: Peridinin chlorophyll protein complex; PM: Particulate matter; PMN: Polymorphonuclear neutrophil; SGJ: Synthetic gastric juice; Sod2: Superoxide dismutase 2; Tnfα: Tumor necrosis factor alpha; Vα14: V alpha 14

Acknowledgements

The authors thank Bruno Mallet.

Funding

This work was supported by the Hauts-de-France Region and the Ministère de l'Enseignement Supérieur et de la Recherche (CPER Climibio), the European Fund for Regional Economic Development, and Digestscience (European Research Foundation on Intestinal Diseases and Nutrition).

Authors' contributions

MD, FD, CW performed the animal exposure, acquired and analyzed the data. CV, MP and MBM interpreted the results of animal experiments. LYA, EP, AOA performed the particulate matter collect and analysis, and interpreted the results of these experiments. MBM drafted the manuscript. CV and MBM shared study supervision. CG and PD participated in manuscript writing. All authors read and approved the final manuscript.

Authors' information

Not applicable

Competing interests

The authors declare they have no competing financial interests.

Author details

[1]Inserm, CHU Lille, U995-LIRIC-Lille Inflammation Research International Center, Univ. Lille, F-59000 Lille, France. [2]Inserm U1019, CNRS UMR 8204, Institut Pasteur de Lille– CIIL – Center for Infection and Immunity of Lille, Univ. Lille, F-59000 Lille, France. [3]SAGE - Département Sciences de l'Atmosphère et Génie de l'Environnement, IMT Lille Douai, Univ. Lille, 59000 Lille, France.

References

1. Anderson JO, Thundiyil JG, Stolbach A. Clearing the air: a review of the effects of particulate matter air pollution on human health. J Med Toxicol. 2012;8:166–75.
2. Chen B, Kan H. Air pollution and population health: a global challenge. Environ Health Prev Med. 2008;13:94–101.
3. Badyda A, Gayer A, Czechowski PO, Majewski G, Dąbrowiecki P. Pulmonary function and incidence of selected respiratory diseases depending on the exposure to ambient PM10. Int J Mol Sci. 2016, 1954;17
4. Beamish LA, Osornio-Vargas AR, Wine E. Air pollution: an environmental factor contributing to intestinal disease. J. Crohns Colitis. 2011;5:279–86.
5. Kaplan G. Air pollution and the inflammatory bowel diseases. Inflamm Bowel Dis. 2011;17:1146–8.
6. Kaplan GG, Dixon E, Panaccione R, Fong A, Chen L, Szyszkowicz M, et al. Effect of ambient air pollution on the incidence of appendicitis. Can Med Assoc J. 2009;181:591–7.
7. Kaplan GG, Szyszkowicz M, Fichna J, Rowe BH, Porada E, Vincent R, et al. Non-specific abdominal pain and air pollution: a novel association. PLoS One. 2012;7:e47669.
8. Orazzo F, Nespoli L, Ito K, Tassinari D, Giardina D, Funis M, et al. Air pollution, aeroallergens, and emergency room visits for acute respiratory diseases and gastroenteric disorders among young children in six Italian cities. Environ Health Perspect. 2009;117:1780–5.
9. Ananthakrishnan AN, McGinley EL, Binion DG, Saeian K. Ambient air pollution correlates with hospitalizations for inflammatory bowel disease: an ecologic analysis. Inflamm Bowel Dis. 2011;17:1138–45.
10. Li R, Navab K, Hough G, Daher N, Zhang M, Mittelstein D, et al. Effect of exposure to atmospheric ultrafine particles on production of free fatty acids and lipid metabolites in the mouse small intestine. Environ Health Perspect. 2015;123:34–41.
11. Kumarathasan P, Blais E, Saravanamuthu A, Bielecki A, Mukherjee B, Bjarnason S, et al. Nitrative stress, oxidative stress and plasma endothelin levels after inhalation of particulate matter and ozone. Part. Fibre Toxicol. 2015;12:28.
12. Martin R, Dowling K, Pearce D, Sillitoe J, Florentine S. Health effects associated with inhalation of airborne arsenic arising from mining operations. Geosciences. 2014;4:128–75.

13. Smith JRH, Etherington G, Shutt AL, Youngman MJA. Study of aerosol deposition and clearance from the human nasal passage. Ann Occup Hyg. 2002;46:309–13.

14. Asgharian B, Hofmann W, Miller FJ. Mucociliary clearance of insoluble particles from the tracheobronchial airways of the human lung. J Aerosol Sci. 2001;32:817–32.

15. Smith JRH, Bailey MR, Etherington G, Shutt AL, Youngman MJ. Effect of particle size on slow particle clearance from the bronchial tree. Exp Lung Res. 2008;34:287–312.

16. Labiris NR, Dolovich MB. Pulmonary drug delivery. Part I: physiological factors affecting therapeutic effectiveness of aerosolized medications. Br J Clin Pharmacol. 2003;56:588–99.

17. Alleman LY, Lamaison L, Perdrix E, Robache A, Galloo J-C. PM10 metal concentrations and source identification using positive matrix factorization and wind sectoring in a French industrial zone. Atmospheric Res. 2010;96:612–25.

18. Mbengue S, Alleman LY, Flament P. Size-distributed metallic elements in submicronic and ultrafine atmospheric particles from urban and industrial areas in northern France. Atmospheric Res. 2014;135–136:35–47.

19. Hamel SC, Buckley B, Lioy PJ. Bioaccessibility of metals in soils for different liquid to solid ratios in synthetic gastric fluid. Environ. Sci. Technol. 1998;32:358–62.

20. Yang A, Jedynska A, Hellack B, Kooter I, Hoek G, Brunekreef B, et al. Measurement of the oxidative potential of PM 2.5 and its constituents: the effect of extraction solvent and filter type. Atmos Environ. 2014;83:35–42.

21. Jacobo-Estrada T, Cardenas-Gonzalez M, Santoyo-Sánchez M, Parada-Cruz B, Uria-Galicia E, Arreola-Mendoza L, et al. Evaluation of kidney injury biomarkers in rat amniotic fluid after gestational exposure to cadmium. J Appl Toxicol JAT. 2016;36:1183–93.

22. Knaapen AM, Shi T, Borm PJA, Schins RPF. Soluble metals as well as the insoluble particle fraction are involved in cellular DNA damage induced by particulate matter. Mol Cell Biochem. 2002;234–235:317–26.

23. Wegesser TC, Last JA. Lung response to coarse PM: bioassay in mice. Toxicol Appl Pharmacol. 2008;230:159–66.

24. Livak KJ, Schmittgen TD. Analysis of relative gene expression data using real-time quantitative PCR and the 2−ΔΔCT method. Methods. 2001;25:402–8.

25. McLennan SM. Relationships between the trace element composition of sedimentary rocks and upper continental crust. Geochem Geophys Geosystems. 2001;2:1021.

26. Tsai M-Y, Hoek G, Eeftens M, de Hoogh K, Beelen R, Beregszászi T, et al. Spatial variation of PM elemental composition between and within 20 European study areas — results of the ESCAPE project. Environ Int. 2015;84:181–92.

27. Sterckeman T, Douay F, Proix N, Fourrier H. Vertical distribution of cd, Pb and Zn in soils near smelters in the north of France. Environ Pollut. 2000;107:377–89.

28. Batonneau Y, Bremard C, Gengembre L, Laureyns J, Le Maguer A, Le Maguer D, et al. Speciation of PM10 sources of airborne nonferrous metals within the 3-km zone of lead/zinc smelters. Environ. Sci. Technol. 2004;38:5281–9.

29. Sobanska S, Ricq N, Laboudigue A, Guillermo R, Brémard C, Laureyns J, et al. Microchemical investigations of dust emitted by a lead smelter. Environ Sci Technol. 1999;33:1334–9.

30. Pakkanen TA, Loukkola K, Korhonen CH, Aurela M, Mäkelä T, Hillamo RE, et al. Sources and chemical composition of atmospheric fine and coarse particles in the Helsinki area. Atmos Environ. 2001;35:5381–91.

31. Maenhaut W, Raes N, Chi X, Cafmeyer J, Wang W, Salma I. Chemical composition and mass closure for fine and coarse aerosols at a kerbside in Budapest, Hungary, in spring 2002. X-Ray Spectrom. 2005;34:290–6.

32. Méndez LB, Gookin G, Phalen RF. Inhaled aerosol particle dosimetry in mice: a review. Inhal Toxicol. 2010;22:1032–7.

33. Blesa S, Cortijo J, Mata M, Serrano A, Closa D, Santangelo F, et al. Oral N-acetylcysteine attenuates the rat pulmonary inflammatory response to antigen. Eur Respir J. 2003;21:394–400.

34. Pichavant M, Rémy G, Bekaert S, Le Rouzic O, Kervoaze G, Vilain E, et al. Oxidative stress-mediated iNKT-cell activation is involved in COPD pathogenesis. Mucosal Immunol. 2014;7:568–78.

35. Charrier JG, McFall AS, Richards-Henderson NK, Anastasio C. Hydrogen peroxide formation in a surrogate lung fluid by transition metals and quinones present in particulate matter. Environ. Sci. Technol. 2014;48:7010–7.

36. Huang S, Hu H, Sánchez BN, Peterson KE, Ettinger AS, Lamadrid-Figueroa H, et al. Childhood blood lead levels and symptoms of attention deficit hyperactivity disorder (ADHD): a cross-sectional study of Mexican children. Environ Health Perspect. 2016;124:868–74.

37. Liao LM, Friesen MC, Xiang Y-B, Cai H, Koh D-H, Ji B-T, et al. Occupational lead exposure and associations with selected cancers: the shanghai Men's and Women's health study cohorts. Environ Health Perspect. 2016;124:97–103.

38. Querol X, Viana M, Alastuey A, Amato F, Moreno T, Castillo S, et al. Source origin of trace elements in PM from regional background, urban and industrial sites of Spain. Atmos Environ. 2007;41:7219–31.

39. Wiseman CLS, Zereini F. Characterizing metal(loid) solubility in airborne PM10, PM2.5 and PM1 in Frankfurt, Germany using simulated lung fluids. Atmos Environ. 2014;89:282–9.

40. Stayner L, Smith R, Thun M, Schnorr T, Lemen RA. Dose–response analysis and quantitative assessment of lung cancer risk and occupational cadmium exposure. Ann Epidemiol. 1992;2:177–94.

41. Dervan PA, Hayes JA. Peribronchiolar fibrosis following acute experimental lung damage by cadmium aerosol. J Pathol. 1979;128:143–9.

42. Breton J, Daniel C, Vignal C, Body-Malapel M, Garat A, Plé C, et al. Does oral exposure to cadmium and lead mediate susceptibility to colitis? The dark-and-bright sides of heavy metals in gut ecology. Sci Rep. 2016;6:19200.

43. Celik I, Gallicchio L, Boyd K, Lam TK, Matanoski G, Tao X, et al. Arsenic in drinking water and lung cancer: a systematic review. Environ Res. 2008;108:48–55.

44. Lu K, Abo RP, Schlieper KA, Graffam ME, Levine S, Wishnok JS, et al. Arsenic exposure perturbs the gut microbiome and its metabolic profile in mice: an integrated metagenomics and metabolomics analysis. Environ Health Perspect. 2014;122:284–91.

45. Monn C, Becker S. Cytotoxicity and induction of Proinflammatory cytokines from human monocytes exposed to fine (PM2.5) and coarse particles (PM10–2.5) in outdoor and indoor air. Toxicol Appl Pharmacol. 1999;155:245–52.

46. Bollati V, Marinelli B, Apostoli P, Bonzini M, Nordio F, Hoxha M, et al. Exposure to metal-rich particulate matter modifies the expression of candidate MicroRNAs in peripheral blood leukocytes. Environ Health Perspect. 2010;118:763.

47. Williams AE, Perry MM, Moschos SA, Larner-Svensson HM, Lindsay MA. Role of miRNA-146a in the regulation of the innate immune response and cancer. Biochem Soc Trans. 2008;36:1211–5.

48. Ghorpade DS, Sinha AY, Holla S, Singh V, Balaji KN. NOD2-Nitric Oxide-responsive MicroRNA-146a Activates Sonic Hedgehog Signaling to Orchestrate Inflammatory Responses in Murine Model of Inflammatory Bowel Disease. J Biol Chem. 2013;288:33037–48.

49. World Health Organization. WHO | Exposure to ambient air pollution [Internet]. WHO. 2016 [cited 2016 Dec 29]. Available from: http://www.who.int/gho/phe/outdoor_air_pollution/exposure/en/

50. Brook RD, Franklin B, Cascio W, Hong Y, Howard G, Lipsett M, et al. Air pollution and cardiovascular disease a statement for healthcare professionals from the expert panel on population and prevention science of the American Heart Association. Circulation. 2004;109:2655–71.

51. Charron A, Harrison RM. Fine (PM2.5) and coarse (PM2.5-10) particulate matter on a heavily trafficked London highway: sources and processes. Environ. Sci. Technol. 2005;39:7768–76.

52. Gurjar BR, Ravindra K, Nagpure AS. Air pollution trends over Indian megacities and their local-to-global implications. Atmos Environ. 2016;142:475–95.

53. Huang K, Zhuang G, Lin Y, Wang Q, JS F, Fu Q, et al. How to improve the air quality over megacities in China: pollution characterization and source analysis in shanghai before, during, and after the 2010 world expo. Atmospheric Chem Phys. 2013;13:5927–42.

54. Schins RPF, Lightbody JH, Borm PJA, Shi T, Donaldson K, Stone V. Inflammatory effects of coarse and fine particulate matter in relation to chemical and biological constituents. Toxicol Appl Pharmacol. 2004;195:1–11.

55. Cho S-H, Tong H, McGee JK, Baldauf RW, Krantz QT, Gilmour MI. Comparative toxicity of size-fractionated airborne particulate matter collected at different distances from an urban highway. Environ Health Perspect. 2009;117:1682–9.

56. Wegesser TC, Last JA. Mouse lung inflammation after instillation of particulate matter collected from a working dairy barn. Toxicol Appl Pharmacol. 2009;236:348.

57. Farina F, Sancini G, Mantecca P, Gallinotti D, Camatini M, Palestini P. The acute toxic effects of particulate matter in mouse lung are related to size and season of collection. Toxicol Lett. 2011;202:209–17.

58. Saravia J, You D, Thevenot P, Lee GI, Shrestha B, Lomnicki S, et al. Early-life exposure to combustion-derived particulate matter causes pulmonary immunosuppression. Mucosal Immunol. 2014;7:694–704.

59. Breznan D, Karthikeyan S, Phaneuf M, Kumarathasan P, Cakmak S, Denison MS, et al. Development of an integrated approach for comparison of in vitro and in vivo responses to particulate matter. Part Fibre Toxicol. 2016;13:41.

60. van Voorhis M, Knopp S, Julliard W, Fechner JH, Zhang X, Schauer JJ, et al. Exposure to atmospheric particulate matter enhances Th17 polarization through the aryl hydrocarbon receptor. PLoS One. 2013;8:e82545.

61. Pichavant M, Goya S, Meyer EH, Johnston RA, Kim HY, Matangkasombut P, et al. Ozone exposure in a mouse model induces airway hyperreactivity that requires the presence of natural killer T cells and IL-17. J Exp Med. 2008;205:385–93.

62. Montbarbon M, Pichavant M, Langlois A, Erdual E, Maggiotto F, Neut C, et al. Colonic inflammation in mice is improved by cigarette smoke through iNKT cells recruitment. PLoS One. 2013;8:e62208.

63. Kish L, Hotte N, Kaplan GG, Vincent R, Tso R, Gänzle M, et al. Environmental particulate matter induces murine intestinal inflammatory responses and alters the gut microbiome. PLoS One. 2013;8:e62220.

64. Salim SY, Kaplan GG, Madsen KL. Air pollution effects on the gut microbiota: a link between exposure and inflammatory disease. Gut Microbes. 2014;5:215–9.

65. Sinagra E, Pompei G, Tomasello G, Cappello F, Morreale GC, Amvrosiadis G, et al. Inflammation in irritable bowel syndrome: myth or new treatment target? World J Gastroenterol. 2016;22:2242.

66. Morris G, Berk M, Carvalho AF, Caso JR, Sanz Y, Maes M. The role of microbiota and intestinal permeability in the pathophysiology of autoimmune and Neuroimmune processes with an emphasis on inflammatory bowel disease type 1 diabetes and chronic fatigue syndrome. Curr Pharm Des. 2016;22:6058–75.

67. Viennois E, Merlin D, Gewirtz AT, Chassaing B. Dietary emulsifier-induced low-grade inflammation promotes colon carcinogenesis. Cancer res. 2016:canres1359.2016.

68. Winer DA, Luck H, Tsai S, Winer S. The intestinal immune system in obesity and insulin resistance. Cell Metab. 2016;23:413–26.

69. Chassaing B, Gewirtz AT. Gut microbiota, low-grade inflammation, and metabolic syndrome. Toxicol Pathol. 2014;42:49–53.

70. Severance GE, Tveiten DH, Lindström LH, Yolken RL, Reichelt K. The gut microbiota and the emergence of autoimmunity: relevance to major psychiatric disorders. Curr Pharm Des. 2016;22:6076–86.

71. Xin X, Dai W, Wu J, Fang L, Zhao M, Zhang P, et al. Mechanism of intestinal mucosal barrier dysfunction in a rat model of chronic obstructive pulmonary disease: an observational study. Exp. Ther. Med. 2016;12:1331–6.

72. Pardo M, Porat Z, Rudich A, Schauer JJ, Rudich Y. Repeated exposures to roadside particulate matter extracts suppresses pulmonary defense mechanisms. Resulting in lipid and protein oxidative damage. Environ. Pollut. Barking Essex 1987. 2015;210:227–37.

73. Shang Y, Zhang L, Jiang Y, Li Y, Airborne LP. Quinones induce cytotoxicity and DNA damage in human lung epithelial A549 cells: the role of reactive oxygen species. Chemosphere. 2014;100:42–9.

74. Lu S, Li Y, Zhang J, Zhang T, Liu G, Huang M, et al. Associations between polycyclic aromatic hydrocarbon (PAH) exposure and oxidative stress in people living near e-waste recycling facilities in China. Environ Int. 2016;94:161–9.

75. Dianat M, Radmanesh E, Badavi M, Goudarzi G, Mard SA. The effects of PM10 on electrocardiogram parameters, blood pressure and oxidative stress in healthy rats: the protective effects of vanillic acid. Environ Sci Pollut Res. 2016;23:19551–60.

76. Bertazzi PA, Cantone L, Pignatelli P, Angelici L, Bollati V, Bonzini M, et al. Does enhancement of oxidative stress markers mediate health effects of ambient air particles? Antioxid Redox Signal. 2013;21:46–51.

77. Samuni Y, Goldstein S, Dean OM, Berk M. The chemistry and biological activities of N-acetylcysteine. Biochim Biophys Acta. 2013;1830:4117–29.

78. Jin HM, Zhou DC, HF G, Qiao QY, SK F, Liu XL, et al. Antioxidant N-acetylcysteine protects pancreatic β-cells against aldosterone-induced oxidative stress and apoptosis in female db/db mice and insulin-producing MIN6 cells. Endocrinology. 2013;154:4068–77.

79. Lin H, Liu X, Yu J, Hua F, Antioxidant HZ. N-acetylcysteine attenuates hepatocarcinogenesis by inhibiting ROS/ER stress in TLR2 deficient mouse. PLoS One. 2013;8:e74130.

80. Amrouche-Mekkioui I, Djerdjouri BN. Acetylcysteine improves redox status, mitochondrial dysfunction, mucin-depleted crypts and epithelial hyperplasia in dextran sulfate sodium-induced oxidative colitis in mice. Eur J Pharmacol. 2012;691:209–17.

81. Ebrahimi F, Esmaily H, Baeeri M, Mohammadirad A, Fallah S, Abdollahi M. Molecular evidences on the benefit of N-acetylcysteine in experimental colitis. Open. Life Sci. 2008;3:135–42.

82. Lorber A, Baumgartner WA, Bovy RA, Chang CC, Hollcraft R. Clinical application for heavy metal-complexing potential of N-acetylcysteine. J Clin Pharmacol. 1973;13:332–6.

83. Banner W, Koch M, Capin DM, Hopf SB, Chang S, Tong TG. Experimental chelation therapy in chromium, lead, and boron intoxication with N-acetylcysteine and other compounds. Toxicol Appl Pharmacol. 1986;83:142–7.

84. Ercal N, Treeratphan P, Hammond TC, Matthews RH, Grannemann NH, Spitz DR. Vivo indices of oxidative stress in lead-exposed C57BL/6 mice are reduced by treatment with meso-2,3-Dimercaptosuccinic acid or N-acetylcysteine. Free Radic Biol Med. 1996;21:157–61.

85. Flora SJ. Arsenic-induced oxidative stress and its reversibility following combined administration of N-acetylcysteine and meso 2,3-dimercaptosuccinic acid in rats. Clin Exp Pharmacol Physiol. 1999;26:865–9.

86. Tulic MK, Vivinus-Nébot M, Rekima A, Medeiros SR, Bonnart C, Shi H, et al. Presence of commensal house dust mite allergen in human gastrointestinal tract: a potential contributor to intestinal barrier dysfunction. Gut. 2016;65:757–66.

87. Trompette A, Gollwitzer ES, Yadava K, Sichelstiel AK, Sprenger N, Ngom-Bru C, et al. Gut microbiota metabolism of dietary fiber influences allergic airway disease and hematopoiesis. Nat Med. 2014;20:159–66.

88. Wang J, Li F, Wei H, Lian Z-X, Sun R, Tian Z. Respiratory influenza virus infection induces intestinal immune injury via microbiota-mediated Th17 cell-dependent inflammation. J Exp Med. 2014;211:2397–410.

89. Schuijt TJ, Lankelma JM, Scicluna BP, de Sousa E, Melo F, Roelofs JJTH, de Boer JD, et al. The gut microbiota plays a protective role in the host defence against pneumococcal pneumonia. Gut. 2016;65(4):575–83.

90. Allais L, Kerckhof F-M, Verschuere S, Bracke KR, De Smet R, Laukens D, et al. Chronic cigarette smoke exposure induces microbial and inflammatory shifts and mucin changes in the murine gut. Environ Microbiol. 2016;18:1352–63.

91. Zuo L, Li Y, Wang H, Wu R, Zhu W, Zhang W, et al. Cigarette smoking is associated with intestinal barrier dysfunction in the small intestine but not in the large intestine of mice. J Crohns Colitis. 2014;8:1710–22.

Detection of titanium particles in human liver and spleen and possible health implications

M. B. Heringa[1*], R. J. B. Peters[2], R. L. A. W. Bleys[3], M. K. van der Lee[2], P. C. Tromp[4], P. C. E. van Kesteren[1], J. C. H. van Eijkeren[1], A. K. Undas[2], A. G. Oomen[1] and H. Bouwmeester[2,5]

Abstract

Background: Titanium dioxide (TiO_2) is produced at high volumes and applied in many consumer and food products. Recent toxicokinetic modelling indicated the potential of TiO_2 to accumulate in human liver and spleen upon daily oral exposure, which is not routinely investigated in chronic animal studies. A health risk from nanosized TiO_2 particle consumption could not be excluded then.

Results: Here we show the first quantification of both total titanium (Ti) and TiO_2 particles in 15 post-mortem human livers and spleens. These low-level analyses were enabled by the use of fully validated (single particle) inductively coupled plasma high resolution mass spectrometry ((sp)ICP-HRMS) detection methods for total Ti and TiO_2 particles. The presence of TiO_2 in the particles in tissues was confirmed by Scanning Electron Microscopy with energy dispersive X-ray spectrometry.

Conclusions: These results prove that TiO_2 particles are present in human liver and spleen, with ≥24% of nanosize (< 100 nm). The levels are below the doses regarded as safe in animals, but half are above the dose that is deemed safe for liver damage in humans when taking into account several commonly applied uncertainty factors. With these new and unique human data, we remain with the conclusion that health risks due to oral exposure to TiO_2 cannot be excluded.

Keywords: Titanium dioxide, Quantification, Human liver, Human spleen, Tissue level, Nanoparticle, Risk assessment, Sp-ICP-HRMS

Background

Titanium dioxide (TiO_2) is produced as titanium white at high production volumes, up to 6 million tons per year [1]. It is incorporated in many products, such as in food (additive E171), toothpaste, supplements and medicines, as well as in applications like paints, plastics, and cosmetics [1]. Food grade TiO_2 contains a fraction of particles in the nanosize range, which is around 10% number-based [2, 3]. No acceptable daily intake (ADI) for oral ingestion of TiO_2 has been derived in the past due to the absence of observed toxic effects in the available chronic rodent study [4], the generally assumed negligible

uptake of TiO_2 following ingestion [5], and the assumed insolubility and inertness of the material [6, 7]. Recent human volunteer studies, however, show elevated blood Ti levels (and indications of TiO_2 particles) 6 h after ingestion of food grade TiO_2 [8], confirming earlier reports of increased blood Ti-levels after ingestion of 160 nm and 380 nm TiO_2 particles [9]. Upon evaluating food grade TiO_2, the European Food Safety Agency (EFSA) acknowledged that TiO_2 is absorbed after oral application, albeit to a low extent, and transported to various organs [10]. Recently, very low oral (0.02 and 0.6%) absorption of TiO_2 nanoparticles has been shown in rats, with a retention of these particles in mainly the liver and spleen [11, 12]. This calls for (nano)particle biokinetic studies in humans [13].

* Correspondence: minne.heringa@rivm.nl
[1]National Institute for Public Health and the Environment (RIVM), Bilthoven, The Netherlands
Full list of author information is available at the end of the article

Toxicokinetic modelling of TiO_2 levels in human organs, based on animal studies and accounting for accumulation, has recently led to the conclusion that a human health risk from the oral intake of TiO_2 nanoparticles cannot be excluded [14]. Although most accumulation was seen in spleen, in the final risk assessment, a potential risk was found for the liver. It remained uncertain whether the modelled levels of TiO_2 nanoparticles for human liver and spleen are accurate, which is best verified by measurements. Although total-Ti has been detected before in human tissues like liver and spleen [15, 16], there currently are no data on the presence of TiO_2 (nano)particles in human tissues from people without titanium implants [17, 18]. Here, we present the first *quantitative* measurements of particles, both in size and concentration, in post-mortem liver and spleen of 15 human subjects (see Table 1) with a corresponding assessment of the risks that can potentially be associated with the observed total Ti and TiO_2 particle concentrations in these tissues.

Methods

Firstly, we determined the total-Ti content in human liver and spleen samples using a fully validated procedure that included the acid digestion of the formaldehyde-fixed homogenized human tissues and ICP-HRMS detection (Peters RJB, Undas A, Memelink J, van Bemmel G, Munniks S, Bouwmeester H, et al.: Development and validation of a method for the detection of titanium dioxide particles in human tissue, submitted). Next, a new, independent subsample was prepared to quantitatively determine the presence of TiO_2 particles in these tissues.

Table 1 Overview of human subjects involved in this study

Subject number	Gender (F/M)	Age (years)	Ethnicity	Ti implants
1	F	80	Caucasian	No
2	F	92	Caucasian	No
3	M	64	Caucasian	Yes
4	M	86	Caucasian	No
5	M	87	Caucasian	No
6	M	79	Caucasian	No
7	F	94	Asian	No
8	F	77	Caucasian	No
9	F	86	Caucasian	No
10	M	77	Caucasian	Yes
11	F	104	Caucasian	No
12	F	96	Caucasian	No
13	F	91	Caucasian	No
14	F	94	Caucasian	No
15	M	56	Caucasian	No

For this, highly sensitive and selective spICP-HRMS was used [2, 19–21]. The enzymatic and gentle chemical sample clean-up and detection method for Ti in tissues and organs was recently fully validated (Peters RJB, Undas A, Memelink J, van Bemmel G, Munniks S, Bouwmeester H, et al.: Development and validation of a method for the detection of titanium dioxide particles in human tissue, submitted). The sample preparation is known not to affect the presence and size of particles [2].

Samples and sample preparation

The inertness of TiO_2 allowed the use of livers (15) and spleens (15) obtained from bodies that were donated to the Department of Anatomy of the University Medical Centre Utrecht for educational and research purposes (Table 1). All ethical regulations concerning the use of these organs were followed, and approval for this specific scientific use was obtained from the board of University Medical Center Utrecht. The bodies, 6 men and 9 women who died at the age of 56 to 104 years, had been fixed in 4% formaldehyde. From these persons written informed consent was obtained during life that allowed the use of their entire bodies for educational and research purposes. While there is no information about their diets, it is known that all persons involved are of Caucasian ethnicity except one who was of Asian ethnicity. All have lived in the Netherlands their entire life and it is therefore assumed that most followed a Dutch diet [22]. Of the 15 persons involved, 2 received titanium implants during their lifetime. For sample preparation, each organ was cut into small pieces and grinded to a size of 0.5–1 mm diameter. To investigate potential sample contamination, all materials that had been in contact with the organs were collected. The total-Ti concentrations in these materials or released by these materials were determined. The average of the analytical results of those blank materials were calculated and subtracted from the sample results if they were above the limit of detection (LOD).

Determination of total-Ti content

An analytical sample of 1 g was collected from each grinded and homogenized sample and brought into a perfluoroalkoxy (PFA) microwave digestion tube to which 6 mL of nitric acid (70% HNO_3) and 2 mL of hydrofluoric acid (40% HF), were added. All subsamples were digested for 55 min in a MARS microwave system (CEM Corporation, Matthews, NC, USA). The temperature program was as follows: at 1600 W power from 20 to 120 °C in 15 min, then to 160 °C in 10 min, and then to 210 °C in 30 min and hold for 1 min. Following digestion and cooling to room temperature, ultra-pure water was added to a total volume of 50 mL. The extracts were shaken manually, diluted 2 times, and analysed with ICP-HRMS.

Quantification was based on ionic titanium standards diluted in the same acidic matrix as the samples. Method blanks were determined by performing the complete procedure, however, without the addition of a sample. The total-Ti content in the blanks was below the method LOD.

Determination of TiO$_2$ particles

For the determination of particle-TiO$_2$, a digestion procedure is followed to liberate the particles. This digestion procedure consists of two steps. In the first step, the tissue in the formaldehyde-fixed sample is depolymerized, while in the second step, a standard enzymatic digestion is performed. An analytical sample of 200 mg was collected from the grinded subsamples and brought into a 12-mL PE tube. In the first step, 4 mL of the digestion buffer was added and the sample was vigorously vortexed for 30 s. The digestion buffer was prepared by dissolving 300 mg of Tris buffer, 92.5 mg EDTA, 5 mg SDS and 3 g NaCl in 100 mL of Milli-Q water. Next, 4 g of glycine are added to the solution and mixed with a magnetic stirrer until complete dissolution. This solution was diluted with Milli-Q water to a final volume of 250 mL.

The tube was heated for 3 h. at 100 °C to depolymerize the formaldehyde-fixed tissue. In the second step, and after cooling to room temperature, 910 μL of proteinase K (2.5 mg/ml) was added. The tube was incubated for 16 h. at 37 °C in a shaking water bath. After cooling to room temperature, the digest was diluted with ultra-pure water and analyzed using spICP-HRMS.

Instrumental analysis with ICP-HRMS

A Thermo Finnigan Element 2 (Thermo Fisher Scientific GmbH, Bremen, Germany), a sector-field based high resolution ICP-MS, was used to measure total-Ti in acidic extracts in standard mode and TiO$_2$ particles in single-particle mode (also called time resolved analysis mode). Single-particle ICP-HRMS is a method for the detection and characterization of (nano-)particles [19, 21]. The Thermo Finnigan Element 2 was operated at a forward power of 1300 W and the argon gas flows were at the following settings; plasma, 15.4 L/min; nebulizer, 1.063 L/min; auxiliary, 1.2 L/min. The sample flow rate to the nebulizer was set at 0.5 mL/min. Data acquisition was done in standard mode and in time resolved analysis mode with titanium measured at m/z 46.95 in medium resolution mode to avoid interferences from $^{36}Ar^{12}C$, $^{32}S^{16}O$ and ^{48}Ca. In standard and time resolved mode the dwell time was 250 and 2 ms respectively, with a total acquisition time of 60 s. The transport efficiency was determined by the analyses of a 50 ng/L diluted aqueous RM8013 (60 nm gold nanoparticle) suspension under the same instrumental conditions as the samples but monitoring m/z 197 for gold. Finally, single-particle data were exported as csv file and processed in a dedicated spreadsheet for the calculation of particle sizes, particle size distributions, and particle number and mass concentrations. Details about this spreadsheet and the calculation of the parameters can be found elsewhere [19]. Method blanks were determined by performing the complete procedure, however, without the addition of a sample. The mass-based TiO$_2$ particle concentrations in the blanks were below the method LOD. Since the blanks of the sampling materials were below the LOD of the total-Ti method they were not involved in the particle analysis.

LOD

For the total-Ti determination the LOD is calculated as 3 times the standard deviation in the results of a blank sample or a sample with a total-Ti content close to the expected LOD. This sample is analysed on each of the validation days. The LOD is calculated as follows:

$$LOD = 3 \times \sqrt{\frac{\sum_{i=1}^{k}(y_i - m)^2}{k-1}}$$

where k is the number of samples, y$_i$ is the result of a single sample and m is average result of the single samples.

For particle-TiO$_2$ there are two LOD values, one for the number- and mass-based concentration (LOD$_C$), and one for particle size (LOD$_S$). LOD$_C$ equals the minimum number of particle peaks in the time scan that differentiates a sample from a blank. A way to determine LOD$_C$ is by the IUPAC recommended approximation (Poisson) described as [23],

$$LOD_C = 3.29 \times \sqrt{N} + 2.72$$

where N is the number of particle peaks observed in the time scan of a blank. The particle number LOD$_C$ can be converted into mass units if the size and density of the particle are known. The determination of the LOD$_S$ is described by Lee et al. and can be estimated as follows [24],

$$LOD_S = \sqrt[3]{\frac{6 \times 3\sigma_m}{R \times f_a \times \rho \times \pi}}$$

where σ$_m$ is the standard deviation in the background noise in the time scan, R is the ICP-MS response (cps/μg), f$_a$ is the mass fraction of analysed element in the nanoparticle and ρ is the density of the nanoparticle material (g/cm^3). The upper size limit of detection is estimated to be around 1500 nm.

Confirmation of TiO₂ particles wit SEM-EDX

Two subsamples of the grinded sample material of both the livers and the spleens were studied using scanning electron microscopy with energy dispersive X-ray detection (SEM-EDX) to confirm the presence of TiO_2 particles in human liver and spleen. The samples with the highest TiO_2 concentrations (as determined with ICP-HRMS) were selected for confirmation with SEM-EDX. Typically, subsamples of > 100 tissue grains were collected on a sampling stub and dried to remove water. These subsamples were analysed with a high resolution field emission gun scanning electron microscopy in combination with energy dispersive X-ray analysis (FEG-SEM/EDX). Approximately 500 images for each sample were viewed at different magnifications (5.000–100.000 X) to identify TiO_2 particles. For each sample, approximately 10 TiO_2 particles (single nanoparticles as well as aggregates/agglomerates) were detected. The surface of the grains was systematically analysed for TiO_2 particles

using the backscattered electron imaging mode. After detection of particles in a field of view, X-ray spectra from the detected particle and surrounding matrix were acquired to determine the identity. Subsequently, plasma-ashing was applied to remove the lipid fraction and obtain a sharper image of the TiO_2 particle.

Results

All tissue levels are given as wet organ weights as obtained after fixation in formalin.

Total Ti measurements

As shown in Table 2, the total-Ti content in the liver ranged from 0.02 to 0.09 mg Ti/kg tissue with an average value of 0.04 ± 0.02 mg Ti/kg tissue[1]. For spleen, the total-Ti content ranged from 0.02 to 0.4 mg Ti/kg tissue with an average value of 0.08 ± 0.1 mg Ti/kg tissue[1]. In the sparsely available literature on human data, liver and spleen concentrations ranging between 0.2 and 1.9 mg Ti/kg tissue have been detected. These

Table 2 Ti and TiO_2 particles in human (post mortem 4% formaldehyde fixed) liver and spleen

Human subject	Tissue	Total Ti mg/kg	TiO₂ (Particles) size range nm	TiO₂ (Particles) number of particles 10⁹/kg tissue	Ti in particles[a] min - max mg/kg tissue	Tissue	Total Ti mg/kg	TiO₂ (Particles) size range nm	TiO₂ (Particles) number of particles 10⁹/kg tissue	Ti in particles[a] min - max mg/kg tissue
1	Liver	0.04	85–320	2.3–7.2	0.01–0.04	Spleen	0.1	90–580	5.7–18	0.06–0.2
2	Liver	0.09	90–440	6.6–21	0.08–0.3	Spleen	0.4	90–420	18–56	0.1–0.4
3	Liver	< LODt	< LODs	< LODn	< LODc	Spleen	0.02	85–370	1.2–3.8	0.01–0.04
4	Liver	0.05	85–550	1.4–4.4	0.03–0.1	Spleen	0.09	85–320	2.8–8.8	0.01–0.02
5	Liver	< LODt	< LODs	< LODn	< LODc	Spleen	0.03	85–520	1.5–4.7	0.02–0.07
6	Liver	0.03	85–380	2.1–6.6	0.01–0.04	Spleen	0.02	85–350	1.3–4.1	0.01–0.04
7	Liver	< LODt	85–370	1.3–4.1	0.01–0.02	Spleen	0.02	< LODs	<LODn	< LODc
8	Liver	0.02	< LODs	< LODn	< LODc	Spleen	< LODt	< LODs	<LODn	< LODc
9	Liver	< LODt	< LODs	< LODn	< LODc	Spleen	0.2	85–410	9.3–29	0.08–0.3
10	Liver	< LODt	< LODs	< LODn	< LODc	Spleen	0.02	85–360	2.1–6.6	0.01–0.04
11	Liver	0.04	85–450	2.6–8.1	0.02–0.07	Spleen	0.03	90–420	3.2–10	0.02–0.07
12	Liver	0.02	< LODs	< LODn	< LODc	Spleen	0.04	90–720	2.1–6.6	0.05–0.2
13	Liver	< LODt	90–440	1.0–3.1	0.03–0.1	Spleen	0.02	90–390	2.3–7.2	0.03–0.10
14	Liver	< LODt	< LODs	< LODn	< LOD	Spleen	0.03	90–430	2.7–5.3	0.03–0.1
15	Liver	< LODt	< LODs	< LODn	< LODc	Spleen	0.04	90–500	2.4–7.5	0.03–0.1
	n > lod	7	7–7	7–7	7–7		14	13–13	13–13	13–13
	average	0.04[b]	86–421	2–8	0.03–0.1		0.08[c]	88–445	4–13	0.04–0.1
	mode	0.04	85–440	–	0.01–0.04		0.02	85–420	2–7	0.01–0.04
	stdev	0.02	2–74	2–6	0.02–0.1		0.1	3–110	5–15	0.03–0.11
	min	0.02	85–320	1–3	0.01–0.02		0.02	85–320	1–4	0.01–0.02
	max	0.09	90–550	7–21	0.08–0.3		0.4	90–720	18–56	0.1–0.4

Particle TiO_2 concentrations are reported as measured (min) and after correction for the analytical recovery (max). All concentrations are corrected for total concentrations in blanks (0.05 mg/kg). LODt (total-Ti) = 0.01 mg/kg; LODs (size) = 85 nm; LODn (number) = 0.8 × 10⁹/kg; LODc (calculated Ti in particles) = 0.005 mg/kg; [a]calculated Ti in particle, calculated according to Laborda et al. [21] and Peters et al. [b] if calculated with ½ LOD for samples below LOD, average total-Ti = 0.02 mg/kg;[c]if calculated with ½ LOD for samples below LOD, average total-Ti = 0.07 mg/kg concentrations have been measured using X-ray fluorescence and neutron activation analysis, while we used HR-ICPS [25, 26].

The blank-corrected limit of detection $(LOD)_{total\ Ti}$ was 0.01 mg/kg tissue, while the analytical recovery for total-Ti was 112 ± 34%, which is in the range of accepted analytical standards [20]. None of the specific steps in the tissue and sample preparation contributed to the blank total-Ti. Two human subjects carried a titanium implant, the total-Ti content in liver and spleen of these subjects was comparable to those observed in the liver and spleen in other subjects.

Particle measurements

The presence of TiO_2 particles in the tissues is evidenced by the characteristic spikes in the time scans of the spICP-HRMS analysis of liver and spleen samples (Fig. 1a, b). TiO_2 particles were detected in 7/15 liver and 13/15 spleen samples (Table 2). The smallest TiO_2 particle that can be detected with this method (LOD_{size}) in these tissues is 85 nm. The number-based TiO_2 particle size distributions in liver and spleen were comparable and had a size range of 85–550 and 85–720, respectively (Table 2 and Fig. 1c). SpICP-HRMS does not allow a further characterisation of the particles being

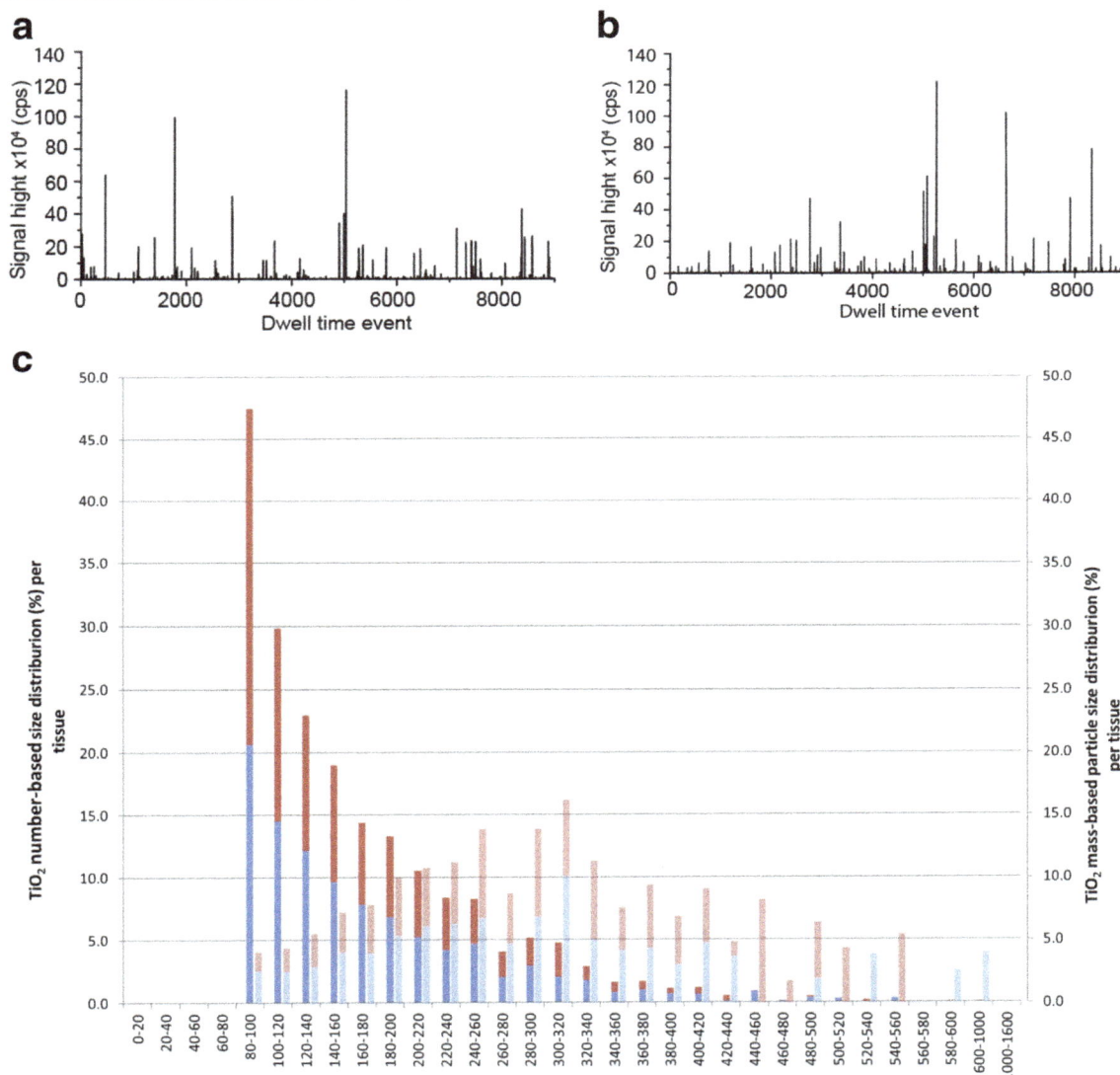

Fig. 1 TiO_2 particles in human (post mortem) liver and spleen. Time scans of the spICP-HRMS analyses of a liver sample (**a**) and spleen sample (**b**). The number of spikes in the time scan is directly proportional to the number of particles in the sample. The signal height of the peaks is directly proportional to the particle's mass from which the equivalent spherical particle size is calculated [22, 23]. **c** The calculated number-based particle size distribution (left axis and dark colours) and the calculated mass-based particle size distribution (right axis and light colours). Since the particle size distribution in liver (red bars) and spleen (blue bars) are very similar, they are stacked

present as agglomerates, aggregates or primary particles. In the tissues, 24% of the TiO_2 particles in the number-based size distribution was < 100 nm, but this fraction may be underestimated considering the LOD_{size} of 85 nm.

The TiO_2 particle mass concentration in liver ranged from 0.01 to 0.3 mg Ti/kg tissue (1.0×10^9 to 21×10^9 TiO_2 particles/kg tissue) (Table 2). In spleen, this concentration ranged from 0.01 to 0.4 mg Ti/kg tissue (1.2×10^9 to 56×10^9 TiO_2 particles/kg tissue). The $LOD_{particle-number}$ in the tissue matrix is 0.8×10^9 particles per kg tissue. The analytical recovery of TiO_2 particles by enzymatic digestion of the matrix is $32 \pm 7\%$. This low analytical recovery is in accordance with best international practices for this sample preparation and detection technique [27]. Because of the low analytical recovery, the Ti concentration of the particles is presented both as a minimum (not corrected for analytical recovery), and a maximum (corrected for analytical recovery) (see Table 2).

The total-Ti values are in general within this Ti concentration range in the particles, Furthermore, tissues with high total-Ti concentrations also contained high TiO_2 particle concentrations, and vice versa. Based on the maximum Ti concentration values in particles, on average minimally 51% (liver) and 67% (spleen) of total Ti is present in these tissues as particle. Taking into account the analytical recovery ($32 \pm 7\%$) and the LOD_{size} (85 nm) for the particles measurements, we assume all total Ti is present as particles.

We did not observe a correlation in the abundance of the TiO_2 particles in liver and spleen from the same subjects, while this would be expected based on the shared external exposure. The reason for this lack of correlation may be related to inter-individual differences in the various involved biodistribution processes.

Lastly, small tissue grains of liver and spleen from two subjects were analysed using SEM-EDX to visualize the TiO_2 particles. As shown in Fig. 2, the observed particles are composed of Ti and oxygen and are present as an aggregate or agglomerate, consisting of smaller primary particles of 75–150 nm. Presence of Ti was also confirmed semi-quantitatively by EDX analysis in dry-ashed liver and spleen samples (Fig. 2d).

Together, these analyses show that approximately all TiO_2 is present as particles in human liver and spleen, with sizes ranging 85–550 and 85–720, respectively (upper size limit of detection was > 1.5 μm). Probably also smaller particles are present, however these cannot be detected with the current methods. The SEM analysis of the particles suggests that the larger particles consist of smaller primary particles. Therefore, for the purpose of risk assessment, we assume that all Ti is ultimately present as TiO_2 nanoparticles.

Risk assessment

In a next step, the total TiO_2 levels in liver and spleen were compared to the toxicologically safe tissue levels for TiO_2 (0.14 mg/kg for spleen and

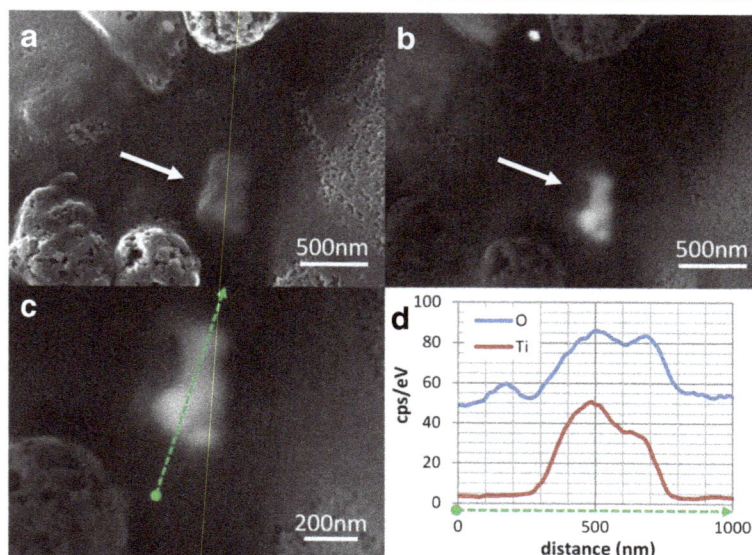

Fig. 2 SEM characterization of detected TiO_2 particles in a dried liver sample. **a** The secondary electron microscope image shows a TiO_2 agglomerate below the surface of the liver tissue (arrow). **b** The backscattered electron image reveals the spherically shaped primary particles within the agglomerate (arrow), with diameters between 75 and 150 nm; (**c**) illustrates the path of the EDX line scan across the aggregate in the same image at higher magnification; (**d**) demonstrates the presence of TiO_2 based on the corresponding increase of response for Ti (red line) and oxygen (blue line) at the position of the particle. This forms a clear indication that the detected particle is indeed TiO_2

0.008 mg/kg for liver), as reported earlier [14]. For liver, the measured TiO_2 concentrations are all below the level where effects occurred in animals, which were the occurrence of liver edema and liver enzyme level changes. However, the seven measurements >LOD are above the level at which effects may occur in humans (Fig. 3). For the estimation of the safe level in humans, interspecies differences were considered and sensitive subpopulations were accounted for, which would include children, elderly, and diseased people   (see also Additional file 1). It can therefore not be excluded that the observed liver levels lead to adverse effects in humans, such as a liver functioning less well, leading to e.g. less detoxification of substances in the blood, and less albumin production. For spleen, it is unlikely that adverse effects will occur in humans as the measured levels are distributed around the estimated safe levels (please note that in the key toxicological study [28], no adverse effects were reported, thus the highest tested dose was used here [14] (see also Additional file 2).

Discussion

The TiO_2 particles observed in the human liver and spleens may have entered the body through dermal, inhalatory or oral exposure. No data on exposure, and thus neither on exposure route, of the subjects included in this study during life is available. However, dermal uptake of TiO_2 particles is unlikely, as TiO_2 particles do not penetrate the (intact) human skin [17, 29]. It is likely that inhalatory uptake can be neglected as the chance is small that these people (all) had occupations with TiO_2 exposure through air. In addition, the estimated maximal non-occupational exposure through this route is 4.5 µg Ti/day (with an average of 0.75 µg TiO_2/day; based on the Ti concentrations in non-occupational settings of 0.01–0.1 µg/m^3) [30]. Furthermore, most of these inhaled TiO_2 particles are eliminated from the lungs by mucociliary clearance in the ciliated part of the lungs, and subsequently swallowed, as seen in some studies [31, 32]. Probably, most human subjects followed a West European diet and used toothpaste, which may result in a mean oral intake of 0.06–5.5 mg TiO_2/kg body weight/day [3, 10, 33, 34]. Recent human volunteer studies indicate the systemic uptake following ingestion of TiO_2 particles [8, 9]. Strikingly, the size range of the TiO_2 particles in the human livers and spleens (i.e. 86–421 and 88–445 nm, respectively) falls within that of the TiO_2 particles in food products (30–600 nm diameter [2]). In conclusion, intestinal exposure, e.g. from food, toothpaste and supplements, but also from any inhaled and swallowed particles, is the most likely source of the Ti and TiO_2 particles as found in the liver and spleens of these 15 subjects. This justifies our comparison with safe tissue levels derived from oral toxicity studies.

The current study shows that both the element Ti and TiO_2 particles are present in post mortem fixed human liver and spleen and that health risks from liver damage due to oral exposure to TiO_2 still cannot be excluded, especially in elderly people. Clearly, some issues as

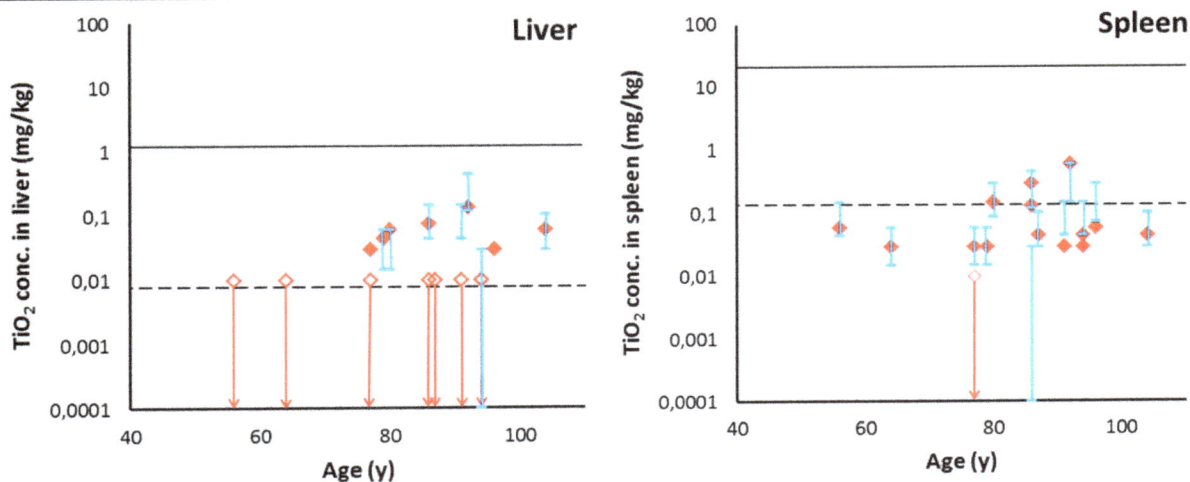

Fig. 3 Observed liver and spleen concentrations compared to toxicological effect levels. Measured total Ti (expressed as TiO_2 to enable comparison, red diamonds) and TiO_2 particle concentrations (blue ranges) in human liver and spleen are plotted against age, together with liver or spleen concentrations that are relevant for risk assessment (black lines). Open diamonds and arrows represent the possible levels in the samples where the Ti level was below the limit of detection (LOD). Measured particle concentrations are given as a range between the minimum possible level (no correction for the analytical recovery) and the maximum possible level (corrected for the analytical recovery). The solid black line represents the organ level at the No Observed Adverse Effect Level (NOAEL) in the animal study, i.e. the highest level at which no adverse effect was observed. The dashed black line represents the organ level below which no effects are expected in humans, considering several uncertainties in the animal data

addressed in Heringa et al. [14] remain unresolved, like the limitations in the toxicological data set and the impact that different forms of TiO_2, with different size [35], surface properties or crystalline structure can have on the observed toxicity. In addition, the available organs for this study were, understandably, limited to relatively older people and their TiO_2 exposure and health condition is not known. Recently, concern has been raised on the potential contribution of TiO_2 on tumor formation in the intestine [36, 37]. More information on the adverse effects of TiO_2 particles, including potential effects on liver as well as on potential carcinogenic induction and promotion in the gastrointestinal tract, would reduce the uncertainties in the current risk assessment.

Conclusion

Using two independent particle characterization techniques, we unequivocally show the presence of TiO_2 particles in (post mortem) human liver and spleen and provide quantitative data on the total human organ burden of TiO_2 particles for the first time. Particles with a size between 85 and 720 nm were found in tissue, of which at least 24% was smaller than 100 nm. This unique study thereby adds another critical piece to the risk assessment puzzle for TiO_2 (nano)particles, showing that health risks related to liver damage (i.e. liver edema and liver enzyme changes) due to TiO_2 particles still cannot be excluded.

Endnotes

[1]Values reported here are based on values above LOD, excluding the values below LOD.

Abbreviations

(FEG-)SEM-EDX: (field emission gun) scanning electron microscopy – energy dispersive X-ray; (sp)ICP-HRMS: (single particle) inductively coupled plasma high resolution mass spectrometry; ADI: Acceptable daily intake; EDTA: Ethylenediaminetetraacetic acid; EFSA: European Food Safety Authority; HF : Hydrofluoric acid; HNO_3: Nitric acid; IUPAC: International Union of Pure and Applied Chemistry; LOD: Limit of detection; NaCl: Sodium chloride; NOAEL: No observed adverse effect level; PE : Polyethylene; PFA: Perfluoroalkoxy; SDS: Sodium dodecyl sulphate; Ti: Titanium; TiO_2: Titanium dioxide

Acknowledgements

Our deep respect goes to the 15 people who donated their bodies to science post mortem and thus enabled these analyses. We thank J. Castenmiller and D. van Aken of the NVWA and K. Planken of the Ministry of Health, Welfare and Sport for their support and fruitful discussions. We thank P. Nobels and W. Schuurmans of Wageningen University Research for their assistance with the ICP-HRMS analysis. Rob Vandebriel (RIVM) is acknowledged for his help on evaluating the spleen effects reported in recent studies, Wim de Jong, Adrienne Sips and Joke Herremans (RIVM) for their useful comments on the paper.

Funding

The research was commissioned and financed by The Netherlands Food and Consumer Product Safety Authority (NVWA) and the Ministry of Economic Affairs.

Authors' contributions

MH, RP, AO, PvK, and HB conceived and designed the experiments. RB contributed sample materials. RP, MvdL, and AU supervised and analysed experiments and data. PT performed SEM-EDX measurements. JvE made the kinetic models for the risk assessment. MH and AO performed the risk assessment. MH, RP, MvdL, AO, and HB co-wrote the paper. All authors read and approved the final manuscript.

Competing interests

The authors declare that they have no competing interests.

Author details

[1]National Institute for Public Health and the Environment (RIVM), Bilthoven, The Netherlands. [2]RIKILT, Wageningen University & Research, Wageningen, The Netherlands. [3]Department of Anatomy, University Medical Center Utrecht, Utrecht, The Netherlands. [4]TNO Earth, Life and Social Sciences, Utrecht, The Netherlands. [5]Present address: Division of Toxicology, Wageningen University, Wageningen, The Netherlands.

References

1. Piccinno F, Gottschalk F, Seeger S, Nowack B. Industrial production quantities and uses of ten engineered nanomaterials in Europe and the world. J Nanopart Res. 2012;14(9):1109.
2. Peters RJ, van Bemmel G, Herrera-Rivera Z, Helsper HP, Marvin HJ, Weigel S, et al. Characterization of titanium dioxide nanoparticles in food products: analytical methods to define nanoparticles. J Agric Food Chem. 2014;62(27):6285–93.
3. Rompelberg C, Heringa MB, van Donkersgoed G, Drijvers J, Roos A, Westenbrink S, et al. Oral intake of added titanium dioxide and its nanofraction from food products, food supplements and toothpaste by the Dutch population. Nanotoxicology. 2016;10(10):1404–14.
4. (NCI) NCI. Bioassay of titanium dioxide for possible carcinogenicity, Carcinogenesis Technical Report Series. Maryland: Bethesda. p. 1979.
5. Warheit DB, Donner EM. Risk assessment strategies for nanoscale and fine-sized titanium dioxide particles: recognizing hazard and exposure issues. Food Chem Toxicol. 2015;85:138–47.
6. FAO. Titanium Dioxide. In: Chemical and Techncial assessment; 2006.
7. JECFA. Specifications for the identity and purity of food additives and their toxicological evaluation. Some food colours, emulsifiers, stabilizers, anticaking agents, and certain other substances. 13th report of the JECFA. In: World Health Organisation Techncial Report Series, No 445; FAO Nutrition Meetings Report Series, No 46. Rome; 1970.
8. Pele LC, Thoree V, Bruggraber SF, Koller D, Thompson RP, Lomer MC, et al. Pharmaceutical/food grade titanium dioxide particles are absorbed into the bloodstream of human volunteers. Part Fibre Toxicol. 2015;12:26.
9. Bockmann J, Lahl H, Eckert T, Unterhalt B. Blood titanium levels before and after oral administration titanium dioxide. Pharmazie. 2000;55(2):140–3.
10. EFSA. Re-evaluation of titanium dioxide (E 171) as a food additive. EFSA J. 2016;14(9)
11. Kreyling WG, Holzwarth U, Schleh C, Kozempel J, Wenk A, Haberl N, et al. Quantitative biokinetics of titanium dioxide nanoparticles after oral application in rats: part 2. Nanotoxicology. 2017;11(4):443–53.
12. Geraets L, Oomen AG, Krystek P, Jacobsen NR, Wallin H, Laurentie M, et al. Tissue distribution and elimination after oral and intravenous administration of different titanium dioxide nanoparticles in rats. Part Fibre Toxicol. 2014;11:30.
13. Bello D, Warheit DB. Biokinetics of engineered nano-TiO2 in rats administered by different exposure routes: implications for human health. Nanotoxicology. 2017;11(4):431–3.
14. Heringa MB, Geraets L, van Eijkeren JC, Vandebriel RJ, de Jong WH, Oomen AG. Risk assessment of titanium dioxide nanoparticles via oral exposure, including toxicokinetic considerations. Nanotoxicology. 2016;10(10):1515–25.
15. Snyder WS, Cook MJ, Nasset ES, Karhausen LR, Parry Howells G, Tipton IH. Report of the task group of reference man. A report prepared by a task group of committee 2 of the international commission on radiological protection: The international Comission on Radiological Protection, Oxford; 1992.
16. Yukawa M, Suzuki-Yasumoto M, Amano K, Terai M. Distribution of trace elements in the human body determined by neutron activation analysis. Arch Environ Health Int J. 1980;35(1):36–44.

17. Shi H, Magaye R, Castranova V, Zhao J. Titanium dioxide nanoparticles: a review of current toxicological data. Part Fibre Toxicol. 2013;10:15.

18. Powell JJ, Faria N, Thomas-McKay E, Pele LC. Origin and fate of dietary nanoparticles and microparticles in the gastrointestinal tract. J Autoimmun. 2010;34(3):J226–33.

19. Peters R, Herrera-Rivera Z, Undas A, van der Lee M, Marvin H, Bouwmeester H, et al. Single particle ICP-MS combined with a data evaluation tool as a routine technique for the analysis of nanoparticles in complex matrices. J Anal Atomic Spectrom. 2015;30(6):1274–85.

20. Tassinari R, Cubadda F, Moracci G, Aureli F, D'Amato M, Valeri M, et al. Oral, short-term exposure to titanium dioxide nanoparticles in Sprague-Dawley rat: focus on reproductive and endocrine systems and spleen. Nanotoxicology. 2014;8(6):654–62.

21. Laborda F, Bolea E, Jimenez-Lamana J. Single particle inductively coupled plasma mass spectrometry: a powerful tool for nanoanalysis. Anal Chem. 2014;86(5):2270–8.

22. van Rossum CTM, Fransen HP, Verkaik-Kloosterman J, Buurma EM, Ocké MC. Dutch National Food Consumption Survey 2007–2010: diet of children and adults aged 7 to 69 years. Bilthoven: National Institute for Public Health and the Environment (RIVM); 2011.

23. Currie LA. Nomenclature in evaluation of analytical methods including detection and quantification capabilities (IUPAC recommendations 1995). In: Pure Appl Chem, vol. 671995: 1699.

24. Lee S, Bi X, Reed RB, Ranville JF, Herckes P, Westerhoff P. Nanoparticle size detection limits by single particle ICP-MS for 40 elements. Environ Sci Technol. 2014;48(17):10291–300.

25. Yukawa M, Amano K, Suzuki-Yasumoto M, Terai M. Distribution of trace elements in the human body determined by neutron activation analysis. Arch Environ Health. 1980;35(1):36–44.

26. National Research Council. Mineral tolerance of animals. second revised ed. Washington: National Academies Press; 2005.

27. Loeschner K, Braband MS, Sloth JJ, Larsen EH. Use of alkaline or enzymatic sample pretreatment prior to characterization og gold nanoparticles in animal tissue by single particle ICPMS. Anal Bioanal Chem. 2014;16:3845–51.

28. Wang Y, Chen Z, Ba T, Pu J, Chen T, Song Y, et al. Susceptibility of young and adult rats to the oral toxicity of titanium dioxide nanoparticles. Small. 2013;9(9–10):1742–52.

29. SCCS, Chaudhry Q. Opinion of the scientific committee on consumer safety (SCCS) – revision of the opinion on the safety of the use of titanium dioxide, nano form, in cosmetic products. Regul Toxicol Pharmacol. 2015;73(2):669–70.

30. IPCS (International Programme on Chemical Safety). Environmental Health Criteria 24_Titanium. Geneva: WHO; 1982. ISBN 92 4 154084 2.

31. Pujalte I, Dieme D, Haddad S, Serventi AM, Bouchard M. Toxicokinetics of titanium dioxide (TiO2) nanoparticles after inhalation in rats. Toxicol Lett. 2017;265:77–85.

32. Kreyling WG, Holzwarth U, Haberl N, Kozempel J, Wenk A, Hirn S, et al. Quantitative biokinetics of titanium dioxide nanoparticles after intratracheal instillation in rats: part 3. Nanotoxicology. 2017;11(4):454–64.

33. Sprong C, Bakker M, Niekerk M, Venneman F. Exposure assessment of the food additive titantuim dioxide (E 171) based on use levels provided by the industry. Bilthoven: RIVM; 2015.

34. Weir A, Westerhoff P, Fabricius L, Hristovski K, von Goetz N. Titanium dioxide nanoparticles in food and personal care products. Environ Sci Technol. 2012;46(4):2242–50.

35. Laurent A, Harkema JR, Andersen EW, Owsianiak M, Vea EB, Jolliet O. Human health no-effect levels of TiO2 nanoparticles as a function of their primary size. J Nanopart Res. 2017;19(4):130.

36. Urrutia-Ortega IM, Garduno-Balderas LG, Delgado-Buenrostro NL, Freyre-Fonseca V, Flores-Flores JO, Gonzalez-Robles A, et al. Food-grade titanium dioxide exposure exacerbates tumor formation in colitis associated cancer model. Food Chem Toxicol. 2016;93:20–31.

37. Bettini S, Boutet-Robinet E, Cartier C, Comera C, Gaultier E, Dupuy J, et al. Food-grade TiO2 impairs intestinal and systemic immune homeostasis, initiates preneoplastic lesions and promotes aberrant crypt development in the rat colon. Sci Rep. 2017;7:40373.

Suppression of PTPN6 exacerbates aluminum oxide nanoparticle-induced COPD-like lesions in mice through activation of STAT pathway

Xiaobo Li[1], Hongbao Yang[2], Shenshen Wu[1], Qingtao Meng[1], Hao Sun[1], Runze Lu[1], Jian Cui[1], Yuxin Zheng[3], Wen Chen[4], Rong Zhang[5], Michael Aschner[6] and Rui Chen[1,7*]

Abstract

Background: Inhaled nanoparticles can deposit in the deep lung where they interact with pulmonary cells. Despite numerous studies on pulmonary nanotoxicity, detailed molecular mechanisms of specific nanomaterial-induced lung injury have yet to be identified.

Results: Using whole-body dynamic inhalation model, we studied the interactions between aluminum oxide nanoparticles (Al_2O_3 NPs) and the pulmonary system in vivo. We found that seven-day-exposure to Al_2O_3 NPs resulted in emphysema and small airway remodeling in murine lungs, accompanied by enhanced inflammation and apoptosis. Al_2O_3 NPs exposure led to suppression of PTPN6 and phosphorylation of STAT3, culminating in increased expression of the apoptotic marker PDCD4. Rescue of PTPN6 expression or application of a STAT3 inhibitor, effectively protected murine lungs from inflammation and apoptosis, as well as, in part, from the induction of chronic obstructive pulmonary disease (COPD)-like effects.

Conclusion: In summary, our studies show that inhibition of PTPN6 plays a critical role in Al_2O_3 NPs-induced COPD-like lesions.

Keywords: Aluminum oxide nanoparticles; PTPN6, Experimental COPD, Inflammation

Background

Airborne nanoparticle-induced pulmonary toxicity has been widely reported. This toxicity is largely dependent on the chemical and physical characteristics of specific nanoparticles. Pulmonary inflammation plays a critical initial event in metal oxide nanoparticle-induced respiratory disorders [1–3].

Aluminum oxide nanoparticles (Al_2O_3 NPs) have been widely used in the chemical, industrial and medical fields [4]. Al_2O_3 NPs represent one of the most abundantly produced nanosized particles, accounting for approximately 20% of the 2005 world market of nanoparticles [5]. The limit values for inhaled aluminum (Al) compounds remain relatively high. For instance, the United States Occupational Safety and Health Administration (OSHA) has set a legal limit (PEL) of 15 mg/m^3 (total dust) and 5 mg/m^3 (respirable fraction) for alumina in dusts averaging over an 8 h work day [6]. In total alumina dusts, nano-scaled particles exhibit a slower precipitation in air than the bulk, therefore increasing exposure duration in humans [7]. It is noteworthy that asthma has been recognized as one of the most prevalent pulmonary diseases in the aluminum exposure occupational setting [4]. In addition, insoluble Al compounds appear to be biopersistent in lung tissues. As demonstrated in rat intratracheal instillation model, only ~9% of Al_2O_3 was cleared from the lungs during a 19-week period following weekly instillation for 20 weeks [8]. Considering the high discharge levels during the

* Correspondence: rui.chen@seu.edu.cn
[1]Key Laboratory of Environmental Medicine Engineering, Ministry of Education, School of Public Health, Southeast University, Dingjiaqiao 87, Nanjing 210009, China
[7]Institute for Chemical Carcinogenesis, Guangzhou Medical University, Guangzhou 511436, China
Full list of author information is available at the end of the article

manufacturing process [7], concern over the biosafety of Al$_2$O$_3$ NPs is warranted.

In term of toxic mechanisms, exposure to Al$_2$O$_3$ NPs has been shown to cause mitochondrial dysfunction in a dose-dependent manner in human fetal lung fibroblasts (HFL1) [9] and human bronchial epithelia HBE [10]. Other studies have shown the number of macrophages in bronchoalveolar lavage fluid (BALF) of Al$_2$O$_3$ nanowhisker-exposed mice to be two-fold higher than in control mice [11]. A series of studies by Pauluhn have further suggested pulmonary inflammation induced by high dose (28 mg/m^3) Al exyhydroxides nanoparticles exposure [12, 13]. Taken together, these studies suggest a possible toxic mechanism involving oxidative stress and inflammation; however, detailed molecular mechanisms by which Al$_2$O$_3$ NPs interact with the pulmonary system have yet to be defined.

Our previous in vitro study suggested that suppression of protein tyrosine phosphatase, non-receptor type 6 (PTPN6) expression level in A549 cells plays a key role in Al$_2$O$_3$ NPs-induced cellular toxicity [14]. PTPN6 has been shown to be a critical negative regulator of intracellular signaling; it is predominantly expressed in hematopoietic cells and epithelia [15, 16]. Suppression of PTPN6 augments oxidative stress and exacerbates chronic inflammatory airway diseases [17]. Activation of the STAT3 pathway is involved in development of pulmonary inflammatory disease [18, 19], and PTPN6 has been recognized in multiple cell lines as a negative regulator of STAT3 [20–22]. In addition, up-regulation of PTPN6 has been shown to inhibit phosphor-STAT3 and mitigate activation of STAT3 in A549 cells [23]. Accordingly, we hypothesized that aberrant expression of PTPN6 might be involved in pulmonary disorders induced by Al$_2$O$_3$ NPs in vivo. To address this hypothesis, mice were exposed to Al$_2$O$_3$ NPs by dynamic inhalation to observe the alterations in lung function and pathology. We subsequently delineated the function of PTPN6 in Al$_2$O$_3$ NPs-related pulmonary disorders by integrating cellular assays with experimental mouse models. Notably, we show that rescue of PTPN6 expression levels significantly alleviates Al$_2$O$_3$ NPs-induced pulmonary inflammation as well as COPD-like lesions in murine lung tissues.

Results
Al$_2$O$_3$ NPs exposure increases levels of inflammatory mediators in mouse lung tissues
Specific airway resistance (sRAW) (an index used to identify acute bronchial response [24]) was measured in conscious mice one day before Al$_2$O$_3$ NPs-exposure and on exposure days 3 and 7. The sRAW in 2 mg/m^3 Al$_2$O$_3$ NPs-treated mice was significantly increased on day 3 and day 7 of exposure. In mice exposed to 0.4 mg/m^3

Al$_2$O$_3$ NPs, a significant increase in sRAW was noted on exposure day 7 when compared with FRA control (Fig. 1a). Based on the findings that low levels of Al$_2$O$_3$ NPs exposure caused phenotype alteration on the 7th day of exposure, all the following experiments were carried out for 7 days.

The aluminum (Al) burdens in lungs of mice were 411 ± 68, 1238 ± 110 and 2951 ± 234 ng/g for the control (filtered-room air, FRA), 0.4 and 2 mg/m^3 Al$_2$O$_3$ NPs-exposed groups, respectively. The 2 mg/m^3 Al$_2$O$_3$ NPs-exposed groups had a 3-fold greater Al burden in the lungs compared to those exposed to 0.4 mg/m^3 Al$_2$O$_3$ NPs. This may be related to greater damage to the lung in response to the higher dose, reflecting altered aggregation and deposition patterns.

Compared to FRA exposed mice, Al$_2$O$_3$ NPs-exposed mice had higher concentrations of bronchoalveolar lavage fluid (BALF) interleukin (IL)-6 (a cytokine associated with decline in lung function [25]) and BALF IL-33 (a cytokine induces chronic airway inflammation [26, 27]) (Fig. 1b). Next, we assayed the total number of cells, number of monocytic cells and neutrophils in BALF. Compared with controls, the percentages of increased levels of IL-6 were 76% and 113%; increased IL-33 levels were 65% and 72.5; increased total cell numbers were 33% and 64%; increased monocytic cells were 34% and 57%, increased numbers of neutrophils were 130% and 250% in the 0.4 and 2 mg/m^3 Al$_2$O$_3$ NPs exposed murine lungs, respectively. All of the above airway inflammatory indices were elevated in an Al$_2$O$_3$ dose-dependent manner when compared to FRA controls (Fig. 1c). Figure 1 d to g depict representative images of inflammatory infiltration in murine lung tissues, noting infiltration of inflammatory cells around small airways (Fig. 2d) (shown by arrow). Figure 1e showed the representative image of alveolar area of control murine lung. Increased infiltrating alveolar neutrophil, lymphocytes and macrophages (Fig. 1f) in response to Al$_2$O$_3$ NPs were also observed (shown by arrows).

Al$_2$O$_3$ NPs exposure induce apoptosis and experimental COPD in mice
The pathological alterations in murine lung tissues were examined by hematoxylin and eosin (H&E) staining. We noted emphysema in the distant alveolar area, characterized by enlarged airspace and increased mean chord lengths (Lm) (established indices of experimental COPD [28]) in lung tissues after Al$_2$O$_3$ NPs exposures compared to FRA control (Fig. 2a and b). The other vital characteristic of experimental COPD, small-airway remodeling, was assayed by Periodic Acid-Schiff (PAS) [27] and Masson's Trichrome staining [29]. Increased mucin glycoprotein secretion was detected by Periodic Acid-Schiff (PAS) staining, and mucus hypersecretion

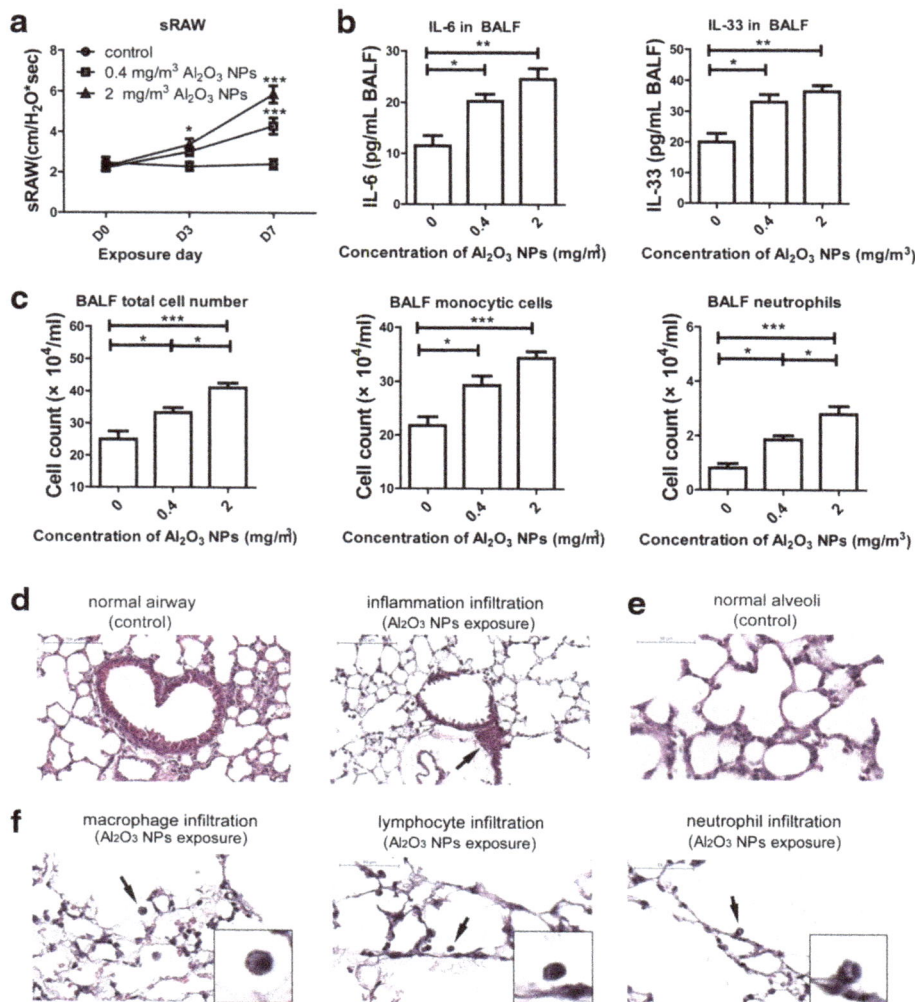

Fig. 1 Pulmonary inflammation induced by Al_2O_3 NPs exposure. **a** sRAW was significantly increased in Al_2O_3 NPs-exposed mice ($n = 10$, *$P < 0.05$, compared with controls; ***$P < 0.001$, compared with control on the same day). **b** Inflammatory mediators were significantly increased in Al_2O_3 NPs-exposed BALF of mice ($n = 4$, *$P < 0.05$, **$P < 0.01$). **c** The total cell number, monocytic cells number and neutrophils number in BALF of Al_2O_3 NPs-exposed mice were significantly increased compared with FRA control ($n = 4$, *$P < 0.05$, ***$P < 0.001$). **d** Representative images of normal airway and airway surrounded by inflammatory cells (showed by arrow). **e** Representative images of distant alveoli (FRA control) **f** Representative images of macrophages, lymphocytes and neutrophil infiltration in alveolar area (Al_2O_3 NPs exposure) (shown by arrow). The images in the right bottom of each panel are magnified of the cell in original images highlighted with black arrows

was observed in airway epithelial cells of Al_2O_3 NPs-exposed mice (Fig. 2c). Masson's Trichrome staining was used to evaluate the deposition of collagen around small airway, a hallmark of airway remodeling. As shown in fig. 2d, the enhanced collagen deposition was enhanced in the lungs of Al_2O_3 NPs-exposed mice when compared with FRA controls. Exposure to ZnO NPs has been reported to lead to emphysema [30]; therefore, ZnO NPs were used as a positive control. It was noted that the major pathologic alterations in murine lungs induced by ZnO NPs occurred in the alveolar areas, characterized by thickened alveolar walls and emphysema (Additional file 1: Figure S1a). However, remodeling of

airways has not been observed (data not shown). These results suggest that different metal oxide NPs exposure leads to varied pathologic alterations in the lungs.

Increased apoptosis of alveolar epithelial and endothelial cells in the lung is a vital upstream event in the pathogenesis of COPD, especially in the development of emphysema [31, 32]. Here, we detected apoptosis in the lungs of mice with the TUNEL assay. As shown in Fig. 2e, the percentage of apoptotic cells was significantly increased in a dose-dependent manner in airway epithelia and alveolar epithelia in the lungs of Al_2O_3 NPs-exposed mice compared with FRA control. Our observation strongly suggests that Al_2O_3 NPs exposure leads to

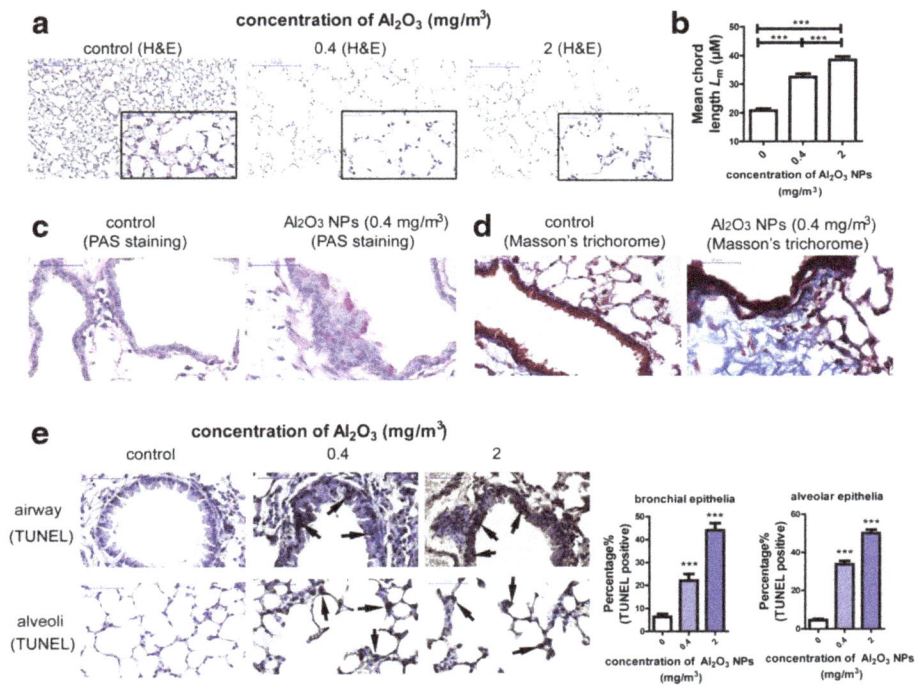

Fig. 2 Exposure to Al$_2$O$_3$ NPs led to experimental COPD in a murine model. **a** Representative images of normal alveolar area and emphysema. The images on the right bottom of each panel are magnified (400) of area from the original one. **b** Lm was significantly increased in Al$_2$O$_3$ NPs-exposed mouse lungs (n = 36, *** P < 0.001). **c** Representative images of PAS staining, the PAS$^+$ cells suggested hypersecretion of airway epithelial cells (shown by arrows). **d** Representative images of Masson's Trichrome staining. Deposit of collagen around airway was stained purple. **e** Representative images of TUNEL staining and percentage of TUNEL$^+$ cells. The TUNEL$^+$ cells were shown by arrows. (n = 30, *** P < 0.001, compared with control group)

inflammation and experimental COPD pathology in murine lungs.

Suppression of PTPN6 resulted in overexpression of apoptosis related gene PDCD4

Our previous study suggested a critical role for PTPN6 in Al$_2$O$_3$ NP-induced lung injury. Bioinformatics analyses demonstrated that PTPN6 interacted with 3 other genes (PDCD4, BAX, and APP) in the transcriptional factor-gene networks. These 4 genes (PTPN6, PDCD4, BAX and APP) were previously shown to be associated with cell death pathway [14]. Consistent with our observations from Al$_2$O$_3$ NPs-exposed cells [14], we found that after Al$_2$O$_3$ NPs exposure lung PTPN6 expression levels were significantly inhibited, and the expression of the other 3 genes (PDCD4, BAX and APP) was significantly increased in a dose-dependent manner (Fig. 3a).

These findings raised the question as to whether the suppression of PTPN6 is only restricted to Al$_2$O$_3$ NPs-exposure. To address this hypothesis, A549 cells were exposed to two types of nanomaterials, zinc oxide (ZnO) NPs and carbon black (CB) NPs, at concentrations of 0, 25 or 100 μg/mL. Expression levels of BAX were significantly increased in ZnO and CB NPs treated A549 cells, suggesting activation of a universal apoptoic pathway.

There were no significant alterations in expression levels of PDCD4, APP or PTPN6 in A549 cells treated by ZnO or CB NPs (Additional file 1: Figure S1b and c). The trends in gene expression levels in ZnO NPs-treated murine lungs were consistent with those noted in ZnO NPs-treated A549 cells (Additional file 1: Figure S1d).

The regulation of PDCD4, BAX and APP by PTPN6 was further validated in two pulmonary cell lines (A549 and HBE). Al$_2$O$_3$ NPs exposure decreased PTPN6 and increased PDCD4, BAX and APP mRNA as well as protein expression levels. However, overexpression of PTPN6 reduced only the expression of PDCD4 to levels statistically indistinguishable from control (Fig. 3b), indicating inhibition of PDCD4 by PTPN6.

To further validate the regulation of PTPN6 to PDCD4 in vivo, we set up a PTPN6 overexpression mouse model employing intranasal instillation of PTPN6 expression lentivirus. The conditional expression of PTPN6 in murine lungs was significantly increased after intranasal instillation (Additional file 1: Figure S2). Conditional overexpression of PTPN6 in murine lungs inhibited the Al$_2$O$_3$ NPs-induced increased expression of PDCD4 to levels indistinguishable from control (Fig. 3c, representative images of negative controls for PDCD4 IHC staining are shown in Additional file 1: Figure S3).

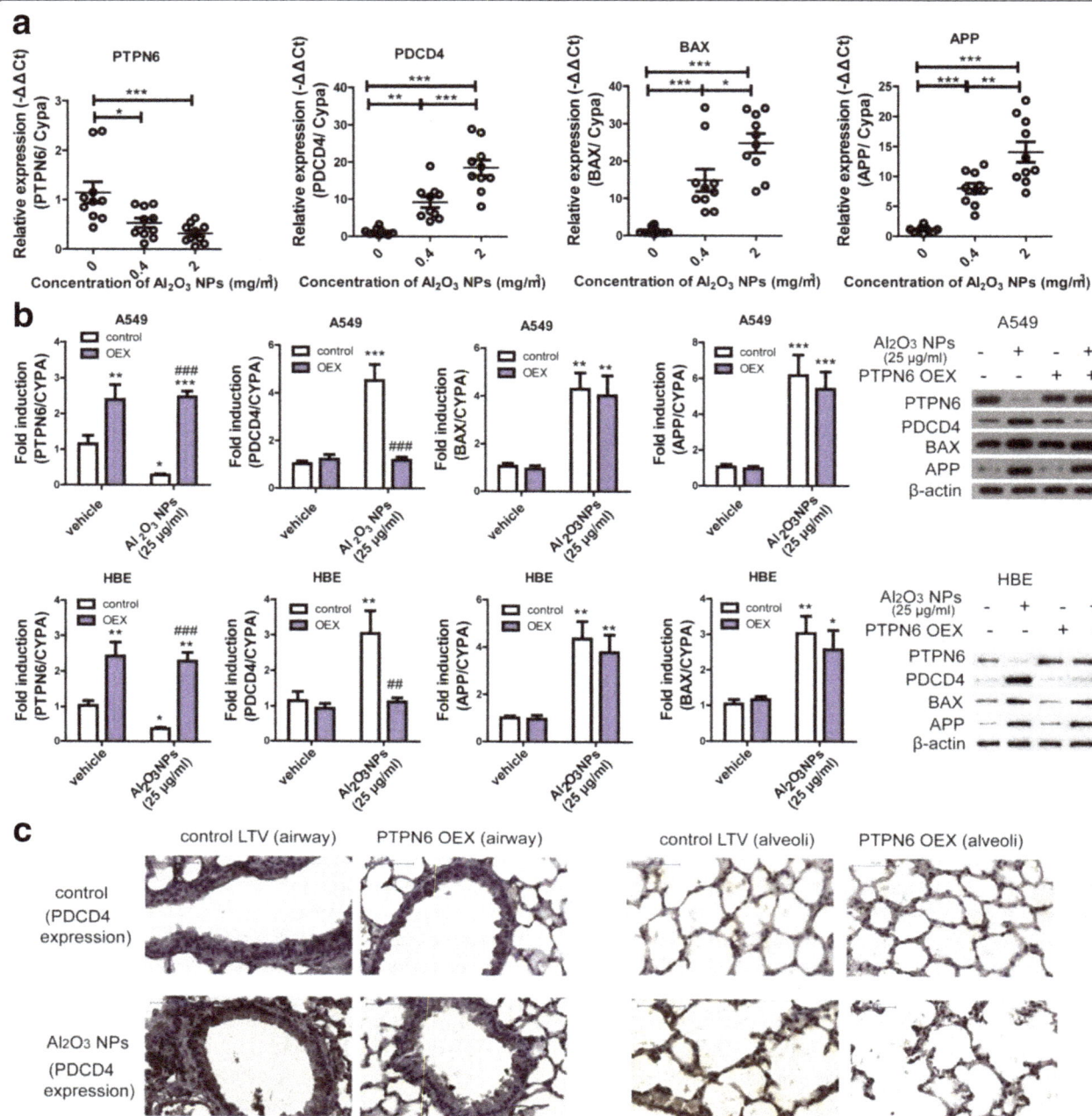

Fig. 3 Overexpression of PTPN6 inhibited PDCD4 expression levels both in vitro and in vivo. **a** expression of PTPN6, PDCD4, BAX and APP in mouse lungs exposed to Al_2O_3 NPs ($n = 10$, [*]$P < 0.05$, [**]$P < 0.01$, [***]$P < 0.001$). **b** mRNA and protein expression levels of PTPN6, PDCD4, BAX and APP in A549 and HBE cells ($n = 6$, [*]$P < 0.05$, compared with vehicle-treated control, [**]$P < 0.01$, compared with vehicle-treated control, [***]$P < 0.001$, compared with vehicle-treated control, [##]$P < 0.01$, compared with vehicle/Al_2O_3 NPs-exposed group, [###]$P < 0.001$, compared with vehicle/Al_2O_3 NPs-exposed group). **c** Representative images of PDCD4 expression in mouse lung tissues. LTV: lentivirus; OEX: overexpression

Thus, the PTPN6/PDCD4 pathway plays a critical role in Al_2O_3 NPs-induced experimental COPD in mice.

Activation of STAT3 mediates Al_2O_3 NPs-induced COPD-like lesions

PTPN6 is a negative regulator to STAT3 signaling [23], and increased PDCD4 expression has been previously shown to be dependent on STAT3 phosphorylation, and subsequently exacerbated inflammation in lung tissues [33]. To address the hypothesis that STAT3 mediated the increased PDCD4 expression induced by PTPN6 inhibition, the expression levels of p-STATs in conditional PTPN6 expression murine lungs were evaluated. As shown in Fig. 4a, expression of p-STAT3 was enhanced

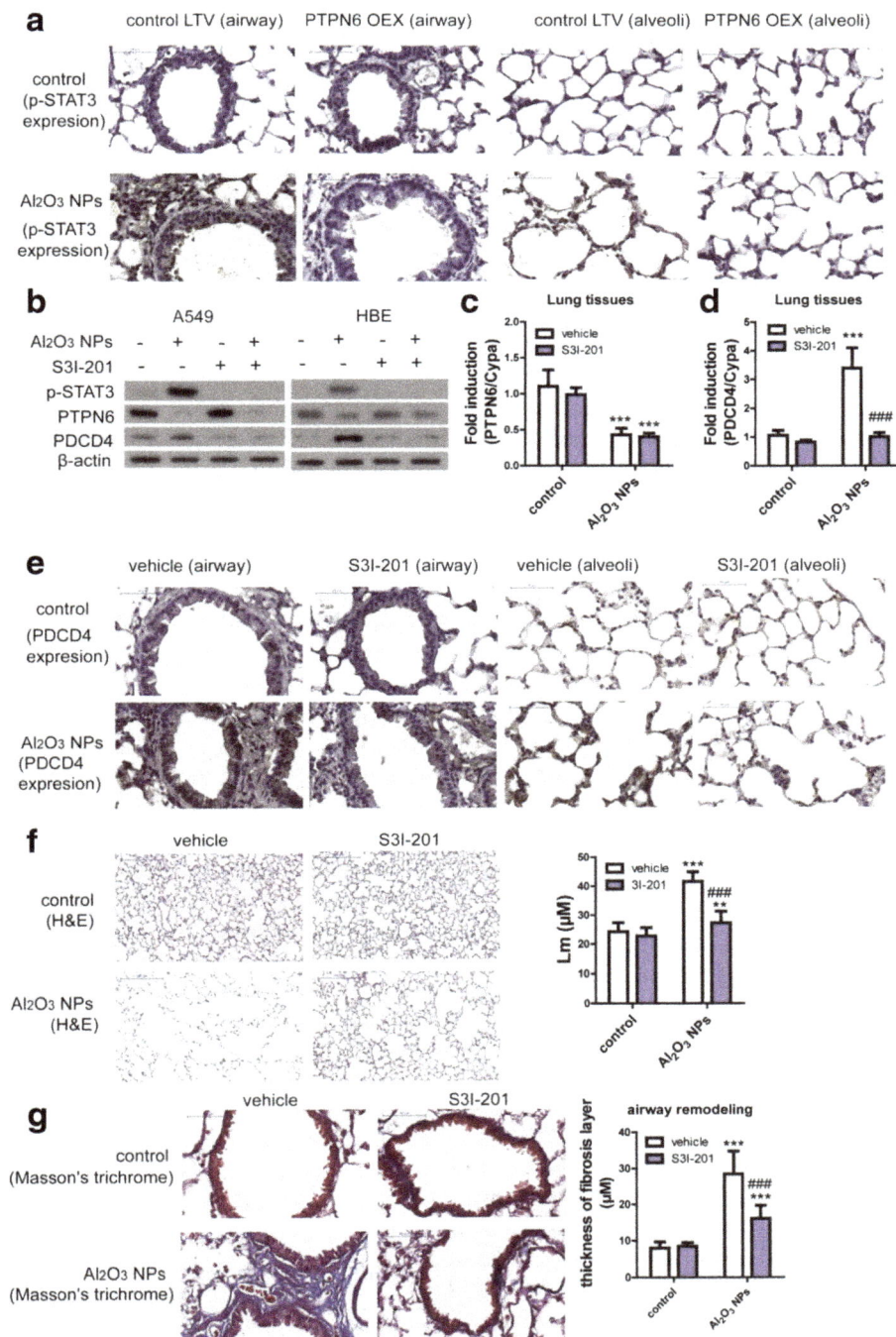

Fig. 4 PTPN6 inhibited PDCD4 expression in a STAT3-dependent manner. **a** Representative images of p-STAT3 in mouse lung tissues. **b** The STAT3 inhibitor (S3I-201) inhibited activation of STAT3 and expression of PDCD4 in A549 and HBE cells. **c** The STAT3 inhibitor (S3I-201) did not inhibit expression of PTPN6 in mouse lung tissues (n = 6, ***$P < 0.001$, compared with vehicle control). **d** The STAT3 inhibitor (S3I-201) inhibited expression of PDCD4 in mouse lung tissues (n = 6, ***$P < 0.001$, compared with vehicle control, ###$P < 0.001$, compared with Al$_2$O$_3$ NPs-treated vehicle mice). **e** Representative images of PDCD4 expression in mouse lung tissues **f** Representative images of emphysema and Lm in mouse lungs (n = 36, **$P < 0.01$, compared with vehicle control, ***$P < 0.001$, compared with vehicle control, ###$P < 0.001$, compared with Al$_2$O$_3$ NPs-exposed vehicle mice). **g** Representative images of airway remodeling and thickness of fibrosis layer around airway in mouse lungs (n = 36, ***$P < 0.001$, compared with vehicle control, ###$P < 0.001$, compared with Al$_2$O$_3$ NPs-exposed vehicle mice)

in both the airway and alveolar areas following Al_2O_3 NPs exposure. Furthermore, PTPN6 overexpression reduced STAT3 phosphorylation. In vitro assays corroborated that an inhibitor of STAT3 activation (S3I-201) effectively inhibited the expression levels of p-STAT3 and PDCD4 following Al_2O_3 NPs exposure (Fig. 4b). The expression levels of PTPN6 were not affected by S3I-201 in murine lungs (Fig. 4c). The results from the in vivo studies corroborate the cellular assays, establishing that murine lung PDCD4 expression both at the mRNA and protein levels were significantly reduced by S3I-201 (Fig. 4d and e). Furthermore, we ascertained that inhibition of STAT3 activation partially ameliorated the Al_2O_3 NPs-induced emphysema and airway remodeling in murine lungs (Fig. 4f and g). Combined, these results demonstrate that suppression of PTPN6 is associated with increased expression of PDCD4 in murine lung tissues, which was dependent upon the activation of STAT3.

Over-expression of PTPN6 protects from COPD-like lesions in mice

As noted above, inhibition of PTPN6 is a critical upstream events in Al_2O_3 NPs-induced COPD-like lesions; therefore, the ability of PTPN6 overexpression to rescue COPD-like effects was addressed. Following PTPN6 overexpression, airway responseness (sRAW), IL-6 and IL-33 levels in BALF were significantly reduced (Fig. 5a and b). Mice were also protected from the Al_2O_3 NPs-induced inury markers previously shown to be associated with emphysema, with levels of matrix metalloproteinase 9 (MMP9) being indistinguishable from those in mice exposed to filtered room air (FRA) [34]. PTPN6-overexpressing mice were resistant to Al_2O_3 NPs-induced changes in the air space enlargement and mean chord length (Fig. 5d), and demonstrated no evidence for small airway remodeling (Fig. 5e). The percentage of apoptotic cells in small airways and alveoli were also accordingly reduced (Fig. 5f). Thus, PTPN6-overexpression protects against emphysema and small airway remodelling, highlighting the functional role of PTPN6 in Al_2O_3 NPs-induced lung injury associated with COPD-like effects.

Key molecular pathway involved in Al2O3 NPs-induced COPD-like lesions

Our results suggest that Al_2O_3 NPs exposure induces emphysema and airway remodeling in murine lungs by suppressing PTPN6 expression and enhancing inflammation. In turn, activation of STAT3 increased PDCD4 expression, leading to apoptosis in lung tissue (Fig. 6). Thus, the PTPN6/STAT3/PDCD4 pathway plays a key role in the pathology of COPD-like lesions induced by Al2O3 NPs exposure.

Discussion

With the wide application of Al_2O_3 NPs in industry, agriculture, consumer product and medicine, concerns exist regarding their potential risk to human health and the environment [4]. Al_2O_3 NPs release into air may occur during the production and application; therefore, inhalation of NPs is of great concern. Here we establish Al_2O_3 NPs dynamic inhalation causes histological alterations, including emphysema and airway remodeling in murine lungs.

In the present study, we noted pulmonary pathology induced by Al_2O_3 NPs was more severe than with other Al_2O_3-based nanowhiskers [11] or aluminum oxyhydroxides nanoparticles [12, 13]. Increased recruitment of macrophages, but no neutrophilic inflammation or cytotoxicity was observed in murine lungs treated by subchronic inhalation of Al_2O_3-based nanowhiskers. In this case, it appeared that macrophages were able to control the aerosol load in the pulmonary system in the absence of cytotoxicity [11]. However, the increased recruitment of macrophages did not sufficiently protect lung tissue from Al_2O_3 NPs-induced injury, as shown in our studies. In other studies, after 4-week inhalation exposure to Al oxyhydroxides nanoparticles, only the high level (28 mg/ m^3) exposure induced similar inflammatory response in rat lungs [12, 13]. These inconsistences between published reports and our results might be attributable to differences in the composition of the Al nanomaterials, exposure duration and experimental animal species. Pauluhn et al. also suggested that acute pulmonary inflammation after nanoparticle exposure appears to be more closely related to the particle surface area and reactivity [4], corroborating that Al_2O_3 NPs, which were used in present study (have higher surface area than nanowhiskers), might cause more severe pulmonary inflammation in comparison to Al_2O_3 nanowhiskers.

Chronic obstructive pulmonary disease (COPD) is characterized by poorly reversible airflow obstruction and abnormal inflammatory responses in the lungs. COPD encompasses a variety of pathologic phenotypes, including airway inflammation, emphysema and remodeling of small airways [35, 36]. Cigarette smoke exposure remains the greatest risk factor for COPD; however, at least one-fourth of patients with COPD are non-smokers. In addition, genetic factors and environmental chemicals are strongly suggested to be related to COPD [37]. Artificial NPs, or airborne nano-scaled particles, have been reported to induce chronic pulmonary disorders. Short-term inhalation exposure to copper oxide (CuO) NPs has been shown to cause dose-dependent lung inflammation, as well as histological alterations characterized by emphysema in rats [38]. An established index of COPD, MMP-9, was increased in lung

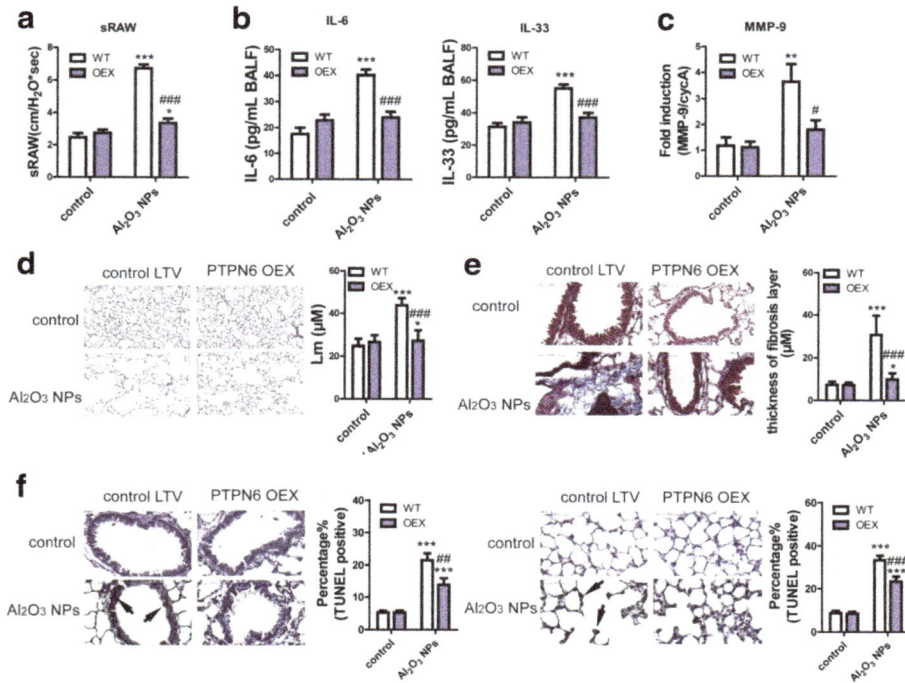

Fig. 5 Overexpression of PTPN6 rescued experimental COPD in mouse model. **a** sRAW of conscious mice (n = 10, *P < 0.05, compared with WT control, ***P < 0.001, compared with WT control, ###P < 0.001, compared with Al_2O_3 NPs-exposed WT mice). **b** Levels of inflammatory mediators in BALF (n = 4, ***P < 0.001, compared with WT control, ###P < 0.001, compared with Al_2O_3 NPs-exposed WT mice). **c** Expression levels of MMP-9 in mouse lungs (n = 6, **P < 0.01, compared with WT control, #P < 0.05, compared with Al_2O_3 NPs-exposed WT mice). **d** Representative images of emphysema and Lm in mouse lungs (n = 36, *P < 0.05, compared with WT control, ***P < 0.001, compared with WT control, ##P < 0.01, compared with Al_2O_3 NPs-exposed WT mice). **e** Representative images of airway remodeling and thickness of fibrosis layer around airway in mouse lungs (n = 36, *P < 0.05, compared with WT control, ***P < 0.001, compared with WT control, ###P < 0.001, compared with Al_2O_3 NPs-exposed WT mice). **f** Representative images of TUNEL staining and percentage of TUNEL+ cells in airway epithelia and alveolar epithelia (n = 30, ***P < 0.001, compared with WT control, ##P < 0.01, ###P < 0.001, compared with Al_2O_3 NPs-exposed WT mice)

homogenates of newborn mice exposed to TiO_2 NPs [39]. Even a single dose of intravenous administration of ZnO NPs induced pulmonary emphysema in mice [40]. Here we report, for the first time, that Al_2O_3 NPs inhalation induced typical pathological alterations characteristic of COPD, including emphysema and small airway remodeling, corroborating that Al_2O_3 NPs represent an environmental risk factor in the etiology of COPD.

The mechanism of COPD remains poorly understood, but involves inflammation and apoptosis [31]. Taking advantage of contemporary bioinformatics approaches, we previously showed that PTPN6 plays a vital role in cellular responses to Al_2O_3 NPs exposure [14]. With respect to the up-stream regulator of PTPN6, activation of pro-inflammatory pathway as well as oxidative stress have been reported to suppress the expression of PTPN6 [41,

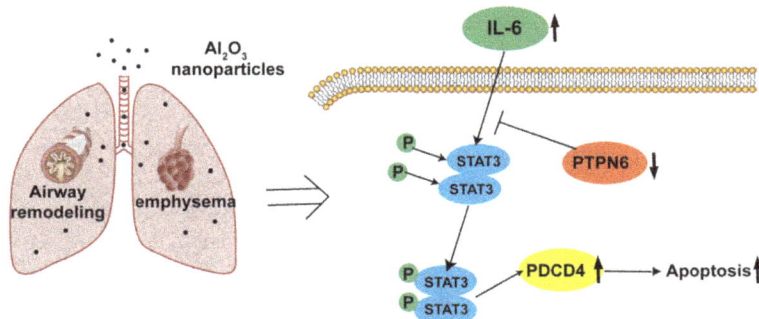

Fig. 6 Key molecular pathway involved in Al_2O_3 NPs-induced COPD-like lesions

42]. Suppression of PTPN6 recruits neutrophil to the injury site and increases neutrophil adhesion in vivo; however, overwhelming accumulation of neutrophils in the tissue may also cause damage [43]. Consistent with our observations, a recent study reported that STAT3 is activated in lung specimen obtained from patients suffering from severe COPD [19]. Aberrant activation of STAT3 pathway is critical for persistent inflammation in lung tissues, and it has been reported that STAT3 activation is negatively regulated by PTPN6 [44]. Accordingly, we examined whether PTPN6 overexpression could alter responses to Al_2O_3 NPs in our experimental COPD model. Overexpression of PTPN6 for the duration of Al_2O_3 NPs-exposure protected mice from airway inflammation (by reducing the numbers of total cell, neutrophil and macrophages; as well as the inflammatory mediator levels in BALF). The mice were also protected from emphysema and airway remodeling by PTPN6 overexpression. The protection afforded with a STAT3 inhibitor was similar to that obtained with PTPN6 overexpression (Fig. 4e to g represent the results of STAT3 inhibitor, Fig. 5d to f represent the results of PTPN6 overexpression).

In addition to Al_2O_3 NPs, cellulose nanocrystals [45], ZnO NPs [30], iron oxide NPs [46] and nanoparticulate carbon black [47] have been reported to induce emphysema in mouse or rat models; however, the mechanisms involved have yet to be defined. A recent study showed that ~1% of wet lung weight (mg/g) nanoparticle carbon black (average particle size 15 nm) exposure led to enlarged alveolar spaces as well as significantly increased numbers of macrophages, neutrophils and lymphocytes in BALF as compared to vehicle controls. Nanoparticle carbon black induced double-stranded DNA break in phagocytes, therefore activating $CD11C^+$ pulmonary antigen presenting cells to secrete pro-T helper 17 cytokines (IL-6 and IL-1β), promoting T helper 17 cell differentiation [47]. Exposures to other metal oxide nanoparticles, such as ZnO and Fe_2O_3, have also been associated with COPD-like lesions [30, 46]. Increased expressions of p53, Ras p21 and JNKs are known to be involved in ZnO-induced cellular responses, consistent with samples from COPD patients [30]. Relatively high doses of iron oxide (Fe_2O_3) NPs exposure induced pulmonary emphysema, interstitial hyperemia and inflammation, accompanied by enhancement of free radicals and reduction in GSH levels in rat lung tissue [46]. Results presented herein support the hypothesis that suppression of PTPN6 and activation of STAT3 pathway is specifically involved in Al_2O_3 NPs-induced COPD-like lesions in mouse model.

Aberrant cell death, such as increased apoptosis, is intensively involved in the pathogenesis of emphysema and small airway remodeling [31, 48]. In Al_2O_3 NPs-induced experimental COPD, we found increased

PDCD4 expression, a marker of enhanced apoptosis which is associated with macrophage alternative activation and airway remodeling [49]. Under conditions of pulmonary inflammation, PDCD4 is a downstream effector of STAT3 activation [33], corroborating our results. We hypothesize that as a consequence of suppressed expression of PTPN6, STAT3 activation and PDCD4 expression increase in airway and alveolar epithelial cells, leading to apoptosis, inflammation and emphysema in experimental COPD.

Some limitations of our study should be noted. In term of the long-term effects, further time points should be included to explore the clearance of Al_2O_3 NPs exposure or reversibility of mice. The in vivo aerosol characterization could be improved by additional details, such as the particle number concentration or size of the aerosol particles. The effects of Al_2O_3 NPs coated with different polymers were not evaluated in the present study, which should be considered in the future.

Conclusions

Taken together, our novel studies provide invaluable new insights into Al_2O_3 NPs-specific pulmonary injury. Our results show PTPN6 is down-regulated in response to Al_2O_3 NPs-induced experimental COPD. Suppression of PTPN6 may have deleterious effects at the molecular, cellular and tissue levels, leading to initiation of inflammation and apoptosis, ultimately resulting in the development of COPD-like lesions. The molecular cascades of PTPN6/STAT3/PDCD4 play a vital role in Al_2O_3 NPs-involved pulmonary disorders. This study raises the possibility of an increased risk of pulmonary disorder upon exposure to Al_2O_3 NPs, suggesting the necessity of intensive protection for susceptible populations, especially in occupational settings.

Methods
Nanomaterials

Al_2O_3 nanoparticles were purchased from Plasmachem GmbH, Germany (purity >99.8%) and stored as nanopowder. The Al_2O_3 nanopowder was used in the animal experiments.

The average primary particle size is 40 nm, with a full range of particle size from 5 to 150 nm (manufacturer's data). The average diameter of Al_2O_3 NPs suspended in cell culture medium (DMEM with 10% FBS) with concentration of 25 μg/mL was 77.7 nm following 30 min ultrasonication, which was tested by zetasizer (nano-zs90, Malvern Instruments, UK) (Additional file 1: Figure S4a). Al_2O_3 NPs aggregated in a time-dependent manner and the aggregation size of Al_2O_3 NPs with higher concentration was greater than those at lower concentration, as shown in Additional file 1: Figure S4b.

Zinc oxide (ZnO) nanopowders (<100 nm particle size (manufacturer's data)) were purchased from Sigma-aldrich, USA. The average diameter of zinc oxide (ZnO) nanopowders was 86.37 nm, which were suspended in DMEM medium (with 10% FBS) at a concentration of 25 μg/mL and followed 30 min ultra-sonication (Additional file 1: Figure S4c). Aggregation of ZnO NPs within 24 h is shown in Additional file 1: Figure S4d.

Carbon black (CB) nanopowder was purchased from Plasmachem GmbH, Germany, with an average primary particle size of 13 nm (manufacturer's data). When suspending in DMEM medium (with 10% FBS) (25 μg/mL) and following 30 min ultra-sonication, the average diameter of CB NPs was 15.1 nm (Additional file 1: Figure S4e). The aggregation of CB NPs in DMEM medium is shown in Additional file 1: Figure S4f.

Cell culture and lentivirus transduction

HBE or A549 cells were seeded in 6-well plates at a density of about 1×10^6 cells per well with DMEM medium with 10% FBS.

A549 cells were treated with 0, 25 or 100 μg/ml ZnO NPs or CB NPs for 24 h, mRNA were then collected for qRT-PCR analysis.

PTPN6 overexpression lentivirus was generated by co-transfection with packaging plasmids, pSPAX2 and pMD2G. The overexpression lentivirus harbored a target gene coding sequence, which was tagged with c-Myc. A549 or HBE cells were added with lentivirus (MOI = 30) and treated with Blasticidin S for two weeks to obtain a stable transduction A549 or HBE cells. For experiments, A549 or HBE cells were thawed and allowed to grow for three passages before use. The control A549 or HBE cells and lentivirus stable transduction (LST) cells were then treated with 0 (vehicle) or 25 μg/ml Al_2O_3 NPs for 24 h, mRNA and proteins were collected for further analysis.

Animals

Male C57BL/6 mice (20–22 g) were purchased from SLRC Laboratory Animal Co., Ltd., China. Animals were treated humanely and all experimental protocols were approved by Committee on Animal Use and Care of Southeast University, China. All the methods in the present study were performed according to approved guidelines. Five mice were housed in each polycarbonate cage with ad libitum access to food and water. Light cycles were set on a 12/12 h light/dark cycle, and room temperature was set at 22.5 °C.

Animal experiments

The dynamic inhalation exposure chambers were outfitted with air quality monitoring equipment and a dust aerosol generator (Beijing HuiRongHe Technology Co.,

Ltd., China). The dry Al_2O_3 nanopowder was stored in sample reservoir, and the concentration of dust aerosol was adjusted by the rotation speed of the rotary brush outfitted in the dust aerosol generator (HRH-DAG768, Beijing HuiRongHe Technology, Co. Ltd., China). Exposure was carried out in stainless-steel Hinners-type whole-body inhalation chambers; the treatment groups received Al_2O_3 NPs, and the control received high efficiency particulate air (HEPA)-filtered room air (FRA) at the same flow rate as the experimental group. The mass concentrations of Al_2O_3 NPs aerosol in the whole-body chamber were measured by a real-time light scattering dust monitor (CEL-712 Microdust Pro, CASELLA CEL Inc., USA), which was placed at the same height as the top of the animal cages. The dust monitor was calibrated using a gravimetric approach by pulling Al_2O_3 NPs aerosol through a filter and weighing filter before and after, then dividing mass by the volume of air sampled. The mice were exposed to each chamber for 8 h per day (from 9 a.m. to 5 p.m.) for 7 consecutive days and sacrificed 24 h after the 7-day-treatment. Light cycles were set on at 12/12 h light/dark cycle. The temperature in the chambers was set at 22.5 °C.

The first batch of animal experiments included three groups (with 15 C57BL/6 mice in each group): control exposed to filtered room air (FRA); mice exposed to Al_2O_3 NPs with a mean concentration of 0.4 mg/m³; or mice exposed to Al_2O_3 NPs with a mean concentration of 2 mg/m³. The selection of exposure concentration took into account results from a previous inhalation study with Al oxyhydroxides nanoparticles [12], OSHA regulation [6], as well as our previous study [14]. Mice were exposed to Al_2O_3 NPs for 7 concecutive days and sacrificed 24 h after Al_2O_3 NPs exposure. The specific airway resistance (sRAW) was measured after dynamic inhalation on exposure days 3 and 7.

The second batch of mice included two groups (with 10 C57BL/6 mice in each group): control exposed to filtered room air (FRA) and mice exposed to ZnO NPs with a mean concentration of 0.4 mg/m³. Mice were exposed to ZnO NPs for 7 concecutive days and sacrificed 24 h after ZnO NPs exposure. One piece of lung tissues were fix in 4% PFA and the other lung tissues were stored in liquid nitrogen.

The third batch of mice were divided into four groups (with 10 C57BL/6 mice in each group): control mice treated with FRA and control vector lentivirus; mice treated with FRA and PTPN6 vector lentivirus; mice treated with 0.4 mg/m³ Al_2O_3 NPs and control vector lentivirus; and mice treated with 0.4 mg/m³ Al_2O_3 NPs coupled with PTPN6 vector lentivirus. Mice received intranasal treatment with 1×10^8 transducing units (TU)/mouse every three days. Treatment began two days before Al_2O_3 NPs exposure. Mice were exposed to Al_2O_3

NPs for 7 consecutive days and sacrified 24 h after Al$_2$O$_3$ NPs exposure.

The fourth batch of mouse included four groups (with ten C57BL/6 mice in each group): control mice treated with FRA and PBS; mice treated with FRA and STAT3 inhibitor S3I-201; mice treated with 0.4 mg/m^3 Al$_2$O$_3$ NPs and PBS; and mice treated with 0.4 mg/m^3 Al$_2$O3 NPs coupled with S3I-201. The STAT3 inhibitor, S3I-201 (Millipore Sigma, USA), was dissolved in DMSO (0.05% DMSO) and injected intraperitoneally. Mice received S3I-201 with a dose of 5 mg/kg every three day and began two days before Al$_2$O$_3$ NPs exposure (totally four times of injection for each mouse). Mice were exposed to Al$_2$O$_3$ NPs for 7 consecutive days and sacrified 24 h after Al$_2$O$_3$ NPs exposure. The specific airway resistance (sRAW) was measured after dynamic inhalation on exposure day 7.

Mouse airway resistance measurement

The specific airway resistance (sRAW) was evaluated in conscious mice, and was measured using the FinePointe non-invasive airway mechanics (DIS Buxco, USA). Each animal was restrained in a special chamber which allowed for the independent measurement of nasal and thoracic flows. Each mouse was monitored for five consecutive minutes.

Aluminum burden

Five mice from each group of the first batch were euthanized under ether anesthesia 1 h after the end of dynamic Al$_2$O$_3$ NPs exposure on the 7th day. All the mice were decapitated on an iced table. Approximately 0.1 g of lung tissue sample was digested with HNO$_3$ in a boiling water bath for 3 h. The aluminum burdens were quantified using an inductively coupled plasma-mass spectrometry (ICP-MS, Agilent 7700, USA). The aluminum burden was calculated as weight/weight of lung tissue (ng/g).

BALF isolation, cell counts and ELISA

Four mice from each group were euthanized by ether, the lungs were lavaged with 1.0 ml ice-cold PBS for three times. BALF was centrifuged at 500 g for 5 min. The cell pellet was suspended in 500 µl PBS and leukocytes were counted using a hemocytometer. Eighty µl suspensions were removed for after Wright-Giemsa stain. The percentage of monocytic cells and neutrophils were counted in a total of 300 cells. The levels of IL-6 (R&D system, USA) and IL-33 (R&D system, USA) in BALF were measured with commercial ELISA kits.

RNA isolation and quantitative real-time PCR assay

One piece of lung tissue from each mouse was collected and stored in liquid nitrogen for qRT-PCR assay. Total RNA of cells and lung tissues was extracted using a GenElute™ Mammalian Total RNA Miniprep Kit (Sigma, USA) according to the manufacturer's protocol. The mRNA levels for modulated genes were determined by reverse transcription of total RNA followed by qRT-PCR on a Quant Studio 6 Flex System (Applied Biosystems, Life Technologies, USA) using SYBR PCR Master Mix reagent kits (Takara, Japan) following the manufacturer's protocol. Primers were designed and provided in Additional file 1: Tables S1. All experiments were independently performed in triplicate. The mRNA levels provided were normalized to cyclophilin A (CYPA).

Histopathological analysis of mice lung tissue

One piece of lung tissue from 6 mice in each group were stored in PFA for 24 h at 4 °C, embedded in paraffin, serially sectioned (5 µm) and mounted on silane-covered slides. The sections selected from each mouse were stained after dewaxing with hematoxylin and eosin (H&E) and evaluated under a light microscope (400×) to examine the tissue histology.

The mean linear intercept (L(m)) is quantified to characterize the enlargement of airspaces in emphysema. Six random fields from each section at ×10 magnification under microscopy were qualitifed by the indirect stereological methods [50].

Three of lung sections from each group were stained with Masson's Trichrome stain and images scanned using the slide scanner Panoramic SCAN (3DHISTECH, Hungary) to obtain a whole slide image. Panoramic Viewer software (3DHISTECH, Hungary) was used to measure the thickness of the sub-epithelial fibrosis layer stained blue by Masson's Trichrome stain at 12 separate sites around the airway by a blinded experienced pathologist. The mean thickness of the sub-epithelial layer in microns was calculated for airway having a mean internal diameter between 300 and 700 µm [28].

Apoptotic cells in lung tissues were evaluated with terminal-deoxynucleoitidyl transferase mediated nick end labeling (TUNEL) staining by a Roche In Situ Cell Death Detection Kit (Roche, U.S.) according to the suggested protocols. The nuclear stained areas (depicted in dark brown) were identified as TUNEL-positive cell. The proportion of TUNEL-positive cells of alveolar epithelia and bronchial epithelia were estimated by an experienced histologists blinded to treatment conditions. Three to five non-overlapping bronchial tubes and five non-overlapping alveolar areas in each section were counted in high-power fields (HPFS, ×400 magnification) and analyzed. The bronchial tubes or alveolar areas with the maximum number of positive cells were selected for analysis [10].

After dewaxing, IHC staining was performed as previously described [10], and samples were incubated overnight at 4 °C with mouse monoclonal antibodies against PTPN6 (1:100) (ab532559, abcam, USA), p-STAT3 (1:100) (ab76315, abcam, USA) and PDCD4 (ab51495, abcam, USA). Binding to tissue sections was visualized with a biotinylated rabbit anti-mouse IgG antibody (1:400; DAKO) and developed using diamino-benzidine (DAB) as a substrate. For the negative controls, the primary antibodies were omitted.

Data analysis

All statistical tests were two-sided and the significance level was set at $P < 0.05$. Significant differences were determined by one-way analysis of variance (ANOVA), followed by Tukey's multiple comparison tests. Kruskal-Wallis test was used to analyze the mean chord length (Lm) and thickness of fibrosis around small airway. The $2^{-\Delta\Delta Ct}$ method was used to analyze the qRT-PCR results in all experiments. Statistical analysis was performed by SPSS 12.0.

Abbreviations

Al$_2$O$_3$: aluminum oxide; BALF: bronchoalveolar lavage fluid; COPD: Chronic obstructive pulmonary disease; CYPA: Cyclophilin A; DAB: Diaminobenzidine; FRA: Filtered room air; H&E: hematoxylin and eosin; HEPA: High efficiency particulate air; HFL1: Human fetal lung fibroblasts; Lm: Mean chord lengths; MMP9: Matrix metalloproteinase 9; NPs: nanoparticles; PAS: Periodic acid-Schiff; PTPN6: Protein tyrosine phosphatase, non-receptor type 6; sRAW: Specific airway resistance; TUNEL: Terminal-deoxynucleoitidyl transferase mediated nick end labeling;

Acknowledgements

We thank Nanjing Milestone Biotechnology Co., Ltd. for the bioinformatics analysis.

Funding

In this work, RC was financially supported by the State Key Program of National Natural Science Foundation of China(81730088);the Major Research Plan of the National Natural Science Foundation (training program) (91643109); National Natural Science Foundation of China (81472938), Thousand Talent Program for Young Outstanding Scientists and the fund of the distinguished talents of Jiangsu Province (BK20150021). XL was supported by Natural Science Foundation of Jiangsu Province (BK20151418). QM was supported by Fund of the Post-graduate Innovative Talents (KYZZ16_0137). YZ, WC and RZ were supported by Major Research Plan of the National Natural Science Foundation 91,643,203, 91,543,208 and 91,643,108, respectively. MA was supported in part by grants from the national Institute of Environmental health Sciences (NIEHS), R01 ES10563, R01 ES07331 and R01 ES020852.

Authors' contributions

RC and XL conceived, designed and directed the study. XL, HS, RL and JC performed and directed experiments. QM, SW, MA and RL contributed animal experiments. HY, YZ, WC and HS contributed to the pathology analysis. SW and RZ contributed to the statistical analysis. XL and MA prepared the manuscript. All authors approved the final manuscript and contributed critical revisions to its intellectual content

Competing interests

The authors declare no competing financial interest.

Author details

[1]Key Laboratory of Environmental Medicine Engineering, Ministry of Education, School of Public Health, Southeast University, Dingjiaqiao 87, Nanjing 210009, China. [2]Center for New Drug Safety Evaluation and Research, China Pharmaceutical University, Nanjing, China. [3]School of Public Health, Qingdao University, Qingdao 266021, China. [4]Guangzhou Key Laboratory of Environmental Pollution and Health Risk Assessment, Department of Toxicology, School of Public Health, Sun Yat-sen University, Guangzhou 510080, China. [5]Department of Toxicology, School of Public Health, Hebei Medical University, Shijiazhuang 050017, China. [6]Department of Molecular Pharmacology, Albert Einstein College of Medicine, Bronx, NY 10461, USA. [7]Institute for Chemical Carcinogenesis, Guangzhou Medical University, Guangzhou 511436, China.

References

1. Braakhuis HM, Cassee FR, Fokkens PH, de la Fonteyne LJ, Oomen AG, Krystek P, de Jong WH, van Loveren H, Park MV. Identification of the appropriate dose metric for pulmonary inflammation of silver nanoparticles in an inhalation toxicity study. Nanotoxicology. 2016;10:63–73.
2. Ho CC, Lee HL, Chen CY, Luo YH, Tsai MH, Tsai HT, Lin P. Involvement of the cytokine-IDO1-AhR loop in zinc oxide nanoparticle-induced acute pulmonary inflammation. Nanotoxicology. 2017;11:360–70.
3. Sager TM, Wolfarth M, Leonard SS, Morris AM, Porter DW, Castranova V, Holian A. Role of engineered metal oxide nanoparticle agglomeration in reactive oxygen species generation and cathepsin B release in NLRP3 inflammasome activation and pulmonary toxicity. Inhal Toxicol. 2016;28: 686–97.
4. Willhite CC, Karyakina NA, Yokel RA, Yenugadhati N, Wisniewski TM, Arnold IM, Momoli F, Krewski D. Systematic review of potential health risks posed by pharmaceutical, occupational and consumer exposures to metallic and nanoscale aluminum, aluminum oxides, aluminum hydroxide and its soluble salts. Crit Rev Toxicol. 2014;44(Suppl 4):1–80.
5. Chen L, Yokel RA, Hennig B, Toborek M. Manufactured aluminum oxide nanoparticles decrease expression of tight junction proteins in brain vasculature. J NeuroImmune Pharmacol. 2008;3:286–95.
6. Code of Federal Regulations, Title 29, 1910.1000, Table Z-1, U.S. Office of the Federal Register National Archives and Records Administration, Washington, DC, 2000.
7. Kolesnikov capital le C, Karunakaran G, Godymchuk A, Vera L, Yudin AG, Gusev A, Kuznetsov D. Investigation of discharged aerosol nanoparticles during chemical precipitation and spray pyrolysis for developing safety measures in the nano research laboratory. Ecotoxicol Environ Saf. 2017;139: 116–23.
8. Schlesinger RB, Snyder CA, Chen LC, Gorczynski JE, Menache M. Clearance and translocation of aluminum oxide (alumina) from the lungs. Inhal Toxicol. 2000;12:927–39.
9. Zhang XQ, Yin LH, Tang M, YP P. ZnO, TiO(2), SiO(2,) and al(2)O(3) nanoparticles-induced toxic effects on human fetal lung fibroblasts. Biomed Environ Sci. 2011;24:661–9.
10. Li X, Zhang C, Zhang X, Wang S, Meng Q, Wu S, Yang H, Xia Y, Chen R. An acetyl-L-carnitine switch on mitochondrial dysfunction and rescue in the metabolomics study on aluminum oxide nanoparticles. Part Fibre Toxicol. 2016;13:4.
11. Adamcakova-Dodd A, Stebounova LV, O'Shaughnessy PT, Kim JS, Grassian VH, Thorne PS. Murine pulmonary responses after sub-chronic exposure to aluminum oxide-based nanowhiskers. Part Fibre Toxicol. 2012;9:22.
12. Pauluhn J. Pulmonary toxicity and fate of agglomerated 10 and 40 nm aluminum oxyhydroxides following 4-week inhalation exposure of rats: toxic effects are determined by agglomerated, not primary particle size. Toxicol Sci. 2009;109:152–67.
13. Pauluhn J. Retrospective analysis of 4-week inhalation studies in rats with focus on fate and pulmonary toxicity of two nanosized aluminum oxyhydroxides (boehmite) and pigment-grade iron oxide (magnetite): the key metric of dose is particle mass and not particle surface area. Toxicology. 2009;259:140–8.

14. Li X, Zhang C, Bian Q, Gao N, Zhang X, Meng Q, Wu S, Wang S, Xia Y, Chen R. Integrative functional transcriptomic analyses implicate specific molecular pathways in pulmonary toxicity from exposure to aluminum oxide nanoparticles. Nanotoxicology. 2016;10:957–69.

15. Alonso A, Sasin J, Bottini N, Friedberg I, Friedberg I, Osterman A, Godzik A, Hunter T, Dixon J, Mustelin T. Protein tyrosine phosphatases in the human genome. Cell. 2004;117:699–711.

16. Cho YS, SY O, Zhu Z. Tyrosine phosphatase SHP-1 in oxidative stress and development of allergic airway inflammation. Am J Respir Cell Mol Biol. 2008;39:412–9.

17. Jang MK, Kim SH, Lee KY, Kim TB, Moon KA, Park CS, Bae YJ, Zhu Z, Moon HB, Cho YS. The tyrosine phosphatase, SHP-1, is involved in bronchial mucin production during oxidative stress. Biochem Biophys Res Commun. 2010;393:137–43.

18. Huan W, Tianzhu Z, Yu L, Shumin W. Effects of Ergosterol on COPD in mice via JAK3/STAT3/NF-kappaB pathway. Inflammation. 2017;40:884–93.

19. Yew-Booth L, Birrell MA, Lau MS, Baker K, Jones V, Kilty I, Belvisi MG. JAK-STAT pathway activation in COPD. Eur Respir J. 2015;46:843–5.

20. Wang J, Zhang L, Chen G, Zhang J, Li Z, Lu W, Liu M, Pang X. Small molecule 1'-acetoxychavicol acetate suppresses breast tumor metastasis by regulating the SHP-1/STAT3/MMPs signaling pathway. Breast Cancer Res Treat. 2014;148:279–89.

21. Chen KF, Su JC, Liu CY, Huang JW, Chen KC, Chen WL, Tai WT, Shiau CW. A novel obatoclax derivative, SC-2001, induces apoptosis in hepatocellular carcinoma cells through SHP-1-dependent STAT3 inactivation. Cancer Lett. 2012;321:27–35.

22. Kim DJ, Tremblay ML, Digiovanni J. Protein tyrosine phosphatases, TC-PTP, SHP1, and SHP2, cooperate in rapid dephosphorylation of Stat3 in keratinocytes following UVB irradiation. PLoS One. 2010;5:e10290.

23. Hou S, Yi YW, Kang HJ, Zhang L, Kim HJ, Kong Y, Liu Y, Wang K, Kong HS, Grindrod S, Bae I, Brown ML. Novel carbazole inhibits phospho-STAT3 through induction of protein-tyrosine phosphatase PTPN6. J Med Chem. 2014;57:6342–53.

24. Santus P, Radovanovic D, Henchi S, Di Marco F, Centanni S, D'Angelo E, Pecchiari M. Assessment of acute bronchodilator effects from specific airway resistance changes in stable COPD patients. Respir Physiol Neurobiol. 2014;197:36–45.

25. Hubeau C, Kubera JE, Masek-Hammerman K, Williams CM. Interleukin-6 neutralization alleviates pulmonary inflammation in mice exposed to cigarette smoke and poly(I:C). Clin Sci (Lond). 2013;125:483–93.

26. Qiu C, Li Y, Li M, Li M, Liu X, McSharry C, Xu D. Anti-interleukin-33 inhibits cigarette smoke-induced lung inflammation in mice. Immunology. 2013;138: 76–82.

27. Byers DE, Alexander-Brett J, Patel AC, Agapov E, Dang-Vu G, Jin X, Wu K, You Y, Alevy Y, Girard JP, Stappenbeck TS, Patterson GA, Pierce RA, Brody SL, Holtzman MJ. Long-term IL-33-producing epithelial progenitor cells in chronic obstructive lung disease. J Clin Invest. 2013;123:3967–82.

28. Cloonan SM, Glass K, Laucho-Contreras ME, Bhashyam AR, Cervo M, Pabon MA, Konrad C, Polverino F, Siempos II, Perez E, Mizumura K, Ghosh MC, Parameswaran H, Williams NC, Rooney KT, Chen ZH, Goldklang MP, Yuan GC, Moore SC, Demeo DL, Rouault TA, D'Armiento JM, Schon EA, Manfredi G, Quackenbush J, Mahmood A, Silverman EK, Owen CA, Choi AM. Mitochondrial iron chelation ameliorates cigarette smoke-induced bronchitis and emphysema in mice. Nat Med. 2016;22:163–74.

29. Chen J, Yang X, Zhang W, Peng D, Xia Y, Lu Y, Han X, Song G, Zhu J, Liu R. Therapeutic effects of resveratrol in a mouse model of LPS and cigarette smoke-induced COPD. Inflammation. 2016;39:1949–59.

30. Kumar A, Najafzadeh M, Jacob BK, Dhawan A, Anderson D. Zinc oxide nanoparticles affect the expression of p53, Ras p21 and JNKs: an ex vivo/in vitro exposure study in respiratory disease patients. Mutagenesis. 2015;30: 237–45.

31. Demedts IK, Demoor T, Bracke KR, Joos GF, Brusselle GG. Role of apoptosis in the pathogenesis of COPD and pulmonary emphysema. Respir Res. 2006; 7:53.

32. Hou HH, Cheng SL, Liu HT, Yang FZ, Wang HC, Yu CJ. Elastase induced lung epithelial cell apoptosis and emphysema through placenta growth factor. Cell Death Dis. 2013;4:e793.

33. Cohen TS, Prince AS. Bacterial pathogens activate a common inflammatory pathway through IFNlambda regulation of PDCD4. PLoS Pathog. 2013;9: e1003682.

34. Braber S, Koelink PJ, Henricks PA, Jackson PL, Nijkamp FP, Garssen J, Kraneveld AD, Blalock JE, Folkerts G. Cigarette smoke-induced lung

35. Barnes PJ, Shapiro SD, Pauwels RA. Chronic obstructive pulmonary disease: molecular and cellular mechanisms. Eur Respir J. 2003;22:672–88.

36. Hogg JC, Chu F, Utokaparch S, Woods R, Elliott WM, Buzatu L, Cherniack RM, Rogers RM, Sciurba FC, Coxson HO, Pare PD. The nature of small-airway obstruction in chronic obstructive pulmonary disease. N Engl J Med. 2004; 350:2645–53.

37. Guan WJ, Zheng XY, Chung KF, Zhong NS. Impact of air pollution on the burden of chronic respiratory diseases in China: time for urgent action. Lancet. 2016;388:1939–51.

38. Gosens I, Cassee FR, Zanella M, Manodori L, Brunelli A, Costa AL, Bokkers BG, de Jong WH, Brown D, Hristozov D, Stone V. Organ burden and pulmonary toxicity of nano-sized copper (II) oxide particles after short-term inhalation exposure. Nanotoxicology. 2016;10:1084–95.

39. Ambalavanan N, Stanishevsky A, Bulger A, Halloran B, Steele C, Vohra Y, Matalon S. Titanium oxide nanoparticle instillation induces inflammation and inhibits lung development in mice. Am J Physiol Lung Cell Mol Physiol. 2013;304:L152–61.

40. Fujihara J, Tongu M, Hashimoto H, Yamada T, Kimura-Kataoka K, Yasuda T, Fujita Y, Takeshita H. Distribution and toxicity evaluation of ZnO dispersion nanoparticles in single intravenously exposed mice. J Med Investig. 2015;62: 45–50.

41. Pesce M, Franceschelli S, Ferrone A, Patruno A, Grilli A, De Lutiis MA, Pluchinotta FR, Bergante S, Tettamanti G, Riccioni G, Felaco M, Speranza L. The NF-kB regulates the SHP-1 expression in monocytes in congestive heart failure. Front Biosci (Landmark Ed). 2017;22:757–71.

42. Lukens JR, Vogel P, Johnson GR, Kelliher MA, Iwakura Y, Lamkanfi M, Kanneganti TD. RIP1-driven autoinflammation targets IL-1alpha independently of inflammasomes and RIP3. Nature. 2013;498:224–7.

43. Stadtmann A, Block H, Volmering S, Abram C, Sohlbach C, Boras M, Lowell CA, Zarbock A. Cross-talk between Shp1 and PIPKIgamma controls leukocyte recruitment. J Immunol. 2015;195:1152–61.

44. Zhao J, Yu H, Liu Y, Gibson SA, Yan Z, Xu X, Gaggar A, Li PK, Li C, Wei S, Benveniste EN, Qin H. Protective effect of suppressing STAT3 activity in LPS-induced acute lung injury. Am J Physiol Lung Cell Mol Physiol. 2016;311: L868–80.

45. Shvedova AA, Kisin ER, Yanamala N, Farcas MT, Menas AL, Williams A, Fournier PM, Reynolds JS, Gutkin DW, Star A, Reiner RS, Halappanavar S, Kagan VE. Gender differences in murine pulmonary responses elicited by cellulose nanocrystals. Part Fibre Toxicol. 2016;13:28.

46. Sadeghi L, Yousefi Babadi V, Espanani HR. Toxic effects of the Fe2O3 nanoparticles on the liver and lung tissue. Bratisl Lek Listy. 2015;116:373–8.

47. You R, Lu W, Shan M, Berlin JM, Samuel EL, Marcano DC, Sun Z, Sikkema WK, Yuan X, Song L, Hendrix AY, Tour JM, Corry DB, Kheradmand F. Nanoparticulate carbon black in cigarette smoke induces DNA cleavage and Th17-mediated emphysema. elife. 2015;4:e09623.

48. Prakash YS, Pabelick CM, Sieck GC. Mitochondrial dysfunction in airway disease. Chest. 2017;

49. Zhong B, Yang X, Sun Q, Liu L, Lan X, Tian J, He Q, Hou W, Liu H, Jiang C, Gao N, Lu S. Pdcd4 modulates markers of macrophage alternative activation and airway remodeling in antigen-induced pulmonary inflammation. J Leukoc Biol. 2014;96:1065–75.

50. Knudsen L, Weibel ER, Gundersen HJ, Weinstein FV, Ochs M. Assessment of air space size characteristics by intercept (chord) measurement: an accurate and efficient stereological approach. J Appl Physiol (1985). 2010;108:412–21.

Cardiovascular and inflammatory mechanisms in healthy humans exposed to air pollution in the vicinity of a steel mill

Premkumari Kumarathasan[1,2]* ⓘ, Renaud Vincent[1,3]*, Erica Blais[1], Agnieszka Bielecki[1], Josée Guénette[1], Alain Filiatreault[1], Orly Brion[1], Sabit Cakmak[1], Errol M. Thomson[1], Robin Shutt[1], Lisa Marie Kauri[1], Mamun Mahmud[1], Ling Liu[1] and Robert Dales[1]

Abstract

Background: There is a paucity of mechanistic information that is central to the understanding of the adverse health effects of source emission exposures. To identify source emission-related effects, blood and saliva samples from healthy volunteers who spent five days near a steel plant (Bayview site, with and without a mask that filtered many criteria pollutants) and at a well-removed College site were tested for oxidative stress, inflammation and endothelial dysfunction markers.

Methods: Biomarker analyses were done using multiplexed protein-array, HPLC-Fluorescence, EIA and ELISA methods. Mixed effects models were used to test for associations between exposure, biological markers and physiological outcomes. Heat map with hierarchical clustering and Ingenuity Pathway Analysis (IPA) were used for mechanistic analyses.

Results: Mean CO, SO_2 and ultrafine particles (UFP) levels on the day of biological sampling were higher at the Bayview site compared to College site. Bayview site exposures "without" mask were associated with increased ($p < 0.05$) pro-inflammatory cytokines (e.g IL-4, IL-6) and endothelins (ETs) compared to College site. Plasma IL-1β, IL-2 were increased ($p < 0.05$) after Bayview site "without" compared to "with" mask exposures. Interquartile range (IQR) increases in CO, UFP and SO_2 were associated with increased ($p < 0.05$) plasma pro-inflammatory cytokines (e.g. IL-6, IL-8) and ET-$1_{(1-21)}$ levels. Plasma/saliva BET-1 levels were positively associated ($p < 0.05$) with increased systolic BP. C-reactive protein (CRP) was positively associated ($p < 0.05$) with increased heart rate. Protein network analyses exhibited activation of distinct inflammatory mechanisms after "with" and "without" mask exposures at the Bayview site relative to College site exposures.

Conclusions: These findings suggest that air pollutants in the proximity of steel mill site can influence inflammatory and vascular mechanisms. Use of mask and multiple biomarker data can be valuable in gaining insight into source emission-related health impacts.

* Correspondence: premkumari.kumarathasan@canada.ca;
renaud.vincent@canada.ca
[1]Environmental Health Science and Research Bureau, Environmental and Radiation Health Sciences Directorate, HECSB, Health Canada, Ottawa, ON, Canada
Full list of author information is available at the end of the article

Background

Increased air pollution levels are associated with increased cardio-respiratory morbidity and mortality [5, 17, 53]. Air pollution exposures are also known to elevate the risk of stroke, Alzheimer's like pathology, mood disorders, gastrointestinal disorders, and adverse birth outcomes [8, 16, 28, 45, 74]. The global burden of diseases study estimated that exposure to ambient $PM_{2.5}$ led to about 3 million deaths and 84 million disability adjusted life years lost due to ischemic heart disease, acute low respiratory infections and etc. [78].

Toxicity of ambient air particulate matter [1] can be influenced by their physicochemical properties. Source emissions and subsequent atmospheric transformation are determinants of physicochemical characteristics of air particles. It is critical to understand the contribution of different sources to air pollutant toxicity for mitigation purposes. For instance, traffic-related air pollution has been shown to impact on the autonomic control of the heart and heart rate variability [59]. Fixed-site industrial sources have also been linked with adverse health effects. Namely, increased $PM_{2.5}$ emissions from a local steel mill in the Utah Valley were associated with increased hospital admissions for respiratory illness and decreased lung function in children [51, 52]. A strong association between children's respiratory health and air pollution was shown through examination of a Children's cohort in Hamilton, Ontario, where two largest steel mills in Canada are present [55]. Recently, we have shown that air pollution levels in the vicinity of a steel mill can alter pulmonary function and cardiovascular physiology in healthy adults [6, 10, 43, 60]. Moreover, decreased mortality rates have been reported with a copper smelter strike and reduced ambient sulfate particulate matter air pollution [54].

Notwithstanding the strong evidence for adverse health impacts of ambient air pollutants, there remain important knowledge gaps in our understanding of the toxicity mechanisms and the biological plausibility of adverse health outcomes [26]. Such investigations can become challenging due to the complexity of air pollutant mixtures [67].

Squadrito et al., 2001 [65] reported that air particles, namely $PM_{2.5}$ contained abundant persistent semiquinone radicals. These radicals can contribute to redox cycling reactions and thus oxidative stress conditions in vivo. Inhalation exposure to ozone or ozone-particle mixtures can lead to the generation of reactive oxygen and nitrogen species in animal models [33, 35, 36, 38, 42]. Acute inhalation of air particles are reported to trigger oxidative stress, inflammation, autonomic and arrhythmogenic effects in heart failure-prone rats [9]. Similarly, inhalation of ozone and ambient air particles are known to cause increased levels of circulating potent vasoconstrictor peptide endothelin (ET)-1 in rats and humans [3, 7, 36, 38, 72, 75, 76].

The objective of this study was to identify any mechanistic changes relevant to cardiovascular and inflammatory pathways in healthy adults who inhaled ambient air in the vicinity of a steel mill. The subjects from a randomized crossover study who were exposed to air pollution near a steel plant site (Bayview site) and a site (College site) well removed from the fixed source emissions [10] were assessed for biochemical and physiological changes. In addition, a mask was used to filter out many of the criteria pollutants (e.g $PM_{2.5}$, ozone) at the steel plant site, to test for any changes due to relatively reduced air pollutant matrix. We hypothesize that, 1. exposure to increased levels of complex air pollutant mixtures can modify biochemical pathways and thus can affect associated physiological measures; 2. mask, by filtration of most criteria pollutants can reduce the levels and complexity of the air pollutant mixture and can permit the characterization of inter-pollutant interactions. Multiple target proteomic and metabolite markers were measured in saliva and plasma samples. Statistical analyses were conducted to test for exposure site-, mask- and individual air pollutant-related biomarker changes, and to identify any associations between these biomarker levels and physiological measures namely, blood pressure and heart rate. Additional bioinformatic tests using a systems biology approach were conducted to gain insight into source emission exposure-related mechanistic changes at the molecular level.

Methods

Materials

Dulbecco's phosphate-buffered saline (PBS, calcium and magnesium free), ethylenediaminetetraacetic acid (EDTA), diethylenetriaminepentaacetic acid (DETPA), phenylmethylsulfonyl fluoride (PMSF), trifluoroacetic acid (TFA), 3,4-dichloroisocoumarin, molecular weight cut-off filters (30, 50 and 100 kDa) and endothelins (Big ET-1(BET-1), ET-1, ET-2, ET-3) were purchased from Sigma (St. Louis, MO, USA). Reagent-grade acetone, acetonitrile, ethyl acetate, and methanol were from commercial suppliers. Butylated hydroxytoluene (BHT) was from United States Biochemical Corporation (Cleveland, OH, USA). Deionized water (DI water) was obtained from a super-Q plus high purity water system (Millipore, Bedford, MA, USA). UHP-grade compressed nitrogen was supplied by Matheson Gas products (Whitby, ON, Canada). Amber glass vials and screw caps with septa were purchased from Chromatographic specialities Inc. (Brockville, ON, Canada). Antiprotease (Halt protease inhibitor) cocktail was obtained from ThermoFisher (Ottawa, ON, Canada). Polyclonal 8-iso-PGF-2α antibody was purchased from Oxford Biomedical Research (Oxford, MI). The EIA assay kit for free 8-isoPGF-2α analysis was from Cayman Chemical

Company (Ann Arbor, MI). Multiplex kits were purchased from either Millipore (Billerica, MA, USA) or BioRad (Mississauga, ON, Canada).

Study population and design

A randomized cross-over study was conducted in Sault Ste. Marie, Ontario, Canada, in the summer of 2010 as described by Dales et al., 2013 [10]. The study was approved by the Health Canada Research Ethics Board and the ethics board of Algoma University, Ontario, Canada. In brief, subjects were primarily college students recruited in the city of Sault Ste. Marie, Ontario. This study cohort ($n = 52$) consisted of both men and women of 18 to 34 years of age (5th to 95th percentile) who did not use medications that could affect inflammation or cardio-pulmonary function and who did not have a history of chronic disease, specifically cardiovascular, respiratory and metabolic disorders, nor seasonal allergies, were healthy non-smoking, and without cigarette smoke exposure at home, as well as consented to provide blood samples for analysis. Exclusion criteria included: pregnant or breast-feeding women, and subjects living in the residential neighborhood bordering on the steel plant.

Each subject was randomized to spend 5 consecutive 8-h days (between 7:50 am and 5:50 pm) on the periphery of a residential neighborhood (Bayview Site) adjacent to a steel plant within 0.87 km of continuously operating coke ovens, or on a college campus (College site) 4.54 km away from this site or were fitted with a 3 M industrial personal air filter system (3 M Canada Inc., London, ON, Canada) only at the Bayview site (Bayview-Mask). Randomization was done using Excel software based on subject identification number. The exposure design is provided in Table 1.

The filters on the 3 M industrial personal air filter system (Helmet:MP330–105 General-Purpose Headgear Assembly; Motor: Breathe-Easy Turbo 022–00–03;Battery: 3 M 520–01–02R01; Filter: 4530301 OVPF (a combined HEPA and organic vapour filter), removed 98% of ozone, close to 99.9% of NO_2, and 95% of NO, 99% of SO_2, and 99.97% of particles of 0.3 μm size and only 1%

of CO (The filters were tested for their performance in our laboratory and the results were consistent with the company's specifications). Also, in general, these study subjects were crossed over between exposure conditions with a 9-d washout period (starting on Saturday through the week and the accompanying weekend until the Monday exposure). The subjects were sedentary mostly during the exposure period, except for a once daily 30 min period of exercise on an elliptical trainer to increase their heart rate to 60% of their predicted maximum value (scheduled to occur between 10:30 am and 1:40 pm). The subjects were protected from sun exposure and precipitation by an overhead awning at each location.

Exposure assessment

Air pollutant measurements were made hourly between 8 h and 18 h by a fixed site ambient air quality monitor (Air Pointer®, Recordum Messtechnik GmbH, Mödling, Austria). This included analyses of $PM_{2.5}$ (mass median aerodynamic diameter < 2.5 μm) by nephelometry, UFP by a TSI® Model 3007 (0.01–1 μm) Ultrafine particle Counter (http://www.tsi.com/condensation-particle-counter-3007/), sulphur dioxide (SO_2) by ultraviolet fluorescence, nitrogen dioxide (NO_2), nitrogen oxides (NO_x) by chemiluminescence, ozone (O_3) by ultraviolet photometry, temperature and relative humidity, at each location.

Physiological measures

Cardiovascular parameters were measured in the study subjects [43]. Both systolic and diastolic blood pressure and pulse rate measurements were made 2 h-post arrival (morning), immediately–post exercise and 5 h-post arrival (afternoon).

Biological samples

Both saliva and blood samples ($n = 52$) were collected late in the afternoon (between 2 and 5 pm) at the end of the exposure week (Friday) at both College and Bayview sites. Baseline sample was collected for both saliva and blood one week prior (Friday between 2 pm and 5 pm)

Table 1 Sequence of exposure patterns followed in this study for all 4 cohorts

Sequence	1st Exposure (5 days)	Washout Period (days)	2nd Exposure (5 days)	Washout Period (days)	3rd Exposure (5 days)
1	A	9	B	9	C
2	B	9	C	9	A
3	C	9	A	9	B
4	A	9	C	9	B
5	B	9	A	9	C
6	C	9	B	9	A

Note: Cohorts 1–4 were spaced by time and the entire exposure took place from May–August 2010
A Bayview Mask, B Bayview Ambient (without mask) and C College

to the beginning of the sequence of exposures. Saliva samples obtained by rolling two cotton rolls in the mouth, one at a time, for 3 min, were transferred into separate Salivette tubes (Sarstedt part# 51.1534, Sarstedt, QC, Canada) containing PMSF and EDTA. These were centrifuged at 1000 g for 5 min and the paired supernatants were pooled. Time-matched blood samples were collected in vaccutainer tubes containing PMSF (final, 1.7 mg/ml) and EDTA (final, 10 mg/ml) and vortexed to stabilize endothelins a class of vasoconstrictor peptides [34]. Whole blood samples were centrifuged at 1448 x g for 10 min to obtain plasma. Both blood plasma and saliva samples were shipped from the exposure site to our laboratory on dry ice, and stored at $-80\,°C$ until further use.

Frozen plasma samples were thawed on ice and vortexed with 20 μL of aqueous 0.1 M DETPA solution and 20 μL of 0.3 M BHT solution in isopropanol and 10 μL of antiprotease cocktail to prevent any post-processing changes due to autoxidation [37]. Aliquots (250 μL) of plasma were used for 8-iso-PGF2α (8-isoprostane) analysis, while another set was used for analysis of circulating endothelin isoforms (Big ET-1, ET-1$_{1-21}$, ET-2 and ET-3) after treatment with 3,4-dichloroisocoumarin in isopropanol and antiprotease cocktail (10 μL). A third set of plasma samples were analysed for inflammatory cytokines, chemokines, and acute phase proteins. Saliva samples thawed on ice were treated with 3,4-dichloroisocoumarin in isopropanol and antiprotease cocktail (28 μL) for endothelin isoforms analyses. All plasma and saliva biological endpoints analyses were conducted in duplicates.

Salivary endothelin analyses
All endothelin isoform analyses were conducted following the procedure described by Tane et al., 1995 [70] using ELISA kits from Phoenix Airmid Biomedical (Canadian supplier for IBL Japan, Oakville, Ontario, Canada). For ET-1$_{1-21}$, ET-1$_{1-31}$ and ET-3 analyses 100uL aliquots of saliva were used. For BET-1 analysis, samples were diluted 10X. Aliquots of saliva samples and the corresponding lyophilized peptide calibration standards were serially diluted two times and were transferred into separate wells in a primary antibody pre-coated plate, and were incubated overnight (16–24 h) at 4 °C. The plates were then washed with 0.05% Tween20 in 40X phosphate buffer, and were treated with 100 μL of detection antibody and were incubated for 16–24 h at 4 °C. These samples were then washed and treated with 100 μL of chromogen, incubated at room temperature for 30 min, were quenched with 1 N H$_2$SO$_4$ solution and were read at 450 nm using a colorimetric assay reader.

Circulating endothelin isoforms in plasma
This procedure was conducted as described by Kumarathasan et al., 2001b [34]. Stabilized plasma samples

were de-proteinized with acidified acetone, cleaned up using molecular weight cut-off filters (30 kDa), dried under N$_2$ flow, reconstituted in the mobile phase A (composition is given below), and were analyzed by a reversed phase HPLC-Fluorescence system. Initial separation of endothelin isoforms (Big ET-1, ET-1$_{1-21}$, ET-2 and ET-3) were carried out on a LC-318 column (25 cm length, 4.6 mm id, 5 μm particle size; Supelco, Oakville, ON) by gradient elution using water-acetonitrile mobile phase (A-30% acetonitrile (aq); B-90% acetonitrile (aq)) with 0.19% of TFA used as the ion-pair reagent. Analytes were measured by fluorescence detection at excitation and emission wavelengths of 240 nm and 380 nm, respectively.

Affinity-based multiplexed targeted proteomic analyses
Analysis of human plasma samples for acute phase proteins relevant to cardiovascular diseases [C-reactive protein (CRP), haptoglobin, fibrinogen, platelet factor (PF4), adiponectin, vonWillebrand Factor (vWF), α$_2$-macroglobulin (A2M), α-acid glycoprotein (AGP), serum amyloid protein (SAP), L-selectin)], and cytokines [interleukins (IL-1, $-2,-4,-5,-6,-7$, $-8,-10$, -12, -13), tumour necrosis factor (TNF-α), granulocyte macrophage colony-stimulating factor (GMCSF) and interferon gamma (IFN-γ)] were done by affinity-based multiplex protein array assays using Bio-Plex Pro Human panels (Biorad) and Milliplex Map kits (Millipore) with a Bio-plex 100 instrument (Biorad), based on the procedure reported by Kumarathasan et al., 2014 [37].

Plasma 8-iso-PGF-2α
Aliquots of plasma (250 μL) samples were stabilized with DETPA and BHT to prevent any autoxidation during the 8-iso-PGF-2α commonly known as 8-isoprostane (8-ISOP) analysis. These samples were then de-proteinized, clarified with ethyl acetate and affinity purified by using a polyclonal 8-iso-PGF-2α antibody following the procedure described by Bielecki et al., 2012 [2]. Purified plasma samples were then analyzed for 8-iso-PGF-2α using the EIA kit from Cayman chemical (Ann Arbor, Michigan).

Statistical analyses
Descriptive statistics was done for air pollution levels on Fridays at College and Bayview site and the pollution levels averaged over 5 days at these sites. Also, IQR values were determined based on data collected on Fridays, and it is equal to the difference between 75th and 25th percentiles, in other words, between upper and lower quartiles, $IQR = Q_3 - Q_1$. The mean and 95% CI are reported for the mean values. We computed the 95% confidence interval for the mean with the following formula: Lower 95% limit = Mean - T$_{.95}$σ$_M$; Upper 95% limit = Mean + T$_{.95}$σ$_M$. Where, T$_{.95}$ is the number of

standard deviations extending from the mean of a T-distribution required to contain 0.95 of the area and σ_M is the standard error of the mean.

Associations among the various saliva and plasma markers were tested by Spearman Rank Order Correlation analyses for all data. Further statistical analyses using mixed effect model testing were conducted to assess the influence of exposure conditions (College site, Bayview site "with" and "without" mask) and criteria air pollutant (CO, NO, NO_2, NO_x, O_3, $PM_{2.5}$, SO_2, UFP) levels on plasma and saliva endpoints and physiological endpoints (blood pressure BP and heart rate HR), adjusting for various confounders. The types of associations tested using statistical models are as follows. *Test 1.* Biomarker levels for Bayview site (ambient, "without" mask) vs College site exposures (*site only*); *Test 2.* Biomarker levels for Bayview site ("with" mask) vs College site exposures (*site only*); *Test 3.* Biomarker levels for Bayview site (ambient, "without" mask) vs Bayview site ("with" mask) exposures; *Test 4.* Association between individual air pollutant levels (daily average for Fridays) and biomarkers; *Test 5.* Exposure type-related differences in physiological (Friday data) measures (Note: Here, corrections for any changes in these measures (e.g systolic BP) associated due to simply wearing the mask, was removed prior to carrying out these comparisons. For this purpose, profiles of each physiological measure (y axis) for with and without mask exposure conditions were plotted against air pollutant levels (x axis) on all five days/exposure week, for each air pollutant. The curves for "with" and "without" mask exposures at the Bayview site were extended to x = 0, and the difference (Δ) between the two curves were determined to assess the pure "mask" effect on these physiological measures. The pure "mask" effect "Δ" value calculated for each physiological measure was in the same order of magnitude irrespective of the air pollutant, suggesting that it is almost a constant measure and a reasonable estimate of the pure "mask" effect. For each physiological measure, the "Δ" value for all air pollutants were thus averaged, and the "Δ_{avg}" value was subtracted from the physiological measures for the "with" mask exposures (daily average for Fridays), prior to carrying out comparisons of physiological measures by exposure type); *Test 6.* Individual air pollutant levels (daily average for Fridays) vs physiological measures; *Test 7.* Biomarker levels vs physiological measures.

The subject-specific mean air pollution exposures (daily averages, Fridays) were calculated as averages of air pollution levels from time the subject arrived at the study site until time of blood or saliva sample collection. For each saliva and blood endpoint, we conducted descriptive statistics, for the complete dataset and for each exposure level separately. All plasma and saliva markers showed skewness in the data points and were log-transformed prior to modelling to attain normality,

with the exception of physiological endpoints (BP and HR). Mixed effects models with Restricted Maximum Likelihood (REML) estimation were employed in these analyses. The exposures and the air pollution levels were treated as fixed effects, and the study participants were treated as random effects. The subjects with masks were not included in the statistical analyses conducted to identify air pollution-related effects, since air pollutant levels under the mask were not measured. The subjects with masks at the Bayview site were only included when exposure site-related effects were tested. An additional random effect of date was examined to reflect the fact that there were four study cohorts present at the study sites on different sets of days.

The models were adjusted for various sets of candidate covariates: date of exposure, carry-over effect (since the same subjects were exposed to the different conditions after one week wash out period), age, sex, body mass index (BMI), ambient air pressure, humidity and temperature.

Baseline observations for plasma and saliva endpoints prior to the exposure regimen were considered as covariates in the model since air pollution measurements were not available. Blood pressure and heart rate measurements considered in these analyses are medians of five readings taken on Friday afternoons around the time when the plasma samples were obtained as well. Note: Biomarker changes (on Fridays of the exposure week) due to exposure at the Bayview site "without" mask (ambient) or at the Bayview site "with" mask, were tested separately against College site exposures. The Akaike Information Criterion was used to choose the best-fitting models. All data management and modelling were conducted in SAS EG 4.2 (Cary, NC, USA) and R version 2.15.1 (The R Foundation for Statistical Computing). Statistical significance was considered at $p < 0.05$.

We also normalized the biomarker level for each subject at different exposure conditions by the average values for this subject during the study period to adjust for individual variability. This information was used to conduct following bioinformatics analyses. Heat map with hierarchical clustering was employed to visualize differential pattern of plasma marker responses as a result of the different exposure scenario. The analysis was done using the hierarchical clustering option in GenePattern (http://genepattern.broadinstitute.org/gp/pages/login.jsf), and formatted in Java treeview (http://jtreeview.sourceforge.net/). Furthermore, Ingenuity Pathway Analysis (IPA) (Ingenuity Systems, www.ingenuity.com) was used to analyse for protein interaction networks, biofunctions and disease pathways using the normalized data. Fold change values (average marker response at Bayview site (with or without mask)/average marker response at the College site) were used for this purpose, and only the protein markers that were significant based on the above mentioned statistical analyses results were included for this analysis.

Results
Characteristics of the study population
The results described here are from 52 subjects (both males and females) who participated in the entire exposure study, and consented to blood draws. Characteristics of the study subjects are shown in Table 2. Most of the study subjects were Caucasian, and the average age was 23 yrs. Most of the study subjects exhibited normal systolic (< 120 mmHg) and diastolic (< 80 mmHg) blood pressure values. Also, the BMI values suggest that most of the subjects were not obese by definition (< 30 kg/m^2).

Exposure
Temperature, relative humidity and air pressure at the two study sites were similar [10] for Fridays of the week during this study period. Nevertheless, air pollutant levels at the Bayview site especially in terms of SO_2, NO_2, NO_x, CO and UFP levels were different compared to that at the College site as stated in our previous reports (Table 3). Briefly, at the Bayview site SO_2 was increased about four-fold, while CO, NO_x and UFP levels were increased about 2–3 fold compared to that at the College site. These Friday measurements are not statistically significantly different from all other days (Additional file 1: Table S2). We have also provided the Air Quality Health Index (AQHI) values for Canada.

Inter-relationships among different biomarkers
The Spearman Rank Order correlation analysis on plasma and saliva end points to assess the relationships between the different biological endpoints in these subjects revealed associations between salivary and plasma endothelins. Salivary BET-1 was correlated with plasma BET-1 ($p = 0.05$, $r = 0.153$). Plasma BET-1 was seen to be positively associated with circulating lipid oxidation

Table 2 General characteristics of the study subjects

Participant Characteristics	Median
Age (year) (5th- 95th percentile)	23.0 (18–34)
Sex, female/male (number)	28/24
Body Mass Index (kg/m^2) (5th- 95th percentile)	25.3 (19.6–35.5)
Ethnicity, Caucasian/other (number)	44/8
Baseline Systolic Blood Pressure (mmHg) (5th - 95thpercentile)	106.5 (92.5–128.5)
Baseline Diastolic Blood Pressure (mmHg) (5th- 95th percentile)	68.0 (57.9–85.9)
Baseline Heart Rate (bpm) (5th- 95th percentile)	73.2 (58.4–92)

marker 8-ISOP ($p = 0.05$, $r = 0.158$) and plasma ET-1$_{1-21}$ was negatively correlated ($p < 0.05$, $r = 0.225$) with 8-ISOP. Plasma ET-1$_{1-21}$ was also found to be negatively correlated ($p < 0.05$, $r \geq 0.178$) with the acute phase proteins AGP, fibrinogen, SAP and haptoglobin. Plasma BET-1 was positively associated with PF4 ($p < 0.05$, $r = 0.205$). Acute phase proteins AGP, fibrinogen, SAP, PF4, adipsin, vWF and haptoglobin were positively correlated ($p < 0.05$, $r \geq 0.270$) with each other except for adiponectin. The acute phase proteins AGP, fibrinogen, SAP and haptoglobin were positively associated ($p < 0.05$, $r \geq 0.154$) with IL-7, IL-8, IL-12, TNF-α and IFN-γ. These correlation coefficients were weak to modest.

Statistical model results
Biomarker profiles

Bayview "without" mask (ambient) vs college site (site only analyses) Relative changes in the biomarker responses at the two sites (*Test 1*) are shown in Table 4. Bayview site ambient exposures were associated with increased ($p < 0.05$) cytokines (e.g. IL-4, IL-6, TNF-α), saliva/plasma endothelins (e.g. BET-1, ET-1$_{(1-21)}$, ET-3) and adiponectin compared to the College site (Table 4). Whereas, plasma AGP, haptoglobin and vWF are decreased ($p < 0.05$) with exposures at the Bayview site (ambient) compared to the College site. In addition, plasma ET-1$_{(1-21)}$, IL-1β, CRP and saliva ET-3 levels exhibited an increasing trend ($p < 0.1$), while plasma A2M and PF-4 showed a decreasing trend ($p < 0.1$) with exposures at the Bayview site (ambient) compared to the College site.

Bayview "with"mask vs college site (site only analyses) The model results (*Test 2*) showed increased ($p < 0.05$) TNF-α, saliva BET-1, ET-1$_{1-21}$ levels and decreased ($p < 0.05$) levels of AGP, haptoglobin, vWF and IL-2 levels after exposure at the Bayview site (with mask) compared to the College site.(Table 5) In addition, increasing trend ($p < 0.1$) in IFNγ, IL-4, IL-8, plasma ET-1$_{1-21}$, ET-3 and saliva ET-1$_{1-31}$ levels and a decreasing trend ($p < 0.1$) in PF-4 and SAP levels are seen with exposures at the Bayview site (with mask) compared to the College site (Table 5).

Bayview "without"mask (ambient) vs Bayview "with"-mask site Results from biomarker response comparisons for the Bayview site "without" (ambient) vs "with" mask exposures (*Test 3*) are provided in Table 6. Here, increased ($p < 0.05$) levels of IL-1β and IL-2, as well as an increasing trend in the levels of plasma BET-1 are seen with exposures at the Bayview site "without" (ambient) mask relative to "with" mask exposures.

Table 3 Daily average air pollutant levels on Fridays for the two study sites (Bayview and College sites)

Pollutant	College Site (Fridays) Mean (95% CI)	Bayview Site (Fridays) Mean (95% CI)
CO (IQR 0.4 ppm)	0.44 (0.43, 0.45)	1.07 (0.95, 1.19)
NO (IQR 6.7 ppb)	1.52 (1.44, 1.60)	6.93 (6.61, 7.24)
NO_2 (IQR 6.6 ppb)	4.39 (4.19, 4.58)	6.78 (6.49, 7.07)
NO_x (IQR 13.2 ppb)	5.90 (5.65, 6.15)	13.52 (12.98, 14.07)
O_3 (IQR 9.2 ppb)	32.81 (32.19, 33.44)	29.91 (29.38, 30.44)
$PM_{2.5}$ (IQR 11.0 $\mu g/m^3$)	11.48 (10.97, 11.99)	12.95 (12.41, 13.48)
SO_2 (IQR 14.8 ppb)	1.56 (1.39, 1.73)	8.13 (7.28, 8.98)
UFP (IQR 32161 particle/cm^3)	6523 (6080, 6966)	14,830 (13,604, 16,057)

Individual air pollutant-related changes in biomarker levels The best fit model results for the tests of association between individual criteria air pollutant levels and plasma/saliva endpoints (*Test 4*) are provided in Table 7 & Additional file 1: Table S1. In terms of cytokine levels, interquartile (IQR) increase in CO was associated with ca. 4.2, 4.3, 1.6, 7.7 and 4.6% increase ($p < 0.05$) in IL-6, IL-7, IL-8, IL-12 and IL-13 cytokines, respectively; IQR increase in O_3 was associated with 47.6 and 14.3% increase in IL-2 and TNF-α ($p < 0.05$) and with increasing trends (5.3%) of IL-8; IQR increases in NO and NO_x were associated with decreased ($p < 0.05$) IL-8 levels. In terms of endothelin isoforms, increased ($p < 0.05$) plasma Big ET-levels were associated with IQR increases in O_3, but IQR increases in SO_2, and UFP were associated with increased ($p < 0.05$) plasma ET-1_{1-21} levels, and similar association ($p < 0.05$) was seen with $PM_{2.5}$ and saliva ET-1_{1-21} levels. In addition, saliva ET-1_{1-21} levels decreased IQR increases in CO as well as O_3 ($p < 0.05$). Acute phase protein profile results showed that adipsin, AGP, A2M, fibrinogen, haptoglobin, L-selectin and PF4 decreased ($p < 0.05$) with IQR increases in all pollutants, except for an increasing trend ($p < 0.1$) for SO_2. Also, IQR increases in SO_2 and $PM_{2.5}$ were associated with an increasing trend in vWF levels ($p < 0.1$).

Table 4 Comparison between biomarker levels after the Bayview site ("without" mask) vs College site exposures

Biomarker	Bayview ("without" mask) vs College site Ratio (95% CI)
A2M	0.887 (0.755, 1.043)+[a]
Adiponectin	1.184 (1.013, 1.385)*[b]
AGP	0.749 (0.590, 0.952)*[a]
CRP	1.410 (0.887, 2.240)+[a]
Haptoglobin	0.852 (0.734, 0.989)*[a]
IL-1β	1.050 (0.999, 1.104)+[b]
IL-4	1.317 (1.021, 1.699)*[a]
IL-6	1.143 (1.002, 1.305)*[c]
PF4	0.847 (0.709, 1.011)+[a]
Plasma ET-$1_{(1-21)}$	1.497 (0.957, 2.340)+[a]
Plasma ET-3	1.330 (1.037, 1.705)*[a]
Saliva BET-1	1.302 (1.034, 1.641)*[c]
Saliva ET-$1_{(1-21)}$	1.167 (1.031, 1.320)*[b]
Saliva ET-3	1.114 (0.979, 1.267)+[b]
TNF-α	1.076 (1.005, 1.151)*[c]
vWF	0.552 (0.349, 0.875)*[a]

*$p < 0.05$; +$p < 0.1$(not significant, trend only)
[b]Covariates: Treatment period, carry over, age, sex, BMI, atmospheric pressure, temperature, relative humidity
[a]Covariates: Treatment period, carry over
[c]Covariates: Treatment period, carry over, age, sex, BMI

Table 5 Comparison of target biomarker levels after the Bayview site ("with" mask) vs College site exposures

Biomarker	Bayview ("with" mask) vs College site Ratio (95% CI)
Adiponectin	1.133 (0.967, 1.327)+[b]
AGP	0.744 (0.584, 0.949)*[a]
Haptoglobin	0.814 (0.700, 0.947)*[a]
IFNγ	1.134 (0.994, 1.294)+[b]
IL-2	0.782 (0.640, 0.956)*[a]
IL-4	1.229 (0.950, 1.590)+[a]
IL-8	1.049 (0.986, 1.117)+[b]
PF4	0.836 (0.698, 1.001)+[a]
Plasma ET-$1_{(1-21)}$	1.443 (0.917, 2.269)+[a]
Plasma ET-3	1.272 (0.989, 1.636)+[a]
Saliva BET-1	1.367 (1.085, 1.723)*[c]
Saliva ET-$1_{(1-21)}$	1.165 (1.030, 1.318)*[b]
Saliva ET-$1_{(1-31)}$	1.132 (0.974, 1.314)+[c]
SAP	0.770 (0.543, 1.092)+[a]
TNF-α	1.075 (1.004, 1.151)*[c]
vWF	0.622 (0.390, 0.991)*[a]

*$p < 0.05$; +$p < 0.1$(not significant, trend only)
[a]Covariates: Treatment period, carry over, age, sex, BMI, atmospheric pressure, temperature, relative humidity
[b]Covariates: Treatment period, carry over
[c]Covariates: Treatment period, carry over, age, sex, BMI

Table 6 Comparison of target biomarker levels after the Bayview site ("without" mask) vs Bayview site ("with" mask) exposures

Comparison	IL-1β Ratio (95% CI)	IL-2 Ratio (95% CI)	Plasma BET-1 Ratio (95% CI)
Bayview Ambient vs Bayview Mask	1.061 (1.012, 1.112)*	1.153 (1.027, 1.294)*	1.135 (0.959, 1.344)+

*$p < 0.05$; +$p < 0.1$(not significant, trend only)
Note: Covariates: Treatment period, carry over, age, sex, BMI, atmospheric pressure, temperature, relative humidity

Physiological measures

Site-related changes Results on associations between physiological measures systolic/diastolic BPs, HR and exposure conditions (*Test 5*) from the best fit models are shown in Table 8. A decreasing trend in the systolic and diastolic BP values is seen with exposures "with" mask at the Bayview site compared to "without" mask exposures at this site, as well as when compared to College site exposures. In addition, both BP values exhibited decreasing trends after exposures at the College site compared to Bayview site exposures "without" mask. Heart rate values are increased after exposures at the Bayview site "with" mask ($p < 0.05$) relative to the Bayview site "without" mask exposures, as well as the College site exposures. Heart rate after College site exposures exhibit a decreasing trend relative to Bayview site "without" mask exposures.

Individual air pollutant-related changes The relationships between individual air pollutants and the physiological endpoints (BP and HR) from the mixed models (*Test 6*) are illustrated in Table 9. Decreased ($p < 0.05$) systolic BP is seen with IQR increase in O_3. IQR increase in UFP is associated with increased ($p < 0.05$) systolic BP. A decrease in diastolic BP is seen with IQR increases CO, O_3 and $PM_{2.5}$, with similar trends ($p < 0.1$) seen for NO_2, NO_x and UFP. IQR increases in NO, O_3, $PM_{2.5}$ and UFP levels were associated with increased ($p < 0.05$) HR values. IQR increase in NO_x exhibited a similar trend ($p < 0.1$) in HR as well.

Biomarker levels and physiological measures Mixed model results (*Test 7*) for associations between plasma/saliva markers and physiological parameters (BP, HR) showed that saliva BET-1 levels were positively associated ($p < 0.05$), while adipsin and PF4 were negatively associated ($p < 0.05$) to systolic BP levels (Table 10). Diastolic BP levels were positively associated ($p < 0.05$) with saliva BET-1 and negatively associated ($p < 0.05$) to plasma BET-1 and vWF. In addition, CRP levels were positively associated ($p < 0.05$) with heart rates, while IL-6 and IL-12 were negatively associated ($p < 0.05$) with HR.

Bioinformatic analyses

Hierarchical clustering The heat map with hierarchical clustering visually illustrates the distinct patterns of biological responses (up-regulated and down-regulated) specific to the Bayview ("with" and "without" mask) and College site exposures (Fig. 1). Pro-inflammatory cytokines IL-1β, IL-2, IL-6 were upregulated after the Bayview ambient ("without" mask) exposures, compared to the other two exposure conditions. Also, at the Bayview site, IL-1β, IL-2 and plasma BET-1 were increased for "without" mask in contrast to "with" mask exposures. Meanwhile, cytokines IL-7, IL-8, IL-13 were increased "with" mask at the Bayview site compared to "without" mask exposures. However, haptoglobin levels are decreased and anti-inflammatory IL-10 levels are increased for the "with" mask exposures compared to "without" mask exposures at the Bayview site, as well as the College site.

IPA The significant protein interaction network with the highest score was different for Bayview site "with" mask exposures compared to that of Bayview site "without" mask (Fig. 2a-b) exposures based on differentially expressed protein markers as compared separately to the College site levels. The strength of significance of association between canonical pathways for some disease outcomes and site-related exposures were higher for the Bayview site "without" mask compared to "with" mask exposures (Additional file 1: Figure S1).

Discussion

In this study, biomarkers of oxidative stress, inflammation and vascular effects were assessed in healthy humans (Table 2) exposed to air in the proximity of a steel plant site (Bayview, with and without a mask) and at a distant College site, to gain information on source-emission-related effects. Exposure to elevated air pollution levels is linked to adverse health effects including cardiac remodelling [44]. Local inflammatory response in the lung is one of the accepted consequences of air particle exposures and is considered to lead to systemic vascular oxidative stress and inflammation that result in adverse cardiac remodelling. We thus assessed the levels of plasma/saliva target markers relevant to these biological processes. Only the subjects

Table 7 Relative change in target biomarker levels associated with IQR changes in air pollutant levels

Pollutant	Biomarker	Ratio (95%CI)
CO	IL-12	1.077 (1.018, 1.139)*
	IL-13	1.046 (1.009, 1.086)*
	IL-5	1.022 (0.998, 1.047)+
	IL-6	1.042 (1.009, 1.077)*
	IL-7	1.043 (1.007, 1.080)*
	IL-8	1.016 (1.001, 1.032)*
	L Selectin	0.966 (0.934, 1.000)*
	ET 1–21 (saliva)	0.966 (0.933, 1.000)*
	ET 1–31 (saliva)	0.962 (0.920, 1.007)+
	ET 3 (saliva)	1.011 (0.975, 1.047)+
NO	GMCSF	0.910 (0.818, 1.012)+
	IL-4	0.859 (0.718, 1.027)+
	IL-8	0.906 (0.845, 0.972)*
NO$_2$	ET 1–21 (saliva)	1.090 (0.904, 1.314)+
NO$_x$	IL-8	0.915 (0.847, 0.989)*
O$_3$	Adipsin	0.669 (0.433, 1.034)+
	GMCSF	1.170 (0.979, 1.398)+
	IL-2	1.476 (1.120, 1.945)*
	L Selectin	0.794 (0.630, 1.000)+
	Big ET-1 (plasma)	1.417 (1.024, 1.962)*
	Big ET-1 (saliva)	0.616 (0.363, 1.046)+
	ET 1–21 (saliva)	0.776 (0.609, 0.988)*
	SAP	0.672 (0.445, 1.013)+
	TNF-α	1.143 (1.006, 1.299)*
	vWF	0.562 (0.328, 0.963)*
SO$_2$	Haptoglobin	1.080 (0.988, 1.182)+
	PF4	0.914 (0.829, 1.007)+
	ET 1–21 (plasma)	1.401 (1.056, 1.858)*
	vWF	1.265 (0.953, 1.679)+
UFP	A2M	0.543 (0.348, 0.848)*
	Adipsin	0.244 (0.095, 0.627)*
	AGP	0.362 (0.209, 0.626)*
	Fibrinogen	0.504 (0.309, 0.823)*
	Haptoglobin	0.548 (0.359, 0.837)*
	L Selectin	0.684 (0.495, 0.947)*
	PF4	0.464 (0.287, 0.750)*
	ET 1–21 (plasma)	4.405 (1.143, 16.973)*
PM$_{2.5}$	IL-4	0.837 (0.700, 1.000)+
	ET 1–21 (saliva)	1.166 (1.001, 1.344)*
	ET 1–31 (saliva)	1.195 (0.998, 1.430)+
	vWF	1.373 (0.985, 1.912)+

*$p < 0.05$; +$p < 0.1$(not significant, trend only)
Covariates: Treatment period, carry over, Age, sex, BMI, atmospheric pressure, temperature and relative humidity

who consented to blood draws on Fridays of the weeks during this exposure period were included in this work.

The criteria air pollutant levels on Fridays (daily average) varied between exposure sites, especially with increases in SO$_2$, UFP, CO, NO and NO$_x$ at the Bayview site compared to the College site (Table 3), these findings were in line with the weekly average results for these neighborhoods [43]. Steel plant activities are typically expected to generate emissions of CO, SO$_2$, NO$_x$ and particles that can vary with operational conditions [66]. Sioutas et al., 2005 [61] reported that long range transport is usually not a major source of UFP unlike PM$_{2.5}$, since UFP has a short lifetime. It is therefore plausible that increased UFP levels at the Bayview site could be attributed to the local emitters at this site. In terms of UFPs, this was associated with relatively large variation. However, we found that variations in UFPs are statistically significantly associated with all eight biomarkers. If the large variation was due to some random errors we would not find so many significant associations. It is unlikely that so many significant associations happen due to random chance alone.

Our general analysis of target biomarker data showed a positive correlation ($p < 0.05$) between saliva and plasma BET-1 levels consistent with our previous work [21]. The lipid oxidation marker 8-isoprostane (8-ISOP) in plasma, a marker of oxidative stress was positively related to plasma BET-1 ($p = 0.05$), but was negatively associated ($p < 0.05$) with ET-1$_{1-21}$, suggesting that oxidative stress may play a role in mediating BET-1, ET-1 responses [38]. BET-1 is cleaved by the endothelin converting enzyme (ECE) to form a mature peptide ET-1, and thus ECE levels can influence the circulating BET-1 and ET-1 levels [30]. Furthermore, our observation on the relationship between plasma BET-1 and PF4 is in line with previous findings on endothelin-induced stimulation of platelet activating factors [48, 49]. Positive associations between AGP, fibrinogen, SAP and haptoglobin as well as with the pro-inflammatory cytokines such as IL-8, TNF-α, IFN-γ in these subjects are typical immune responses. The strength of the correlations observed in this study may be weak due to the smaller sample size and because the study participants were healthy subjects.

We focussed on significant ($p < 0.05$) mixed effects model results, since we are aware that false associations due to multiple comparisons may occur during statistical analyses on a relatively large dataset. Yet, due to the exploratory nature of this work, we also show trends in some consistent, mechanistically meaningful target biomarkers (did not reach significance, $p < 0.1$) that are known to respond with air pollutant exposures, and the directionality of these markers can be useful in collective biomarker pattern-based mechanistic verification.

Table 8 Change in physiological endpoints by exposure

Site Comparison	Physiological endpoint		
	Systolic BP (mmHg) Change (95% CI)	Diastolic (mmHg) Change (95% CI)	Heart Rate (bpm) Change (95% CI)
Bayview "with" mask vs College site	−0.7439 (− 3.4666, 1.9789)	−0.5652 (− 2.7252, 1.5947)	3.5312 (1.1294, 5.9330)*
Bayview "with" mask vs Bayview "without" mask	−1.2172 (− 3.8714, 1.4370)	− 0.6673 (− 2.7715, 1.4368)	2.3532 (0.0150, 4.6913)*
College site vs Bayview "without" mask	− 0.4733 (− 3.1738, 2.2272)	−0.1021 (− 2.2438, 2.0396)	− 1.1780 (− 3.5589, 1.2029)*

*$p < 0.05$
Covariates: Carry over, age, sex and BMI, sequential order of treatments

Association of study site exposures to biomarker levels exhibited increased ($p < 0.05$) pro-inflammatory cytokines, vasoactive endothelins, and an increasing trend in a known marker of inflammation CRP [14, 32] (Table 4) after Bayview site "without"mask exposures compared to College site exposures, suggesting activation of proinflammatory pathways and alteration in endothelin homeostasis at the Bayview site. Yet, decreased AGP, haptoglobin and vWF levels and increased adiponectin (that is secreted by the adipose tissue) levels, after Bayview site exposures compared to College site exposures suggest probably a transient disturbance in acute phase protein homeostasis. Because this is a short term exposure study and is conducted with healthy subjects, active compensatory feedback mechanisms can be operative.

Although the Bayview site "with mask" exposures were associated with some significantly ($p < 0.05$) altered some inflammatory and vascular function-related biomarker levels as with "without mask" exposures at this site, compared to College site exposures (Table 5), "with mask" exposures only affected less number of biomarkers contributing to the above noted biological processes, implying selective and reduced effects. It was also interesting to note increased ($p < 0.05$) plasma IL-1β and IL-2 levels and an increasing trend ($p < 0.1$) in plasma BET-1 levels after Bayview site "without" mask exposures compared to "with" mask exposures (Table 6) implying only some modifications to biomarker responses

even after filtration of many criteria pollutants by the mask, at this site. Coke oven emissions from steel mills are known to contribute to VOC, SVOCs (e.g. PAHs, benzene, dioxins, furans) in their vicinity, and these pollutants have been associated with inflammatory and cardiovascular effects [13]. The main focus of this study was criteria pollutants and the mask filtered most of them except for CO and UFP < 0.3 μm size, and we assume that the VOC and SVOCs were filtered by the mask.

The mixed effects model results on the associations between single air pollutants and biomarkers identified individual pollutant-specific effects (Table 7 & Additional file 1: Table S1). For instance, IQR increases in O_3 and CO levels were associated with increased proinflammatory cytokines suggesting pollutant-specific activation of pro-inflammatory mechanisms [46]. However, IQR increases in CO and O_3 levels were associated with decreased acute phase proteins L-Selectin and vWF, respectively. Similar association between O_3 and vWF has been reported before [56]. Meanwhile, IQR increases in NO and NOx were associated with decreased IL-8 levels in these subjects. In terms of vascular function-related effects, IQR increases in the gaseous pollutants SO_2, O_3 and CO were associated with (Table 7) pollutant-specific endothelin responses. Plasma and also saliva $ET-1_{1-21}$ levels have been implicated in cardiovascular diseases [11, 15]. Interestingly, the particulate air pollutants UFP and $PM_{2.5}$ fractions were also associated with different

Table 9 IQR changes in air pollutants and associated changes in physiological endpoints

Pollutant	Physiological endpoints Change (95% CI)		
	Systolic BP	Diastolic BP	Heart Rate
CO (ppm)	−0.07 (− 0.34, 0.20)	−0.22 (− 0.45, − 0.002)*	0.13 (− 0.11, 0.36)
NO (ppb)	0.46 (−0.87, 1.79)	0.62 (−0.48, 1.72)	1.75 (0.47, 3.03)*
NO_2 (ppb)	− 0.74 (− 2.73, 1.24)	− 1.64 (− 3.31, 0.030)+	0.60 (− 0.84, 2.03)
NO_x (ppb)	0.31 (− 1.64, 2.25)	−1.64 (− 3.54, 0.25)+	1.89 (− 0.002, 3.78)+
O_3 (ppb)	− 1.48 (− 2.76, − 0.20)*	− 1.82 (− 2.85, − 0.78)*	1.62 (0.49, 2.75)*
$PM_{2.5}$ (ug/m^3)	− 0.97 (−2.31, 0.38)	−1.97 (− 3.04, − 0.89)*	1.52 (0.35, 2.7)*
SO_2 (ppb)	− 0.15 (− 0.70, 1.01)	−0.26 (− 0.96, 0.45)	0.22 (− 0.53, 0.98)
UFP (particle/cm^3)	6.25 (2.79, 9.71)*	− 4.67 (− 9.56, 0.22)+	1.35 (0.29, 2.42)*

*$p < 0.05$; +$p < 0.1$(not significant, trend only)
Covariates: Carry over, age, sex and BMI, sequential order of treatments

Table 10 Change in physiological endpoints associated with IQR changes in target biomarkers

Biomarker	Physiological Parameters Change (95% CI)		
	Systolic BP (mmHg)	Diastolic BP (mmHg)	Heart Rate (bpm)
Adipsin	−1.94 (− 3.62, −0.26)*[a]	0.38 (− 0.81, 1.04)[a]	− 0.06 (− 1.62, 1.51)[a]
CRP	0.40 (− 0.28, 1.08)[a]	0.24 (− 0.27, 0.76)[a]	1.13 (0.56, 1.69)*[b]
IL-10	− 0.01 (− 0.85, 0.82)[a]	− 0.15 (− 0.77, 0.47)[a]	− 0.61 (− 1.33, 0.10)+[a]
IL-12	− 0.07 (− 0.27, 0.14)[a]	− 0.05 (− 0.20, 0.10)[a]	− 0.25 (− 0.42, − 0.08)*[a]
IL-6	0.08 (− 1.00, 1.15)[a]	− 0.09 (− 0.09, 0.73)[a]	− 1.09 (− 2.01, − 0.17)*[a]
IL-7	− 0.14 (− 1.05, 0.76)[a]	− 0.20 (− 0.88, 0.47)[a]	− 0.68 (− 1.45, 0.10)+[a]
PF4	− 1.57 (− 2.95, − 0.19)*[a]	0.19 (− 0.87, 1.26)[a]	0.03 (− 1.17, 1.24)[a]
Plasma BET-1	1.41 (−0.59, 3.41)[a]	− 1.22 (− 2.65, 0.20)*[c]	−0.44 (− 2.17, 1.30)[a]
Saliva BET-1	1.82 (0.64, 3.00)*[a]	1.11 (0.08, 2.14)*[a]	− 0.02 (− 1.21, 1.16)[a]
Saliva ET-1(1−21)	1.78 (−0.25, 3.80)+[a]	0.66 (− 0.94, 2.25)[a]	− 1.01 (− 2.81, 0.80)[a]
vWF	− 0.35 (− 1.25, 0.55)[a]	0.77 (0.08, 1.45)*[c]	−0.39 (− 1.22, 0.43)+[a]

*$p < 0.05$; +$p < 0.1$(not significant, trend only)
[a]Covariates: Treatment period, and carry over
[b]Covariates:Treatment period, carry over, age, sex and BMI
[c]Covariates: Treatment period, carry over, age, sex and BMI, atmospheric pressure, temperature, and relative humidity

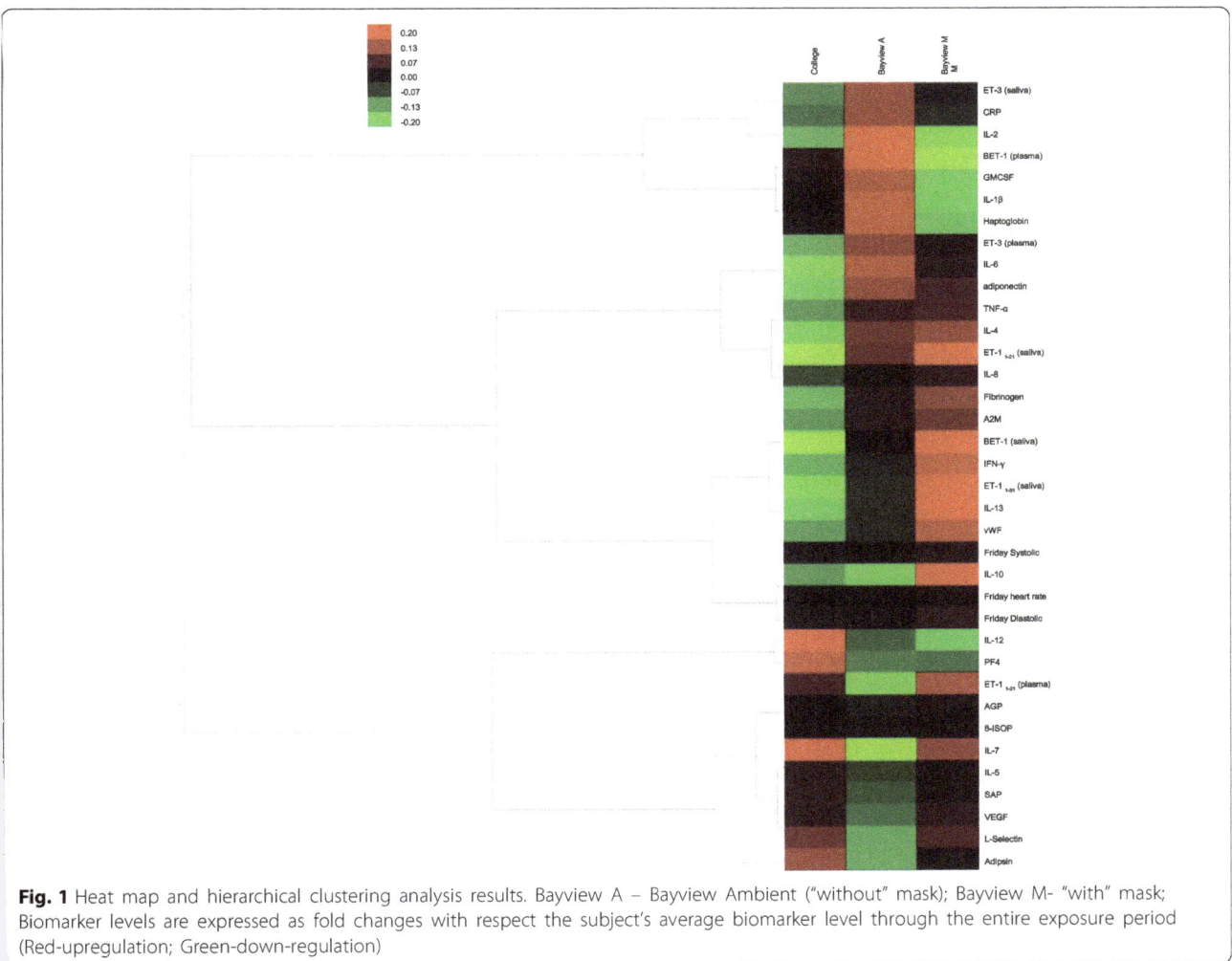

Fig. 1 Heat map and hierarchical clustering analysis results. Bayview A – Bayview Ambient ("without" mask); Bayview M- "with" mask; Biomarker levels are expressed as fold changes with respect the subject's average biomarker level through the entire exposure period (Red-upregulation; Green-down-regulation)

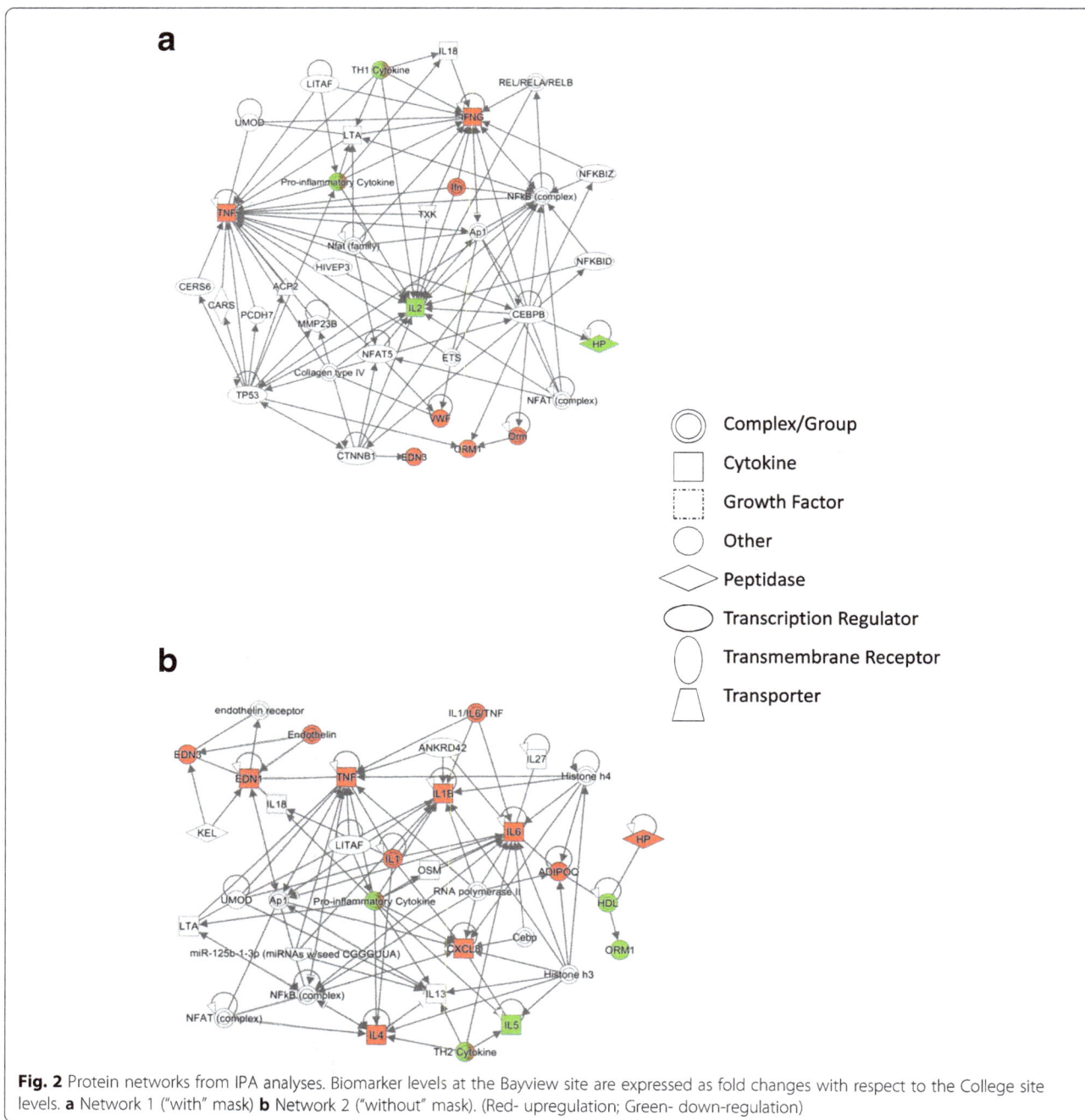

Fig. 2 Protein networks from IPA analyses. Biomarker levels at the Bayview site are expressed as fold changes with respect to the College site levels. **a** Network 1 ("with" mask) **b** Network 2 ("without" mask). (Red- upregulation; Green- down-regulation)

plasma/saliva marker profiles (Table 7 & Additional file 1: Table S1). IQR increase in UFP was associated with increased plasma ET-1_{1-21} and decreased acute phase protein responses, while IQR increases in PM$_{2.5}$ levels are associated with increased saliva ET-1_{1-21} levels, demonstrating PM size-related differences in biomarker profiles. Similar PM-related biomarker responses have been observed previously [23, 50, 63, 69]. It was interesting to note that increasing trend ($p < 0.1$) in vWF levels were observed with IQR increases in SO$_2$ and PM$_{2.5}$ levels.(Table 7) Increased

plasma vWF, a multifunctional glycoprotein is known to be associated with thrombosis [73]. These individual pollutant-related changes in biomarker responses were assessed to get some notion of individual pollutant's contribution to the overall effects, from exposure to three types of air pollutant mixtures (Bayview site "with" and "without" mask, and College site exposures). However, individual air pollutant-specific biomarker responses seemed to only explain very few site-related effects (e.g. IL-6, saliva ET-1_{1-21}), and the remainder of the site-related responses appeared to be influenced by inter-pollutant interactions based on the nature of the air pollutant mixture [38]. As indicated before, the mask used in this study filtered most criteria air pollutants except for CO and < 0.3 µm PM (e.g UFP) at the Bayview site. The increased plasma IL-8, ET-1$_{1-21}$, adiponectin and decreased haptoglobin responses associated "with" mask exposures at this site appeared to be typical responses for IQR increases in CO and UFP (Tables 5, 7) and perhaps associated inter-pollutant interactions including non-criteria pollutants that may have filtered through the mask. Furthermore, the mask appeared to dampen or favour some mechanistic pathways. This observation is similar to a previous report by Karthikeyan et al., 2013 [29] where the use of diesel particle filter increased some biological responses even though it filtered particulate matter effectively, and thus the observed effects were attributed to increased NO$_2$ levels, instead. On the other hand, the use of mask at the Bayview site inadvertently served as a tool for deconstruction of the complex air pollution mixture at this site, and offered an opportunity to assess the effects of select components of the exposure matrix, with insight into inter-pollutant interactions on these simple pollutant mixtures.

In terms of site-related changes on physiological measures (BP and HR), both systolic and diastolic BP values (Fridays) were relatively decreased (not significant) after Bayview site "with" mask exposures compared to the other two exposures (Table 8). Nevertheless, Bayview site "with" mask exposures were associated with relatively increased heart rate compared to Bayview site "without" mask and College site exposures. Also, heart rate was lower after College site exposures relative to Bayview site "without" mask exposures. These findings are consistent with previous reports [43]. Interestingly, the use of mask is shown to improve air pollution exposure-related physiological outcomes [39]. Associations between individual air pollutants and physiological measures, indicated increased ($p < 0.05$) systolic blood pressure (SysBP) with UFP, but not with PM$_{2.5}$ (Table 9). Similar finding was reported by Pieters et al., [50]. Increased ozone and CO levels were associated with decreased BP values. Interestingly exposure to CO is associated with low BP (https://medlineplus.gov/ency/article/002804.htm). Also, IQR increases in PM$_{2.5}$ and UFP were associated with increased heart rate values, and similar relationships were seen with O$_3$, NO and NO$_x$. Increased systolic and diastolic BP values were associated ($p < 0.05$) with increased saliva BET-1 levels in this study (Table 10). This is in line with previous findings in animal models and in humans [4, 20, 75, 76]. In addition, heart rate was positively associated ($p < 0.05$) with plasma CRP (Table 9), consistent with a previous

report by Pope et al., 2004 [53]. In addition, we have previously reported on the impact of increased air pollution levels at the Bayview site on autonomic control of the heart [60]. CRP is associated with cardiovascular disease mechanisms [57]. Overall, these observations imply some perturbations in cardiovascular function at the Bayview site. Nevertheless, increased anti-inflammatory adiponectin levels [27], and decreased haptoglobin the major hemoglobin binding protein associated with Bayview site exposures, support activation of some compensatory mechanisms [31, 40, 41, 47].

Overall, the mixed model results suggest that relatively high levels of air pollutants at the Bayview site may have contributed to elevated levels of some pro-inflammatory markers and endothelins as well as some acute phase protein changes. Even though the use of mask removed many criteria pollutants, CO and UFP fractions filtered through this mask along with any escaped VOCs may have contributed to the relatively decreasing trends in BP and increasing heart rate compared to other exposures. Although, CO X UFP interaction can explain the observed results, since CO exposure is associated with lowering of BP through cGMP pathway [68], it could be considered as the main contributor to the observed BP effect. This is consistent with a positive association (not significant) seen between CO and VEGF, in this work (Additional file 1: Table S1). Meanwhile, in this work UFP is associated with increased plasma endothelin (ET-1) (Table 7) and increasing trend (not significant) in CRP (Additional file 1: Table S1), and ET-1 is known to induce CRP via MAPK signaling in vascular smooth muscle cells and effect vasopressor responses [77]. These results are consistent with the positive associations seen between UFP and heart rate, as well as CRP and heart rate. These findings reveal that the simplification of the air pollutant mix by the use of mask can provide relatively clear information on pollutant-specific molecular changes that can potentially lead to observed physiological effects.

Alternatively, heat map and hierarchical clustering results on normalized biomarker data (to remove the inter-subject variability) also revealed that Bayview and College site exposures elicited distinct inflammatory and endothelinergic responses (Fig. 1) as with the mixed model results. For instance, pro-inflammatory cytokines IL-1β, IL-2, IL-6 and plasma BET-1 were seen to be upregulated after the Bayview ambient ("without" mask) exposures, compared to the other two exposure conditions and this is consistent with the statistical model results (Table 7). However, decreased haptoglobin levels and increased anti-inflammatory IL-10 levels for the "with" mask exposures compared to "without" mask exposures at the Bayview site, as well as the

College site, support the concept of active compensatory mechanisms. (Fig. 1).

Protein interaction networks obtained by conducting Ingenuity Pathway Analyses (IPA) on normalized multiple protein biomarker information (included significant changes) provided mechanistic information [25]. The highest scoring protein networks A and B with highest scores corresponding to "with" and "without" mask exposures at the Bayview site, respectively (Fig. 2a-b) exhibited NF-kB and proinflammatory cytokine nodes in both networks suggesting activation of inflammatory pathways after both these exposures. Nevertheless, the networks related to "with" and "without" mask exposures at the Bayview site appear to be somewhat different (Fig. 2a-b) and suggest Th1 (cell-mediated immunity and inflammation) and Th2 (allergy type inflammation)-like inflammatory responses, respectively [64]. The two types of helper T cells (Th1, Th2) produce cytokines characteristic of the corresponding inflammatory responses. Furthermore, network B corresponding to the Bayview site "without" mask exposures with increased IL-1β, IL-4, IL-6 and ET-1 may suggest some vascular immune responses. Pro-inflammatory changes such as increased IL-6 and TNF-α levels (Tables 5, 5, 6, 7, 8) are known to trigger acute phase protein responses and increase endothelins exhibiting signs similar to endothelial dysfunction [19, 22, 24, 27, 71]. Vascular wall cells, macrophages and Th2 cells can contribute to increased IL-1β, IL-4, IL-6 and ET-1 levels. IL-4 is known to increase IL-6 levels and impact on vascular endothelial cell barrier function [62]. IL-1β is known to induce prepro ET-1 gene by various mechanisms [24]. Moreover, UFP and SO_2 are shown to mediate NFkB-signalling pathway-related inflammatory conditions [12, 58], while exposure to particulate matter is known to trigger Th2 type immune responses and negatively impact on pulmonary vasculature [18]. We have reported on reduced pulmonary function in subjects after exposure at the Bayview site [10], and there are recent findings suggesting airway inflammation (Kauri et al. unpublished results) associated with exposures at this site. Also, these protein interaction networks are consistent with the molecular mechanisms proposed for air pollution exposure-related effects [44]. The canonical pathway analyses by IPA identified various disease functions including cell growth and proliferation, cell-cell signalling, immune cell trafficking, inflammatory response and cardiovascular disease, for Bayview site exposures (Additional file 1: Figure S1).

Despite the strengths of this work, there were some limitations in this study. For instance, masks were used only at the source emission site, the site central to this study and not at the college site, due to budget, timeline and resource constraints-driven 3-type of exposure design. Also, the subjects in this study had to raise the hood of the mask during eating and drinking for very short periods of time, for snacks and lunch. However, the hood was up for a brief period during food intake only, and there still was a flow of cool, clean air over them. Also, the hood was up during the lung function tests [10], yet this was conducted for all subjects for the same time period in a closed cooler relatively clean air system (In a trailer at the Bayview site, and inside the building at the college site). Throughout their participation in the study (including the washout period), participants were asked to refrain from spending time in locations they would be exposed to second hand smoke and from working at locations with increased air pollution. Nevertheless, the reported results should be considered as relative responses. Besides, this is a short-term exposure study with a focus only on healthy subjects. Furthermore, air pollutants other than the criteria pollutants were not measured in this study, as well as the air pollutants under the mask were not measured in this work.

In essence, the multiple biomarker analysis along with the use of mask in this work is a novel approach for the assessment of air pollution-related health effects. Exposure to relatively higher air pollutant levels in the Bayview neighborhood may mediate molecular mechanisms relevant to inflammatory and vascular function-related pathways. Activation of some compensatory mechanisms noticed in these healthy subjects may have played a protective role thus resulting in only subtle physiological changes. Single air pollutant-specific biomarker responses in combination with exposure type-related differences assisted in gaining insight into inter-pollutant interactions. Furthermore, the unique approach of use of mask along with multiple biomarker response information in different biological compartments permitted insight into source emission-associated mechanistic changes related to observed physiological outcomes. Thus, these findings contribute to the advancement of source emission-related risk assessment efforts.

Conclusions

Our findings from multiple biomarker analyses reveal that elevated air pollutant levels at the steel mill site can contribute to perturbations in inflammatory and vascular mechanisms, and perhaps may explain the subtle physiological changes seen in this study and in previous reports. The use of mask can permit experimental deconstruction of complex air pollution mixtures thus simplifying the exposure matrix to gain insight on target pollutant-specific effects as well as inter-pollutant interactions. This work warrants the use of high content biomarker analyses (e.g. proteomic, metabolomic) in combination with the use of mask in future air pollution exposure studies, to advance the understanding on source emission-related adverse outcome pathways.

Abbreviations

8-ISOP: 8-isoprostane; A2M: α_2-macroglobulin; AGP: α-acid glycoprotein; BMI: Body mass index; BP: Blood pressure; CRP: C-reactive protein; ECE: Endothelin converting enzyme; ETs: Endothelins; GMCSF: Granulocyte macrophage colony-stimulating factor; HR: Heart rate; IFN-γ: Interferon gamma; IL: Interleukins; IPA: Ingenuity Pathway Analysis; IQR: Interquartile range; PF4: Platelet factor; REML: Restricted Maximum Likelihood; SAP: Serum amyloid protein; TNF-α: Tumour necrosis factor; UFP: Ultrafine particles; vWF: VonWillebrand Factor

Acknowledgements

The authors would like to acknowledge Ildiko Horvath (Project Site Coordinator), Stephanie Blaney (Assistant Project Site Coordinator), the NORDIK Institute, Algoma University, Sault Ste. Marie, Canada; Lorie Bottos (City Solicitor), City of Sault Ste. Marie; Rod Stewart (District Supervisor) and Blair McLaughlin (Senior Environmental Officer), Ontario Ministry of the Environment; David Trowbridge (Professor), Sault College; Dr. Anne Lee, the GroupHealth Centre, Sault Ste. Marie; Ryan Kulka and Liu Sun, Exposure Assessment Section, Health Canada; Marc Smith-Doiron, Population Studies Division, Health Canada; Sheryl Bartlett, Population Studies Division, Health Canada. We would also like to thank the internal reviewers Drs Bhaja Krushna Padhi and Dharani Das, EHSRB, Health Canada, for their valuable comments.

Funding

This work was funded by the Clean Air Regulatory Agenda at Health Canada, Government of Canada.

Authors' contributions

PK contributed to the study design and deployment and made a substantial contribution to the analysis and interpretation of data, drafted and revised the manuscript. RV contributed to project development, experimental design and manuscript revisions. EB assisted in study deployment and performed biomarker analysis, assisted in data analysis and manuscript preparation. AB performed biomarker analysis and assisted in manuscript preparation. JG contributed to study coordination, deployment and manuscript preparation. AF assisted in study deployment and performed biomarker analysis. OB contributed statistical analysis. SC contributed in statistical analysis. EMT contributed to project development and experimental design, and to manuscript revision. RS contributed to study coordination and to manuscript revision. LMK contributed to study coordination, and manuscript revision. MM contributed to study design, statistical analysis and data evaluation. LL contributed to study design and manuscript revision. RD contributed to the experimental design and manuscript revision. All authors read and approved the final manuscript.

Competing interests

The authors declare that they have no competing interests.

Author details

[1]Environmental Health Science and Research Bureau, Environmental and Radiation Health Sciences Directorate, HECSB, Health Canada, Ottawa, ON, Canada. [2]Interdisciplinary School of Health Sciences, Faculty of Health Sciences, University of Ottawa, Ottawa, ON, Canada. [3]Department of Biochemistry, Microbiology and Immunology, Faculty of Medicine, University of Ottawa, Ottawa, ON, Canada.

References

1. Akhtar US, Rastogi N, McWhinney RD, Urch B, Chowb C, Evans GJ, et al. The combined effects of physicochemical properties of size-fractionated ambient particulate matter on in vitro toxicity in human A549 lung epithelial cells. Toxicol Rep. 2014;1:145–56.

2. Bielecki A, Saravanabhavan G, Blais E, Vincent R, Kumarathasan P. Efficient sample preparation method for high-throughput analysis of 15(S)-8-iso-PGF2α in plasma and urine by enzyme immunoassay. J Anal Toxicol. 2012; 36:595–600.

3. Bouthillier L, Vincent R, Goegan P, Adamson IYR, Bjarnason S, Guenette J, et al. Acute effects of inhaled urban particles and ozone: lung morphology, macrophage activity, and plasma Endothelin-1. Am J Pathology. 1998;153(6): 1873–84.

4. Brook RD, Brook JR, Urch B, Vincent R, Rajagopalan S, Silverman F. Inhalation of fine particulate air pollution and ozone causes acute arterial vasoconstriction in healthy adults. Circulation. 2002;105(13):1534–6.

5. Burnett RT, Brook J, Dann T, Delocla C, Philips O, Cakmak S, et al. Association between particulate-and gas-phase components of urban air pollution and daily mortality in eight Canadian cities. Inhal Toxicol. 2000; 12(4):15–39.

6. Cakmak S, Dales R, Kauri LM, Mahmud M, Van Ryswyk K, Vanos J, et al. Metal composition of fine particulate air pollution and acute changes in cardiorespiratory physiology. Environ Pollut. 2014;189:208–14.

7. Calderón-Garcidueñas L, Mora-Tiscareño A, Fordham LA, Valencia-Salazar G, Chung CJ, Rodriguez-Alcaraz A, et al. Respiratory damage in children exposed to urban pollution. Pediatr Pulmonol. 2003;36(2):148–61.

8. Calderón-Garcidueñas L, Kavanaugh M, Block M, D'Angiulli A, Delgado-Chávez R, Torres-Jardón R, et al. Neuroinflammation, hyperphosphorylated tau, diffuse amyloid plaques, and down-regulation of the cellular prion protein in air pollution exposed children and young adults. J Alzheimers Dis. 2012;28(1):93–107.

9. Carll AP, Haykal-Coates N, Winsett DW, Hazari MS, Ledbetter AD, Richards JH, et al. Cardiomyopathy confers susceptibility to particulate matter-induced oxidative stress, vagal dominance, arrhythmia and pulmonary inflammation in heart failure-prone rats. Inhal Toxicol. 2015;27(2):100–12.

10. Dales R, Kauri LM, Cakmak S, Mahmud M, Weichenthal SA, Van Ryswyk K, et al. Acute changes in lung function associated with proximity to a steel plant: a randomized study. Environ Int. 2013;55:15–9.

11. Denver R, Tzanidis A, Martin P, Krum H. Salivary endothelin concentrations in the assessment of chronic heart failure. Lancet. 2000;355(9202):468–9.

12. Donaldson K, Stone V. 2003. Current hypotheses on the mechanisms of toxicity of ultrafine particles. Ann Ist Super Sanita. 2003;39(3):405–10.

13. Environment and Climate Change Canada. Guidelines, objectives, codes and practice. Sept 18, 2013.

14. Gabay C, Kushner I. Acute phase proteins and other systemic responses to inflammation. The New Eng J Med. 1999;340(6):448–54.

15. Galatius-Jensen S, Wroblewski H, Emmeluth C, Bie P, Haunsø S, Kastrup J. Plasma endothelin in congestive heart failure: a predictor of cardiac death? J Card Fail. 1996;2(2):71–6.

16. Ghosh JK, Wilhelm M, Su J, Goldberg D, Cockburn M, Jerrett M, et al. Assessing the influence of traffic-related air pollution on risk of term low birth weight on the basis of land-use-based regression models and measures of air toxics. Am J Epidemiol. 2012;175(12):1262–74.

17. Goldberg MS, Burnett RT, Valois MF, Flegel K, Bailar JC III, Brook J, et al. Associations between ambient air pollution and daily mortality among persons with congestive heart failure. Environ Res. 2003;91:8–20.

18. Grunig G, Marsh LM, Esmaeil N, Jackson K, Gordon T, Reibman J, Kwapiszewska G, Park S. Perspective: ambient air pollution: inflammatory response and effects on the lung's vasculature. Pulm Circ. 2014;4(1):25–35.

19. Guo Y, Lip GYH, Apostolakis S. Inflammation in atrial fibrillation. J Am College Cardiol. 2012;60(22):2263–70.

20. Gurusankar R, Jetha S, Curtin K, Filiatreault A, MacIntyre D, Guenette J, et al. Inhalation of low levels of ambient air pollutants increases blood pressure in healthy subjects in a randomized, placebo-controlled, single blind, crossover trial. Am J Respir Crit care med 183. 2011;2011:A6387.

21. Gurusankar R, Kumarathasan P, Saravanamuthu A, Thomson E, Vincent R. Correlation between saliva and plasma levels of endothelin isoforms ET-1, ET-2 and ET-3. Int J Pept. 2015;2015:828759.

22. Heinrich PC, Castell JV, Andust T. Interleukin-6 and the acute phase response. Biochem J. 1990;265:621–36.

23. Herder C, Baumert J, Thorand B, Martin S, Lowel H, Kolb H, et al. Chemokines and incident coronary artery disease. Arterioscler Thromb Vasc Biol. 2006;26(9):2147–52.

24. Herman WH, Holcomb JM, Hricik DE, Simonson MS. Interleukin-1 beta induces endothelin-1 gene by multiple mechanisms. Transplant Proc. 1999; 31(1–2):1412–3.

25. Jia P, Kao C, Kuo P, Zhao Z. A comprehensive network and pathway analysis of candidate genes in major depressive disorder. BMC Systems Biology. 2011;5(Suppl 3):S12.

26. Johns DO, Stanek LW, Walker K, Benromdhane S, Hubbell B, Ross M, et al. Practical advancement of multipollutant scientific and risk assessment approaches for ambient air pollution. Environ Health Perspect. 2012;120(9): 1238–42.

27. Jung UJ, Choi M. Obesity and its metabolic complications: the role of Adipokines and the relationship between obesity, inflammation, insulin resistance, dyslipidemia and nonalcoholic fatty liver disease. Int J Mol Sci. 2014;15:6184–223.

28. Kaplan GG, Szyszkowicz M, Fichna J, Rowe BH, Porada E, Vincent R, et al. Non-specific abdominal pain and air pollution: a novel association. PLoS One. 2012;7(10):e47669.

29. Karthikeyan S, Thomson EM, Kumarathasan P, Guénette J, Rosenblatt D, Chan T, Rideout G, Vincent R. Nitrogen dioxide and ultrafine particles dominate the biological effects of inhaled diesel exhaust treated by a catalyzed diesel particulate filter. Toxicol Sci. 2013;135(2):437–50.

30. Kaw S, Hecker M, Vane JR. The two-step conversion of big endothelin 1 to endothelin 1 and degradation of endothelin 1 by subcellular fractions from human polymorphonuclear leukocytes. Proc Natl Acad Sci U S A. 1992; 89(15):6886–90.

31. Kazeem A, Olubayo A, Ganiyu A. Plasma nitric oxide and acute phase proteins after moderate and prolonged exercises. Iran J Basic Med Sci. 2012;15(1):602–7.

32. Koenig W, Sund M, Fröhlich M, Fischer HG, Löwel H, Döring A, et al. C-reactive protein, a sensitive marker of inflammation, predicts future risk of coronary heart disease in initially healthy middle-aged men: results from the MONICA (monitoring trends and determinants in cardiovascular disease) Augsburg cohort study, 1984 to 1992. Circulation. 1999;99(2):237–42.

33. Kumarathasan P, Vincent R, Goegan P, Potvin M, Guenette J. Hydroxyl radical adduct of 5-Aminosalicylic acid: a potential marker of ozone-induced oxidative stress. Biochem Cell Biol. 2001a;79:1–10.

34. Kumarathasan P, Goegan P, Vincent R. An automated high-performance liquid chromatography fluorescence method for the analyses of Endothelins in plasma samples. Anal Biochem. 2001b;299(1):37–44.

35. Kumarathasan P, Vincent R, Goegan P, Bjarnason S, Guenette J. Alteration in lipid oxidation levels and aromatic hydroxylation in ozone exposed fisher 344 rats. Toxicol Mech Methods. 2002;12:195–210.

36. Kumarathasan P, Blais E, Goegan P, Yagminas A, Guenette J, Adamson IYR, et al. 90-day repeated inhalation exposure of SP-C/TNF-α transgenic mice to air pollutants. Int J Toxicol. 2005;24:59–67.

37. Kumarathasan P, Vincent R, Das D, Mohottalage S, Blais E, Blank K, et al. Applicability of a high-throughput shotgun plasma protein screening approach in understanding maternal biological pathways relevant to infant birth weight outcome. J Proteome. 2014;100:136–46.

38. Kumarathasan P, Blais E, Saravanamuthu A, Bielecki A, Mukherjee B, Bjarnason S, et al. Nitrative stress, oxidative stress and plasma endothelin levels after inhalation of particulate matter and ozone. Part Fibre Toxicol. 2015;12:28–45.

39. Langrish JP, Mills NL, Chan JKK, Leseman DLAC, Aitken RJ, Fokkens PHB, Cassee FR, Li J, Donaldson K, Newby DE, Jiang L. Beneficial cardiovascular effects of reducing exposure to particulate air pollution with a simple facemask. Part Fibre Toxicol. 2009;6:8–16.

40. Lee CW, Cheng TM, Lin CP, Pan JP. Plasma haptoglobin concentrations are elevated in patients with coronary artery disease. PLoS one. 2013; 8(10):e76817.

41. Lee SH, Hong HR, Han TK, Kang HS. Aerobic training increases the expression of adiponectin receptor genes in the peripheral blood mononuclear cells of young men. Biol Sport. 2015;32(3):181–6.

42. Liu L, Kumarathasan P, Guenette J, Vincent R. Hydroxylation of salicylate to 2,3-Dihydroxybenzoic acid in the respiratory tract: effects of aging and ozone exposure in fisher 344 rats. Am J Physiology (Lung Cell Mol Physiol). 1996;271:L995–L1003.

43. Liu L, Kauri LM, Mahmud M, Weichenthal S, Cakmak S, Shutt R, et al. Exposure to air pollution near a steel plant and effects on cardiovascular

44. Liu Y, Goodson JM, Zhang B, Chin MT. Air pollution and adverse cardiac remodeling: clinical effects and basic mechanisms. Front Physiol. 2015;6:162.

45. Maheswaran R, Haining RP, Brindley P, Law J, Pearson T, Fryers PR, et al. Outdoor air pollution and stroke in Sheffield, United Kingdom – a small-area level geographical study. Stroke. 2005;36:239–43.

46. Manzer R, Dinarello CA, McConville G, Mason RJ. Ozone exposure of macrophages induces an alveolar epithelial chemokine response through IL-1α. Am J Respir Cell Mol Biol. 2008;38(3):318–23.

47. Moreno LO, Copetti M, Fontana A, Bonis CD, Salvemini L, Trischitta V, Menzaghi C. Evidence of a causal relationship between high serum adiponectin levels and increased cardiovascular mortality rate in patients with type 2 diabetes. Cardiovasc Diabetol. 2016;15:17.

48. Mustafa SB, Gandhi CR, Harvey SA, Olson MS. Endothelin stimulates platelet-activating factor synthesis by cultured rat Kupffer cells. Hepatology. 1995; 21(2):545–53.

49. Neerhof MG, Khan S, Synowiec S, Qu XW, Thaete LG. The significance of endothelin in platelet-activating factor-induced fetal growth restriction. Reprod Sci. 2012;19(11):1175–80.

50. Pieters N, Koppen G, Van Poppel M, De Prins S, Cox B, Dons E, et al. Blood pressure and same-day exposure to air pollution at school: associations with nano-sized to coarse PM in children. Environ Health Perspect. 2015;123(7):737–42.

51. Pope CA. Respiratory disease associated with community air pollution and a steel mill. Utah Valley Am J Public Health. 1989;79:623–8.

52. Pope CA, Dockery DW. Acute health effects of PM10 pollution on symptomatic and asymptomatic children. Am Rev Respir Dis. 1992; 145:1123–8.

53. Pope CA, Burnett RT, Thurston GD, Thun MJ, Calle EE, Krewski D, et al. Cardiovascular mortality and long-term exposure to particulate air pollution: epidemiological evidence of general pathophysiological pathways of disease. Circulation. 2004;109:71–7.

54. Pope CA, Rodermund DL, Gee MM. Mortality effects of a copper smelter strike and reduced ambient sulfate particulate matter air pollution. Environ Health Perspect. 2007;115:679–83.

55. Pouliou T, Kanaroglou PS, Elliott SJ, Pengelly LD. Assessing the health impacts of air pollution: a re-analysis of the Hamilton children's cohort data using a spatial analytic approach. Int J Environ Health Res. 2008;18:17–35.

56. Rich DQ, Kipen HM, Huang W, Wang G, Wang Y, Zhu P, Ohman-Strickland P, Hu M, Philipp C, Diehl SC, Lu S, Tong J, Gong J, Thomas D, Zhu T, Zhang J. Association between changes in air pollution levels during the Beijing Olympics and biomarkers of inflammation and thrombosis in healthy young adults. JAMA. 2012;307(19):2068–78.

57. Ridker PM, Hennekens CH, Buring JE, Rifai N. C-reactive protein and other markers of inflammation in the prediction of cardiovascular disease in women. N Engl J Med. 2000;342:836–43.

58. Sang L, Miller JJ, Corbit KC, Giles RH, Brauer MJ, Otto EA, et al. Mapping the NPHP-JBTS-MKS protein network reveals ciliopathy disease genes and pathways. Cell. 2011;145(4):513–28.

59. Shields KN, Cavallari JM, Hunt MJO, Lazo M, Molina M, Molina L, et al. Traffic-related air pollution exposures and changes in heart rate variability in Mexico City: a panel study. Environ Health. 2013;12:7–21.

60. Shutt RH, Kauri LM, Weichenthal S, Kumarathasan P, Vincent R, Thomson EM, Liu L, Mahmud M, Cakmak S, Dales R. Exposure to air pollution near a steel plant is associated with reduced heart rate variability: a randomised crossover study. Environ Health. 2017;16(1):4–13.

61. Sioutas C, Delfino RJ, Singh M. Exposure assessment for atmospheric ultrafine particles (UFPs) and implications in epidemiologic research. Environ Health Perspect. 2005;113:947–55.

62. Skaria T, Burgener J, Bachli E, Schoedon G. IL-4 causes Hyperpermeability of vascular endothelial cells through Wnt5A signaling. PLoS One. 2016;11(5):e0156002.

63. Smith DA, Irving SD, Sheldon J, Cole D, Kaski JC. Serum levels of the anti-inflammatory cytokine interleukin-10 are decreased in patients with unstable angina. Circulation. 2001;104(7):746–9.

64. Sprague AH, Khalil RA. Inflammatory cytokines in vascular dysfunction and vascular disease. Biochem Pharmacol. 2009;78(6):539–52.

physiology: a randomized crossover study. Int J Hyg Environ Health. 2014; 217(2–3):279–86.

65. Squadrito GL, Cueto R, Dellinger B, Pryor WA. Quinoid redox cycling as a mechanism for sustained free radical generation by inhaled airborne particulate matter. Free Radic Biol Med. 2001;31(9):1132–8.

66. Sridhar K, Mohaideen JA. Environmental impact and forecast of pollutants from coke oven gas and natural gas combustion. Int J Eng Res Dev. 2012;1(1):42–25.

67. Stanek LW, Brown JS, Stanek J, Gift J, Costa DL. Air pollution toxicology-a brief review of the role of the science in shaping the current understanding of air pollution health risks. Toxicol Sci. 2011;120(Suppl 1):S8–27.

68. Stec DE, Drummond HA, Vera T. Role of carbon monoxide in blood pressure regulation. Hypertension. 2008;51:597–604.

69. Szomjak E, Der H, Kerekes G, Veres K, Csiba L, Toth J, et al. Immunological parameters, including CXCL8 (IL-8) characterize cerebro- and cardiovascular events in patients with peripheral artery diseases. Scand J Immunol. 2010; 71(4):283–91.

70. Tane N, Inoue H, Aihara M, Ishida H. The effects of endothelin-1 on flap necrosis. Ann Plast Surg. 1995;35(4):389–95.

71. Tedgui A, Mallat Z. Cytokines in atherosclerosis: pathogenic and regulatory pathways. Physiol Rev. 2006;86:515–81.

72. Thomson E, Kumarathasan P, Goegan P, Aubin R, Vincent R. Differential regulation of the lung endothelin system by urban particulate matter and ozone. Toxicol Sci. 2005;88(1):103–13.

73. van Loon JE, Sonneveld MA, Praet SF, de Maat MP, Leebeek FW. Performance related factors are the main determinants of the von Willebrand factor response to exhaustive physical exercise. PLoS One. 2014; 9(3):e91687.

74. Villeneuve PJ, Chen L, Stieb D, Rowe BH. Associations between outdoor air pollution and emergency department visits for stroke in Edmonton. Canada Euro J Epidemiol. 2006;21:689–700.

75. Vincent R, Kumarathasan P, Goegan P, Bjarnason SG, Guenette J, Berube D, et al. Inhalation toxicology of urban ambient particulate matter: acute cardiovascular effects in rats. Res Rep Health Eff Inst. 2001a;104:5–54.

76. Vincent R, Kumarathasan P, Mukherjee B, Gravel C, Bjarnason S, Urch B, et al. Exposure to urban particles (PM2.5) causes elevations of the plasma vasopeptides endothelin ET-1 and ET-3 in humans. Am J Resp Crit care med. 2001b;163:A313.

77. Wang CJ, Liu JT, Guo F. (–)-epigallocatechin Gallate inhibits Endothelin-1-induced C-reactive protein production in vascular smooth muscle cells. Basic Clin Pharmacol Toxicol. 2010;107:669–75.

78. WHO Report 2016. Ambient air pollution: A global assessment of exposure and burden of disease. p. 1–132. http://apps.who.int/iris/bitstream/10665/250141/1/9789241511353-eng.pdf

Permissions

The contributors of this book come from diverse backgrounds, making this book a truly international effort. This book will bring forth new frontiers with its revolutionizing research information and detailed analysis of the nascent developments around the world.

We would like to thank all the contributing authors for lending their expertise to make the book truly unique. They have played a crucial role in the development of this book. Without their invaluable contributions this book wouldn't have been possible. They have made vital efforts to compile up to date information on the varied aspects of this subject to make this book a valuable addition to the collection of many professionals and students.

This book was conceptualized with the vision of imparting up-to-date information and advanced data in this field. To ensure the same, a matchless editorial board was set up. Every individual on the board went through rigorous rounds of assessment to prove their worth. After which they invested a large part of their time researching and compiling the most relevant data for our readers.

The editorial board has been involved in producing this book since its inception. They have spent rigorous hours researching and exploring the diverse topics which have resulted in the successful publishing of this book. They have passed on their knowledge of decades through this book. To expedite this challenging task, the publisher supported the team at every step. A small team of assistant editors was also appointed to further simplify the editing procedure and attain best results for the readers.

Apart from the editorial board, the designing team has also invested a significant amount of their time in understanding the subject and creating the most relevant covers. They scrutinized every image to scout for the most suitable representation of the subject and create an appropriate cover for the book.

The publishing team has been an ardent support to the editorial, designing and production team. Their endless efforts to recruit the best for this project, has resulted in the accomplishment of this book. They are a veteran in the field of academics and their pool of knowledge is as vast as their experience in printing. Their expertise and guidance has proved useful at every step. Their uncompromising quality standards have made this book an exceptional effort. Their encouragement from time to time has been an inspiration for everyone.

The publisher and the editorial board hope that this book will prove to be a valuable piece of knowledge for researchers, students, practitioners and scholars across the globe.

List of Contributors

Alicia Sanchez, Julio L. Alvarez, Yeranddy A. Alpizar, Julio Alvarez-Collazo and Karel Talavera
Department of Cellular and Molecular Medicine, Laboratory of Ion Channel Research, KU Leuven; VIB Center for Brain & Disease Research, Leuven, Belgium

Kateryna Demydenko
Department of Cellular and Molecular Medicine, Laboratory of Ion Channel Research, KU Leuven; VIB Center for Brain & Disease Research, Leuven, Belgium
Department of Cardiovascular Sciences, Laboratory of Experimental Cardiology, Leuven, KU, Belgium

Carole Jung and Miguel A. Valverde
Department of Experimental and Health Sciences, Laboratory of Molecular Physiology and Channelopathies, Universitat Pompeu Fabra, Barcelona, Spain

Stevan M. Cokic
KU Leuven BIOMAT, Department of Oral Health Sciences, KU Leuven & Dentistry University Hospitals Leuven, Leuven, Belgium

Peter H. Hoet
Department of Public Health and Primary Care, KU Leuven, Leuven, Belgium

L. Lamon, D. Asturiol, A. Richarz, E. Joossens, R. Graepel, K. Aschberger and A. Worth
European Commission, Joint Research Centre, Ispra, Varese, Italy

Rob J. Vandebriel, Jolanda P. Vermeulen, Laurens B. van Engelen, Britt de Jong, Liset J. de la Fonteyne-Blankestijn and Wim H. de Jong
Centre for Health Protection, National Institute for Public Health and the Environment (RIVM), BA, Bilthoven, The Netherlands

Lisa M. Verhagen and Marieke E. Hoonakker
Intravacc, AL, Bilthoven, The Netherlands

Sridhar Jaligama and Asmaa Sallam
Department of Pediatrics, University of Tennessee Health Science Center, Memphis, TN 38103, USA Children's Foundation Research Institute, Le Bonheur Children's Hospital, Memphis, TN 38103, USA

Jeffrey Harding
Department of Pediatrics, University of Tennessee Health Science Center, Memphis, TN 38103, USA Children's Foundation Research Institute, Le Bonheur Children's Hospital, Memphis, TN 38103, USA
Department of Biological Sciences, Louisiana State University, Baton Rouge, LA 70803, USA

Vivek S. Patel and Stephania A. Cormier
Department of Pediatrics, University of Tennessee Health Science Center, Memphis, TN 38103, USA Children's Foundation Research Institute, Le Bonheur Children's Hospital, Memphis, TN 38103, USA
Department of Biological Sciences, Louisiana State University, Baton Rouge, LA 70803, USA
Department of Comparative Biomedical Sciences, Louisiana State University School of Veterinary Medicine, Room 2510, 1909 Freight Dock, Skip Bertman Drive, Baton Rouge, LA 70803, USA

Tammy R. Dugas
Department of Comparative Biomedical Sciences, Louisiana State University School of Veterinary Medicine, Room 2510, 1909 Freight Dock, Skip Bertman Drive, Baton Rouge, LA 70803, USA

Pingli Wang
Department of Respiratory and Critical Care Medicine, Second Affiliated Hospital, Zhejiang University School of Medicine, Hangzhou, China

Matthew Kelley
Department of Pharmacology, Toxicology, and Neuroscience, Louisiana State University Health Sciences Center, Shreveport, LA 71103, USA

Skylar R. Mancuso
St.Joseph's Academy, Baton Rouge, LA 70808, USA

Guohua Qin, Jin Xia, Yingying Zhang and Nan Sang
College of Environment and Resource, Research Center of Environment and Health, Shanxi University, Taiyuan, Shanxi 030006, People's Republic of China

Lianghong Guo
State Key Laboratory of Environmental Chemistry and Ecotoxicology, Research Center for Eco-Environmental Sciences, Chinese Academy of Sciences, Beijing 100085, People's Republic of China

Rui Chen
CAS Key Laboratory for Biomedical Effects of Nanomaterials and Nanosafety& CAS Center for Excellence in Nanoscience, Beijing Key Laboratory of Ambient Particles Health Effects and PreventionTechniques, National Center for Nanoscience & Technology of China, Beijing 100190, People's Republic of China

Nicole C. Roy
Food Nutrition & Health Team, Food & Bio-based Products Group, AgResearch, Grasslands Research Centre, Tennent Drive, Private Bag 11008, Palmerston North 4442, New Zealand
Riddet Institute, Massey University, Private Bag 11222, Palmerston North 4442, New Zealand

Sebastian Riedle
Food Nutrition & Health Team, Food & Bio-based Products Group, AgResearch, Grasslands Research Centre, Tennent Drive, Private Bag 11008, Palmerston North 4442, New Zealand
Riddet Institute, Massey University, Private Bag 11222, Palmerston North 4442, New Zealand
Conreso GmbH, Neuhauser Str. 47, 80331, München, Germany

Don E. Otter
Food Nutrition & Health Team, Food & Bio-based Products Group, AgResearch, Grasslands Research Centre, Tennent Drive, Private Bag 11008, Palmerston North 4442, New Zealand
Center for Dairy Research, University of Wisconsin-Madison, 1605 Linden Drive, Madison, WI 53706-1565, USA

Harjinder Singh
Riddet Institute, Massey University, Private Bag 11222, Palmerston North 4442, New Zealand

Laetitia C. Pele
Biomineral Research Group, MRC Human Nutrition Research, Elsie Widdowson Laboratory, 120 Fulbourn Road, Cambridge CB1 9NL, UK

Rachel E. Hewitt and Jonathan J. Powell
Biomineral Research Group, MRC Human Nutrition Research, Elsie Widdowson Laboratory, 120 Fulbourn Road, Cambridge CB1 9NL, UK
Department of Veterinary Medicine, Biomineral Research Group, University of Cambridge, Madingley Road, Cambridge CB3 0ES, UK

Antonio Anax Falcão de Oliveira, Michelle Francini Dias, Tania Marcourakis and Ana Paula Melo Loureiro
Departamento de Análises Clínicas e Toxicológicas, Faculdade de Ciências Farmacêuticas, Universidade de São Paulo, Av.Prof.Lineu Prestes 580, Bloco 13 B, São Paulo CEP 05508-000, Brazil

Tiago Franco de Oliveira
Departamento de Análises Clínicas e Toxicológicas, Faculdade de Ciências Farmacêuticas, Universidade de São Paulo, Av.Prof.Lineu Prestes 580, Bloco 13 B, São Paulo CEP 05508-000, Brazil
Departamento de Farmacociências, Universidade Federal de Ciências da Saúde de Porto Alegre, Rua Sarmento Leite 245, Porto Alegre, Rio Grande do Sul CEP 90050-170, Brazil

Marisa Helena Gennari Medeiros and Paolo Di Mascio
Departamento de Bioquímica, Instituto de Química, Universidade de São Paulo, Av. Prof. Lineu Prestes 748, São Paulo CEP 05508-000, Brazil

Mariana Veras and Miriam Lemos
Laboratório de Poluição Atmosférica Experimental – LIM05, Hospital das Clínicas, Faculdade de Medicina, Universidade de São Paulo, Av. Dr. Arnaldo 455, São Paulo CEP 01246903,Brazil

Paulo Hilário Nascimento Saldiva
Laboratório de Poluição Atmosférica Experimental – LIM05, Hospital das Clínicas, Faculdade de Medicina, Universidade de São Paulo, Av. Dr. Arnaldo 455, São Paulo CEP 01246903,Brazil
Instituto de Estudos Avançados, Universidade de São Paulo, R. do Anfiteatro, 513, São Paulo CEP 05508060, Brazil

Mingxia Ren, Li Zhao and Dayong Wang
Key Laboratory of Environmental Medicine Engineering in Ministry of Education, Medical School, Southeast University, Nanjing 210009, China

Xuecheng Ding and Qi Rui
College of Life Sciences, Nanjing Agricultural University, Nanjing 210095, China

Natalia Krasteva
Institute of Biophysics and Biomedical Engineering, Bulgarian Academy of Science, 1113 Sofia, Bulgaria

Alaeddin Bashir Abukabda, Carroll Rolland McBride, Thomas Paul Batchelor, William Travis Goldsmith, Elizabeth Compton Bowdridge and Krista Lee Garner
Department of Physiology and Pharmacology, West Virginia University School of Medicine, 64 Medical Center Drive, Robert C. Byrd Health Sciences Center - West Virginia University, Morgantown, WV 26505-9229, USA
Toxicology Working Group, West Virginia University School of Medicine, Morgantown, WV, USA

Timothy Robert Nurkiewicz
Department of Physiology and Pharmacology, West Virginia University School of Medicine, 64 Medical Center Drive, Robert C. Byrd Health Sciences Center - West Virginia University, Morgantown, WV 26505-9229, USA
Toxicology Working Group, West Virginia University School of Medicine, Morgantown, WV, USA
National Institute for Occupational Safety and Health, Morgantown, WV, USA

Sherri Friend
National Institute for Occupational Safety and Health, Morgantown, WV, USA

Ditte Marie Jensen, Daniel Vest Christophersen, Martin Roursgaard, Steffen Loft and Peter Møller
Department of Public Health, Section of Environmental Health, Faculty of Health and Medical Sciences, University of Copenhagen, Øster Farimagsgade 5A, Building 5B, 2nd Floor, DK-1014 Copenhagen K, Denmark

Majid Sheykhzade
Department of Drug Design and Pharmacology, Section of Molecular and Cellular Pharmacology, Faculty of Health and Medical Sciences, University of Copenhagen, Universitetsparken 2, 22, 2100 Copenhagen, Denmark

Gry Freja Skovsted and Jens Lykkesfeldt
Experimental Animal Models, Department of Veterinary and Animal Sciences, Faculty of Health and Medical Sciences, University of Copenhagen, Ridebanevej 9, DK-1870 Frederiksberg C, Denmark

Rasmus Münter
Colloids and Biological Interfaces, Department of Micro- and Nanotechnology, Technical University of Denmark, 2800 Kongens Lyngby, Denmark

Antonio Pietroiusti, Luisa Campagnolo, Andrea Magrini and Leonardo Palombi
Department of Biomedicine and Prevention, University of Rome Tor Vergata, Via Montpellier 1, 00133 Rome, Italy

Enrico Bergamaschi
Department of Sciences and Public Health and Pediatrics, University of Turin, Turin, Italy

Marcello Campagna
Department of Medical Sciences and Public Health, University of Cagliari, Cagliari, Italy

Giuseppe De Palma
Department of Medical and Surgical Specialties, Radiological Sciences, and Public Health, Section of Public Health and Human Sciences, University of Brescia, Brescia,Italy

Sergio Iavicoli
Department of Occupational and Environmental Medicine, Epidemiology and Hygiene, Italian Workers' Compensation Authority (INAIL), Rome, Italy

Veruscka Leso and Ivo Iavicoli
Department of Public Health, University of Naples Federico II, Naples, Italy

Michele Miragoli
Department of Medicine and Surgery, University of Parma, Parma, Italy

Paola Pedata
Department of Experimental Medicine- Section of Hygiene, Occupational Medicine and Forensic Medicine, University of Campania Luigi Vanvitelli, Naples, Italy

Cécile Vignal, Madjid Djouina, Florian Dingreville, Christophe Waxin, Corinne Gower-Rousseau, Pierre Desreumaux and Mathilde Body-Malapel
Inserm, CHU Lille, U995-LIRIC-Lille Inflammation Research International Center, Univ. Lille, F-59000 Lille, France

Muriel Pichavant and Adil Ouali Alami
Inserm U1019, CNRS UMR 8204, Institut Pasteur de Lille- CIIL – Center for Infection and Immunity of Lille, Univ. Lille, F-59000 Lille, France

Laurent Y. Alleman and Esperanza Perdrix
SAGE - Département Sciences de l'Atmosphère et Génie de l'Environnement, IMT Lille Douai, Univ. Lille, 59000 Lille, France

P. C. E. van Kesteren, J. C. H. van Eijkeren, A. G. Oomen and M. B. Heringa
National Institute for Public Health and the Environment (RIVM), Bilthoven, The Netherlands

R. J. B. Peters, M. K. van der Lee and A. K. Undas
RIKILT, Wageningen University & Research, Wageningen, The Netherlands

H. Bouwmeester
RIKILT, Wageningen University & Research, Wageningen, The Netherlands
Division of Toxicology,Wageningen University, Wageningen, The Netherlands

R. L. A. W. Bleys
Department of Anatomy, University Medical Center Utrecht, Utrecht, The Netherlands

P. C. Tromp
TNO Earth, Life and Social Sciences, Utrecht, The Netherlands

Xiaobo Li, Shenshen Wu, Qingtao Meng, Hao Sun, Runze Lu and Jian Cui
Key Laboratory of Environmental Medicine Engineering, Ministry of Education, School of Public Health, Southeast University, Dingjiaqiao 87, Nanjing 210009, China

Rui Chen
Key Laboratory of Environmental Medicine Engineering, Ministry of Education, School of Public Health, Southeast University, Dingjiaqiao 87, Nanjing 210009, China
Institute for Chemical Carcinogenesis, Guangzhou Medical University, Guangzhou 511436, China

Hongbao Yang
Center for New Drug Safety Evaluation and Research, China Pharmaceutical University, Nanjing, China

Yuxin Zheng
School of Public Health, Qingdao University, Qingdao 266021, China

Wen Chen
Guangzhou Key Laboratory of Environmental Pollution and Health Risk Assessment, Department of Toxicology, School of Public Health, Sun Yat-sen University, Guangzhou 510080, China

Rong Zhang
Department of Toxicology, School of Public Health, Hebei Medical University, Shijiazhuang 050017, China

Michael Aschner
Department of Molecular Pharmacology, Albert Einstein College of Medicine, Bronx, NY 10461, USA

Erica Blais, Agnieszka Bielecki, Josée Guénette, Alain Filiatreault, Orly Brion, Sabit Cakmak, Errol M.Thomson, Robin Shutt, Lisa Marie Kauri, Mamun Mahmud, Ling Liu and Robert Dales
Environmental Health Science and Research Bureau, Environmental and Radiation Health Sciences Directorate, HECSB, Health Canada, Ottawa, ON, Canada

Premkumari Kumarathasan
Environmental Health Science and Research Bureau, Environmental and Radiation Health Sciences Directorate, HECSB, Health Canada, Ottawa, ON, Canada
Interdisciplinary School of Health Sciences, Faculty of Health Sciences, University of Ottawa, Ottawa, ON, Canada

Renaud Vincent
Environmental Health Science and Research Bureau, Environmental and Radiation Health Sciences Directorate, HECSB, Health Canada, Ottawa, ON, Canada

Department of Biochemistry, Microbiology and Immunology, Faculty of Medicine, University of Ottawa, Ottawa, ON, Canada

Index

www.ingramcontent.com/pod-product-compliance
Lightning Source LLC
Chambersburg PA
CBHW061250190326
41458CB00011B/3631